CARDIOPULMONARY IMAGING

Each volume of *The Core Curriculum Series* examines one key area in radiology and focuses on the essential information readers need for rotations and later, written board examination. Readers will appreciate the easy-to-follow format, the abundant high-quality illustrations, and the full complement of learning tools—including chapter outlines, bulleted lists, tables, summary boxes, and points for review. Please contact the publisher for additional information on existing and upcoming titles.

Other titles in *The Core Curriculum Series*...

Brant: *Ultrasound*
Cardenosa: *Breast Imaging*
Castillo: *Neuroradiology*
Chew: *Musculoskeletal Imaging*

The Core Curriculum

CARDIOPULMONARY IMAGING

ELLA A. KAZEROONI, MD, MS

Professor and Director of Thoracic Radiology
Department of Radiology
University of Michigan Medical School
Ann Arbor, Michigan

BARRY H. GROSS, MD

Professor of Radiology
Department of Radiology
University of Michigan Medical School
Ann Arbor, Michigan

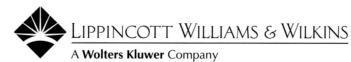

LIPPINCOTT WILLIAMS & WILKINS
A **Wolters Kluwer** Company

Philadelphia • Baltimore • New York • London
Buenos Aires • Hong Kong • Sydney • Tokyo

Developmental Editor: Kerry B. Barrett
Production Editor: Rakesh Rampertab
Manufacturing Manager: Benjamin Rivera
Cover Designer: QT Design
Compositor: Lippincott Williams & Wilkins Desktop Division
Printer: Maple Press

© 2004 by LIPPINCOTT WILLIAMS & WILKINS
530 Walnut Street
Philadelphia, PA 19106 USA
LWW.com

Library of Congress Cataloging-in-Publication Data

Kazerooni, Ella A.
    Cardiopulmonary imaging / Ella A. Kazerooni, Barry H. Gross.
        p. ; cm.—(The core curriculum)
    Includes bibliographical references and index.
    ISBN 0-7817-3655-2
        1. Cardiopulmonary system—Imaging. 2. Cardiopulmonary
    system—Diseases—Diagnosis. 3. Diagnostic imaging. I. Gross, Barry H.
    II. Title. III. Series.
    [DNLM: 1. Thoracic Diseases—diagnosis. 2. Diagnostic Imaging—methods.
    3. Radiography, Thoracic—methods. WF 975 K23c 2003]
    RC702.K396 2003
    616.1′0754—dc21

                                                            2003052176

To my husband Chuck, and our children Charlie, Isabel and John—thank you for your patience, encouragement, good humor, and unconditional love. You are the constant shining lights in my life. Thank you for being you.

To my father, who passed away from pancreatic cancer when I was fifteen years old. I hope you would have been proud. To my mother who kept the family together—thanks for believing in and supporting me.

To all my mentors, teachers, colleagues, and students. This book is drawn from experiences with each of you. Thank you.

—Ella Kazerooni

Age 50, first (? last) book, many to thank—particularly:
Parents: You made me who I am.
Mentors: Ben Felson, Roy Filly, and Bill Martel.
Colleagues: Gary Glazer (mentor, too), David Spizarny, and Phil Cascade.
Children: Lauren, Carrie, and Paul—you are my pride and joy.
Mostly, my wife: Thank you Susan for the unbounded joy of being together.

—Barry Gross

CONTENTS

Preface   ix

Acknowledgments   xi

1.   Basic Thoracic Anatomy and Physiology   1

2.   Imaging Modalities and Applications   25

3.   Approach to the Chest Radiograph   49

4.   Radiographic Report   69

5.   Pneumonia in the Immunocompetent Host   79

6.   Infections in the Immunocompromised Host   117

7.   Lung Cancer   143

8.   Other Thoracic Neoplasms   165

9.   Radiology of Mediastinal Masses   197

10.   Thoracic Imaging in the Critically Ill   217

11.   Lines, Tubes, and Devices   255

12.   Thoracic Trauma   295

13.   Pulmonary Manifestations of Systemic Diseases   323

14.   Diffuse Lung Disease   357

15.   Obstructive Lung Disease   401

16.   The Central Airways   429

17.   Radiology of the Pleura   457

18.   The Thoracic Aorta   483

19.   Adult Congenital Heart Disease   513

20.   Acquired Cardiac Disease   545

21.   Pulmonary Vascular Disease   581

22.   Thoracic Interventional Techniques   617

Subject Index   635

PREFACE

When I was first approached about the possibility of writing this *Core Curriculum: Cardiopulmonary Imaging* textbook, I felt it was an honor, but also realized I could not do it alone. I knew immediately that it would only be possible with the expertise, wisdom, and editorial excellence that Dr. Barry Gross possesses, and am very grateful that he agreed to coauthor this text. My first month as a resident was on thoracic radiology, and his teachings at the alternator still echo in my mind when I work with students, residents and fellows to this day. (In fact, recently I was listening to him work with a resident and students at the PACS workstation, and wished I could sit there again!) Not long after my chest rotation many of the faculty that I worked with left the university, and the difference this made in the quality of the educational experience was striking. Fortunately, by my second month on thoracic radiology, Dr. William Martel had recruited Dr. Melvin Figley to spend a few months here while the chest group was rebuilt. Another outstanding month! I was sold on thoracic radiology as a career! I hope, with this textbook, similarly to "sell" thoracic radiology to radiology residents in training (and even to medical students who haven't yet chosen radiology as a career!).

We begin this textbook with normal thoracic anatomy and basic physiology, illustrated predominantly with multi-detector CT reconstructions. This is followed by material on the imaging modalities that are commonly applied to the thorax. Given the complexity of the modern CT and MR machines of today, an understanding of how they work, and how changes in acquisition parameters impact the end product (images) are critical to obtaining high quality examinations that are not just general examinations, but are tailored to the clinical question. In 10 years we have gone from having 2 or 3 thoracic CT protocols, to over a dozen. An understanding of our complex imaging equipment comes before instruction in how to recognize normal and abnormal, as well it should. We also emphasize how to recognize imaging artifacts that may simulate disease and how to protocol and monitor examinations for quality. Still, even in 2003 it all comes back to the chest radiograph. We provide practical tips on how to approach the interpretation of the chest radiograph as well as guidance on preparing radiology reports, which are the tangible product of what we do as radiologists and (we hope) a true reflection of what we found and what it may mean. Chest radiographic examinations (or images now that we nearly a fully digital department) are the most common single radiologic test performed, with estimates that 30 to 70 percent of radiologic exams are chest radiographs depending on the practice setting. They are the most commonly interpreted examinations by radiologists. One of the most common ways that radiologists interact with referring physicians is through the reports and consultations generated by these examinations. While on the surface chest radiographs appear to be "simple" to interpret, interpretation may involve subtle displacement of a line, interface or shadow, subtle opacity, or slight change from a prior study. In contrast, on examinations such as CT and MR the anatomy and abnormalities are displayed with greater anatomic resolution and less overlap of structures, and can be viewed not only axially, but with multiplanar and advanced processing techniques, making them in some ways easier to interpret.

Thoracic radiology has come a long way in the last ten to fifteen years, when it was dominated by the hard copy chest radiograph. Today, HRCT, helical CT for pulmonary emboli, CT and MR angiography and cardiac imaging, and PET scanning for lung nodules and cancer staging are mature techniques, widely disseminated in practice. Ten years ago we did perhaps eight to ten dedicated chest CT scans a day. Now, it is not unusual to do thirty to forty in a day. Thoracic radiology is also better known as cardiopulmonary radiology. In fact, the American Board of Radiology uses the term "cardiopulmonary" for one of the ten examination sections of the oral board examination in diagnostic radiology. In recognition of this, we chose to call this textbook *Cardiopulmonary Imaging*. We have included not only traditional thoracic radiology topics, such as lung cancer, thoracic infections, mediastinal masses, the airway, pleural disease and interstitial and obstructive lung diseases, but also have included the cardiovascular radiology aspects of cardiopulmonary radiology, in recognition of how important this material is to "thoracic" radiology. This material can be found within general thoracic chapters such as ICU imaging, and also within dedicated chapters on adult manifestations of congenital heart disease, acquired heart disease, pulmonary vascular disease, and the thoracic aorta.

This textbook, which we hope you will enjoy, learn from and refer to, could not have been completed without many important people. This was a group effort, and we would like to thank every member of the Thoracic Radiology Division at the University of Michigan, Ann Arbor, Michigan, who contributed to the chapters. Those people are Naama Bogot, Philip Cascade, Paul Cronin, Benoit Desjardins, David Jamadar, Aine Kelly, Uwada Murray, Smita Patel, Perry Pernicano, Leslie Quint, and Michael Sneider.

We also want to thank our physician colleagues for their collegial interaction and multidisciplinary approach. We would especially like to recognize Fernando Martinez in Pulmonary Medicine and Mark Orringer, Mark Iannettoni, and Michael Deeb in Thoracic and Cardiothoracic Surgery.

Lastly, we want to thank all the students, residents, and fellows, past and present, who have rotated through thoracic radiology for the excitement, questions and ideas that they bring with them every day, and for sharing in the fun.

—Ella Kazerooni

ACKNOWLEDGMENTS

We would like to thank the following *contributing authors*, our colleagues, in the Thoracic Radiology Division of the Department of Radiology at the University of Michigan, who all helped to write this book, and without whom this text could not have been completed:

Naama R. Bogot, MD
Lecturer

Philip N. Cascade, MD, FACR, FACC, FACCP
Professor

Paul Cronin, MBBCh, MRCPI, FRCR
Lecturer

Benoit Desjardins MD, PhD
Lecturer

Aine M. Kelly, MBBCh, MRCPI, FRCR
Lecturer

David A. Jamadar MD
Clinical Assistant Professor

Uwada Murray, MD
Lecturer

Smita Patel, MBBS, MRCP, FRCR
Clinical Assistant Professor

Perry G. Pernicano, MD
Clinical Assistant Professor

Leslie E. Quint, MD
Professor

Michael B. Sneider, MD
Clinical Assistant Professor

Erica L. Thwaite, MBBS, MRCP, FRCR
Consultant Radiologist
University Hospital Aintree

We wish to extend our gratitude also to the many clinical colleagues with whom we worked at the University of Michigan, especially those in the Divisions of Pulmonary and Critical Care Medicine and Hematology and Oncology within the Department of Internal Medicine, the Sections of Thoracic and Cardiac Surgery within the Department of Surgery, and the Department of Radiation Oncology. In particular, we would like to thank Fernando Martinez, MD.

Thanks to those who helped bring this book to fruition. Sarah Abate, our department's media coordinator, who transformed everyone in the division into Adobe Photoshop users (and that was no easy task). Robert Combs, our departmental photographer for two decades, who was overwhelmed with digital photography requests, but always kept his cool. Mary Crossett, Dottie French, Ayana Murray, Dawn Reed, and Cynthia Sims-Holmes gave their assistance and patience during manuscript preparation. A special thank you to Diane Williams, who did her best to keep me (Ella) on schedule, adjusted image quality, and prepared the materials to be sent to the publisher. Special appreciation also goes to Dr. Sandro Cinti for his help with several illustrations. Lastly, we thank the publication team at Lippincott, Williams & Wilkins, including Joyce-Rachel John and Kerry Barrett, for the opportunity as well as their patience shown along the way. And thanks Nestor!

Cardiopulmonary Imaging

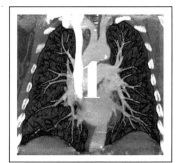

BASIC THORACIC ANATOMY AND PHYSIOLOGY

- Chest Wall
- Diaphragm
- Mediastinum
- Pleura and Fissures
- Airway
- Lungs
- Pericardium
- Heart
- Aorta and Arteries
- Veins
- Lymphatic System

An understanding of thoracic imaging requires knowledge of the anatomy being imaged, as described in this chapter, as well as the imaging techniques applied to the thorax, covered in Chapter 2. Table 1.1 lists the major anatomic structures within the thorax that are discussed. The anatomic illustrations are presented as either line drawings or as computed tomography (CT) renderings of thoracic anatomy generated from 16-row multidetector CT examinations of the thorax at thin collimation.

CHEST WALL

The thoracic contents are bounded by the chest wall, providing both the shape of the thorax and protection for the intrathoracic contents (Table 1.2). The skin, subcutaneous tissues, and muscles that surround the rib cage and shoulder girdle appear radiographically indistinguishable from each other, whereas on CT the skin, fat, and muscles are recognized by their difference in attenuation. The hard endoskeleton of the thorax is comprised primarily of the ribs, sternum, and spine anchored to the shoulder girdle by the clavicles, scapulae, and surrounding muscles (Fig. 1.1).

Ribs

The obliquely oriented ribs are slanted anteriorly in a downward direction laterally to medially (Figs. 1.2A and 1.3A), whereas the posterior ribs are slanted in an upward direction from laterally to medially (Figs. 1.2B and 1.3B) (1). On the inferior inner surface is a costal groove, in which an intercostal artery, vein, and nerve run. Posteriorly, the ribs articulate with the spine, and anteriorly the costochondral cartilages (first to seventh) are attached to the sternum and a cartilaginous bridge (eighth to twelfth). Anteriorly, the costochondral cartilages are radiolucent in childhood through young adulthood, gradually calcifying with advancing age. There are gender-specific patterns by which this cartilage calcifies. In women the central portion calcifies first, whereas in men the upper and lower borders calcify first (2). The first costochondral cartilage is often particularly bulky and

In women the central portion of the costochondral cartilage calcifies first; in men the upper and lower borders calcify first.

Table 1.1: Thoracic Anatomy Overview

Chest wall
Diaphragm
Mediastinum
Pleura
Airway
Lungs
Pericardium
Heart
Aorta and arterial structures
Vena cava and venous structures
Lymphatic system

Table 1.2: The Chest Wall

Nonosseous	Osseous
Skin	Ribs
Subcutaneous fat	Sternum
Muscles	Shoulder girdle
	Spine

The "big-rib sign" on a lateral radiograph is used to identify the right ribs.

can mimic an underlying pulmonary nodule, particularly when asymmetric. The right ribs can be differentiated from the left ribs on a lateral radiograph using the *"big-rib sign"* (Fig. 1.3B) (3). By convention, lateral images are taken with the left side against the radiographic plate; the right ribs are therefore further from the radiographic plate and appear to be magnified or bigger because of divergence of the x-ray beam. The most common supernumerary or accessory rib is a *cervical rib* arising from the seventh cervical vertebra as an enlarged costal element. They occur in approximately 0.5% to 1.5% of the population, are usually bilateral, are more common in women, and may be a cause of thoracic outlet syndrome (1,4,5). Occasionally, ribs may be congenitally fused or bifid in appear-

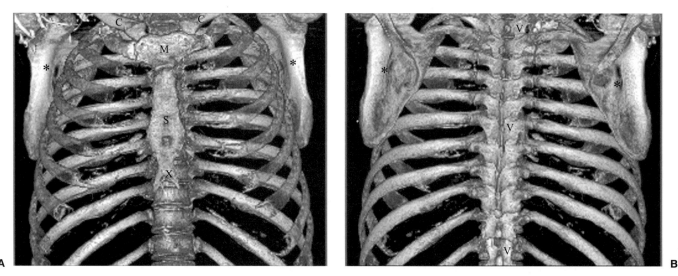

A   B

Figure 1.1 Normal thoracic endoskeleton. Three-dimensional computed tomography reconstructions in the (*A*) anterior and (*B*) posterior projections. Asterisk, scapulae; C, clavicles; M, manubrium; S, sternal body; V, vertebrae; X , xiphoid.

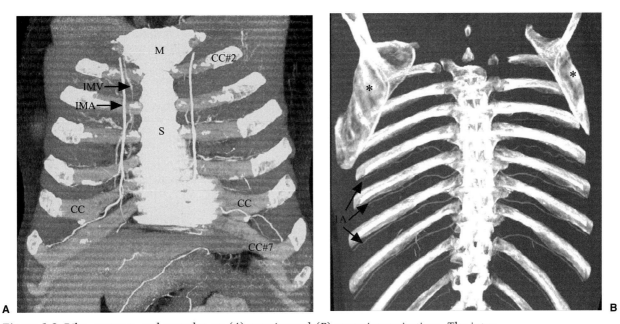

Figure 1.2 Ribs, sternum, and scapulae on (A) anterior and (B) posterior projections. The intercostal arteries (IA) are seen running immediately inferior to the ribs. Note the downward slant of the anterior ribs from the lateral to medial direction. The partially calcified costochondral cartilages (CC) extend from the anterior rib ends to the sternum. The second costochondral cartilage extends to the sternomanubrial angle (CC#2). The seventh costochondral cartilage (CC#7) extends medially to the xiphoid process. The internal mammary arteries (IMA) and veins (IMV) parallel the lateral borders of the sternum. Note the upward slant of the posterior ribs from the lateral to medial direction. Asterisk, scapulae; M, manubrium; S, sternal body.

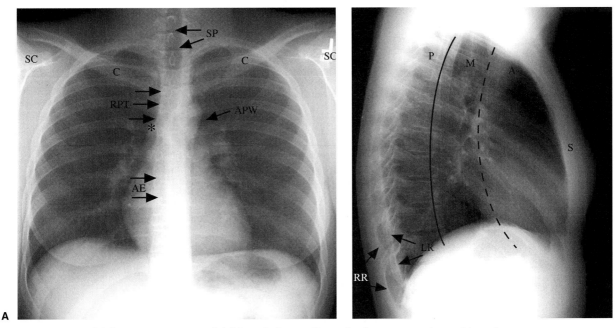

Figure 1.3 Normal (A) posteroanterior and (B) lateral chest radiographs demonstrate the position of the anterior and posterior ribs. The *dashed vertical line* separates the anterior and middle mediastinum, and the *solid vertical line* separates the middle and posterior mediastinum. Note the *"big rib"* sign on the lateral radiograph (larger more posterior appearing ribs are the right ribs [RR] versus the smaller left ribs [LR]). SC, scapulae; A, anterior mediastinum; AE, azygoesophageal recess; APW, aortopulmonary window; C, clavicles; M, middle mediastinum; P, posterior mediastinum; RPT, right paratracheal stripe; S, sternum; SP, spinous processes; v, vertebral bodies; Asterisk, azygos vein.

ance. Usually, the thorax is wider in transverse dimension than in the anteroposterior dimension. A *"barrel-shaped"* chest refers to a thorax that is equally wide in both dimensions and is a sequela of chronic obstructive lung disease, such as emphysema. Along the inferior border of the first and second ribs, 1 to 5 mm thick "companion shadows" are seen on radiographs in approximately one-third of individuals and are due to adjacent fat (6,7); they should not be mistaken for a pneumothorax (Chapter 17).

On axial CT images, only a portion of each rib is seen because of their oblique orientation. Counting the ribs on CT can be done using three anatomic landmarks: clavicular heads (rib 1), sternal angle (rib 2), and xiphoid process (rib 7). The first rib can be found behind the medial third of the clavicle (8). This is the method we generally use, acknowledging this is tedious when counting down to the lower most ribs. The second costochondral cartilage anteriorly is located at the sternal angle; this method can also be used on a lateral radiograph. Finally, the seventh costochondral cartilage can be found at the xiphoid process (1); this landmark is less consistent (Fig. 1.2A).

Counting the ribs on CT can be done using three landmarks, from which successive ribs can be counted in the posterior direction.

Sternum

The sternum forms the midline anterior portion of the thoracic cage and is made up of the manubrium (the thickest portion; articulates with the clavicles), the sternal body, and the xiphoid process (Figs. 1.1A, 1.2A, and 1.4). The sternal notch, also known as the jugular notch, is at the upper manubrium border; palpating this area reveals the trachea. The sternal angle is formed by the manubrium and sternal body and is also known as the angle of Louis. On a chest radiograph it is at the T-4 vertebral body level. The xiphisternal articulation is at the T-9 vertebral body level. Seven costochondral cartilages articulate with the sternum. Deformities of the sternum occur in 1 in 300 people and are usually of little clinical consequence, other than being aesthetically unattractive; when severe, respiratory symptoms may occur (9). The most common is *pectus excavatum*, also known as *"funnel chest"*; it represents depression of the sternum from its normal location, easily recognizable on lateral radiographs. On a frontal radiograph it may cause blurring of the right heart border, mimicking a right middle lobe process, with displacement of the heart to the left, and exaggerated anterior angulation of the ribs. Pectus carinatum or *"pigeon breast"* represents abnormal protrusion of the sternum; the middle and lower sternum are most commonly involved (9,10). There may be an association with congenital heart disease in up to 10% of individuals. A sternal foramen is an incidental focal defect in ossification or failure

On a posteroanterior radiograph, the sternal angle is at the T-4 vertebral body level.

Pectus excavatum creates an ill-defined right heart border on a posteroanterior radiograph.

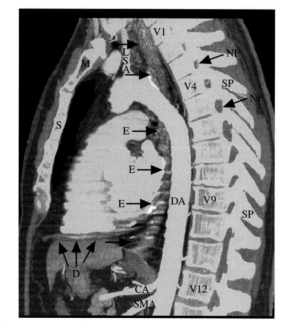

Figure 1.4 Midline sagittal reconstruction demonstrates the vertically oriented esophagus (E) anterior to the descending thoracic aorta (DA). CA, celiac axis; D, diaphragm; LSA, left subclavian artery; M, manubrium; NF, neural foramina; S, sternum; SMA, superior mesenteric artery; SP, spinous processes; V, vertebra by thoracic number.

of union of embryonic elements that form the sternum, readily visible on CT as a hole in the sternum. Although the sternum is difficult to evaluate on chest radiographs, particularly on the frontal views, it can be evaluated in great detail with CT.

Shoulder Girdle

Together the clavicles and scapulae, otherwise know as collar bone and shoulder blades, form the shoulder girdle (Figs. 1.1, 1.2, and 1.3). The clavicle is a double-curved bone that medially articulates with the sternum and laterally with the acromion of the scapula; both are synovial joints. Numerous ligaments anchor the clavicle as well, including the costoclavicular and sternoclavicular ligaments medially and the acromioclavicular and coracoclavicular ligaments laterally. The rhomboid fossa is a notch that is occasionally seen radiographically on the undersurface of the medial clavicle 1 to 2 cm from the sternal articulation and is the location from which the costoclavicular ligament arises. The interspace between the first and second ribs anteriorly can be palpated immediately below the medial clavicle.

The scapulae are thin flat bones with a thick ridge or spine projecting posteriorly. The costal surface of the scapula faces the ribs and is concave, containing the subscapularis muscle, whereas the dorsal surface is convex and contains the supraspinatus and infraspinatus muscles above and below the spinal ridge, respectively. Laterally the spine continues into the acromion. The superolateral aspect of the scapula is concave, forming the glenoid fossa. Superiorly there is a small scapular notch. Sprengel's deformity, or high-riding scapula, is an uncommon congenital abnormality (11).

Spine

There are 12 thoracic vertebrae (Figs. 1.1B, 1.3B, and 1.4). There is less variation in the number of thoracic vertebral bodies than in the lumbosacral spine. Each vertebra is made up anteriorly of a body or corpus designed for weight-bearing, connected posteriorly to the vertebral arches that are made up of the pedicles and laminae. The cross-sectional anatomy of a thoracic vertebra is illustrated in Fig. 1.5. Progressively lower thoracic vertebrae are larger than the one above it. The bodies of adjacent vertebra articulate with each other through a cartilaginous joint containing a fibrocartilaginous intervertebral disc. The corpus and arches surround the vertebral foramen, which contains the spinal cord. The primary function of the arches is to protect the spinal cord. The spinous processes project posteriorly and inferiorly from the arches. The transverse processes project laterally from the arches. The superior and inferior articular processes project upwardly and downwardly from the laminae, respectively, to form the synovial facet joints. Spinous processes and lamina of adjacent vertebra articulate across fibrous joints. Each vertebra articulates with a pair of ribs; the rib head articulates with the upper aspect of vertebra of the same number, the tubercle with the inferior aspect. At many levels the rib head also articulates with the rib at the next lower segmental level. The space between the pedicles of two adjacent vertebra form the intervertebral foramen, through which the intercostal nerves exit the spinal canal (Fig. 1.4). The upper four thoracic vertebrae may have features of cervical vertebra, the middle four are typically thoracic, and the lower four may have features of lumbar vertebrae. There is normally kyphosis to the thoracic spine. A loss of thoracic kyphosis results in a straight thoracic spine. This "straight-spine" or "straight-back" syndrome may include thoracic scoliosis, pectus excavatum, and is associated with mitral valve prolapse (12,13).

The 12 thoracic vertebral bodies form the normal kyphosis of the posterior chest wall.

DIAPHRAGM

The diaphragm is a dome-shaped convex-upward musculotendinous structure that separates the thoracic and abdominal cavities; it is divided into three portions. The *sternal portion* is the smallest and arises from the xiphoid process. The *costal portion* is the largest, arising from the seventh through twelfth ribs. The vertebral (a.k.a. lumbar) portion arises

The muscular diaphragm plays a major role in inspiration by moving caudally, generating negative intrathoracic pressure and therefore airflow into the lungs.

from the lateral aspects of the L1-4 vertebrae in the form of two crura; the right crus is thicker and longer than the left. The *fibrous component* of each portion extends centrally to form the *central tendon*. The right hemidiaphragm is usually half an interspace higher than the left, with its upper border at the fifth anterior rib through the sixth to seventh anterior rib interspace level on the posteroanterior radiograph (4,14). There are two possible explanations: The liver below the hemidiaphragm on the right elevates it or the heart above the left hemidiaphragm pushes it down.

Three openings in the diaphragm allow passage of structures between the thorax and abdomen. The *foramen for the inferior vena cava* is located in the central tendon at the T8-9 intervertebral disc level to the right of midline. The midline *esophageal hiatus* arises within fibers of the right crus, contains the esophagus and vagus nerve, and is located at the T-10 vertebral body level. The *aortic hiatus* is located at the T12-L1 intervertebral disc level just to the left of midline and contains the aorta, azygos and hemiazygos veins, and thoracic duct. It actually lies behind the crura of the diaphragm where they join. A tendinous arch joins the crura together anterior to the hiatus, known as the median arcuate ligament. Where the diaphragm overlies the psoas muscles and quadratus lumborum, there is a thickening in the fascia that forms the medial and lateral arcuate ligaments, respectively. In attaching to the diaphragm, they seal the abdominal contents below the diaphragm. The diaphragm is inseparable from the abdominal structures on radiographs. On CT it is visible as a soft tissue attenuation band-like structure (Fig. 1.4).

The common congenital hernias of the diaphragm arise from failure of portions of the diaphragm to fuse. Ninety percent of these are *Bochdalek hernias*, which arise posterolaterally due to failure of the costal and vertebral portions of the diaphragm to fuse; these are more common on the left than the right because of the protective effect of the liver posteriorly and are usually diagnosed in neonates and young children. Although an acute hernia can be life threatening in adults because of bowel strangulation, small incidental Bochdalek hernias are common on CT, particularly in patients with long-standing obstructive lung disease (15). *Morgagni hernias* arise anteromedially from failure of the sternal and costal portions to fuse; these are more common on the right.

MEDIASTINUM

The mediastinum is bounded laterally by the mediastinal pleura, inferiorly by the diaphragm, and superiorly by the thoracic inlet. It is divided into compartments. Anatomists, surgeons, and radiologists often use different definitions of these compartments. The definitions used here are based on the classification of Dr. Benjamin Felson. Many have said that the specification of "compartment" is artificial today, because the use of cross-sectional imaging makes discrete localization of abnormalities possible. However, the compartments convey information on anatomic localization, imply differential diagnoses, and are very applicable when interpreting chest radiographs. The easiest way to describe these compartments is by drawing two vertical lines on a lateral radiograph (Fig. 1.3B). The *anterior mediastinum* is everything anterior to the line drawn along the anterior aspect of the trachea, continuing inferiorly along the posterior heart border. The *posterior mediastinum* is everything posterior to the line drawn one-third of the vertebral body width behind the anterior border of the spine. Everything between these two lines is the *middle mediastinum*. Many classifications (but not this one) place the heart in the *middle mediastinum*. The *aortopulmonary window* is that part of the mediastinum that is between the main pulmonary artery and the aortic arch and is normally concave to flat on the posteroanterior radiograph (Figs. 1.3A and 1.5). The left recurrent laryngeal nerve runs in the aortopulmonary window; hence, masses in this location may be associated with left vocal cord paralysis and hoarseness. The contents of the mediastinal compartments are listed in Table 1.3. The borders of the cardiopericardial silhouette and mediastinum are described in Chapter 3.

The left recurrent laryngeal nerve runs in the aortopulmonary window; new hoarseness or vocal cord paralysis may be due to a mass in this location.

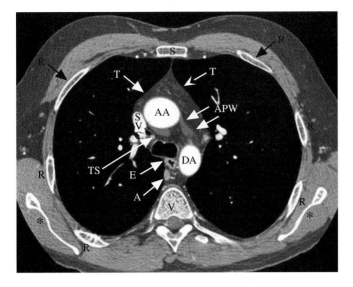

Figure 1.5 Axial computed tomography image through the thymus gland (T) and the aortopulmonary window (APW). The thymus gland drapes over the ascending aorta and aortopulmonary window. In this 52 year old it is almost completely of fat attenuation. A, azygos vein; AA, ascending aorta; DA, descending aorta; E, esophagus; R, ribs; S, sternal body; TS, transverse sinus of the pericardium; Asterisk, scapulae.

Esophagus

The esophagus is a vertically oriented structure that runs the length of the middle mediastinum, anterior to the spine, just to the left of midline, posterior to the airway, and to the right of the descending thoracic aorta (Figs. 1.4 and 1.5). The esophagus is divided into thirds. The proximal 5 cm long cervical esophagus begins at the cricoid cartilage at the C-6 vertebral body level and ends at the thoracic inlet. The middle third of the esophagus begins at the thoracic inlet and ends at the tracheal carina, whereas the lower third extends from the carina to the gastric fundus at the gastroesophageal junction, located at the T-11 vertebral body level (16). The reflection of the right mediastinal pleura against the vertically oriented esophagus and azygos vein forms the *azygoesophageal recess* below the level of the azygos arch (Fig. 1.3A). Smooth indentations are noted on the esophagus at the level of the aortic arch and the left main bronchus during an esophagram. The esophagus is a muscular organ made up of striated muscle proximally and smooth muscle distally, the primary function of which is the propulsion of food. The resting state of the esophagus is collapsed, becoming distended transiently when liquid or solid material is swallowed. The esophageal wall has mucosal, submucosal, and muscular layers, but unlike the stomach and intestines does not possess an adventitia or covering serosal layer. This permits the spread of esophageal malignancy directly into the mediastinum.

Displacement of the azygoesophageal recess to the right in the subcarinal region indicates a subcarinal mass, such as a bronchogenic cyst or lymph node mass. Displacement just above the diaphragm is most commonly due to a hiatal hernia.

Unlike the rest of the gastrointestinal tract, the esophagus has no outer adventitial layer to impede the spread of malignancy.

Table 1.3: Mediastinal Compartments and Their Contents

Anterior	Middle	Posterior
Thymus	Airway	Nerve roots
Heart	Aortic arch	Descending aorta
	Esophagus	
	SVC	
	Aygos/Hemiazygos veins	
	Thoracic duct	
Lymph nodes	Lymph nodes	Lymph nodes
	Phrenic/vagus nerves	

SVC, superior vena cava.

Thymus

The thymus is a bilobed gland located in the superior portion of the anterior mediastinum behind the manubrium, anterior to the trachea, aortic arch, great vessels, and the brachiocephalic veins, extending caudally onto the surface of the pericardium (Fig. 1.5). It is comprised predominantly of lymphocytes and has a connective tissue capsule. T-lymphocytes are produced in the thymus gland and migrate to other lymphoid organs in the body for maturation. This quadrilateral shaped structure is readily visible on the chest radiographs of children, reaching its largest size at age 2 (16). Over time the thymus involutes and becomes replaced with fat; more than one-half of individuals over 40 years of age have a completely fatty thymus on CT (17). On CT, the soft tissue attenuation of the thymus can be located in all individuals under 30 years of age, but in only 17% of adults over 49 years of age. By 60 years of age the thymus gland weighs less than 50% of what it weighed before 19 years of age (18). With thymic hyperplasia the thymus may be abnormally enlarged. Rebound thymic hyperplasia often occurs in children and young adults after chemotherapy or corticosteroid treatment. In contrast, follicular or lymphoid thymic hyperplasia occurs with conditions such as myasthenia gravis.

> The bilobed quadrilaterally shaped thymus reaches peak size at age 2, gradually involuting with fatty replacement through the fifth decade of life.

PLEURA AND FISSURES

The pleura is comprised of a single cell layer of mesothelial cells, with submesothelial connective tissue containing a rich network of lymphatics. The lungs are enclosed within the pleural space, as if the lungs were a fist that was pushed into a balloon until the opposing sides of the balloon meet, with the balloon (pleura) almost completely surrounding the fist except at the wrist, analogous to the hilum of the lung. The *parietal pleura* lines the thoracic cage, and the *visceral pleura* is adherent to the lungs. Parietal pleura is named according to that portion of the thoracic cage that is adhered by the surrounding endothoracic fascia, hence *cervical pleura* over the apex of the lung, *costal pleura* along the ribs, diaphragmatic, and *mediastinal pleura*, respectively. The parietal pleura and visceral pleura are inseparable at the hila of the lungs. At the upper border of the hila they are directly contiguous. At the lower border of the hila there is a redundancy where the visceral and parietal meet, known as the *inferior pulmonary ligament*. This runs caudally from the inferior pulmonary vein through the lungs as the *inter-sublobular septum,* ending on the surface of the diaphragm. It is the thickness of two layers of pleura, anchors the lung to the diaphragm, and is a potential pleural space in which fluid or air may appear loculated (19). A small amount of fluid within the pleural space provides lubrication during respiration, as the parietal pleura moves with the chest wall, whereas the visceral pleura moves with the lung. The caudal extent of the parietal pleura is much greater than the visceral pleura, with the costodiaphragmatic recesses extending caudally by several interspaces or approximately 5 cm in quiet respiration.

> Parietal and visceral pleura blend at the hilum of each lung; redundancy inferior to this creates the inferior pulmonary ligament.

> The caudal edge of the pleural space is several centimeters lower than the edge of the lung, particularly posteriorly.

The fissures are invaginations of visceral pleura into the lungs, dividing the lungs into lobes (Figs. 1.6 and 1.7). The normal fissures include a *major (or oblique) fissure* that runs obliquely through each lung and separates the upper and lower lobes and a dome-shaped *minor (or horizontal)* fissure that runs horizontally through in the right lung at the level of the fourth anterior rib and separates the right upper and middle lobes. On radiographs, the major fissures begin posteriorly at the T-5 vertebral level and run caudally and anteriorly downward, touching the diaphragm a few centimeters behind the anterior chest wall. On radiographs, the pleural surfaces are not visible, except for the fissures. On thick-section CT the fissures appear as avascular planes. With thin collimation CT the fissures themselves are seen, as is the parietal pleura, particularly if there is abundant extrapleural fat. Although we think of fissures as complete structures that prevent the spread of disease such as pneumonia from one lobe to another, the use of thin collimation CT routinely reveals that in 83% of right lungs and 50% of left lungs the fissures are incomplete (20).

> Pleural fissures are commonly incomplete.

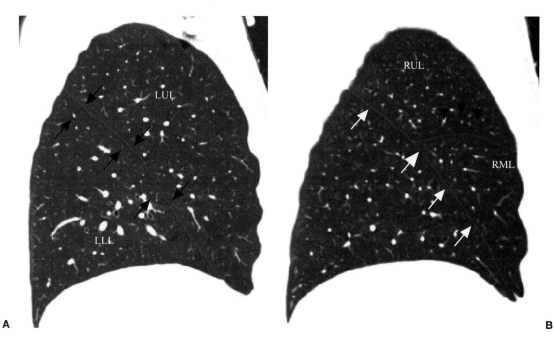

Figure 1.6 Sagittal computed tomography reconstructions demonstrate the pleural fissures. *A.* Oblique course of the left major fissure (*arrows*). *B.* Oblique course of the right major (*arrows*) is slightly less vertical than the left; horizontal course of the minor fissure (*arrowheads*). LLL, left lower lobe; LUL, left upper lobe; RLL, right lower lobe; RML, right middle lobe; RUL, right upper lobe.

Accessory fissures are extra fissures that can be seen on approximately 10% of chest radiographs, 20% of conventional CTs, and with higher frequency on thinner multidetector CT acquisitions. Detail on specific accessory fissures, including the *azygos fissure*, the *inferior accessory fissure,* the *superior accessory fissure*, and other accessory fissures is given in Chapter 17 (21–23). There are many more accessory fissures seen on gross pathologic examination and with thin-section CT, most of which are unnamed (24).

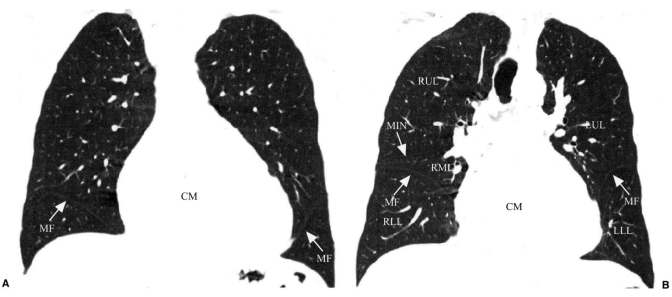

Figure 1.7 Coronal computed tomography reconstructions demonstrate the pleural fissures. *A.* Anterior: the caudal extent of the major fissures (MF) is anterior. CM, cardiopericardial silhouette. *B.* Middle: minor (MIN) and major fissures on the right.

(continued on next page)

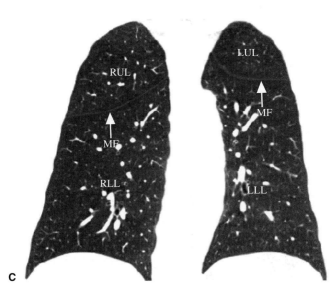

Figure 1.7 (continued) C. Posterior: the cephalad extent of the major fissures (MF) is highest posteriorly. LLL, left lower lobe; LUL, left upper lobe; RLL, right lower lobe; RUL, right upper lobe.

AIRWAY

The airway conducts air from the larynx to and from the alveoli of the lungs for the purpose of gas exchange with blood in the pulmonary capillary circulation. The *trachea* and large *bronchi* are rigid and noncollapsible because of the presence of cartilaginous c-shaped rings or plates and are thick enough so that there is no gas exchange across their walls, their primary function being to conduct air. They are lined by pseudostratified ciliated columnar epithelium that facilitates the clearing of small particulate matter from the airways in an upward direction toward the oropharynx. Glands within the subepithelial connective tissue secrete mucus. Bronchioles do not contain cartilage in their walls and are of two types. *Terminal (a.k.a. membranous) bronchioles* measure approximately 0.6 mm in diameter and conduct air like the trachea and bronchi. The smaller *respiratory bronchioles* have alveoli arising from their walls, and both conduct air as well as exchange gas (25).

Trachea and Main Bronchi

Airway anatomy is illustrated in Fig. 1.8. The trachea extends from the larynx at approximately the C-6 vertebral level to the T-5 level where it bifurcates at the carina (26). It extends above and below the sternal notch, above which it can be directly palpated. The trachea is generally a midline structure, normally deviating to the right at the level of the aortic arch and with a gradual slant from the anterior to posterior direction as it extends caudally from the larynx. This rightward slant explains why aspirated material more readily reaches the right lung than the left. The trachea contains 16 to 20 c-shaped cartilage rings that are horizontal and parallel to each other, that prevent airway collapse during expiration. Posteriorly, the membranous (noncartilaginous) wall may be convex outward, flat, or convex inward; the latter usually indicates expiration on imaging studies. The right main bronchus has six to eight cartilage rings and is shorter and more horizontal than the left main bronchus, arising at a 25-degree angle. The left main bronchus is 4 to 5 cm long, contains 9 to 12 cartilage rings, and is more oblique in orientation, arising at a 45-degree angle (26). The right main bronchus is the *eparterial bronchus*, that is, the bronchus sits above the right pulmonary artery, whereas the left main bronchus is the *hyparterial bronchus*, positioned below the left pulmonary artery. The right main bronchus divides into the right upper lobe bronchus and the 3 to 4 cm long bronchus intermedius, the latter then dividing into the right middle and right lower lobe bronchi. The left main bronchus divides into the left upper lobe bronchus, lingular bronchus, and left lower lobe bronchus. Additional details on tracheal and main bronchus diameter and length and

On a posteroanterior radiograph, the carina is at the T-5 vertebral body level.

A concave posterior membranous wall of the trachea on CT is usually an indication that the image was obtained during expiration.

The right main bronchus is eparterial. The left main bronchus is hyparterial.

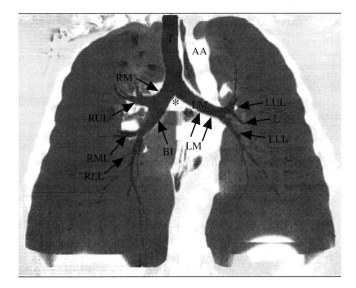

Figure 1.8 Coronal minimum intensity projection of the central airways. Asterisk, carina; AA, aortic arch; BI, bronchus intermedius; L, lingula; LLL, left lower lobe bronchus; LM, left main bronchus; LUL, left upper lobe bronchus; RLL, right lower lobe bronchus; RM, right main bronchus; RML, right middle lobe bronchus; RUL, right upper lobe bronchus; T, trachea.

common variants of anatomy, such as the *tracheal* or *"pig" bronchus*, the *"bridging" bronchus* , and the *"paracardiac" bronchus*, can be found in Chapter 16 (27).

The *right paratracheal stripe* is formed by the reflection of mediastinal pleura against the right wall of the trachea (Fig. 1.3A). The esophagus lies immediately posterior to the trachea and slightly to the left; with disease such as esophageal cancer, care must be taken to exclude airway invasion when the tumor is in direct contiguity with the airway. Small mucous pseudotumors are estimated to appear in the central tracheobronchial tree on CT in approximately 2% of examinations; with coughing and repeat image these should be cleared (28).

Intrapulmonary Bronchi

Lobar bronchi divide into the segmental bronchi, as listed in Table 16.1. The lobar bronchi are 1 to 2 cm in length; the lingular bronchus is 2 to 3 cm long. The azygos vein arches over the right upper lobe bronchus from the posterior to anterior direction; on a posteroanterior radiograph it is seen end-on as a biconvex structure 1 cm or smaller in size in the tracheobronchial angle (Fig. 1.3A). Of note, the right middle lobe bronchus arises anterolaterally at the same level that the right lower lobe superior segment bronchus arises and heads directly posteriorly. In the lower lobes the superior segments arise first, followed by a basilar stem that gives rise to the segmental bronchi, as listed in Table 1.4. The basilar bronchi arise in the order they are listed; as seen on CT they arise counterclockwise in the right lower lobe and clockwise in the left lower lobe. The medial and anterior segments are generally anterior to the inferior pulmonary veins and the lateral and posterior segments posterior to the inferior pulmonary vein. Although most bronchi run

"M.A.L.P." is the branching order of the lower lobe segmental bronchi in a clockwise direction in the left lower lobe and the counterclockwise direction in the right lower lobe. M, medial; A, anterior; L, lateral; P, posterior.

Table 1.4: Pulmonary Lobar and Segmental Bronchi

Lobar	Segmental
Right upper lobe	Anterior Posterior Apical
Right middle lobe	Medial Lateral
Right lower lobe	Superior Medial Anterior Lateral Posterior
Left upper lobe	Anterior Apicoposterior
Lingula	Superior Inferior
Left lower lobe	Superior Anteromedial Lateral Posterior

obliquely or perpendicular to the CT axial sections and are therefore seen in cross-section, bronchi such as the lingular bronchus and its segmental bronchi and the segmental bronchi of the right middle lobe run in the axial plane of CT and are seen in the axial CT plane. Ten generations of bronchi divide in a generally dichotomous manner, decreasing in diameter from 12.2 mm centrally to 1.3 mm peripherally (29).

LUNGS

Normal lung attenuation on inspiratory CT ranges from approximately −800 to −850 HU.

Distal to the respiratory bronchioles are approximately four generations of *alveolar ducts* lined with *alveoli*, the last divisions of which measure approximately 0.4 mm (29). The primary function of the lungs is gas exchange, and the largest part of the lungs is made up of the gas within the 300 million alveoli found in the lungs, with a total surface area of 140 m^2 (30). As estimated in rats, the alveolar portion of the lung comprises approximately 87% of total lung volume, whereas the nonalveolar portion of the lungs, including bronchioles and larger airways, comprises the remaining 13%. Of the alveolar volume, only 6% is comprised of tissue versus 13% of the nonalveolar lung; the remainder is gas (31). The large percentage of lung volume comprised of air, with relatively little tissue, explains why the lungs are lucent on radiographs and have a very low attenuation number on CT. Normal lung attenuation on inspiratory CT ranges from approximately −800 to −850 Hounsfield units (HU). There is an attenuation gradient from the anterior nondependent lung to the posterior dependent lung that may vary between 40 and 60 HU, the more dependent lung having the higher attenuation value. With increasing expiration, lung attenuation increases as the air component of the lung decreases. Between 90% and 10% of vital capacity, attenuation increases by approximately 160 HU (32). Physically, the right lung is larger than the left because of the presence of the heart on the left side.

The lungs are very vascular structures and enhance intensely with intravenous contrast when they are collapsed and emptied of air.

Gas exchange occurs across the alveolar walls. The common wall of adjacent alveoli is called the *interalveolar septum*. Alveolar walls contain a rich capillary network, making the lungs a very vascular structure and explaining why atelectatic lung enhances intensely with intravenous contrast on CT. Inhaled air and capillaries are separated by epithelium, interstitium, and vascular endothelium for a distance of approximately 0.2 μm (30). Oxygen and carbon dioxide are exchanged through the alveolar walls, into and out of the circulating red blood cells. At any one time, red blood cell volume in the capillaries alone is 0.2 L. Over 90% of the alveolar surface is lined by type I pneumocytes. The remainder is made up of the type II pneumocytes that produce surfactant. Type I cells are much larger than type II cells; in total there are twice as many type II cells than type I cells. Surfactant is made up of phospholipids, the predominant one being dipalmitoyl phosphatidylcholine. The primary property of surfactant is to reduce alveolar surface tension, which prevents alveolar collapse with expiration and allows for ease of reexpansion with subsequent inspiration.

The central/axial interstitium surrounds the bronchovascular bundles. The peripheral interstitium includes the interlobular septa.

The connective tissue network of the lungs is divided into two compartments. The *central or axial compartment* surrounds the bronchovascular bundles and extends centrally from the hila to the opening of the alveoli. The *peripheral or septal interstitium* arises from the visceral pleural connective tissue and includes the interlobular septa, known better as "*Kerley B*" lines on chest radiographs in the setting of interstitial edema. These septa contain pulmonary veins and lymphatics. Details of the secondary pulmonary lobule anatomy can be found in Chapter 14 and Fig. 14.26.

Another major function of the lungs is immune surveillance and the clearance of particulate matter inhaled with air (33). This function is served both by the ciliated airway lining and alveolar macrophages; the latter are found in much greater abundance in the lungs of smokers than nonsmokers (34). Approximately 9% of the cells in the lungs are macrophages. Most inhaled particulate matter is either quickly phagocytosed by macrophages or expelled through the airway within 24 hours (35).

PERICARDIUM

The pericardium is to the heart what the pleura is to the lungs. The pericardial space surrounds the heart and normally contains 20 to 25 mL of serous fluid for lubrication during cardiac motion (36). *Visceral pericardium* is attached to the myocardium by fat-containing subepicardial connective tissue, whereas the *parietal pericardium* is a thick fibrous layer that blends with the adventitia of great vessels as they enter and exit the heart. Like the pleura, the pericardium is lined by mesothelial cells. Sternopericardial ligaments connect the heart anteriorly to the xiphisternal junction and manubrium. The upper border of the pericardial sac is at approximately the sternal angle where pericardium blends with the aorta, pulmonary arteries, and superior vena cava. Caudally, the parietal pericardium is adherent to the central tendon of the diaphragm. The normal "potential" capacity of the pericardial sac is approximately 300 mL. Rapid accumulations of greater than this amount of fluid impairs cardiac function, largely by reduced systemic venous return and compression of the lower pressure right-sided cardiac chambers. Larger volumes of fluid may be physiologically adjusted for when accumulation occurs slowly. Congenital partial or complete absence of the pericardium is rare, resulting in communication of the pericardial and pleural spaces; when focal it is most common over the left atrial appendage and left atrium, which can herniate through the defect. Most such defects are incidental.

> The cephalad border of the pericardium is at the level of the sternal angle.

The normal pericardium measures 1 to 2 mm on cross-sectional imaging, such as CT and magnetic resonance imaging (MRI) (Fig. 1.9) (37). Pericardium is most visible anterior to the right ventricle on CT and MRI where there is adjacent fat. Several pericardial recesses are readily visible with cross-sectional imaging (38–40). The *transverse sinus* of the pericardium is posterior to the ascending aorta and main pulmonary artery, seen on imaging as a fluid-filled, usually curved structure immediately posterior the ascending aorta (Fig. 1.5). It can be confused for a lymph node or an aortic dissection flap. High-riding recesses can extend into the right paratracheal area and anterior to the aortic arch in the prevascular space, and should not be confused for underlying pathology.

> Normal pericardium measures 1 to 2 mm in thickness on CT and MRI.

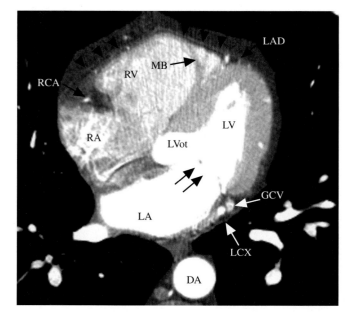

Figure 1.9 Axial computed tomography four-chamber image of the heart. Note the thin pericardium (*arrowheads*) seen anteriorly. DA, descending thoracic aorta; gCV, great cardiac vein; LA, left atrium; LAD, left anterior descending coronary artery; LV, left ventricle; LVot, left ventricular outflow tract; LCX, left circumflex coronary artery; MB, moderator band; RA, right atrium; RCA, right coronary artery; RV, right ventricle; *arrows*, mitral valve.

HEART

Cardiac anatomy is often not covered or is only minimally covered in thoracic radiology texts. However, the heart is an important part of thoracic radiology, whether it is the heart "shadow" in the middle of every chest radiograph or the detailed anatomic or functional information available from MRI and CT. Cardiac imaging evaluates not only anatomy, the basis of radiologic interpretation, but also cardiac function, perfusion, metabolism, and tissue characterization.

The human heart is a four-chamber conical structure predominantly located within the left hemithorax (Figs. 1.10, 1.11, 1.12, and 1.13). The heart has an *apex* at the infero-lateral margin of the left ventricle and a *base* posteriorly at the left atrium. Nonoxygenated blood from the superior and inferior vena cavae (systemic venous return) and the coronary sinus (the cardiac venous return) passes into *right atrium*, through the tricuspid valve into the *right ventricle*, and then through the pulmonic valve into the *pulmonary artery*, which carries the blood into the lungs for gas exchange. The openings of the inferior vena cava and coronary sinus into the right atrium are adjacent to each other on the inferior margin of the heart and contain valves known as the *eustachian* and *thebesian valves*, respectively. Oxygenated blood exits the lungs through the *pulmonary veins* into the *left atrium*, passes through the mitral valve into the *left ventricle*, after which it passes through the aortic valve into the ascending thoracic aorta (41). There are usually four pulmonary veins that drain into the left atrium, each receiving three to five major venous tributaries from the lungs (Fig. 1.10). The four pulmonary veins are the *right superior and inferior pulmonary veins* and the *left superior and inferior pulmonary veins*. Sometimes two veins may join together before draining into the left atrium, such as the left superior and inferior pulmonary veins. In other cases there is an extra vein draining directly into the left atrium, such as an additional right middle lobe vein. Anomalous pulmonary venous return creates a left-to-right shunt and is discussed in Chapter 19.

The right ventricle is the most anterior cardiac chamber, forms most of the anterior heart border on a posteroanterior radiograph, and is prone to contusion during blunt force trauma to the anterior chest wall.

Cardiac chambers, heart borders and changes with chamber enlargement are discussed in Chapters 3 and 20. Figures 1.9 and 1.11A are axial CT images demonstrating the cardiac chambers. The *right atrial appendage* lies anterior and superior to the right atrium. The right ventricle is the most anterior chamber, residing immediately behind the sternum. As such, it is prone to contusion when blunt force is applied to the anterior chest wall during trauma, such as a steering wheel injury during a motor vehicle accident or a crush injury while playing football. The right ventricle is heavily trabeculated. A distinct structure seen on cross-sectional imaging within the right ventricular

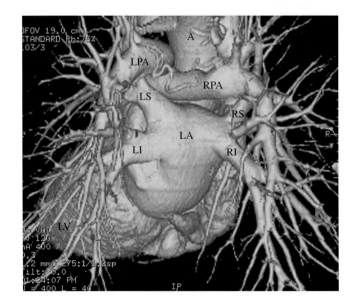

Figure 1.10 Shaded surface display of the left atrium and pulmonary veins in the posterior projection from electrocardiogram-gated 16-row multidetector computed tomography. A, aorta; LA, left atrium; LI, left inferior pulmonary vein; LPA, left pulmonary artery; LS, left superior pulmonary vein; LV, left ventricle; RI, right inferior pulmonary vein; RPA, right pulmonary artery; RS, right superior pulmonary vein.

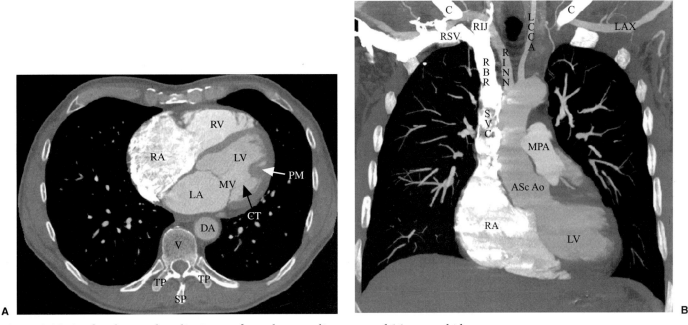

Figure 1.11 Axial and coronal cardiac images from electrocardiogram-gated 16-row multidetector computed tomography (CT) of the heart. In contrast to the non–electrocardiogram-gated image in Fig. 1.9, note the greater detail in both the axial plane and the coronal reconstruction, the latter possible due to the isotropic voxels of 16-row MDCT. *A.* Axial CT image illustrates the four cardiac chambers. Note the mitral valve (MV) with leaflets in the open position, because this image represents ventricular diastole. Chorda tendina (CT) is seen attaching to a papillary muscle (PM). DA, descending aorta; LA, left atrium; LV, left ventricle; RA, right atrium; RV, right ventricle; SP, spinous process; TP, transverse process; V, vertebral body. *B.* Coronal CT image. AscAo, ascending aorta; C, clavicle; LAX, left axillary artery; LCCA, left common cartoid artery; MPA, main pulmonary artery; RBR, right brachiocephalic vein; RIJ, right internal jugular vein; RINN, right innominate artery; RSV, right subclavian vein; SVC, superior vena cava.

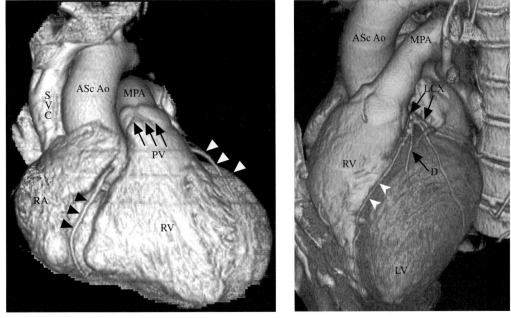

Figure 1.12 Cardiac surface anatomy from electrocardiogram-gated 16-row multidetector computed tomography in the (*A*) anterior projection and (*B*) long-axis projection. Note the right coronary artery (*black arrowheads*) in the right atrioventricular groove and left anterior descending coronary artery (*white arrowheads*) that runs in the interventricular groove; both are epicardial vessels. AscAo, ascending aorta; D, first diagonal; LCX, left circumflex coronary artery; MPA, main pulmonary artery; RA, right atrium; RV, right ventricle; SVC, superior vena cava; *small arrows* indicate the pulmonic valve.

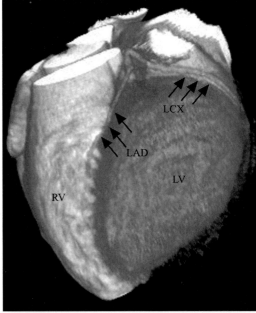

A

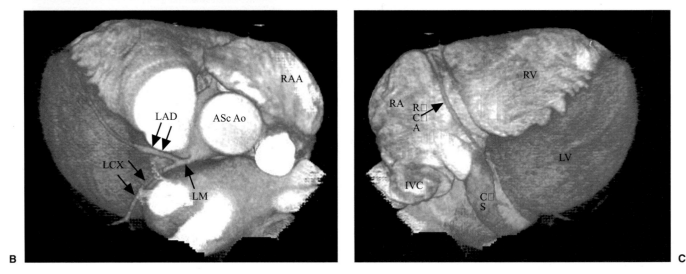

B
C

Figure 1.13 Cardiac surface anatomy and the coronary arteries. *A.* Projection along the interventricular groove demonstrates the right (RV) and left ventricles (LV) with the left anterior descending coronary artery (LAD) in the interventricular groove and the left circumflex coronary artery (LCX) in the more posterior left atrioventricular groove. *B.* Left main (LM) coronary artery as it arises from the left coronary cusp of the ascending aorta (AscAo). Left circumflex (LCX) and left anterior descending coronary arteries (LAD) on a projection from above the heart. *C.* View of the inferior surface of the heart demonstrates the inferior most aspect of the right coronary artery, as well as the coronary sinus (CS) and inferior vena cava (IVC) draining into the inferior aspect of the right atrium. RAA, right atrial appendage.

The right atrium forms most of the right heart border on a posteroanterior radiograph, whereas the left atrium forms most of the posterior heart border on a lateral radiograph.

apex is the *moderator band.* The left atrium forms most of the posterior cardiac border and the right atrium most of the right heart border. The wall of the left ventricle is thicker and more muscular than the right ventricle. The cardiac chambers are lined internally by endocardium, beneath which the myocardium made up of cardiac muscle fibers resides. The *left atrial appendage* lies anterior and superior to the left atrium and is longer and narrower than the right atrial appendage (Fig. 1.14). The *atrial septum* between the right and left atrium is thin and translucent; it contains a depression on the right atrial side known as the *fossa ovalis,* a remnant of the foramen ovale through which blood passed from right atrium to left atrium before birth. The *ventricular septum* separates the right and left ventricles and is thicker and more muscular. The *aortic, tricuspid,* and *pulmonic valves* are normally three-leaflet valves, whereas the *mitral valve* is a two-leaflet valve. *Papillary muscles* in the right and left ventricles are connected by chordae tendineae to the tricuspid and mitral valves, respectively, as illustrated in Fig. 1.11A.

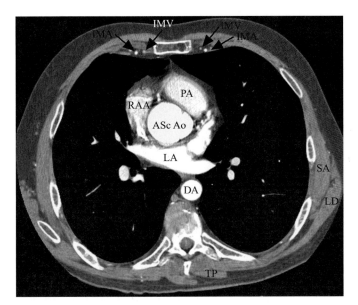

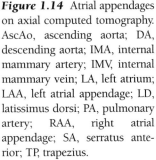

Figure 1.14 Atrial appendages on axial computed tomography. AscAo, ascending aorta; DA, descending aorta; IMA, internal mammary artery; IMV, internal mammary vein; LA, left atrium; LAA, left atrial appendage; LD, latissimus dorsi; PA, pulmonary artery; RAA, right atrial appendage; SA, serratus anterior; TP, trapezius.

The papillary muscles prevent prolapse of the valves into their respective atria during ventricular contraction during systole (41,42).

The heart is supplied by two coronary arteries that arise from the aortic root (Figs. 1.12 and 1.13). The right coronary artery arises from the right anterolateral aspect of the aortic root and runs anteriorly and inferiorly in the right atrioventricular groove. In addition to supplying the right atrium, right ventricle, and atrial septum, it usually supplies the sinoatrial and atrioventricular nodes. As it extends under the inferior surface of the heart, it becomes the posterior descending coronary artery. The left main coronary artery arises from the left lateral aspect of the aortic root, is 0.5 to 1.5 cm long, and quickly bifurcates into the left anterior descending coronary artery and the left circumflex coronary artery. The left main coronary artery supplies the left atrium, left ventricle, and the ventricular septum. The left anterior descending coronary artery runs left anterolaterally into the interventricular groove, whereas the left circumflex coronary artery runs posterolaterally and inferiorly in the left atrioventricular groove. Acute marginal branches arise from the right coronary artery, diagonal arteries from the left anterior descending coronary artery, and obtuse marginal branches from the left circumflex coronary artery. Anomalous coronary artery origins are discussed in Chapter 19. All these coronary arteries are epicardial, as they reside on the surface of the heart. Septal and muscular perforating arteries arise from the epicardial arteries and dive into the cardiac wall (42). Most cardiac blood supply occurs during diastole. Cardiac venous drainage parallels the arterial blood supply, with epicardial veins paralleling the epicardial arteries, that together drain into the coronary sinus on the inferior/posterior aspect of the heart, adjacent to the left circumflex coronary artery. The gold standard method for evaluating the coronary arteries is direct catheterization and contrast injection. Both CT and MRI are used to map the pulmonary veins and left atrium and cardiac veins for electrophysiologic ablation procedures and planning for biventricular pacemaker placement in which a lead is placed into the coronary sinus (43). CT and MRI are also making strides in the mapping and evaluation of the coronary arteries as well.

Central and cardiac pressure measurements vary throughout the cardiac cycle. Alterations in cardiac physiology and how that relates to the development of pulmonary edema are described in Chapter 10.

The coronary arteries are epicardial, that is they lie on the surface of the heart.

AORTA AND ARTERIES

The thoracic aorta is divided into the ascending aorta, the aortic arch, and the descending thoracic aorta. At the root of the aorta there are three aortic sinuses, right, left, and non-coronary, the first two giving rise to their respective coronary arteries. The aorta exits the left ventricle at the aortic valve, approximately at the third left costochondral cartilage in the parasternal region. It then extends anteriorly to the right and in the cephalad direction for approximately 5 cm, ending in the aortic arch. The ascending aortic diameter is approximately 3 cm; greater than 4 cm is considered abnormal. The aortic arch gives rise to the great vessels in the following order: *right innominate artery, left common carotid artery, left subclavian artery* (Figs. 1.15 and 1.16). The right innominate artery is approximately 4 to 5 cm long and gives rise to the right subclavian and right common carotid arteries. Common variants include the *bovine aortic arch*, in which the left common carotid artery arises from the right innominate artery (Figs. 1.15) and direct origin of the left vertebral artery from the aortic arch, rather than from the left subclavian artery (44,45). Common congenital anomalies of the aortic arch are described in Chapter 19. On a radiograph, the junction of ascending aorta and aortic arch is at the right half of the sternal angle, where the aorta emerges from the pericardial sac. The arch continues cephalad, before turning posterior and leftward behind the lower half of the manubrium. The under-surface of the aortic arch is at the level of the sternal angle. The *ligamentum arteriosum* is the remnant of the ductus arteriosus that closes at birth, having permitted the passage of blood from the main pulmonary artery to the aorta during fetal development. In adults it is an approximately 1.5-cm long fibrous band. On radiographs, the aortic knob is formed by the posterior leftward course of the aortic arch.

At approximately the T4-5 intervertebral disc level, the aortic arch becomes the descending thoracic aorta. The latter gives rise to intercostal arteries and to three bronchial

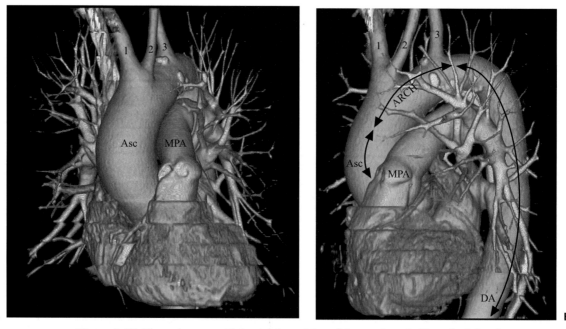

Figure 1.15 Thoracic aorta with bovine branching of the aortic arch. Note the left pulmonary artery extends posteriorly from the main pulmonary artery as a "mini-arch" under the aortic arch. *A.* Anterior projection. *B.* Oblique sagittal projection. 1, right innominate artery; 2, left common carotid artery; 3, left subclavian artery; ARCH, aortic arch; Asc, ascending aorta; DA, descending aorta; MPA, main pulmonary artery.

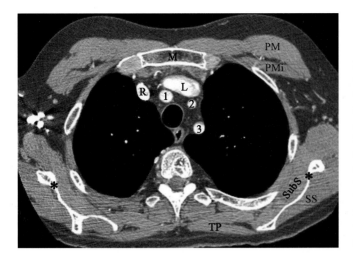

Figure 1.16 Great vessels and chest wall at the level of the upper mediastinum on axial computed tomography image. Asterisk, scapula; 1, right innominate artery; 2, left common carotid artery; 3, left subclavian artery; L, left brachiocephalic vein; M, manubrium; PM, pectoralis major; PMi, pectoralis minor; R, right brachiocephalic vein; SS, supraspinatus; SubS, subscapularis; TP, trapezius.

arteries (two left and one right) with variable origins near the T-5 level (16). At the aortic hiatus of the diaphragm, the descending thoracic aorta passes into the abdomen as the abdominal aorta. Uncommonly, an artery arising from the descending thoracic aorta supplies the blood flow to an isolated portion of lower lobe lung parenchyma, known as a *sequestration*. Intrapulmonary sequestrations are contained within the normal pleura of the lower lobe, whereas extrapulmonary sequestrations have their own pleural lining and are more commonly associated with additional congenital anomalies (46).

Other arterial structures of note include the *internal mammary arteries* that arise from the subclavian arteries and run vertically in the right and left parasternal regions (Figs. 1.2A and 1.14). The subclavian arteries become the *axillary arteries* when they course over the first anterior ribs at the lateral margin of the thoracic cage (Fig. 1.11B). The *lateral thoracic arteries* arise from the proximal axillary arteries and descend vertically in the anterolateral chest wall. The *inferior thyroidal arteries* are now commonly seen with fast thin-section CT arising from the thyrocervical trunk off of the subclavian artery in the superior mediastinum above the thoracic inlet.

VEINS

The veins parallel the arteries described above. The *internal jugular veins* parallel the common carotid arteries. The *subclavian veins* parallel the subclavian arteries. The internal jugular and subclavian veins join to form the *brachiocephalic veins* behind the medial heads of the clavicles. They join together to form the valveless superior vena cava behind the right first costochondral cartilage (Fig. 1.11B). The valveless brachiocephalic veins are 2.5 cm long on the right and 6 cm long on the left, the greater length of the left vein because of its oblique downward course across the mediastinum to the right-sided superior vena cava (16). The *superior vena cava* is 7.5 cm long, forms the upper right border of the mediastinum, and drains into the right atrium. The lower portion of the superior vena cava is contained within the pericardial sac and is immediately anterior to the right main bronchus. Uncommonly, individuals may have both left- and right-sided vena cavae; an isolated left superior vena cava is rare. When present, the left-sided vena cava usually still communicates with the right-sided superior vena cava across a left brachiocephalic vein. Left-sided superior venae cavae usually drain directly into the coronary sinus of the heart (47).

The azygos vein courses vertically along the right anterior aspect of the thoracic spine from the abdomen up to the superior vena cava, where it enters posteriorly at the T-4 ver-

The internal jugular and subclavian veins join to form the brachiocephalic veins behind the medial heads of the clavicles.

A left superior vena cava is usually a dual system accompanied by a right superior vena cava; rarely, it is isolated.

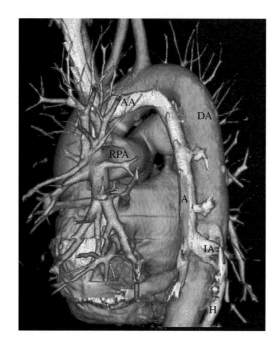

Figure 1.17 Azygos vein anatomy on an oblique sagittal CT reconstruction viewed from the right. A, azygos vein; AA, azygos arch; H, hemiazygos vein; IA, interazygos vein; RPA, right pulmonary artery; DA, descending aorta.

tebral body level (Figs. 1.17 and 1.18). It is formed at the diaphragm by the ascending lumbar vein and the right subcostal vein. Unlike the superior vena cava and brachiocephalic veins, the azygos vein does contain valves. The hemiazygos vein similarly runs vertically along the left anterior aspect of the thoracic spine, crossing rightward and draining into the azygos vein at the T-9 level. An interazygos vein often communicates between the azygos and hemiazygos veins. The intercostal veins, esophageal veins, and bronchial veins drain into the azygos/hemiazygos system (16).

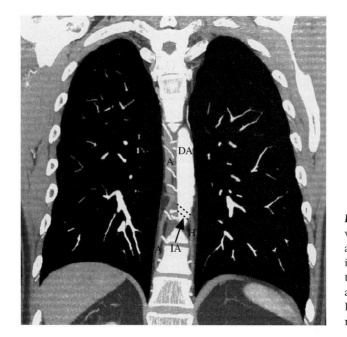

Figure 1.18 Azygos vein runs vertically to the right of midline, anterior to the spine. Note the intercostal arteries arising from the descending aorta (DA). A, azygos vein; H, hemiazygous vein; IA, interazygos vein runs posterior to the aorta.

LYMPHATIC SYSTEM

The large lymphatic structure that is responsible for most of the lymph return from the thorax, abdomen, pelvis, and lower extremities is the *thoracic duct*. It is the thoracic continuation of the abdominal cisterna chyli after it enters the thorax through the diaphragm at the aortic hiatus. The thoracic duct is a vertically oriented structure that runs anterior to the thoracic vertebral bodies to the right of the descending thoracic aorta. At the T6-7 level the duct deviates from midline toward the left, draining into the left internal jugular vein. The pleural layers contain an extensive network of lymphatics. Lymph flows medially from the visceral pleura to the hilar lymph nodes through the axial/bronchovascular and peripheral/interlobular septal interstitium of the lungs. Occasionally, *small intrapulmonary lymph nodes* are visible in the subpleural lung as 5 to 12 mm, smoothly marginated, round or ovoid, soft tissue attenuation nodules on CT; these are not uncommon in smokers (48).

> The thoracic duct runs anterior to the spine, toward the right side of the descending aorta below the T6-7 level, and to the left side above that level.

Normal lymph nodes are not visible on chest radiographs but are seen as round to ovoid soft tissue attenuation structures on CT, sometimes with a fatty hilum. By convention, lymph nodes 1 cm and larger in short axis are considered abnormally enlarged and in the setting of malignancy suspicious for tumor spread. Short axis is used because it is more consistent than long axis. However, we know that tumor cells may reside in lymph nodes less than 1 cm in size, and nodes larger than 1 cm may be hyperplastic. Most tracheobronchial mediastinal nodes and pulmonary lymph nodes are classified by the American Thoracic Society Classification scheme (Fig. 1.19). Although the most common use

> Small intrapulmonary lymph nodes may appear as 5- to 12-mm, noncalcified, smooth, round or ovoid nodules in the subpleural lung and are common in smokers.

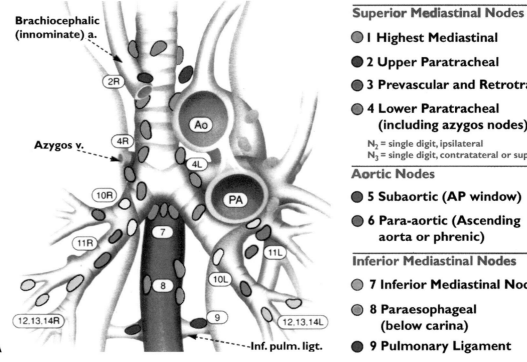

A

Superior Mediastinal Nodes

- **1 Highest Mediastinal**
- **2 Upper Paratracheal**
- **3 Prevascular and Retrotracheal**
- **4 Lower Paratracheal (including azygos nodes)**

  N₂ = single digit, ipsilateral
  N₃ = single digit, contrataeral or supraclavicular

Aortic Nodes

- **5 Subaortic (AP window)**
- **6 Para-aortic (Ascending aorta or phrenic)**

Inferior Mediastinal Nodes

- **7 Inferior Mediastinal Nodes**
- **8 Paraesophageal (below carina)**
- **9 Pulmonary Ligament**

N₁ Nodes

- **10 Hilar**
- **11 Interlobar**
- **12 Lobar**
- **13 Segmental**
- **14 Subsegmental**

B

Figure 1.19 Lymph node mapping scheme for lung cancer. *A.* Drawing. *B.* Table defining node stations. (Courtesy of Dr. JP Ko.)

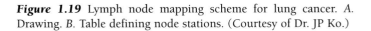

of this scheme is for the staging of lung cancer, it can be used for the description of lymph nodes due to any disease process. Other lymph node groups visible with thoracic imaging include internal mammary lymph nodes adjacent to the arteries and veins of the same name, in a parasternal location; they drain the breast tissue and anterior chest wall. Cardiophrenic lymph nodes are found adjacent to the heart at the level of the xiphoid. Anterior mediastinal lymph nodes are found anterior to the superior vena cava, left innominate artery, and ascending aorta behind the sternum. Nodes are also located along the esophagus and descending aorta, termed paraesophageal and paraaortic nodes, respectively.

REFERENCES

1. Kurihara Y, Yakushiji YK, Matsumoto J, et al. The ribs: anatomic and radiologic considerations. *Radiographics* 1999;19:105–119; 151–152.
2. Sanders CF. Sexing by costal cartilage calcification. *Br J Radiol* 1966;39:233.
3. Naidich JB, Naidich TP, Hyman RA, et al. The big rib sign: localization of basal pulmonary pathology in lateral projection utilizing differential magnification of the two hemithoraces. *Radiology* 1979;131:1–8.
4. Felson B. *Chest roentgenology.* Philadelphia: WB Saunders, 1973.
5. Remy-Jardin M, Remy J, Masson P, et al. Helical CT angiography of thoracic outlet syndrome: functional anatomy. *AJR Am J Roentgenol* 1997;174:1667–1674.
6. Gluck MC, Twigg HL, Ball MF, et al. Shadows bordering the lung on radiographs of normal and obese persons. *Thorax* 1972;27:232–238.
7. Felson B. A review of over 30,000 normal chest radiograms. In: *Chest roentgenology.* Philadelphia: WB Saunders, 1973:494–501.
8. Bhalla M, McCauley DI, Golimbu C, et al. Counting ribs on chest CT. *J Comput Assist Tomogr* 1990;14:590–594.
9. Haje SA, Harcke HT, Bowen JR. Growth disturbance of the sternum and pectus deformities: imaging studies and clinical correlation. *Pediatr Radiol* 1999;29:334–341.
10. Fonkalsrud EW, Beanes S. Surgical management of pectus carinatum: 30 years' experience. *World J Surg* 2001;25:898–903.
11. Khairouni A, Bensahel H, Csukonyi Z, et al. Congenital high scapula. *J Pediatr Orthopaed B* 2002;11:85–88.
12. Kumar UK, Sahasranam KV. Mitral valve prolapse syndrome and associated thoracic skeletal abnormalities. *J Assoc Phys India* 1991;39:536–539.
13. Dhuper S, Ehlers KH, Fatica NS, et al. Incidence and risk factors for mitral valve prolapse in severe adolescent idiopathic scoliosis. *Pediatr Cardiol* 1997;18:425–428.
14. Lennon EA, Simon G. The height of the diaphragm in the chest radiograph of normal adults. *Br J Radiol* 1965;38:937–943.
15. Mullins ME, Stein J, Saini SS, et al. Prevalence of incidental Bochdalek's hernia in a large adult population. *AJR Am J Roentgenol* 2001;177:363–366.
16. Woodburne RT. *Essentials of human anatomy*, 7th ed. New York: Oxford University Press, 1983.
17. Francis IR, Glazer GM, Bookstein FL, et al. The thymus: reexamination of age-related changes in size and shape. *AJR Am J Roentgenol* 1985;145:249–254.
18. Baron RL, Lee JK, Sagel SS, et al. Computed tomography of the normal thymus. *Radiology* 1982;142:121–125.
19. Berkmen YM, Drossman SR, Marboe CC. Intersegmental (intersublobar) septum of the lower lobe in relation to the pulmonary ligament: anatomic, histologic, and CT correlations. *Radiology* 1992;185:389–393.
20. Otsuji H, Uchida H, Maeda M, et al. Incomplete interlobar fissures: bronchovascular analysis with CT. *Radiology* 1993;187:541–546.
21. Felson B. The azygos lobe: its variation in health and disease. *Semin Roentgenol* 1989;24:56–66.
22. Godwin JD, Tarver RD. Accessory fissures of the lung. *AJR Am J Roentgenol* 1985;144:39–47.
23. Felson B. The lobes and interlobar pleura: fundamental roentgen considerations. *Am J Med Sci* 1955;230.
24. Berkmen T, Berkmen YM, Austin JH. Accessory fissures of the upper lobe of the left lung: CT and plain film appearance. *AJR Am J Roentgenol* 1994;162:1287–1293.
25. Horsfield K. Diameters, generations, and orders of branches in the bronchial tree. *J Appl Physiol* 1990;68:457–461.

26. Gray H. *Gray's anatomy*. Norwich, CT: Longman, 1973.
27. Wu JW, White CS, Meyer CA, et al. Variant bronchial anatomy: CT appearance and classification. *AJR Am J Roentgenol* 1999;172:741–744.
28. Westra D, Verbeeten B Jr. Some anatomical variants and pitfalls in computed tomography of the trachea and mainstem bronchi. I. Mucoid pseudotumors. *Diagn Imag Clin Med* 1985;54: 229–239.
29. Weibel ER. *Morphometry of the human lung*. New York: Academic Press, 1963.
30. Gehr P, Bachofen M, Weibel ER. The normal human lung: ultrastructure and morphometric estimation of diffusion capacity. *Respir Physiol* 1978;32:121–140.
31. Stone KC, Mercer RR, Freeman BA, et al. Distribution of lung cell numbers and volumes between alveolar and nonalveolar tissue. *Am Rev Respir Dis* 1992;146:454–456.
32. Verschakelen JA, Van Fraeyenhoven L, Laureys G, et al. Differences in CT density between dependent and nondependent portions of the lung: influence of lung volume. *AJR Am J Roentgenol* 1993;161:713–717.
33. Geiser M, Cruz-Orive LM, Im Hof V, et al. Assessment of particle retention and clearance in the intrapulmonary conducting airways of hamster lungs with the fractionator. *J Microsc* 1990;160: 75–88.
34. Crapo JD, Barry BE, Gehr P, et al. Cell number and cell characteristics of the normal human lung. *Am Rev Respir Dis* 1982;126:332–337.
35. Gehr P, Geiser M, Im Hof V, et al. Surfactant and inhaled particles in the conducting airways: structural, stereological, and biophysical aspects. *Microsc Res Techn* 1993;26:423–436.
36. Dudiak CM, Olson MC, Posniak HV. Abnormalities of the azygos system: CT evaluation. *Semin Roentgenol* 1989;24:47–55.
37. Delille JP, Hernigou A, Sene V, et al. Maximal thickness of the normal human pericardium assessed by electron-beam computed tomography. *Eur Radiol* 1999;9:1183–1189.
38. Olson MC, Posniak HV, McDonald V, et al. Computed tomography and magnetic resonance imaging of the pericardium. *Radiographics* 1989;9:633–649.
39. Choi YW, McAdams HP, Jeon SC, et al. The "high-riding" superior pericardial recess: CT findings. *AJR Am J Roentgenol* 2000;175:1025–1028.
40. Groell R, Schaffler GJ, Rienmueller R. Pericardial sinuses and recesses: findings at electrocardiographically triggered electron-beam CT. *Radiology* 1999;212:69–73.
41. Hollinshead WH. The thorax. In: *Textbook of anatomy*. Philadelphia: Harper & Row, 1974: 491–556.
42. Gedgaudas E, Moller JH, Castaneda-Zuniga WR, Amplatz K. Embryology and anatomy of the heart: acquired vascular disease. In: *Cardiovascular radiology*. Philadelphia: WB Saunders, 1985:1–16.
43. Cascade PN, Sneider MB, Koelling TM, et al. Radiographic appearance of biventricular pacing for the treatment of heart failure. *AJR Am J Roentgenol* 1447;177:1447–1450.
44. Oh E, Quint DJ, Gross BH. Identification of vertebral arteries on CT of the chest. *Br J Radiol* 2001;74:328–330.
45. Felson B. Aortic arch anomalies: a few facts and a lot of speculation. *Semin Roentgenol* 1989;24: 69–74.
46. Ko SF, Ng SH, Lee TY, et al. Noninvasive imaging of bronchopulmonary sequestration. *AJR Am J Roentgenol* 2000;175:1005–1012.
47. Cormier MG, Yedlicka JW, Gray RJ, et al. Congenital anomalies of the superior vena cava: a CT study. *Semin Roentgenol* 1989;24:77–83.
48. Bankoff MS, McEniff NJ, Bhadelia RA, et al. Prevalence of pathologically proven intrapulmonary lymph nodes and their appearance on CT. *AJR Am J Roentgenol* 1996;167:629–630.

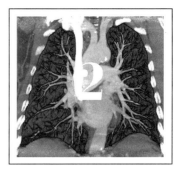

Imaging Modalities and Applications

■ Chest Radiograph
■ Fluoroscopy, Conventional Tomography, and Bronchography
■ Computed Tomography
■ Magnetic Resonance Imaging
■ Nuclear Medicine
■ Angiography
■ Ultrasonography

Over the past three decades, the introduction of new imaging modalities has had a profound impact on the practice of cardiopulmonary radiology. Many of the new modalities have not only complemented but replaced the classic imaging arsenal (1). For example, conventional planar tomography and bronchography have been replaced by computed tomography (CT) with multiplanar reconstructions. No other imaging modality matches the level of detail of the lungs provided by CT. Dynamic imaging of the heart was markedly changed with the introduction of echocardiography and is currently again being transformed by cardiac magnetic resonance imaging (MRI) and CT. Fluoroscopy has become an almost completely lost art. In this chapter, we introduce the main imaging modalities in clinical use and elaborate on their principles and applications.

CHEST RADIOGRAPH

Its origins going back to 1895, the plain radiograph still represents the cornerstone of modern cardiopulmonary radiology. Depending on the practice setting, around 30% to 60% of all radiologic examinations performed in the clinical practice of radiology are plain radiographs of the chest. These are simple, quick, cheap, and provide useful clinical information for diagnostic and follow-up purposes. The major indications for chest radiography are listed in Table 2.1 (2).

The basic principles of chest radiography are relatively simple (Fig. 2.1); a patient is placed between an x-ray source and a detector. A point source emits photons with energies in the x-ray range toward the patient. These photons penetrate the patient, are attenuated (mostly by scattering and absorption), and those that come out of the patient are captured by the detector. This generates a single projection image of attenuation properties of the patient onto the detector (Fig. 2.2). Lungs contain mostly air and thus show little attenuation of the photons traversing them. Other tissues, like the heart, great vessels, and chest wall, are denser and show greater attenuation of the x-ray beam.

The point source is an x-ray tube that emits radiation in the "diagnostic" x-ray range, which is between 60 and 150 keV. Photons with energies at the upper end of that range have better penetrance in the body and are therefore less attenuated. Photons with energies at the lower end of the range are more attenuated by the soft tissues and osseous struc-

The single most commonly performed radiologic examination is the chest radiograph.

Radiation in the diagnostic range is 60 to 150 keV.

Table 2.1: Indications for Chest Radiograph

Diagnostic
    Cardiopulmonary symptoms
        Cough, hemoptysis, shortness of breath, chest pain, etc.
    Preoperative for thoracic surgery
    Preoperative if known cardiopulmonary limitations
    Staging of thoracic tumors and extrathoracic malignancies
    Infection
        Pleural, parenchymal, mediastinal
Follow-up
    Previously diagnosed cardiopulmonary disease
        Pneumonia resolution to exclude endobronchial lesion
        Pulmonary edema
    Monitoring of intensive care unit patients
        Lung disease
        Pleural disease
        Lines and tubes positions
    Monitoring of postoperative patients

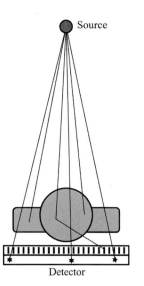
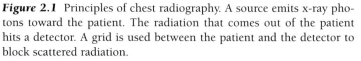

Figure 2.1 Principles of chest radiography. A source emits x-ray photons toward the patient. The radiation that comes out of the patient hits a detector. A grid is used between the patient and the detector to block scattered radiation.

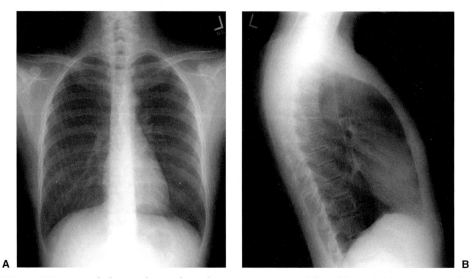

Figure 2.2 Normal chest radiograph in the posteroanterior (A) and lateral (B) positions. The radiograph has wide latitude and can represent lung structures, cardiac and vascular structures, soft tissues of the chest wall, and ribs. Metallic nipple markers are used here.

tures of the chest. Tube voltage, measured in peak kilovoltage (kVp), determines the maximum energy of the emitted photons. Tube current, measured in milliampere (mA), combined with exposure time in seconds, determines the total number of photons emitted. Both kVp and mA are controlled by the operator. Typical values for a chest radiograph are 120 kVp and 5 mA.

The simplest type of detector is a plastic film covered with a light-sensitive emulsion, silver halide. Films alone have very limited sensitivity to x-rays; therefore, an amplifying screen must be placed against the film to produce multiple visible photons for each incident x-ray. Plain films can display a wide range of attenuations (wide latitude). More modern detectors are digital in nature (3). In computed radiography, the detector is a plate of phosphor or selenium phosphor, which captures x-rays. Once exposed, the plate is scanned point by point by a laser beam. Each point emits a radiation of intensity that is quantified and is proportional to the x-ray energy captured at that specific point on the plate. Computed radiography offers greater latitude than the screen–film combination. In direct radiography, the plate is usually made of a grid of tiny elements called charged coupled devices (like sensors in most modern digital cameras) or thin-film transistors (like flat screens for computers). These elements can directly record and quantify the number of photons striking each point of the plate without the need to scan the plate point by point with a laser beam. It is therefore much faster to process than computed radiography. With all types of detectors, grids and filters are usually used to block scattered photons and eliminate photons of too low energy, respectively.

The position of the patient with respect to the detector can vary. In the most common technique, posteroanterior and lateral views of the chest are obtained (Fig. 2.2). The patient is placed in the upright position, 180 cm (6 feet) from the source, facing the detector so the radiation crosses the patient from the back to the front (posteroanterior) and then with the left side facing the detector (lateral). These two projections allow a gross three-dimensional estimate of the structures in the chest. In bedridden patients, the x-ray plate or detector is typically inserted under the patient, and the radiation crosses the patient in a front to back direction (anteroposterior). The distance between the source and the patient is often decreased to 100 to 125 cm, which produces a larger magnification of anatomic structures in the anterior aspect of the chest, particularly the heart and superior mediastinum (Fig. 2.3). If the patient is placed on a table lying on their side, a lateral decu-

Tube voltage (kVp) determines maximum energy of the x-ray photons.

Tube current (mA) × time (seconds) determines the number of photons emitted (mA).

Decubitus images are useful for evaluation of pleural fluid (free flowing or not), pneumothorax (when patient cannot sit upright), and air trapping (failure of dependent lung to collapse).

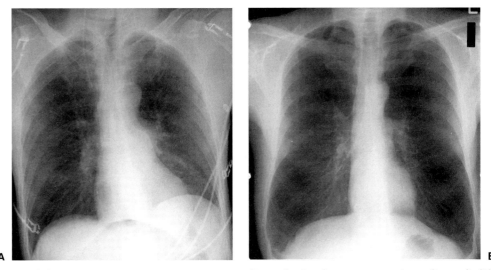

A   **B**

Figure 2.3 Posteroanterior vs. anteroposterior radiograph. On the anteroposterior radiograph *(A)* of this normal patient, the detector is against the back of the patient. A combination of decreased distance between the source and the patient and increased distance between the detector and the anterior mediastinal structures compared with the posteroanterior radiograph *(B)* leads to magnification of the heart.

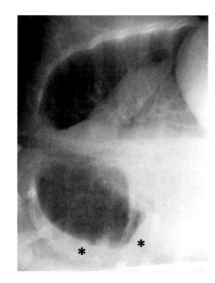

Figure 2.4 Lateral decubitus. The patient is positioned with their side against a table, and a radiograph is taken across the table. A free-flowing right pleural effusion is demonstrated (asterisk).

bitus view is obtained. This is useful to assess for a pleural effusion (Fig. 2.4) (4) or air trapping on the dependent side and pneumothorax on the nondependent side. Oblique views with the patient at an angle to the film can be obtained to eliminate superposed structures. A common angled view is the apical lordotic view, with photons crossing the patient from a low anterior to a high posterior position. This provides a better view of the lung apices (5) by projecting the clavicles above them (Fig. 2.5).

In most cases, the radiograph is taken with the patient in full inspiration. Several respiratory maneuvers can be performed by the patient immediately before radiographic exposure. A radiograph with the patient in expiration may demonstrate air trapping. Radiographs taken while the patient is performing a Valsalva or a Müller maneuver can also be taken to assess changes in vascular structures or masses.

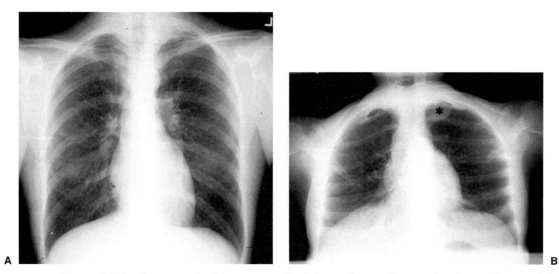

Figure 2.5 Lordotic view. In this patient with a left apical neurofibroma, the abnormality is subtle on the posteroanterior radiograph (A), but the lordotic view (B) improves visualization of the lung apices, and the neurofibroma (asterisk) becomes more apparent.

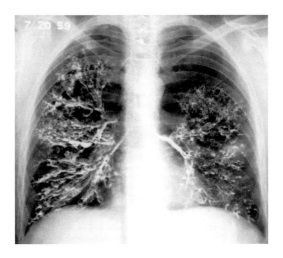

Figure 2.6 Bronchography, circa 1950. An endobronchial inhaled contrast agent was used to demonstrate the presence of bronchiectasis.

FLUOROSCOPY, CONVENTIONAL TOMOGRAPHY, AND BRONCHOGRAPHY

Fluoroscopic imaging is largely a dead or dying art. In the past it had been used to evaluate pulmonary nodules and mediastinal vasculature. It is still occasionally used to assess diaphragmatic motion ("sniff test"). This test involves dynamic evaluation of the simultaneous motion of the two hemidiaphragms during normal breathing and forced rapid inspiration (a "sniff"). If there is paralysis of one hemidiaphragm, it will not move as well as the contralateral part (Fig. 2.6) and may show paradoxical motion during rapid inspiration.

Bronchography is also an obsolete technique involving the administration of iodinated contrast via inhalation to coat the surface of the tracheobronchial tree and to evaluate the presence and extent of bronchiectasis. This has been completely replaced by high resolution CT.

Conventional tomography is an obsolete technique that used simultaneous movement of a source of x-ray and a detector in opposite directions with respect to a specific plane of imaging, to blur all the structures out of that plane of imaging. This has been replaced by CT (6).

COMPUTED TOMOGRAPHY

Invented in 1972 by Hounsfield, CT is the imaging modality of choice for evaluating the thorax, after the chest radiograph, because the level of anatomic detail is unmatched by anything else in radiology. Indeed, the only other imaging modality that offers more extensive anatomic detail than CT is direct tissue examination under a microscope by a pathologist (which is much more invasive than CT). Note that whereas the in-plane spatial resolution of CT is 5 times lower than that of plain radiography (Table 2.2), the contrast resolution (the depiction of subtle differences in contrast) is 10 times greater than that of chest radiography. This improved contrast resolution, in combination with the tomographic nature of CT, enables CT to provide much better anatomic detail than plain radiography, despite the lower spatial resolution. The indications for chest CT are indicated in Table 2.3 (7).

The basic principles of CT are relatively simple (Fig. 2.7) and are an extension of plain film radiography. The point source of x-ray photons and the detectors are placed on opposite sides of the patient on a ring-like structure, called the gantry. The gantry rotates around the patient, located on a table at its center. Photons are emitted toward the patient,

After the chest radiograph, CT is the method of choice for most advanced imaging of the thorax.

Table 2.2: Spatial Resolution and Effective Radiation Dose of Thoracic Imaging Modalities

Modality	Resolution (mm)	Dose (mSv)
CXR	0.08	0.02 (PA)
		0.04 (lateral)
DR	0.17	0.02 (PA)
		0.04 (lateral)
CT	0.4	8
		0.6–1.2 (screening)
MRI	1.0	0
Planar nuclear medicine	7.0	0.4 (Xe)–18 (Ga)
PET	3.0	7
Angiography	0.13	12
US	0.3	0
Background radiation	n/a	3 per year

CXR, chest radiography; DR, digital radiography; CT, computed tomography; MRI, magnetic resonance imaging; PET, positron emission tomography; US, ultrasound.
From Bushberg JT, et al. *The essential physics of medical imaging*, 2nd ed. Philadelphia: Lippincott, Williams & Wilkins, 2002, with permission.

Table 2.3: Indications for Thoracic Computed Tomography

Thoracic
  Further characterize CXR abnormality (e.g., nodule, mediastinal mass)
  Detection and follow-up of neoplastic disease (e.g., metastatic sarcoma, lymphoma)
  Characterization of lung nodules
    Benign vs. indeterminate
  Parenchymal lung disease (e.g., emphysema, interstitial lung disease, infection)
  Airway disease
    Central and peripheral airways
  Pleural disease
    Empyema, metastasis, mesothelioma
  Postsurgical complications
  Percutaneous biopsy guidance
  Localization for VATS
Cardiac
  Cardiac abnormalities on CXR
  Cardiac anatomy
  Coronary arteries
    Calcification, patency with CTA
    Aberrant coronary arteries
  Postcardiac bypass grafting complications
    Mediastinitis
Vascular
  Aorta: aneurysm, trauma, dissection, coarctation
  Pulmonary arteries: embolus, pulmonary hypertension
  Venous: SVC/brachiocephalic vein thrombus or obstruction

VATS, video-assisted thoracoscopic surgery; CXR, chest radiography; CTA, CT angiography; SVA, superior vena cava.

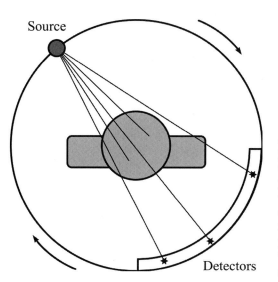

Source

Detectors

Figure 2.7 Principles of computed tomography. The source of x-rays and the detectors are on opposite sides of the gantry with the patient at the center of the gantry. Radiation that crosses the patient is detected, producing a projection of attenuation information. By rotating the gantry around the patient, multiple projections are obtained, which are then used to mathematically reconstruct tomographic attenuation images.

penetrate the patient, and are captured by one or more detectors. This generates a series of projection images of attenuation properties of the patient. Images representing photon attenuation at each point in the volume traversed by the photons can then be mathematically reconstructed from the different projections (Fig. 2.8).

The source of radiation, the x-ray tube, rotates continuously around the gantry, using a slip-ring technology in more modern scanners. Collimation is used at the source. The x-ray tube voltage in CT is usually 120 kVp, similar to that of a plain chest radiograph. However, CT uses a longer exposure time, 1 second per gantry rotation, with combined tube current–exposure time value of 200 mA, which increases the radiation dose.

CT scanner technology has gone through several generations of refinements (8). Early scanners used incremental table displacement and produced one set of axial projections at each table position. Modern scanners use continuous table displacement while the gantry rotates and produce helical projections, with a stationary 360-degree array of detectors around the entire gantry. The latest scanners have multiple rows of detectors in the direction of slice thickness. An entire CT of the chest using a multislice CT scanner takes only a few seconds. The recorded projections are helical in nature, and planes of imaging are interpolated from the helical projection data. In single-row detectors, collimation deter-

Fast helical CT scanners can image the entire thorax in seconds, reducing respiratory motion artifact.

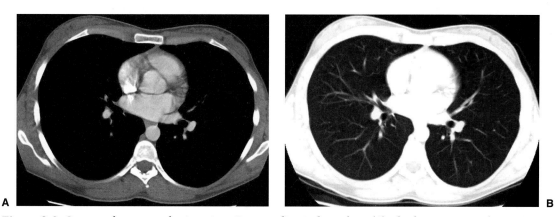

A   B

Figure 2.8 Computed tomography imaging. On a mediastinal window (A), the lungs are mostly black and the mediastinum and chest wall are emphasized. On a lung window (B), these structures are white and the fine structures of the lungs are emphasized.

Beam pitch is table travel per gantry rotation divided by beam collimation.

Data pitch is table travel per gantry rotation divided by normal slice width. This is the preferred definition for multislice CT.

mines slice thickness, whereas it is determined by detector configuration and reconstruction algorithm in multiple row scanners. The table travel per complete rotation of the gantry with respect to x-ray beam collimation is called the "beam pitch." In multislice scanners, the table travel per complete rotation of the gantry with respect to the data slice thickness is called the "data pitch."

Several postprocessing steps can be performed when the slices are reconstructed from the projections. Tissue-specific algorithms, such as "soft tissue" or "lung," are available to more accurately reconstruct the CT projection data based on assumptions of x-ray photon energy and tissue attenuation. The projection data represent attenuation of multiple points through a volume of the chest. In practice, the projection data are used to reconstruct entire axial slices of the patient or only a subset of each slice, called the "field of view." But one is far from limited to reconstructing axial images. One of the most powerful features of CT is the ability to reformat the image data into multiplanar and three-dimensional images. Axial and helical data can be reformatted to produce simple images in the coronal or sagittal planes (Fig. 2.9). To improve visualization, volumetric data can also be combined into a single image representing for each pixel the maximum or minimum value of that pixel through the volume (Fig. 2.10). Powerful algorithms can also produce three-dimensional images with shaded surface display (Fig. 2.11) or even endobronchial images (virtual bronchoscopy) (Fig. 2.12) (9,10).

The reconstructed images represent a range of attenuations of different points in a slice of the patient. CT image values are typically scaled to 4,096 different levels of attenuation recorded, measured in "Hounsfield units" (HU). By convention, air has a value of −1,000 HU and water a value of 0 HU. Hounsfield units in medical CT typically range from −1,000 and +3,000. Modern monitors cannot display the full range of attenuation values, because they are typically limited to 256 levels of gray. Moreover, the radiologist's eyes can only distinguish between 30 to 90 levels of gray. The operator can choose to map any range of attenuation values into the displayed 256 levels of gray. The center of this range of displayed attenuation values is called the "window level" and the width of this range is called the "window width." A soft tissue window typically displays attenuation levels in the range of −400 to +200 HU and emphasizes structures in the mediastinum, whereas a lung window displays attenuation levels in the range of −1,000 to −300 HU and emphasizes structures in the lung (Fig. 2.8).

Different window and level combinations are used to evaluate structures of different attenuation, such as lung, soft tissue, and bone windows settings.

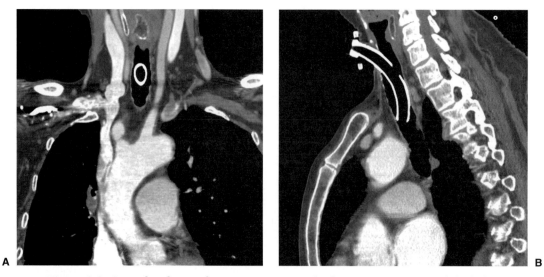

A   **B**

Figure 2.9 Coronal and sagittal reconstructions. Multiplanar reconstruction of the helical projection data in the coronal (*A*) and sagittal (*B*) planes can be performed. This improves visualization of some structures, such as the lung apices and the great vessels.

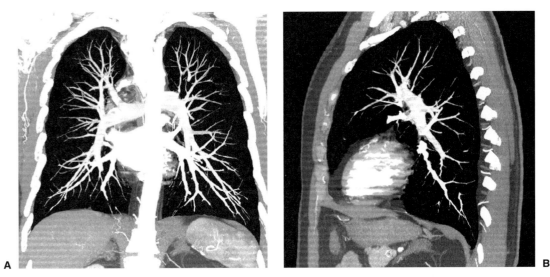

A   B

Figure 2.10 Maximal intensity projection reconstructions. Information from a stack of images representing a volume can be combined into a single image representing for each pixel the maximum value of that pixel through the volume, shown here in the coronal (*A*) and sagittal (*B*) planes.

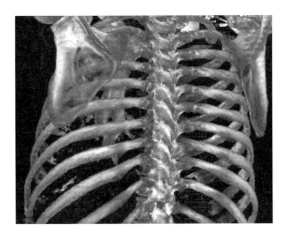

Figure 2.11 Three-dimensional reconstructions. Data can be further processed to produce three-dimensional images with shaded surface of any chest structure, such as the heart, mediastinum, lungs or ribs.

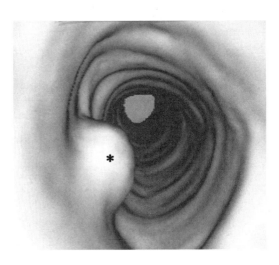

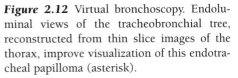

Figure 2.12 Virtual bronchoscopy. Endoluminal views of the tracheobronchial tree, reconstructed from thin slice images of the thorax, improve visualization of this endotracheal papilloma (asterisk).

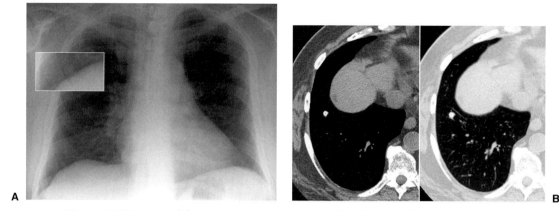

Figure 2.13 Lung nodule on computed tomography. The faint nodule projecting at the right lung base near the diaphragm (A) was further investigated by Computed Tomography, which revealed a calcified granuloma (B).

CT angiography requires a faster rate of intravenous contrast administration than routine CT.

In general, for cardiopulmonary imaging, the patients lay still in a supine position on the table and hold their breath for the duration of the CT acquisition. Scanning can be performed at end-inspiration and end-expiration and also in the prone or decubitus positions. Furthermore, intravenous contrast can be administered to the patient before scanning to emphasize vascular structures and to modify the attenuation properties of different parts of the body. For routine chest CT, contrast is injected at 2 mL/s, whereas for CT angiogram (CTA) contrast is injected at 4 mL/c.

Different scanning protocols are used to answer different clinical questions (Figs. 2.13 and 2.14). Table 2.4 illustrates common CT protocols. In general, thicker slices (5 mm) provide enough anatomic detail for diagnosis of most cardiopulmonary disease. Thinner (1 to 1.5 mm) slices are used in three different contexts. For interstitial lung disease (11), thin slices are used with 10-mm spacing between slices. This covers only 10% of the chest but provides improved pulmonary parenchymal detail while minimizing radiation dose. For CT angiography, thin continuous slices are used to provide fine detail of the entire vascular tree of concern (12). For screening, thin continuous slices at very low doses are used to detect small lung nodules (13).

CT acquisition parameters should be optimized to obtain diagnostic images without unnecessary radiation exposure to patients.

With multislice CT scanners and protocols involving thin continuous slices, radiation dose per examination has become a concern (14). Total effective dose for a chest CT equals up to 200 to 400 plain chest radiographs (15), which is quite high. The dose for a screening CT is, however, equal to only 30 to 60 plain chest radiographs (Table 2.2). Manufacturers are including several optimizations to their scanners to lower the dose, and scanning protocols are designed to use the lowest possible radiation doses that will provide an answer to clinical problems.

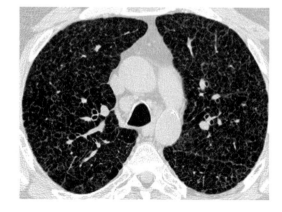

Figure 2.14 High resolution computed tomography allows exquisite visualization of the fine detail of the lung parenchyma in this patient with Langerhan's cell histiocytosis.

Table 2.4: Thoracic Computed Tomography Protocols

Name	Slice Thickness (mm)	Pitch	Start	End	mA	Intravenous Position	Intravenous Contrast
Lung nodule	5	1.5–2	Lung apices	Lung bases	Low	Supine	No
	1.25	1.0	Top of nodule	Bottom of nodule	Regular	Supine	No
Routine chest	5	1.5–2	Lung apices	Lung bases	Regular	Supine	Yes
Lung cancer	5	1.5–2	Lung apices	Adrenal glands	Regular	Supine	Yes
High resolution	1–1.5	10-mm spacing	Lung apices	Lung bases	Regular	Inspiration Expiration Prone Supine	No
Trachea	1–1.5	1.5–2	7 cm below carina	Above epiglottis	Regular	Inspiration Expiration Supine	Yes
Pulmonary veins	1–1.5	1.5–2	Lung bases	Lung apices	Regular	Supine	Yes
SVC	2.5	1.5–2	Lung apices	Lung bases	Regular	Supine	Yes
Pulmonary embolus	1–1.5	1.5–2	2 cm below diaphragm	Lung apices + legs	High	Supine	Yes
Thoracic aorta	2.5	1.5–2	2 cm above arch	Diaphragm	Regular	Supine	Yes
Cardiac	1–1.5	1.5–2	Aortic	Diaphragm	Regular	Supine	Yes
Lung cancer screening	1–1.5	1.5–2	Apex	Lung bases	Low	Supine	No

SVC, Superior vena cava.

MAGNETIC RESONANCE IMAGING

MRI for cardiopulmonary disease has been in clinical use since the 1980s (Fig. 2.15). It has proven extremely valuable to evaluate abnormalities of the chest wall, diaphragm, and mediastinum (Table 2.5) (16–18). MRI is also important for both anatomic and functional assessment of the heart, aorta, and pulmonary arteries (19,20). Its clinical value to assess lung disease is currently limited. Several experimental techniques are under active development, including pulmonary imaging using hyperpolarized gases (21).

MRI is particularly useful for evaluation of cardiovascular and posterior mediastinal structures within the thorax.

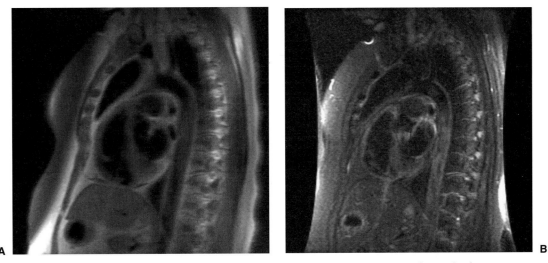

A   B

Figure 2.15 Magnetic resonance imaging of the chest. Magnetic resonance provides multiplanar imaging emphasizing different tissue contrast information. A T1-weighted sagittal image (A) provides excellent anatomic detail, whereas a T2-weighted image (B) can reveal increased water content, and thus increased signal, found in many pathologies.

Table 2.5: Indications for Thoracic Magnetic Resonance Imaging

Thoracic
  Chest wall neoplasm (especially superior sulcus tumors)
  Mediastinal tumors (e.g., bronchogenic cysts)
  Lung parenchyma: limited, experimental
  Thoracic outlet and brachial plexus
Cardiac
  Congenital heart disease: shunts, complicated anatomy
  Myocardium
    Cardiomyopathy
    Ischemic disease
    Hypertension
    Right ventricular dysplasia
  Pericardium: thickening, effusion, tamponade, pericardial cyst
  Masses: thrombus, tumors
  Valves (limited): stenosis, regurgitation
Vascular
  Aorta: aneurysm, trauma, dissection, coarctation
  Pulmonary arteries: embolus, pulmonary hypertension
  Venous: SVC thrombus or obstruction

SVC, superior vena cava.

Only enough physics to understand the basic principles of MRI is discussed here (22). In terms of MRI, the atomic nucleus is a system that has two important properties (Fig. 2.16). First, the nucleus has a "magnetic moment" represented by a small magnetization vector along its axis. Second, the nucleus has an "angular momentum" or a "spin" that can be thought of as a rotation about its axis. Only nuclei with an odd number of protons or an odd number of neutrons possess angular momentum. When an object possessing a magnetic moment is placed under a strong external magnetic field (B_0, typically 10,000 times greater than the earth's magnetic field), it experiences a force to align it with the external magnetic field, like a compass. If the object also has angular momentum, it experiences a force called a "torque" that generates a motion of "precession" of its magnetic moment at a specific angle around the direction of the external magnetic field (or around its opposite direction), similar to the motion of a spinning top (Fig. 2.17A). The frequency of the precession, called the "Larmor frequency," is directly proportional to the intensity of the external magnetic field around the object.

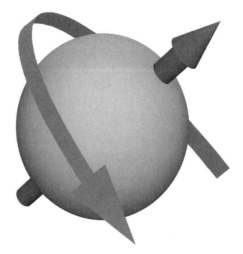

Figure 2.16 Magnetic properties of nucleus. A hydrogen nucleus has two important magnetic properties: a magnetic moment, represented by an *arrow* along its axis, and an angular momentum or spin.

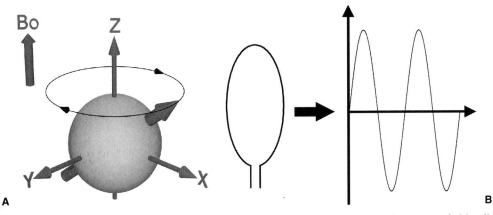

Figure 2.17 Precession. A precessing magnetic moment *(A)* under an external magnetic field will generate a signal in a coil *(B)* that is too small to measure. It is the signal from trillions of precessing magnetic moments that is measured in practice.

A precessing magnetization vector induces an electric current in an external loop of wire (a "coil") and therefore produces a nuclear magnetic resonance signal (Fig. 2.17B). This signal is proportional to the component of the magnetization vector perpendicular to the external magnetic field. The current induced by the magnetic moment of a single precessing nucleus is too small to measure. Under a strong magnetic field, there is a small excess of nuclei precessing around B_0 compared with those precessing in the opposite direction (few per million). If there is a sufficiently large number of precessing spins such that there is a dominant direction of alignment of magnetic moments, the "net magnetization M_0" (Fig. 2.18) is measurable as long as it too is precessing. At equilibrium, there is no component of M_0 perpendicular to B_0; thus, no signal is available. To detect M_0, one needs to disturb the equilibrium and apply a second smaller external magnetic field, B_1, which rotates around the B_0 field at the Larmor frequency (Fig. 2.19). This exerts two effects on the precessing magnetic moments of a large number of nuclei: It will synchronize their phase of precession and exert another force, or "torque," that rotates the net magnetization away from the direction of B_0. An effective means to generate a rotating B_1 field is by application of radiofrequency

In MRI, the signal is generated by the induction of an electric current in a coil (longitudinal relaxation; local tissue environment) and T2 (vertical relaxation; rejects local spin dephasing).

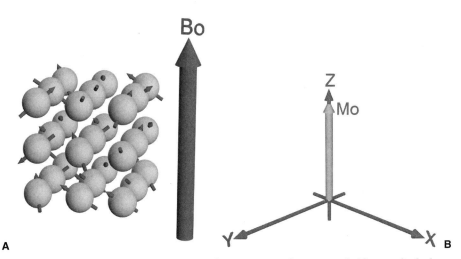

Figure 2.18 Net magnetization vector. When an external magnetic field is applied, there is a small excess of spins pointing toward the external magnetic field compared with those pointing in the opposite direction *(A)*. The net difference (trillions of atoms) will produce a non-zero net magnetization, M_0, pointing toward the external magnetic field *(B)*.

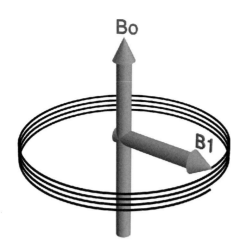

Figure 2.19 Rotating B_1 field. To produce a non-zero net transverse magnetization, a small second rotating field, B_1, is applied orthogonal to the external magnetic field. This synchronizes spins and creates an additional torque on the net magnetization away from the external field.

MR images are generated using gradients (varying magnetic fields) and pulse sequences (external pulses).

energy. Both effects of the B_1 field increase the component of M_0 perpendicular to B_0, M_{xy}, and therefore increases the signal induced by M_0.

Once the B_1 field is stopped, the net magnetization returns slowly to its equilibrium state in the direction of B_0, a phenomenon called "relaxation" (Fig. 2.20A). Relaxation of the magnetization vector of each tissue is different and is most influenced by two important quantities (Fig. 2.20B): T_1 characterizes the relaxation of the component of the magnetization vector that is parallel to the B_0 field (longitudinal relaxation), and T_2 characterizes the relaxation of the component that is perpendicular to the B_0 field (transverse relaxation). T_1 reflects local tissue environment, whereas the much shorter T_2 reflects local spin dephasing. The latter can be partly reversed (and thus signal recovered) using a refocusing technique by a 180-degree pulse perpendicular to B_0 (spin refocused echo).

MRI is a technique that generates images of the human body, using these basic physical principles together with spatially varying magnetic fields, called "gradients," and complex sequences of external pulses, called "pulse sequences." These gradients encode spatial positional information. Pulse sequences are constructed to generate images that emphasize one or more aspects of these T_1 and T_2 components (Fig. 2.15). In these sequences, preparatory pulses are occasionally used. Examples of such preparatory pulses are an inversion 180-degree pulse, which is used to eliminate signal from a specific tissue (fat, blood, myocardium), and a chemical saturation pulse to eliminate the signal of fat. The signal of blood is affected by its motion in and out of the imaging plane, a characteristic that many sequences take into account to image blood vessels.

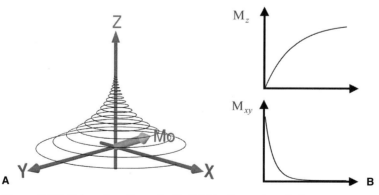

Figure 2.20 Relaxation. Once the B_1 field is discontinued, the net magnetization vector slowly returns to its state of equilibrium (*A*). The temporal variations of the longitudinal, M_z, and transverse, M_{xy}, components (*B*) of that magnetization vector are, respectively, determined by the T_1 and T_2 values of the local tissue environment.

Table 2.6: Sample Thoracic MRI Protocols

Name	Sequence 1	Sequence 2	Sequence 3	Sequence 4	Sequence 5	Sequence 6
Chest mass	Localizer	Axial T1	Axial T2	Multiplanar T1 post-Gd		Optional sequences
Thoracic outlet	Localizer	Sagittal T1	Sagittal gradient	Axial T2		Optional sequences
Cardiac mass	Localizer	Multiplanar bright blood	Multiplanar black blood	Axial T1	Axial T1 post-Gd	Optional sequences
RV dysplasia	Localizer	Multiplanar bright blood	Axial black blood	Axial black blood with fat-sat		Optional sequences
Pericarditis	Localizer	Multiplanar bright blood	Multiplanar black blood	Axial T1	Coronal T2	Optional sequences
Cardiac viability	Localizer	Multiplanar bright blood	Short-axis perfusion post-Gd	Multiplanar delayed hyperenhancement		Optional sequences
Aorta	Localizer	Black blood axial	3D gradient sagittal oblique post-Gd	3D gradient oblique coronal post-Gd		Optional sequences

MRI, magnetic resonance imaging; RV, 3D, three-dimensional; fat-sat, fat saturation.

An MRI protocol is simply a set of pulse sequences, chosen to emphasize a specific structure or pathologic process under consideration. Sample cardiopulmonary MRI protocols are illustrated in Table 2.6. For cardiac imaging, spin-echo sequences produce dark signal in the blood and are commonly called "black-blood sequences." Gradient-echo sequences produce high signal in the blood and are called "bright-blood sequences" (Fig. 2.21). MRI is often performed using the intravenous administration of a gadolinium-based contrast agent to better visualize vascular structures, such as the aorta (Fig. 2.22A) (19) and the pulmonary arteries (Fig. 2.22B); to better characterize masses; and to characterize myocardial perfusion and viability. Cardiac MRI is now considered the gold standard for the assessment of left ventricular ejection fraction (20).

The length of an MRI examination is 30 to 60 minutes, much longer than the few seconds of a CT examination. MRI offers much better tissue contrast than CT but typically has lower in-plane spatial resolution. Contraindications to MRI examinations include patients with pacemakers, aneurysm clips, metal fragments in the eyes, or some metallic

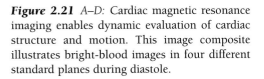

A,B **C,D**

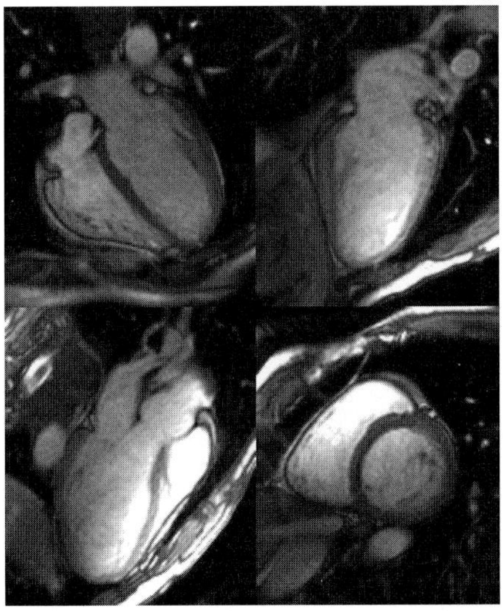

Figure 2.21 *A–D:* Cardiac magnetic resonance imaging enables dynamic evaluation of cardiac structure and motion. This image composite illustrates bright-blood images in four different standard planes during diastole.

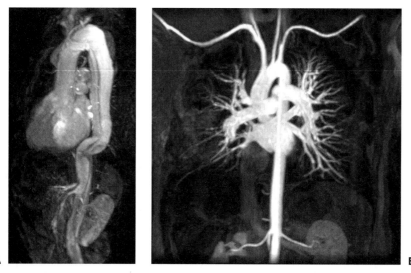

A   B

Figure 2.22 Magnetic resonance angiography. Magnetic resonance angiography of the aorta and its branches is useful to evaluate aortic dissection (*A*). Magnetic resonance angiography of the pulmonary arteries enables good visualization of the pulmonary arteries (*B*) and can be used to rule out pulmonary embolism.

implants. Pregnant patients are often scanned, usually without the administration of intravenous contrast.

NUCLEAR MEDICINE

In nuclear medicine imaging, a radioactive agent is administered to a patient and images are detected based on emission and radioactive decay.

In chest radiography and CT, the source of radiation is located outside the patient. In nuclear medicine studies, the source of radiation is administered to the patient in the form of a radiopharmaceutical, either via inhalation or intravenous injection. Once properly distributed into the body, the source emits radiation by radioactive decay, which is then captured by detectors outside the patient (Fig. 2.23).

A radiopharmaceutical is a complex made up of two parts: a molecule or aggregate of molecules that has a specific biological function and a radionuclide that is the source of radiation. In chest radiology, the radionuclide is either a gamma emitter or a positron emitter. Corresponding detectors for these are, respectively, a gamma camera and a positron emission tomography (PET) camera. A gamma camera records a projection of the radiopharmaceutical distribution in the patient. This is called planar imaging. Information from multiple projections can also be combined into volumetric data and produce tomographic

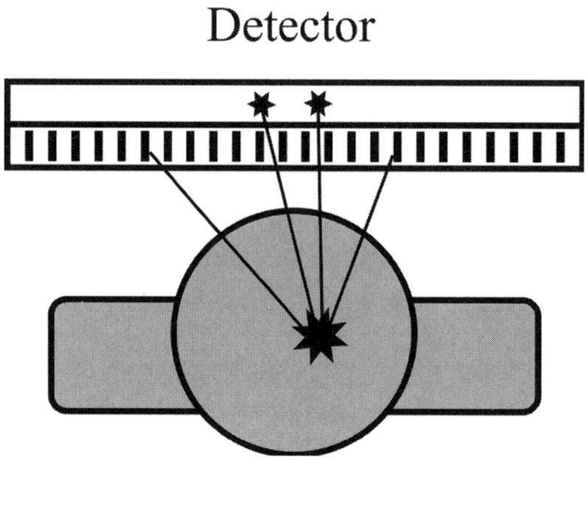

Detector

Figure 2.23 Principles of planar radionuclide imaging. The source of radiation is located inside the patient. Radiation that leaves the patient is captured by the detector, which produces projection images of the distribution of the radiotracer in the patient.

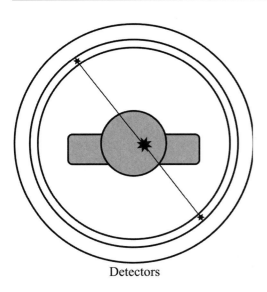

Detectors

Figure 2.24 Principles of positron emission tomography. Emitted positrons quickly collide with tissue electrons, and their annihilation produces two collinear photons in opposite directions, which are captured by the detectors. The position of the photon pair and difference in timing between the two detections allow determination of position of the emitter.

images. This is called single photon emission CT. A PET camera is made of a ring of detectors surrounding the patient (Fig. 2.24), similar to CT. These detect collinear photons in opposite directions emitted by the annihilation of a positron–electron pair and can therefore pinpoint with relative precision the position of origin of the pair of photons in the body and produce tomographic imaging.

The main clinical indications for radionuclide imaging in radiology are indicated in Table 2.7. The most common radionuclide examinations for cardiopulmonary disease are discussed.

Lung Perfusion Scan
Technetium-99m labeled human albumin microspheres or microaggregated albumin are complex aggregates that measure from 10 to 150 μm in size. They are administered via a peripheral vein and lodge themselves into precapillary arterioles in the lungs after going through the heart. The distribution of radioactivity throughout the lungs reflects the distribution of perfusion. In thromboembolic disease, part of the arterial vascular supply to the

Perfusion scintigraphy reflects relative, not absolute, perfusion of the lungs.

Table 2.7: Indications for Thoracic Radionuclide Imaging
Pulmonary
Ventilation/perfusion
Pulmonary embolus (acute and chronic)
Assessment of split function for surgical planning
Emphysema surgery patient selection
PET, SPECT
Cancer staging and follow-up
Indeterminate pulmonary nodule
Gallium scan
Infection (HIV)
Neoplasm (lymphoma)
Fever of unknown origin
Cardiac
Cardiac perfusion
Ischemia and infarct characterization
Ejection fraction
Wall motion
PET, positron emission tomography; SPECT, single position emission computed tomography; HIV, human immunodeficiency virus.

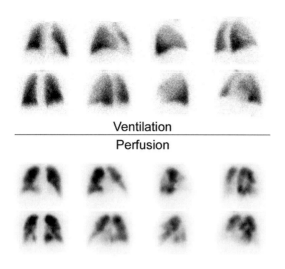

Ventilation

Perfusion

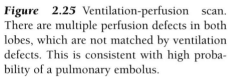

***Figure* 2.25** Ventilation-perfusion scan. There are multiple perfusion defects in both lobes, which are not matched by ventilation defects. This is consistent with high probability of a pulmonary embolus.

lungs is compromised and cannot be reached by the radiopharmaceutical. These regions will show absence of or decreased radioactivity (Fig. 2.25). This examination is very sensitive but not very specific for pulmonary emboli (23), because many etiologies of lung pathology can cause a decrease in lung perfusion, including malignancy and infection.

Lung Ventilation Scan

To improve specificity for pulmonary emboli, a lung perfusion scan is combined with a lung ventilation scan. In the latter, xenon (^{133}Xe) or a ^{99m}Tc radiolabeled aerosol is administered to the patient via inhalation into a closed system. Xenon requires a special ventilation system, so technetium is generally preferred. Detectors measure radioactivity in the lungs during the wash-in, equilibrium, and wash-out phases of the examination. Classically, thromboembolic disease manifests as normal ventilation in areas of abnormal perfusion (Fig. 2.25), whereas other lung diseases typically show both abnormal ventilation and perfusion in the affected areas. However, in many cases of pulmonary emboli, matched defects can be seen (23).

Gallium Scan

Gallium (^{67}Ga) citrate is administered to the patient intravenously. Gallium will distribute slowly throughout the body, accumulating mainly in the liver, spleen, bone marrow, nasopharynx, lachrymal glands, thymus, and breasts. Imaging is performed more than 24 hours after injection. Uptake of gallium in the lungs is increased in infection and inflammation and in neoplastic processes. It may be used to follow disease activity in lymphoma (Fig. 2.26) (24) and to differentiate between active tumor and residual fibrosis when soft tissue remains after treatment. It is also used in human immunodeficiency virus infection to detect lung disease in a setting of a normal chest radiograph.

The exact mechanism by which gallium uptake occurs is not well understood.

Positron Emission Tomography

A glucose analogue, ^{18}FDG(fluorodeoxyglucose)-6-phosphate, is administered intravenously. FDG distributes in the body and localizes to different organs proportionally to the local glucose uptake and metabolism. Other less commonly used PET agents include ^{13}N-ammonia, L-methyl-^{11}C-methionin, and ^{18}F- fluoromisonidazole. The two main organs of distribution of FDG are the brain and the heart. FDG also localizes to active tumor. It can detect tumors as small as 7 mm in size, which is better than single photon emission CT using thallium or ^{99m}Tc sestamibi, which has poor sensitivity for tumors below 2 cm in size (25). For the heart, FDG allows assessment of local myocardial viability (26). PET lacks the spatial resolution of CT but enables the distinction between metabolically active and silent tissues, which CT cannot do. For the lungs, it enables distinc-

A negative PET in a patient with a lung nodule greater than 7 mm in diameter is a strong indicator of a benign lesion. However, some tumors, such as bronchoalveolar cell carcinoma, are known to yield false-negative PETs.

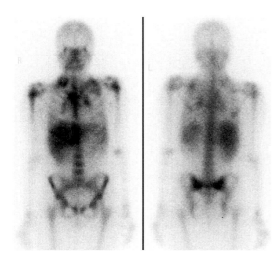

Figure **2.26** Gallium scan. There is increased gallium uptake in the multiple lymphoma lesions in the chest of this patient, the largest in the right supraclavicular area. (Courtesy of Dr. C. Bui, Ann Arbor, Michigan.)

tion between benign and malignant tumor and between recurrent tumor and postoperative changes (Fig. 2.27) (27,28). In combination with CT, images of both modalities can be registered and provide a combination of anatomic detail and metabolic activity (29). Combined CT–PET scanners now permit simultaneous acquisition for better anatomic registration.

Cardiac Perfusion Scan

Thallium chloride (^{201}Tl) is a potassium analogue that distributes in tissues with an intact sodium-potassium pump. Technetium sestamibi distributes in tissues by passive diffusion, whereas teboroxime is avidly extracted by the myocardium. Either radiopharmaceutical can be used to assess local myocardial perfusion (30) by quantifying local differences in extraction of the radiopharmaceutical by the myocardium in the rest and stress states (Fig. 2.28). The stress state is induced either by exercise or by the administration of a drug like dipyridamole or adenosine, which increases heart rate and blood pressure. This study can also assess ventricular wall motion.

Cardiac Function

Red blood cell labeling multiple gated acquisition studies (MUGA) is performed by different techniques involving technetium (^{99m}TcO$_4^-$). Gating is used to assess differences in

A positive PET in a patient with a lung nodule indicates a metabolically active lesion, such as a lung cancer, and also infection, such as tuberculosis.

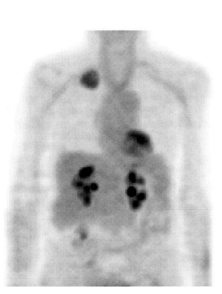

Figure **2.27** Positron emission tomography. Active tumor at the right lung apex shows increased metabolic rate and thus increased uptake of 18-fluorodeoxyglucose.

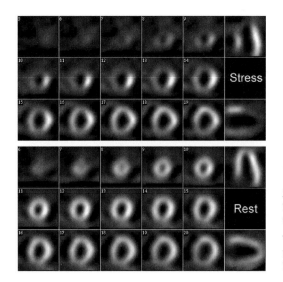
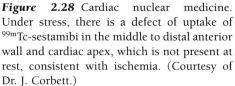

Figure 2.28 Cardiac nuclear medicine. Under stress, there is a defect of uptake of ^{99m}Tc-sestamibi in the middle to distal anterior wall and cardiac apex, which is not present at rest, consistent with ischemia. (Courtesy of Dr. J. Corbett.)

blood pool activities within the left ventricle, between systole and diastole. From these values, a left ventricular ejection fraction is determined. Wall motion can also be assessed by this study.

Infarct Scan

Pyrophosphate (99mTc-pyrophosphate) parallels calcium metabolism and binds to denaturated proteins in damaged myocardium. Increased update of the radiopharmaceutical is seen in myocardial infarction, as well as cardiomyopathies and myocardial injury.

ANGIOGRAPHY

Fluoroscopic imaging is similar in principle to standard radiography, except that the detector is inherently digital, records dynamic information of temporal change in attenuation, and displays the information in real time. It is therefore equivalent to a rapid movie-like sequence of simple radiographs using the same projection, although the dose of radiation per image is lower. Angiography is the use of fluoroscopic imaging before, during, and after administration of intravenous iodinated contrast agents for the purpose of visualizing vascular structures. Contrast is administered either via a peripheral vein or by a catheter placed directly into the vessels of the thorax, including the aorta, coronary arteries, pulmonary arteries, bronchial arteries, or the heart. Although the risks related to angiography used to be significant, the introduction of pigtail catheters and low osmolarity contrast agents has significantly decreased these risks (31).

Angiography most often uses a digital subtraction approach for imaging (Fig. 2.29) (32,33). This involves two sets of images, respectively, without and with the intravascular contrast agent, that are subtracted from each other. If patient motion between the two sets of images is minimal, then the subtracted image will display mostly intravascular contrast and will minimize background structures.

Clinical indications for angiography are indicated in Table 2.8. In cardiopulmonary radiology, angiographic examinations for the lungs include pulmonary angiography (Fig. 2.30) (32) and bronchial artery angiography. For the heart and great vessels, aortography (33,34), coronary angiography, and ventriculography are performed. Aortography and pulmonary angiography are slowly being replaced by noninvasive techniques, like CT or MR angiography. Both CT and MR angiography are commonly performed for diagnosis before percutaneous interventional procedures like aortic stent grafts (35). Angiography is useful in emergency situations or when the results of noninvasive examinations are equivocal.

Many simple diagnostic angiography studies have been replaced by CT angiography and MR angiography. Thoracic angiography studies are now more often coupled to an intervention, such as embolization, stent-graft, and thrombolysis, than in the past.

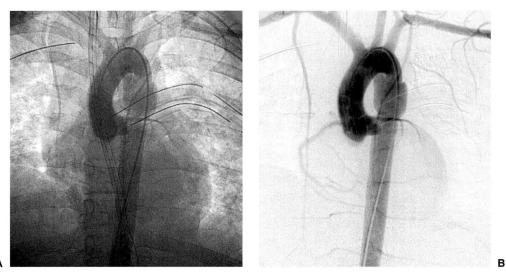

A   B

Figure 2.29 Subtraction technique. The injury to the thoracic aorta is difficult to assess given the cardiac and rib shadows (*A*). If the background, the same image without contrast, is subtracted from the image with contrast, then the aortic injury becomes more conspicuous (*B*). (Courtesy of Dr. K. Cho, Ann Arbor, Michigan.)

Table 2.8: Indications for Thoracic Angiography

Pulmonary arteries
   Pulmonary embolism (acute or chronic)
   Pulmonary hypertension
      Chronic PE
      Extrinsic compression
      Mediastinal fibrosis
   Congenital abnormalities
      AVMs, hypoplastic, stenosis, anomalous venous drainage
Aorta
   Traumatic injury
   Ruptured aneurysm or dissection
   Stent graft placement
Cardiac
   Coronary artery disease
   Valvular disease

PE, pulmonary embolism; AVMs, arteriovenous malformations.

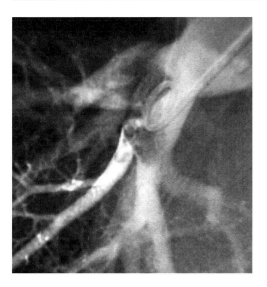

Figure 2.30 Pulmonary angiogram. There are filling defects in branches of the pulmonary arteries, consistent with pulmonary emboli. (Courtesy of Dr. K. Cho, Ann Arbor, Michigan.)

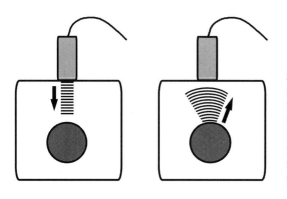

Figure 2.31 Principles of ultrasonography. Sound waves are emitted by a transducer, are reflected at tissue interfaces, and the reflected waves are captured by the same transducer. The intensity of the reflected signal and the time at which the signal was received are used to determine the exact position of the sonographic interfaces.

ULTRASONOGRAPHY

Diagnostic ultrasound waves are in the 1- to 20-MHz range (audible sound range is 20 Hz to 20 kHz).

The basic principles of ultrasonography are as follows. A hand-held transducer containing a piezoelectric crystal is put into direct contact with the part of the body to be imaged and produces a narrow beam of sound waves, which travel through a physical medium by inducing compressions and rarefactions in that medium. These sound waves are in the ultrasound range from 1 to 20 MHz in medical applications and are beyond the audible range for humans (from 20 Hz to 20 kHz). These sound waves are either reflected back to the transducer, refracted, scattered, or attenuated at tissue interfaces. The waves that are reflected back to the transducer are recorded and produce a signal that, once processed, indicates the different interfaces in the penetrated tissues and their respective depths (Fig. 2.31). By rapidly changing the orientation of the beam of sound waves, two-dimensional imaging of a section of the body can be performed.

Ultrasound is mostly used for cardiac imaging, not pulmonary imaging (36). Echocardiography is largely the province of cardiology in the United States and so is only covered briefly here. Because of its good spatial resolution and its exquisite temporal resolution, echocardiography is the first modality of choice in clinical practice for the anatomic and functional assessment of heart disease (Fig. 2.32). Its main clinical indications are listed in Table 2.9. It can be performed by either a transthoracic approach or a transesophageal approach. Doppler echocardiography can be used to quantify blood velocity through the different cardiac chambers and valves.

Ultrasound is most commonly used by diagnostic radiologists for the evaluation and treatment of pleural disease.

Ultrasound has a very limited diagnostic role in the chest outside the heart. It is commonly used to distinguish between pleural effusions and pleural masses (37,38) (although this is mostly done by CT) (Fig. 2.33) and to assess motion of the diaphragm (39). Ultrasound has a somewhat greater role in invasive procedures (40), including thoracentesis guidance and to guide a biopsy needle for chest wall masses and pulmonary masses adjacent to the chest wall. Most other lung biopsies are routinely performed under CT guidance.

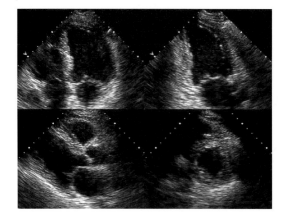

Figure *2.32* Cardiac echocardiography. Echocardiographic imaging shows normal appearance of the heart in four standard planes. (Courtesy of Dr. W. Armstrong, Ann Arbor, Michigan.)

Table 2.9: Indications for Thoracic Ultrasound

Thoracic
  Pleural effusions
  Pleural masses
  Diaphragm
  Interventional procedures (guidance or localization)
Cardiac
  Congenital heart disease: shunts, complicated anatomy
  Myocardium
    Cardiomyopathy
    Ischemic disease
    Hypertension
  Pericardium: thickening, effusion, tamponade
  Cardiac masses: thrombus, tumors
  Valves: stenosis, regurgitation, prosthetic, vegetations
Vascular
  Aorta: dilatation, dissection
  Pulmonary arteries: pulmonary hypertension

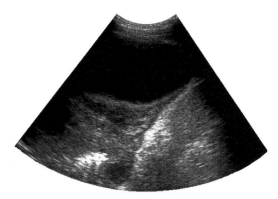

Figure **2.33** Pleural effusion. A large anechoic area above the left hemidiaphragm is consistent with a left pleural effusion.

REFERENCES

1. Fraser RS, Müller NL, Colman N, et al., eds. *Fraser and Pare's diagnosis of diseases of the chest.* St. Louis: WB Saunders, 1999.
2. American College of Radiology. ACR standard for the performance of pediatric and adult chest radiography. Reston, VA: American College of Radiology, 1997.
3. Yaffe MJ, Rowlands JA. X-ray detectors for digital radiography. *Phys Med Biol* 1997;42:1.
4. Rigler LG. Roentgen diagnosis of small pleural effusion: a new roentgenographic position. *JAMA* 1931;96:104.
5. Rundle FF, Delambert RM, Epps RG. Cervicothoracic tumors: a technical aid to their roentgenologic localization. *AJR Am J Roentgenol* 1959;81:316.
6. Grenier P, Maurice F, Musswet D, et al: Bronchiectasis: assessment by thin section CT. *Radiology* 1986;161:95–99.
7. American College of Radiology. ACR standard for the performance of pediatric and adult thoracic computed tomography (revised). Reston, VA: American College of Radiology, 1998.
8. Bushberg JT, et al. *The essential physics of medical imaging*, 2nd ed. Philadelphia: Lippincott, Williams & Wilkins, 2002.
9. Remy-Jardin M, Remy J, Artaud D, et al. Volume rendering of the tracheobronchial tree: clinical evaluation of bronchographic images. *Radiology* 1998;208:761–770.
10. Higgins WE, Ramaswamy K, Swift RD, et al. Virtual bronchoscopy for three dimensional pulmonary image assessment: state of the art and future needs. *Radiographics* 1998;18:761–768.
11. Webb WR, Müller NL, Naidich DP, eds. *High resolution CT of the lung.* New York: Lippincott-Raven, 1996.

12. Mayo JR, Remy-Jardin M, Müller NL, et al. Pulmonary embolism: prospective comparison of spiral CT with ventilation-perfusion scintigraphy. *Radiology* 1997;205:447–452.
13. Henschke CI, Yankelevitz DF. CT screening for lung cancer. *Radiol Clin North Am* 2000;38:487.
14. Slovis TL. CT and computed radiography: the pictures are great, but is the radiation dose greater than required? *AJR Am J Roentgenol* 2002;179:39–41.
15. Wall BF, Hart D. Commentary: revised radiation doses for typical x-ray examinations. Report of a recent review of doses to patients from medical x-ray examinations in the UK by NRPB. *Br J Radiol* 1997;70:437–439.
16. Naidich DP, Zerhouni EA, Siegelman SS, eds. *Computed tomography and magnetic resonance of the thorax*. New York: Raven Press, 1991.
17. Fortier MV, Mayo JR, Swensen SJ, et al. MR imaging of chest wall lesions. *Radiographics* 1994;14:597.
18. Heelan RT, Demas BE, Caravelli JF, et al. Superior sulcus tumor: CT and MR imaging. *Radiology* 1989;170:637.
19. Kersting-Sommerhoff BA, Higgins CB, White RD, et al. Aortic dissection: sensitivity and specificity of MR imaging. *Radiology* 1988;166:651–655.
20. Manning WJ, Pennell DJ, eds. *Cardiovascular magnetic resonance*. New York: Churchill Livingstone, 2002.
21. Kauczor HU. Current issues in hyperpolarized gases in MRI: biomedical investigations and clinical applications. *NMR Biomed* 2000;13:173.
22. Brown MA, Smelka RC. *MR: basic principles and applications*. New York: John Wiley & Sons, 1995.
23. The PIOPED Investigators. Value of the ventilation/perfusion scan in acute pulmonary embolism. *JAMA* 1990;263:2753–2759.
24. Front D, Israel O. The role of Ga-67 scintigraphy in evaluating the results of therapy of lymphoma patients. *Semin Nuclear Med* 1995;25:60–71.
25. Goldsmith SJ, Kostakoglu L. Nuclear medicine imaging of lung cancer. *Radiol Clin North Am* 2000;38:511.
26. Mesotten L, Maes A, Vande Werf F, et al. PET radiopharmaceuticals used in viability studies in acute myocardial infarction: a literature survey. *Eur J Nucl Med Mol Imag* 2002;29:3–6.
27. Sazon DAD, Santiago SM, Hoo GWS, et al. Fluorodeoxyglucose-positron emission tomography in the detection and staging of lung cancer. *Am J Respir Crit Care Med* 1996;153:417.
28. Chinn R, Ward R, Keyes JW, et al. Mediastinal staging of non-small-cell cancer with positron emission tomography. *Am J Respir Crit Care Med* 1995;152:2090.
29. Wahl RL, Quint LE, Greenough RL, et al. Staging of mediastinal non-small cell lung cancer with FDG PET, CT and fusion images: preliminary prospective evaluation. *Radiology* 1994;191:371.
30. Hachamovitch R. Clinical application of rest thallium-201/stress technetium-99m sestamibi isotope myocardial perfusion single-photon emission computed tomography. *Cardiol Rev* 1999;7:83.
31. Hudson ER, Smith TP, McDermott VG, et al. Pulmonary angiography performed with iopamidol: complications in 1434 patients. *Radiology* 1996;198:61–65.
32. van Rooij WJ, den Heeten GJ, Sluzewski M. Pulmonary embolism: diagnosis in 211 patients with use of selective pulmonary digital substraction angiography with a flow-directed catheter. *Radiology* 1995;195:793.
33. Guthaner DF, Miller DC. Digital substraction angiography of aortic dissection. *AJR Am J Roentgenol* 1983;141:157.
34. Davies ER, Roylance J. Aortography in the investigation of traumatic mediastinal haematoma. *Clin Radiol* 1970;21:297.
35. Thurnher SA, Dorffner R, Thurnher MM, et al. Evaluation of abdominal aortic aneurysm for stent-graft placement: comparison of gadolinium-enhanced MR angiography versus helical CT angiography and digital subtraction angiography. *Radiology* 1997;205:341–352.
36. Otto CM. *Textbook of clinical echocardiography*. St. Louis: WB Saunders, 2000.
37. McLoud TC, Flower CDR, Hadfield JW. Ultrasound of the pleura: sonographic, CT and MR imaging. *AJR Am J Roentgenol* 1991;156:1145–1153.
38. Yang PC, Luh KT, Chang DB, et al. Value of sonography in determining the nature of pleural effusion: analysis of 320 cases. *AJR Am J Roentgenol* 1992;159:29–33.
39. Gottesman E, McCool FD. Ultrasound evaluation of the paralyzed diaphragm. *Am J Respir Crit Care Med* 1997;155:1570–1574.
40. O'Moore PV, Mueller PR, Simeone JF, et al. Sonographic guidance in diagnostic and therapeutic interventions in the pleural space. *AJR Am J Roentgenol* 1987;149:1–5.

Approach to the Chest Radiograph

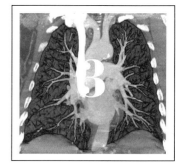

- Approach to the Radiograph
- Approach to the Radiograph in the Picture Archiving and Communication System (PACS) Era

Especially for neophyte interpreters of radiographs, it is essential to approach the images in the proper way. For $29.95 we will send you the ancient secret approach to the chest radiograph discovered by Leonardo da Vinci. It not only improves your interpretation of chest radiographs, it helps you to win friends and influence people.

In reality, only the first sentence of the last paragraph is true. Any approach to the chest radiograph is likely to be successful if it results in a reproducible systematic scheme for evaluating radiographs. We detail one such approach that may help you to keep things organized. You are welcome to use this or to adapt it or to create your own system.

The key thing to avoid, especially as you begin to look at radiographs, is the "gestalt" approach. By gestalt we mean looking at the radiograph and hoping to receive an overall impression in a mysterious way (perhaps via radiowaves, ESP, or ESPN). We confess that as we have become more experienced at interpreting chest radiographs, we do make an initial rapid scan of a study and often come up with a quick gestalt of normal or abnormal. Even so, we supplement this initial impression with a more systematic review of the image for a more complete diagnosis. This initial gestalt is not always correct, but with experience it has been reassuring how often relatively small or subtle abnormalities on a radiograph will, in essence, announce their presence, calling attention to themselves even at the first cursory review of the image. This is presumably what experience does for a radiologist. Many years of experience do not decrease the necessity for a formal review scheme that reduces errors of carelessness. Still, it is probably nice to realize that image interpretation will not always be a purely mechanical exercise, that there will be an element of art as the image itself "talks to you." We now present a recommended approach.

APPROACH TO THE RADIOGRAPH

The approach is based on the observation that many inexperienced film readers think of a chest radiograph as a lung radiograph. This leads to interesting errors of perception, such as missing major abnormalities completely when the lungs are normal and missing key extrapulmonary abnormalities that completely elucidate the diagnosis when the lungs are abnormal.

For that reason, we recommend saving the lungs for last. One way to make this easier to accomplish is to start on the periphery of the radiograph and work one's way in. Thus, we recommend beginning the assessment of the chest radiograph by examining the bones and soft tissues of the chest wall and also by assessing the neck and the upper abdomen. Next come the pleural spaces bilaterally. We then skip across the lungs to examine the mediastinum, followed by the heart and great vessels. With all that out of the way, the lungs are finally assessed. A more detailed examination of this approach follows.

A Brief Consideration of Position and Projection

Before we get into the detailed approach to the radiograph, a brief discourse on position and projection is advisable. Because radiographs are generally two-dimensional representations of three-dimensional anatomy, we recommend two right-angle projections of a structure for best depiction of that structure. In the chest, this means that we try to obtain a frontal chest radiograph, either posteroanterior (PA) (x-ray beam enters the patient from behind and emerges through the front, where the x-ray cassette or digital plate awaits) or anteroposterior (AP) (beam from in front traverses the anterior thorax and emerges through the back) and a lateral radiograph. We prefer a PA radiograph when the patient's condition permits, in part to limit the portion of the radiograph obscured by the soft tissues of the heart; anterior structures like the heart are more magnified on an AP view than on a PA view. We similarly prefer a left lateral radiograph (beam enters via the patient's right side and emerges from the left side), which also limits the magnification of the heart. A standard chest radiograph is obtained with a distance of 72 inches from the x-ray source to the cassette or digital plate and with the patient in the upright position, taking and holding a deep inspiration.

This idealized version of reality is not always reproducible in real life. Some patients are unable to follow instructions (language barrier, decreased mentation) or unable to take a deep breath (dyspnea, pleuritic chest pain). Acutely ill patients may be unable to stand; semiupright radiographs can sometimes be obtained with the patient in bed, but supine radiographs are another potential outcome. Patients who cannot come to our department for radiographs can be examined with portable equipment but almost always in the AP projection and seldom with a lateral view. The distance from x-ray source to image may have to be less than 72 inches, resulting in magnification of the entire chest. These technical modifications have consequences with regard to visualization and diagnosis of thoracic abnormalities.

Outside the Thorax: Soft Tissues

Assess symmetry of breasts.

Assess symmetry of neck soft tissues.

Assess for soft tissue calcifications, gas, or metal.

Careful assessment of the extrathoracic soft tissues occasionally plays a critical role in the evaluation of the chest. One of the most important things to which we try to pay attention is symmetry of the soft tissues of the neck and the breasts (Fig. 3.1). This is because asymmetry may indicate prior surgery, and this may in turn indicate prior cancer.

You might believe that interest in prior cancer is based on generating a differential diagnosis for abnormalities that are subsequently detected. You would be only partly right. The differentiation of normal from abnormal is, in our opinion, the single most important job of the chest radiologist and also the single hardest job of the chest radiologist. Although malpractice attorneys paint a picture of missed abnormalities as "obvious," such abnormalities do not come prospectively labeled (except in textbooks such as this). In many instances a question arises as to whether a finding is an overlap of normal structures, a normal variant, a benign abnormality, or a more important finding.

Pretest probability is an important factor in deciding whether a finding is real or artifact and important or unimportant. Experience teaches that pre-employment chest radiographs on patients in their twenties are virtually certainly normal. Chest radiographs on "twenty-somethings" with chest pain are almost as frequently normal. In such a setting, a questionable nodule is virtually never a real nodule, and we almost never bring up the

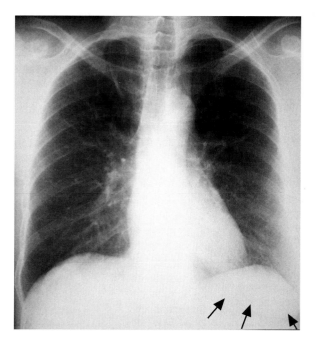

Figure 3.1 Prior right mastectomy. Left breast outline is visible *(arrows)*, and there is also asymmetric lucency over the right lung base laterally.

need for follow-up radiographs or oblique radiographs or limited thin-section computed tomography or positron emission tomography.

But what if the patient has been treated for cancer? Although cancer is not commonly found in such young patients, we do occasionally see breast cancer in that age group, which could result in mastectomy. We do occasionally see thyroid cancer in that age group, which could result in neck dissection. So the observation of asymmetric neck or breast soft tissues could change the pretest probability significantly and could make us read the radiograph and interpret the questionable abnormalities very differently.

Of course, the patient is certainly aware that he or she has had previous breast or thyroid cancer. Unfortunately, for studies like chest radiographs we as interpreting radiologists almost never see the patients. The referring physician is also certainly aware of this diagnosis. You may be tempted to believe it is ridiculous that a radiologist's knowledge of such diagnoses would have to rely on his or her ability to make observations on the radiograph. All we can say is, "Just wait until you start looking at radiographic requisitions." The best we can often hope for is clinical history that is not out-and-out incorrect or frankly misleading. Many requisitions are completed by overworked clerks who know very little medicine. If they are told to order chest radiographs, they write a history like "rule out infiltrate." Even an accurate history that details symptoms and current clinical concerns may not include relevant past information thought not to be of current clinical concern (such as remote breast cancer).

The bottom line is that observations such as previous mastectomy are important, clinically relevant, influential in deciding whether a study is normal or abnormal, and critical to differential diagnosis of abnormalities. It is likely that many health systems will go to a computerized order entry system in the not-so-distant future. One day, it may be easy to retrieve all relevant clinical information for every ordered radiograph. Until that day, the systematic approach to the radiograph requires an assessment of the symmetry of neck and breast soft tissues.

OUTSIDE THE THORAX: ABDOMEN

A complete consideration of abdominal diseases is outside the scope of this text. Nevertheless, some observations are relevant. Because of the centering of an upright chest radiograph and its technique, it is often far better than an upright abdominal radiograph at

Assess lucent structures: bowel gas pattern, free intraperitoneal gas, bowel wall gas, and other extraintestinal gas (retroperitoneal, biliary, etc.).

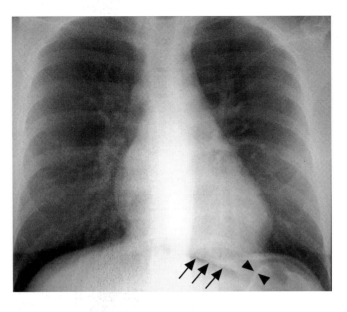

Figure 3.2 Upright free intraperitoneal gas. The central tendon of the diaphragm is visible (*arrows*), and there is also visualization of inner and outer walls of left upper quadrant bowel (Rigler's sign) (*arrowheads*).

depicting free intraperitoneal gas (Fig. 3.2), usually under the right hemidiaphragm. Although larger amounts of gas are required, supine chest radiographs can also be evaluated for intraperitoneal gas (Fig. 3.3).

Assess soft tissue structures: organomegaly and soft tissue masses.

Splenomegaly can be an important finding for explaining intrathoracic abnormalities. It may raise the possibility of leukemia or lymphoma, helping to explain mediastinal and hilar lymph node enlargement or thoracic opportunistic infection. In a trauma patient it may indicate splenic hematoma or laceration, tying in with left pleural effusion or pneumothorax. It may go along with hepatomegaly and/or ascites in a patient with liver disease, elucidating right pleural effusion. Splenomegaly is generally diagnosed via medial displacement of gas in the stomach and caudal displacement of gas in the splenic flexure along with mass-like soft tissue in the left upper quadrant of the abdomen (Fig. 3.4).

Assess opaque structures: skeletal abnormalities, calculi, and metallic foreign bodies.

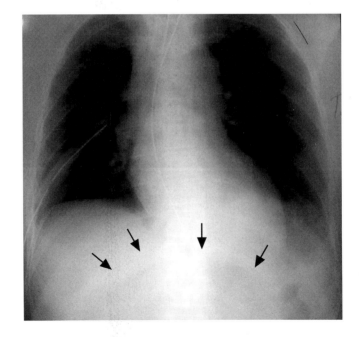

Figure 3.3 Supine free intraperitoneal gas. There is a large central lucency in the upper abdomen (*arrows*).

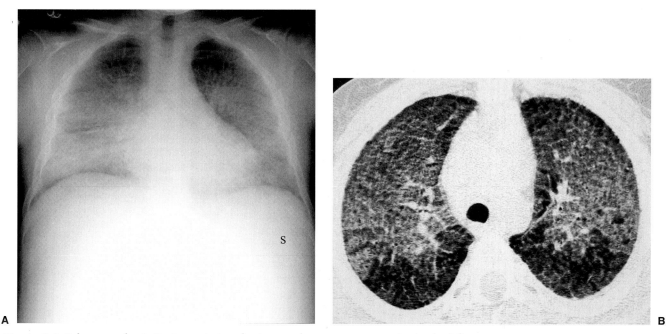

Figure 3.4 Splenomegaly. *A.* Posteroanterior chest x-ray: homogeneous opacity in the left upper quadrant of the abdomen (S). *B.* High resolution chest computed tomography: diffuse parenchymal abnormality, largely ground glass opacity and interlobular septal thickening. Young patient + splenomegaly + diffuse lung disease = storage disease; this is Niemann-Pick disease.

Although most bowel gas will be outside the field of view of a chest radiograph, inspection of the bowel contained in a chest radiograph may yield evidence of bowel obstruction, infarction, or other abnormalities. At a minimum, this can lead the alert chest radiologist to recommend standard abdominal radiographs for better evaluation. Similarly, patients with lower thoracic or shoulder pain may actually be experiencing referred pain from upper abdominal disease. Such abnormalities may result in mass effect on upper abdominal bowel.

Outside the Thorax: Bones
As with abdominal findings, skeletal findings could constitute a separate textbook entirely. Nevertheless, a few observations are in order. One is that it is very difficult to detect skeletal abnormality without careful examination of individual bones; look at the trees, forget the forest. Especially when there is chest pain, try to compare the ribs from side to side, one by one. Trauma is another setting where painstaking inspection of visualized bones can prevent important mistakes.

It is interesting to note that the absence of a structure usually seen may be much harder to detect than the presence of abnormality of that structure (Fig. 3.5). Similarly, inexperienced interpreters may have difficulty distinguishing between variants of normal and abnormalities. Side-to-side comparison is particularly helpful in these settings; unlike abnormalities, normal variants are often bilateral and are reasonably symmetric.

With abnormalities at the periphery of the chest, it may be difficult to distinguish between those originating in the pleura and those arising in the chest wall (extrapleural). Shape of the lesion may be helpful (Chapter 17), but adjacent skeletal abnormality is absolute proof that the lesion is in the extrapleural space.

Compare for symmetry of bilateral structures.

If there are two views, assess both (sternum and spine better seen on lateral view).

Evaluate all the way to the edge of the radiograph.

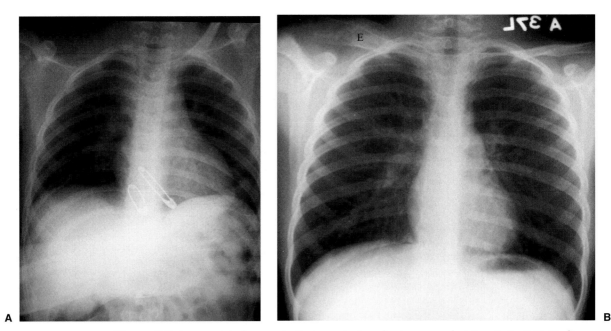

Figure 3.5 Asymmetric bones. *A.* Posteroanterior chest x-ray: what is missing? *B.* Earlier posteroanterior chest x-ray in same patient: expansile neoplasm of distal right clavicle (E) is Ewing sarcoma and right clavicle is surgically absent in *A*.

PLEURA

Concentrate on thoracic apex and base.

The pleural spaces are potential spaces at the periphery of the lungs. For the purposes of this chapter the key pleural abnormalities we want to detect are pneumothorax and pleural effusion. Both illustrate the importance of patient position on the radiographic appearance of abnormality. Air and fluid in the pleura migrate in opposite directions; fluid moves to the dependent aspect of the space, whereas air moves to the nondependent aspect. With a patient upright, we look for pneumothorax at the thoracic apex and for pleural effusion in the caudal hemithorax (Fig. 3.6). However, many patients being examined for these findings are hospitalized critically ill patients. They may be unable to assume the upright position, in which case fluid will spread out along the posterior aspect of the chest (Fig. 3.7) and air will rise to the anterior aspect of the chest. Leading to more confusion, such patients may be quickly propped upright for a radiograph without allowing air or fluid the few minutes it may take to redistribute as expected.

Supplement liberally with decubitus radiography.

Fortunately, a solution is available. Even very ill patients are often able to assume the lateral decubitus position. For suspected pleural effusion, we put the side of presumed abnormality down to get fluid to layer along the inner aspect of the ribs (Fig. 3.7). For suspected pneumothorax we put the side of presumed abnormality up to get air to rise under the inner aspect of the ribs. This also works for free intraperitoneal gas. In that setting we do a left side down decubitus radiograph so that intraperitoneal gas rises over the hepatic margin.

Look carefully for the lung edge.

The key observation in the diagnosis of pneumothorax is visualization of the lung edge. When the potential pleural space contains no gas or fluid, the lung edge is so closely applied to the inner aspect of the chest wall that it cannot be visualized. Gas in the pleural space displaces this edge and provides good contrast for its visualization (the gas is black, the edge is white). Especially in supine patients (but even sometimes in upright patients) we need to look for gas in the caudal aspect of the chest, the least dependent portion of the pleural space in the supine position (Fig. 3.8).

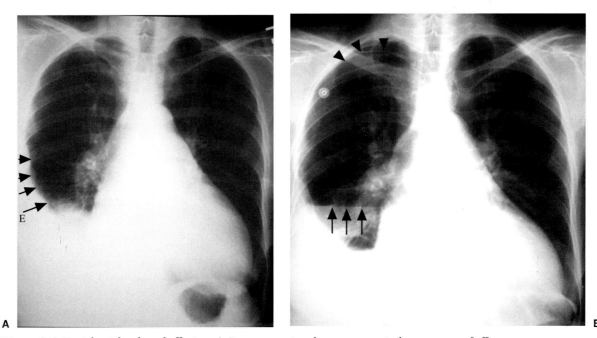

A   B

Figure 3.6 Upright right pleural effusion. *A.* Posteroanterior chest x-ray: typical appearance of effusion (E), with meniscus appearance in right lateral costophrenic angle *(arrows). B.* Posteroanterior chest x-ray after thoracentesis: there is now an air-fluid level *(arrows)*, indicating hydropneumothorax. The right lung edge is visible in the more cephalad pleural space *(arrowheads)*.

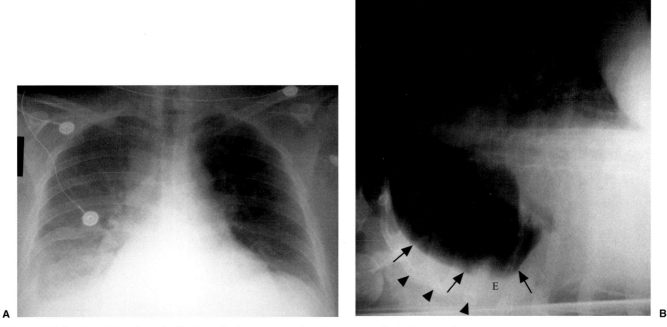

A   B

Figure 3.7 Supine right pleural effusion. *A.* Anteroposterior chest x-ray: hazy increased opacity throughout the right hemithorax, despite which right lung vessels are easily visualized. *B.* Right lateral decubitus radiography: effusion (E) layers between the lung edge *(arrows)* and the inner margins of the ribs *(arrowheads)*.

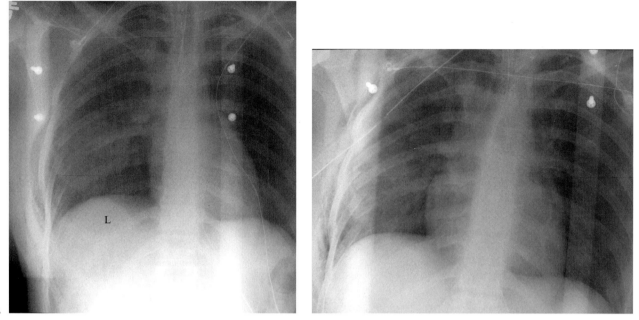

Figure 3.8 Supine right pneumothorax. *A.* Anteroposterior chest x-ray: lucency (L) at the base of the right hemithorax and overlying the right upper quadrant of the abdomen. *B.* Anteroposterior chest x-ray after chest tube placement: lucency has resolved.

Pleural effusion classically produces a "meniscus" appearance of soft tissue opacity (fluid), displacing the lung away from the lateral and posterior costophrenic sulci (Fig. 3.6A). Because the posterior costophrenic sulcus is the most dependent portion of the upright pleural space, blunting of the normally sharp posterior costophrenic angle on the lateral radiograph is the best indicator of a small effusion. On the frontal radiograph the lateral costophrenic sulcus is often evaluated, but subpulmonic effusion can leave that angle unblunted (Fig. 3.9). In such cases we need to look for three signs

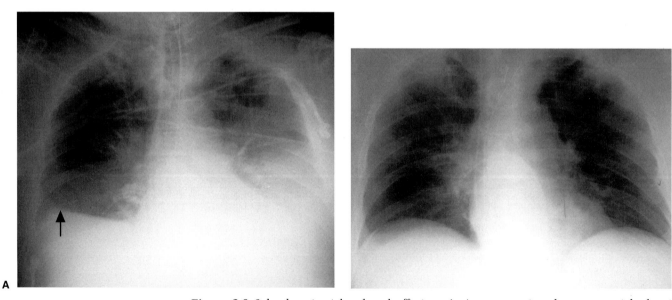

Figure 3.9 Subpulmonic right pleural effusion. *A.* Anteroposterior chest x-ray: right hemidiaphragm is uniformly opaque, with lateral displacement of apparent dome *(arrow)*. *B.* Anteroposterior chest x-ray after effusion resolved: normal gradation of diaphragmatic opacity and more medial diaphragmatic dome.

of effusion: uniform opacity of the ipsilateral hemidiaphragm, instead of the usual gradation of opacity from very white in the upper abdomen to very dark in the lower lung; loss of visualization of the posterior lung vessels through the hemidiaphragm on the frontal radiograph; and displacement of the apparent dome of the hemidiaphragm, usually found one-third of the way from the midline to the lateral chest wall, more laterally.

MEDIASTINUM

Skipping past the lungs, we evaluate the midline space between the two lungs (the mediastinum). One important indicator of mediastinal abnormality is widening of the mediastinum. It would be very helpful to identify as abnormal any mediastinum wider than a given measurement. Unfortunately, it is very difficult to come up with such a measurement. Mediastinal width depends on projection (wider on AP views than PA views), x-ray source to image distance (wider with shorter distance), depth of inspiration (wider with poorer inspiration), patient rotation (the aorta is more prominent when the patient is rotated in the left anterior oblique projection), and patient age (atherosclerotic unwinding of the aorta, common with increasing patient age, accentuates mediastinal width), among other factors. Although it is sometimes obvious that a mediastinum is too wide (Fig. 3.10), that is not always the case. As in most cases of trying to distinguish normal from abnormal, experience is very helpful (another way of saying that you can expect to be poor at making such distinctions when you first begin to interpret chest radiographs).

Assess normal contours.

Mediastinal contours may also be helpful. Focal contour bulges can be important clues to the presence of mediastinal abnormality. Such contour abnormalities may be surprisingly subtle (Fig. 3.11), and bitter experience teaches that mediastinal masses of astounding size are sometimes virtually invisible.

It can be useful to evaluate normal mediastinal structures for displacement, which may allow diagnosis of noncontour deforming mediastinal abnormalities. The trachea is usually in the midline in the upper thorax (Fig. 3.12) and usually deviates slightly to the right at the level of the aortic arch. Rightward deviation tends to increase with atherosclerotic aortic disease. Tracheal deviation can be simulated by patient rotation; this is best evaluated by comparing the position of the medial clavicles (anterior structures) against that of the spinous processes of the vertebrae (posterior structures). The clavicles should

Evaluate for deviation of normal structures.

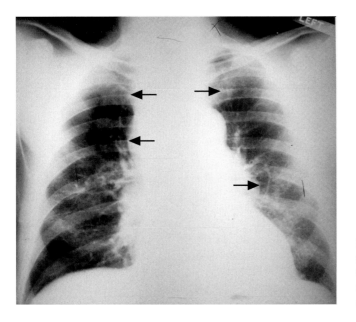

Figure 3.10 Unequivocal mediastinal widening (*arrows*). This should call to mind lymphoma or metastatic disease but actually represents amyloidosis.

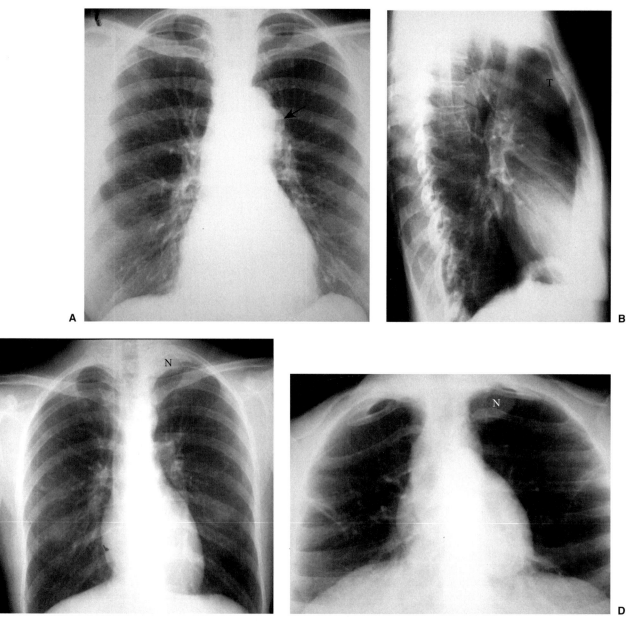

Figure 3.11 Subtle contour abnormalities. *A.* Posteroanterior chest x-ray: small bump *(arrow)* over aortopulmonary window. *B.* Lateral chest x-ray: surprisingly large anterior mediastinal mass (T) is thymoma. *C.* Posteroanterior chest x-ray in a different patient: soft tissue mass at apex of left hemithorax (N). *D.* Apical lordotic radiography demonstrates mass (N), a neurofibroma, to better advantage.

Assess for calcifications, gas, or metal.

be equidistant from the spinous processes. Head turning can also be misleading and is evaluated by following the spinous processes up into the neck and by assessing chin position. Similarly, evaluating a contrast-filled esophagus for deviation may allow diagnosis of an aberrant right subclavian artery coursing between the esophagus and the spine; other periesophageal abnormalities can be similarly demonstrated, but oral contrast is virtually always required.

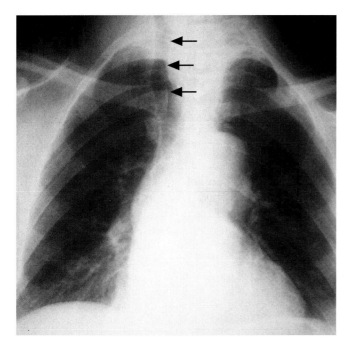

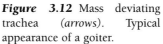

Figure 3.12 Mass deviating trachea *(arrows)*. Typical appearance of a goiter.

CARDIOPERICARDIAL SILHOUETTE

Analysis of the mediastinum readily leads to evaluation of the heart. Note the intentional use of the term "cardiopericardial silhouette"; this reminds us that enlargement of this structure may be seen with a normal heart but with significant pericardial abnormality. In some instances a large pericardial effusion has a distinctive appearance (described as a "water bottle" shape) (Fig. 3.13), but the differentiation of cardiomegaly from pericardial effusion by shape is seldom easy. Pericardial effusion

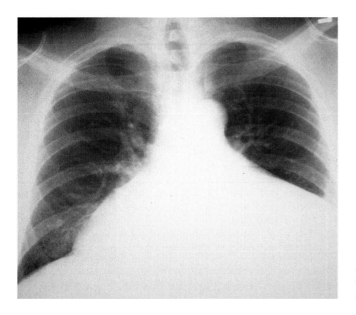

Figure 3.13 Pericardial effusion with classic "water bottle" configuration.

Assess size and shape (two views are helpful for both).

Assess normal contours.

deserves special consideration when the cardiopericardial silhouette enlarges rapidly (Fig. 3.14) or when catheters or pacemakers are displaced from the apparent edge of the silhouette (Fig. 3.15).

Cardiomegaly is also a diagnostic challenge. As a rough rule of thumb we often measure the maximum transverse cardiac diameter and compare it with the maximum transverse thoracic diameter; a ratio of greater than 0.5 is used to indicate cardiomegaly. Inexperienced observers tend to rely on this parameter; those of us with more experience have been disappointed too often. The cardiothoracic ratio is influenced by rotation, position, and projection; the heart will be magnified on an AP view of the chest, and the cardiac apex may project further laterally on a relatively lordotic view of the chest. The transverse cardiac diameter also appears larger on an expiratory view or in diastole. It is preferable to use both views (when a frontal and lateral are obtained) to get a handle on cardiac size. Even then, a research project in the 1980s convinced us that experienced chest radiologists looking at radiographs in patients who had concurrent echocardiography were not reliably able to distinguish normal from abnormal heart size. If there is a question about cardiac size, presence or absence of pericardial effusion, or even ejection fraction, echocardiography amplifies our diagnostic capabilities enormously.

It is also important to view the cardiac margins for evidence of specific chamber enlargement. The normal right heart border is formed by the right atrium and the superior vena cava, with a variable contribution from the aging ascending aorta. The normal left heart border is formed by the aortic knob, the main and left pulmonary artery, and the left ventricle. Even when the overall transverse cardiac diameter is normal, the so-called fourth mogul (an additional left heart contour) and the double density sign below the right hilum may indicate left atrial enlargement (Fig. 3.16). Other signs of left atrial enlargement include splaying of the carina, increased subcarinal opacity, and posterior displacement of the mid-portion of the heart border on the lateral radiograph. Left ventricular enlargement results in more caudal posterior dis-

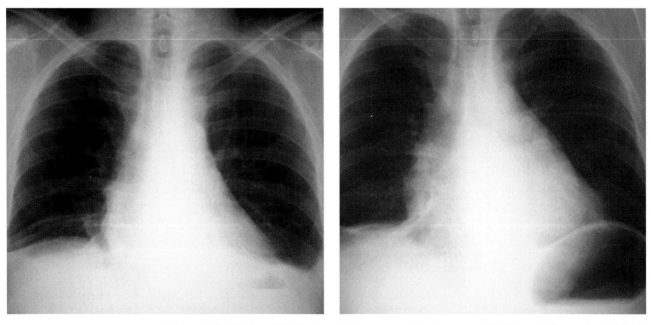

A   **B**

Figure 3.14 Pericardial effusion. *A.* Anteroposterior chest x-ray 12-20: typical postsurgical findings after mitral valve repair. *B.* Anteroposterior chest x-ray 12-30: larger cardiopericardial silhouette; patient in distress. Echocardiography confirmed pericardial effusion, clinically causing pericardial tamponade.

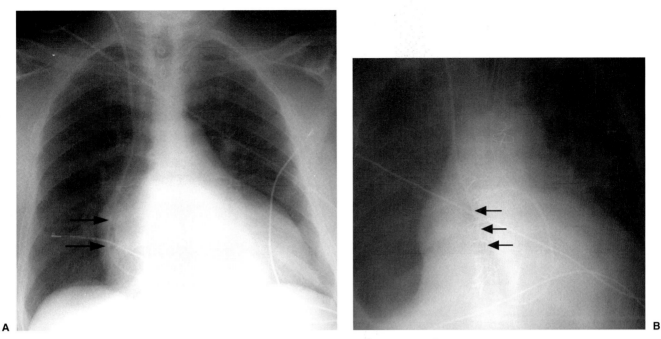

A   B

Figure 3.15 Pericardial effusion diagnosed by catheter position. *A.* Anteroposterior chest x-ray in patient without pericardial effusion: enlarged cardiopericardial silhouette reflects known cardiomyopathy, but pulmonary artery catheter *(arrows)* is not deviated from right cardiac margin. *B.* Anteroposterior chest x-ray in a different patient with large pericardial effusion. Note displacement of pulmonary artery catheter *(arrows)*.

placement of the heart border on the lateral view. This may be particularly evident when comparing the position of the posterior heart border with that of the inferior vena cava. Although left atrial enlargement has useful signs, we remain unimpressed by the ability to predict specific chamber enlargement (based on the 1980s research project discussed previously).

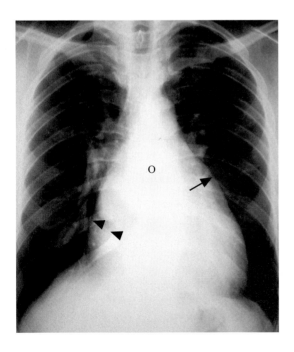

Figure 3.16 Cardiomegaly with left atrial enlargement. Diagnostic signs include fourth mogul *(arrow)*, increased subcarinal opacity (O), and double density sign *(arrowheads)*.

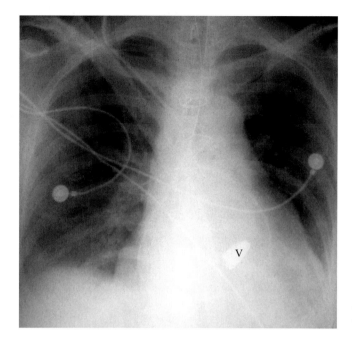

Figure 3.17 Confusing location of prosthetic valves on anteroposterior chest x-ray. Patient with previous placement of prosthetic mitral and aortic valves (V), which are completely superimposed.

Assess for calcifications.

Intracardiac calcifications may indicate cardiac abnormality even in the absence of cardiopericardial silhouette enlargement (Chapter 20). When frontal and lateral views are available, differentiating between calcified aortic and mitral valves is not generally challenging. However, on isolated frontal views (especially in postsurgical patients) this may be surprisingly difficult (Fig. 3.17).

GREAT VESSELS

Assess aortic contour, size, and calcification.

As noted above, aortic size and configuration change with age. Gross enlargement (aneurysm) may be evident but is generally better evaluated by thoracic computed tomography or magnetic resonance imaging. Nevertheless, it is important to evaluate the aorta for certain particular signs of aortic dissection, especially in patients with chest pain or pain radiating to the back. Dissection may result in an irregular aortic margin (Fig. 3.18). It occasionally results in displacement of intimal calcification away from the aortic edge, although this sign is difficult to evaluate with chest radiographs because apparent displacement may only reflect our two-dimensional representation of a structure moving through space both from front to back and from right to left. Many patients with aortic dissections have a normal chest x-ray appearance of the aorta, reminding us that with appropriate symptomatology, any chest x-ray is suspicious for dissection.

Assess distinctness of pulmonary vessels and other signs of interstitial pulmonary arteries.

Evaluation of pulmonary vascular abnormalities is covered at greater length in Chapter 21. In this setting we consider the diagnosis of congestive heart failure in very simplistic terms. Although pulmonary vascular redistribution (relative enlargement of upper lobe pulmonary veins, which are usually smaller than lower lobe veins because of gravity) can be an important sign of pulmonary venous hypertension in ambulatory patients, those are not the patients we are usually asked to assess for congestive heart failure. Pulmonary vascular redistribution is not helpful in patients who spend most of their time supine or semisupine, where the gravitational effect makes posterior veins bigger than anterior veins (on a frontal radiograph, who knows which are which?). We are therefore far more concerned with signs of interstitial pulmonary edema, such as pulmonary vascular indistinctness, fissural thickening, and septal lines (Fig. 3.19);

Assess size and symmetry of central pulmonary arteries.

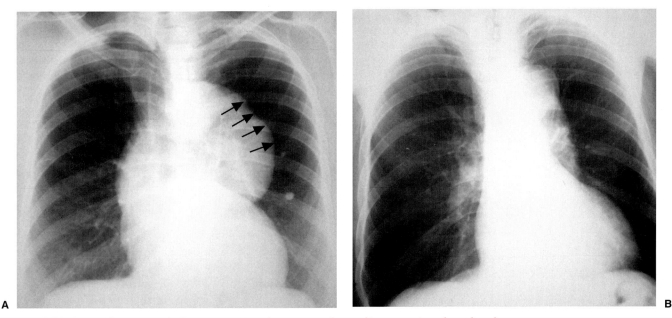

A

B

Figure 3.18 Aortic dissection. *A*. Posteroanterior chest x-ray: descending aorta is enlarged and irregular in contour *(arrows)*. *B*. Posteroanterior chest x-ray in a different patient: descending aortic contour irregularity is more subtle.

pleural effusion can be an important accompanying finding. It is a mistake to think of fissural thickening as being a result of pleural effusion. Instead, it is generally a manifestation of subpleural interstitial edema; when subpleural lung on either side of a fissure develops edema, we do not resolve this as a perifissural abnormality but as fissural thickening.

Assess size and symmetry of peripheral pulmonary arteries.

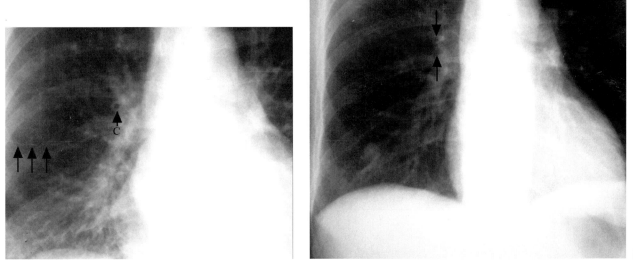

A

B

Figure 3.19 Interstitial pulmonary edema. *A*. Posteroanterior chest x-ray with patient in congestive heart failure: peribronchial cuffing (C), fissural thickening *(arrows)*, and vascular indistinctness. *B*. Posteroanterior chest x-ray after heart failure resolved: resolution of findings, with return of bronchial wall thickness to normal *(arrows)*.

LUNGS

Compare side to side.

Assess for focal or diffuse lucency or opacity.

Inspect closely but also from afar.

Supplement with additional views (oblique, lordotic) as needed.

After you have waited so patiently for so long, here is disappointing news: You have to read most of the rest of the book to learn how to diagnose lung disease at chest radiography (you probably thought that one chapter would do the trick, didn't you?). For the beginning observer, it is useful to think of lung diseases as focal or diffuse and to look at focal diseases as nodular or non-nodular and diffuse diseases as alveolar or interstitial. Nodular or non-nodular is relatively easy: Does it look like a mass? Does it look like it has well-defined margins? If you had tweezers or tongs, could you easily lift it out of the chest? Would you even want to?

As for alveolar and interstitial disease, their characteristics are described in Chapter 14. Instead of describing specific lung abnormalities here, we conclude this section with a description of selected signs in chest radiography:

Silhouette Sign

Loss of visualization of a normal anatomic landmark (such as the left hemidiaphragm) indicates an abnormality in the immediately adjacent lung (in this instance, the left lower lobe) that would otherwise outline that landmark. Similarly, loss of visualization of the right heart border indicates disease in the medial segment of the right middle lobe (Fig. 3.20). Not all silhouette signs are equally reliable; disease that overlaps both the right heart border and the right hemidiaphragm and silhouettes neither is in the right lower lobe. The longer contact between right lung and hemidiaphragm than between left lung and hemidiaphragm, because of the heart, means that right lower lobe disease will not always silhouette the right hemidiaphragm.

Hilum Overlay Sign

In differentiating an enlarged main, left, or right pulmonary artery from an overlying mediastinal mass, the demonstration of pulmonary vessels converging medial to the apparent lateral margin of the "mass" indicates that it is not the artery (Fig. 3.21). The converse, the hilum convergence sign, suggests that when pulmonary vessels converge to the edge of a "mass" (but not medial to it), the mass is pulmonary artery.

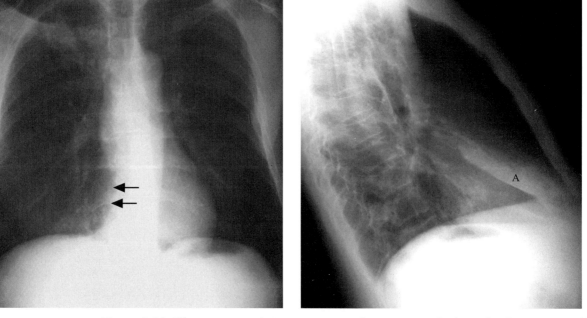

Figure 3.20 Silhouette sign. A. Posteroanterior chest x-ray: right heart border is not visible (*arrows*). B. Lateral chest x-ray: middle lobe air-space disease (*A*) is responsible.

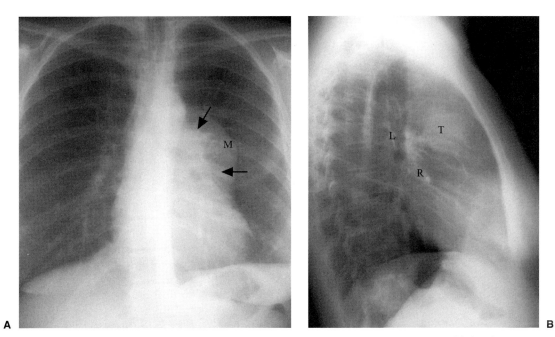

A

B

Figure 3.21 Hilum overlay sign. *A.* Posteroanterior chest x-ray: mass (M) overlies main and left pulmonary artery, but arteries converge medial to edge of mass *(arrows)*. *B.* Lateral chest x-ray: mass is teratoma (T) anterior to right (R) and left (L) pulmonary arteries.

Air Bronchogram

When alveoli are filled with blood, pus, water, or cells, air-filled bronchi may stick out as branching black structures against a white backdrop (Fig. 3.22); otherwise, the walls of bronchi are generally too thin to allow demonstration of the bronchi. Air bronchograms thus indicate that a given abnormality is alveolar; in addition, they prove that an abnormality on the chest radiograph is parenchymal (e.g., not pleural or extrapleural).

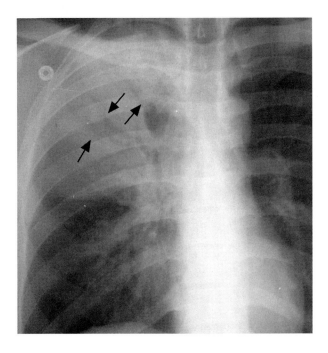

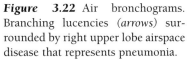

Figure 3.22 Air bronchograms. Branching lucencies *(arrows)* surrounded by right upper lobe airspace disease that represents pneumonia.

Superior Triangle Sign, Inferior Triangle Sign, and Luftsichel

These are signs of lobar atelectasis or collapse. When the right lower lobe collapses, the superior vena cava may rotate laterally, producing a triangular configuration (superior triangle sign). In contradistinction, upper lobe collapse may produce a triangular configuration at the diaphragmatic dome (inferior triangle sign). With left upper lobe collapse, the hyperinflated left lower lobe adjacent to the aortic arch results in a crescent-like configuration known by its German name (luftsichel) (Fig. 3.23).

Golden S Sign

A collapsed lobe occurring in the absence of a central mass often has a concave border. When there is a central mass associated with atelectasis there is often a resultant focal convexity that results in an "S" shape (or more often, a backward S) (Fig. 3.24).

Comet-Tail Sign

Rounded atelectasis is a mass-like lesion of collapsed lung, typically occurring after a pleural effusion or other pleural abnormality. Lung seemingly becomes adherent to the adjacent pleural abnormality, so that when pleural disease recedes, the lung may twist into a rounded configuration. The diagnosis is aided considerably by demonstration of vessels and bronchi that supply the atelectatic portion of lung "swirling" into the lung with a comet-tail configuration (Fig. 3.25).

Cervicothoracic and Thoracoabdominal Signs

Because there is no anterior lung above the level of the clavicles, a lesion that extends above that level and remains sharply outlined must be located posteriorly in the chest. This does not apply only to lesions in the lung, because this sign can be seen with posterior mediastinal and pleural lesions as well. A lesion that simply disappears at the level of the clavicle is generally anterior. This is the cervicothoracic sign. Similarly, the posterior costophrenic sulcus of lung extends far more caudally than anterior basilar lung. Therefore, a lesion that extends below the dome of the diaphragm and remains sharply outlined

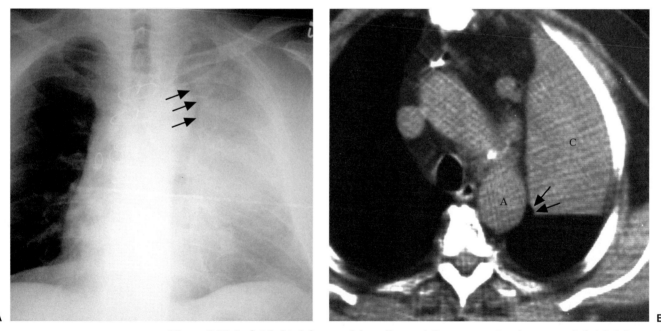

A   B

Figure 3.23 Luftsichel in left upper lobe collapse. *A.* Posteroanterior chest x-ray: luftsichel (*arrows*) outlines aortic knob. *B.* Computed tomography: collapsed left upper lobe (C) with sliver of expanded left lower lobe (*arrows*) insinuating adjacent to posterior aortic arch (*A*).

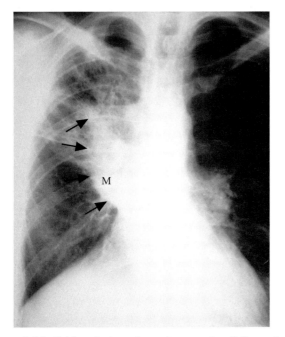

Figure 3.24 Golden S sign. Central convexity (M) results in backward S shape of elevated minor fissure (*arrows*).

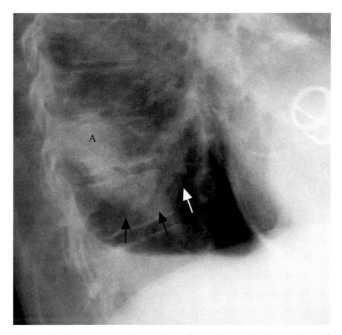

Figure 3.25 Comet-tail sign. Vessels and bronchi (*arrows*) swirl into area of round atelectasis (A).

must be in the posterior chest, whereas a lesion that abruptly terminates at the dome of the diaphragm must be anterior (thoracoabdominal sign).

APPROACH TO THE RADIOGRAPH IN THE PICTURE ARCHIVING AND COMMUNICATION SYSTEM ERA

In general, interpreting chest images on monitors instead of chest radiographs on alternators necessitates no change in the approach to the study. A reproducible systematic approach remains of the utmost importance. However, experience with viewing studies on the monitor leads to the following recommendation: Always take the time to view digital images in a magnified mode. This tends to slow the interpreter down (at least a little), but there are definitely lesions that cannot be seen without magnifying the image. Do not use optical magnification (magnifying glass in many systems), because it results in visual distortion.

An added advantage of viewing images this way is that it automatically gets the viewer out of gestalt mode, requiring immersion in the local details of the image. It also forces one to scrutinize the entire image carefully. We do not only view the image in a magnified form. We liken this to the practice (when viewing radiographs on alternators) of leaning forward and looking closely at the films, using a high intensity light as necessary, but also leaning back in an effort to see the forest for the trees before signing off on a case. The magnified image at the monitor is the correlate of leaning forward, but a final survey of the restored original image is like leaning back for the overview.

One other helpful tool for viewing images at the monitor is an image-sharpening algorithm (bone reconstruction or large edge or the like). This is very helpful for questionable pneumothorax and for location of a difficult-to-visualize catheter tip.

RADIOGRAPHIC REPORT

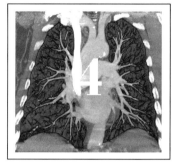

- Information
- Style
- Communication
- Pet Peeves
- Standards of Practice for Radiology Reporting
- More Pet Peeves

It is hard to overemphasize the importance of the radiographic report. The essence of radiologic diagnosis is the correct observation and interpretation of radiographic findings, but even correct observations and interpretations are inadequate if they are not conveyed appropriately. Among the critical elements are information, style, and communication.

It would be wrong to suggest that there is only one correct way to convey what is gleaned from the radiograph. To reinforce that point, two of us have teamed up to air our views on the subject. We begin with comments from Barry Gross.

INFORMATION

Let me begin by expressing my understanding of how difficult it is to dictate radiographic reports. My experience indicates that success in the preclinical years of medical school helps to prepare you for success in the clinical years. Success in the clinical years improves your likelihood of success as a clinical intern. However, nothing in my previous experience prepared me for the first few months of my radiology residency. The responsibility for interpretation of images was daunting enough. Even more unforgettable was the literally painful exercise of trying to dictate a small stack of chest radiographs for the first time. I remember sitting with dictaphone in hand, struggling to put into words what needed to be said.

There are two times when it is particularly important to consider the information content of your radiographic reports: when you first start dictating and all the time after that. It is helpful to remember that the referring clinician reading your report may not have images to view at the time the report is read. You should try to put yourself into that clinician's place, making sure the descriptions you provide will be meaningful even to someone not looking at the radiograph.

In addition, be sure your report says what you intend. We conduct a very instructive teaching conference with our residents from time to time. One resident is positioned in a far corner of the room, unable to view the radiographs being presented. A second resident has to describe the findings on the radiographs so that the first resident is able to make a correct diagnosis. It is eye-opening to the residents to see what erroneous diagnoses their initial descriptors evoke and just as instructive to find out how easily many diagnoses can be made with a few well-chosen phrases. Dictators of radiographic reports should be sure they are choosing phrases in this fashion.

Here are a few questions to consider. Have you made it clear what is abnormal (if there is an abnormality)? Does your description indicate where the abnormality resides? If there is a possible abnormality, have you indicated your degree of certainty that the finding is abnormal? If there is uncertainty, have you suggested how it can be resolved?

I do not mean to imply that a definitive diagnosis can always be made. I also suspect that the more difficult cases for diagnosis are also often the more difficult cases for dictation. A good radiographic report is not always a report that gives the answer; sometimes it is simply a report that clarifies what further questions need to be addressed. However, clarity is an important feature of a good report. When a clinician finishes reading a good radiographic report, there ought to be a sense of understanding about whether the radiograph is normal, abnormal, or possibly abnormal; about what the abnormality does or might represent; and about how remaining uncertainties can be addressed (1).

STYLE

To coin a phrase, "Brevity is the soul of wit." Brief accurate reports are far more helpful to clinicians than long accurate reports. Brief reports are far more likely to be read in their entirety. Residents sometimes like to run through long lists of pertinent negatives in their reports as proof that they have looked at a variety of structures in the chest. My advice is to keep the search pattern but do not feel compelled to mention everything you have looked at. Truly pertinent negatives are great (if the clinical history is rule out pneumothorax, it is advisable to say "no pneumothorax"). Otherwise, my personal favorite report is "normal."

There are a number of ways to organize reports. Some radiologists like to dictate findings and then separately to dictate conclusions. This is certainly an acceptable way to organize a report, but there is a huge pitfall to avoid. A frequent outcome of this reporting style is as follows:

> Findings: The heart is enlarged. There are thickened fissures and septal lines as well as vascular indistinctness. There are bilateral pleural effusions. Impression: Cardiomegaly with fissural thickening, septal lines, and pleural effusions.

The problem is that the "impression" is seldom an impression; it is more often a rehash of what has already been said. This style works well if the report above is redone as follows:

> Findings: The heart is enlarged. There are thickened fissures and septal lines as well as vascular indistinctness. There are bilateral pleural effusions. Impression: Congestive heart failure.

Dictation pointer: Be brief.

My current preference is to avoid redundancy by dictating only impressions. To encourage brevity I do not adhere to strict grammatical correctness, instead using phrases. The report described above might look like this:

> Impression: Cardiomegaly with interstitial pulmonary edema manifested by fissural thickening, septal lines, vascular indistinctness, and bilateral pleural effusions. This most likely indicates congestive heart failure.

Some of my colleagues prefer to dictate findings and impressions for computed tomography (CT) reports because there are usually more findings. I adhere to the impressions-only style for CT, although I add a technique section that describes what area was scanned, what sort of contrast was administered, and what field of view was used (so it can be used again for follow-up studies). A typical example of such a technique section would be as follows:

> Scanning was performed from the lung apices through the caudal aspects of the adrenal glands with uncomplicated administration of oral and bolus nonionic intravenous contrast. DFOV (displayed field of view) = 36.

My favorite CT report is the same as my favorite chest x-ray report (as noted above, it is "normal").

Whatever I am dictating, I try to maintain a balance between appropriate modesty and inappropriate uncertainty. In other words, I am quick to acknowledge that I do not know what every finding represents or what its significance may be in a particular patient (in one memorable dictation, at least to me, I included the phrase, "I have no idea what this is"). Nevertheless, I hate to see uncertainty creep into every report. Referring clinicians already complain (and joke) about the tendency of radiologists to hedge (i.e., to couch their interpretations in so many layers of doubt that they can never be pinned down to a specific diagnosis). Why add unnecessary fuel to this fire?

In particular, I seldom refer to pacemaker lead tips, for example, as being "projected over the right ventricle," even when I only have a frontal radiograph to evaluate. I believe that for most vascular catheters, we know where the tips are because the catheters are following the course of the vascular tree, just as they have in the other 22,000 catheter placements we previously reviewed. In almost every instance, that course could only be duplicated by a catheter taped to the skin surface, a highly unlikely alternative. I only allow uncertainty to enter my report if the catheter follows an atypical course or if there has been interval development of a potential complication that could indicate catheter malposition (such as mediastinal widening). The same applies to enteric and endotracheal tube placements. I make no similar claims for chest tubes; because the tube is not in a conducting structure like the vascular tree or the gastrointestinal tract, I do not know if it is in the pleura, lung, chest wall, or somewhere else.

With regard to style, I encourage you to find your own voice. I do not believe my personal style is the only acceptable one; it is simply the best one. Still, I do not require all reports dictated by residents under my supervision to be in my personal style. I try to encourage diverse styles as long as they do not include words, phrases, or errors that are anathema to me.

Dictation pointers: Be clear, confident, but not overweening. Correct your reports as needed. Call results frequently.

COMMUNICATION

We must keep in mind the ultimate purpose of having radiologists to interpret various imaging studies. It is not merely to have highly trained and capable interpreters of those images. We move closer to our true purpose when we better understand the nature of the examinations being ordered and their impact on patient care. The key question for any study is "how will this advance the care of this particular patient?" Although I do not advocate sorting through the chest radiographic requisitions for a particular day to decide which ones should and should not be done, I believe that mindset is important and perfectly appropriate for studies such as chest CT and magnetic resonance imaging (MR). My objective is not to refuse to do examinations so that my life will be easier; it is to recognize that our tests are not always completely benign, and even tests that do not endanger the patient may still have significant costs to the patient, especially financial costs. The bottom line is that there must be communication to the radiologist about the motive behind a proposed study, and communication back to the referring clinician is sometimes essential (and surprisingly welcomed by our clinical colleagues) when there is a better way to approach the given problem.

We get closer still to our ultimate purpose when we understand that communication does not end there. The report itself is a critical element in communicating with the clinicians, especially if it is structured properly. Even if your report is brief, accurate, and to the point, consider these questions:

- What if it is lost in the mail (or cyberspace)?
- What if the referring clinician left for a month-long vacation yesterday and will not see your report for quite some time?
- What if everything in your system works well (in which case I hope you will call me to tell me how it is done) and the referring clinician gets your report in 1 to 3 days: How will that delay impact the particular patient whose abnormalities you have detected?

Although the finely crafted radiologic report often suffices to convey what we want it to, that still may not be enough. I try to call reports to referring clinicians at least 5 to 10 times a day. It is obvious enough that this needs to be done with emergent life-threatening findings (such as tension pneumothorax) and equally obvious that it should be our practice for unexpected potentially ominous findings (preoperative chest for hernia repair showing a noncalcified lung mass). There are many times during the course of a radiologist's day when it is unclear if a report needs to be called or not. My advice is that if you are not sure, call. I call most times when I detect pneumonia in an outpatient. I call most times when a patient with an extrathoracic neoplasm has what I believe is the first evidence of intrathoracic metastases. I call most times when a catheter or tube placement goes astray or may have caused a complication. I call most times when an immunocompromised host has potential evidence of an opportunistic infection.

Ultimately, we need to realize that although many of us no longer do physical examinations or prescribe routine patient medications or discuss findings and prognosis with patients, our real job is to take care of patients. Communication is a critical part of that job. Some of our communication should be with the patient, especially with the patient who is ill and frightened and in pain. We can reduce patient distress by explaining the more invasive procedures that we do (such as percutaneous biopsies) in sympathetic tones and by making sure that we medicate patients appropriately to limit suffering.

Most of our communication will probably be with the referring physicians. We still make a crucial contribution to patient care when we convey important information promptly and directly and when we make sure that the diagnostic workup does not make unnecessary detours caused by lack of knowledge on the part of the referring physicians. That is where we can be champions of patient care.

An important element of communication is the recommendation of subsequent workup for questionable findings. I believe it is sometimes our responsibility to tell the clinician what should come next. When I find a small noncalcified lung nodule in a patient without old radiographs at my institution, I typically note that comparison with outside old radiographs could be helpful, but if there are none available, chest CT might be appropriate. If there is a questionable nodule adjacent to the right first costochondral junction, I often suggest apical lordotic radiography. In most such instances, I try hard not to tie the clinician's hands. I specifically try to include the phrase "if clinically indicated" in most such recommendations. This acknowledges that there may be circumstances of which I am unaware (the availability to the clinician of outside medical records, or a patient request for no further tests, as two examples) that eliminate the need for further evaluation. I do not want the subsequent record to imply that the clinician failed to do something when only I thought it was necessary. In summary, my recommendations are to be confident in your approach and direct in sharing your expertise but without treating the referring clinician as a complete idiot.

Dictation pointers: Make recommendations for additional views (oblique, lordotic), additional diagnostic studies, and, above all, comparison with outside old radiographs. Leave the clinician an out ("if clinically indicated").

PET PEEVES

Although I have hundreds of pet peeves, with regard to the radiographic report I want to emphasize two. The first is the appearance of the finished product. I have on several occasions addressed the following question to our radiology residents: "What is the tangible product of your work?" If you are a carpenter and you build a set of bookshelves, you have an obvious tangible product. If you are an author and you write a collection of essays, you have a similarly obvious tangible product. The tangible product of a radiologist's work is less evident.

The essence of our work is patient care, but our specific contributions are often difficult to tease out. In fact, it is both amusing and distressing to read patient charts for evidence of our work, even when we have interpreted studies correctly and (unbelievably enough) even when we have communicated our findings directly to the patient care team. There are still occasions where the daily notes, discharge summaries, and subsequent care plans do not seem to acknowledge the findings we have worked so hard to convey to the referring service.

Even the actual interpretation of images does not really result in a tangible product. The most tangible result of what we do is the finished radiographic report. That being the case, why would you want this end product to be sloppy, rife with misspellings, and full of easily correctable errors? I am always on the lookout for superfluous words and incorrect usage. As an example of the former, I virtually never use the word "sided" (right-sided chest tube is not preferable to right chest tube, in my opinion). With regard to the latter, a typical grammatical example I avoid is "the remainder of the lungs are normal." The subject of this sentence (remainder) is singular, so it really should be "the remainder of the lungs is normal." This is so awkward that no one can possibly use it; instead, say something like "the lungs are otherwise normal." A typical anatomic example I avoid is "there is a pneumothorax in the left lower lobe." As pneumothorax is a pleural abnormality, it obviously occurs outside of the lung. These examples are not intended to be all-inclusive; I suspect that each dictating radiologist can, with a little thought, come up with individual opportunities for improvement.

I will not tolerate even minor stylistic flaws such as split infinitives because I believe they undermine my authority (I believe the clinician reader wonders whether my sloppiness in reporting extends to sloppiness in interpreting). However, I should note that I go through my checkbook looking for the mathematical error if my bank statement is off by 1 cent (not for the 1 cent, just to satisfy my need to know where I went wrong). You may be able to live with a report that says "study of 1-7-02 compared with prior study of December 22, 2001." Even so, how can you sign off on a report that notes a right lung nodule in the findings but calls it a left lung nodule in the impression? How can your report include an obvious typing or voice-recognition error resulting in a word that is bizarrely out of context? How can your report include comparison with a prior study whose date is still in the future?

It is clear that many reports are signed in haste, with egregious errors included. I used to dictate "short of breath," but somehow our typists often translated this as "short of breast." This is the type of error that simply cannot be included in a final report—and yet this is the type of error that does make its way into our "finished products." (I now invariably dictate "dyspnea" instead.) Would you want a carpenter in your employ to leave similar flaws in the finished product? Our reports have an extended life of their own and will ultimately be the longstanding evidence of our careers in radiology. Please treat them with the care they deserve.

The other pet peeve I want to address is the inability to communicate findings. I am incredibly sympathetic to the problem of reaching the person who can manage the important information you are trying to convey. A brief list of some of the involved problems would include the following: no referring physician listed on the requisition, wrong referring physician listed on the requisition, illegible referring physician listed on the requisition, referring physician out of town, referring physician unavailable by telephone, services changed since the study was ordered, referring physician was only cross-covering, patient was subsequently transferred or discharged, and "someone ordered that study using my name, and I do not know the patient." I frequently get frustrated, and I do not like to make more than two or three phone calls to communicate a given finding.

However, conversely there are more ways than ever to communicate. You can E-mail, alphanumeric page, leave a voice mail message, or call the referring physician's cell phone. You can leave a message with the referring physician's secretary, ensuring that someone will be able to pass the message along. These are all appropriate for messages that should not be lost but need not be communicated right away (such as a noncalcified lung mass in a preoperative patient). For more urgent messages, you can call the nurse taking care of the patient. You can call the resident covering that patient. For outpatients you can call the clinic coordinator from the referring service. You can call the emergency room physician in charge for an emergency room patient. Obviously, the solution you choose will be tailored to the setting in which you work. Just as obviously, there *is* usually a solution.

Both of these pet peeves boil down to time. I am personally reading more studies per day than ever before. For those of us in academic medical centers, the amount of protected time for research, teaching, and administration is shrinking. Financial pressures in both academic medical centers and private practices are resulting in diminished support—fewer clerks and secretaries result in more nonphysician jobs being done by radiologists. Referring physicians want us there more hours per day than ever before. We still want to give time to our outside interests, and many of us are particularly eager to have time to spend with our families.

So at the end of the day (or throughout the day) it must be tempting to just sign off reports without reading them carefully. It must be tempting to call reports only when we believe we will be sued if we fail to do so. It must be tempting to give up after one attempt to reach a referring physician. (Somehow, it apparently is not tempting to make our reports shorter, which would actually be a good thing!)

I advise you, I urge you, I implore you, do not give in to the temptation. Despite the time pressures that we face, nonradiologists are not sympathetic to our plight—and they are right! We are incredibly well compensated for what we do. Compared with most physicians we work surprisingly short hours and have many vacation and meeting days per year. Our call burdens are generally relatively minor. But that is not really the issue. Even if all our time concerns were valid, that would still not justify shoddy or sloppy work. We are professionals, and we must perform as such. That requires excellent radiographic reports in every sense of the word, with timely communication of important radiographic findings.

Now, for another slant on the radiographic report, I am turning it over to our alternate sponsor, Phil Cascade.

I begin my comments in a somewhat serious vein, by discussing the medical–legal implications of the American College of Radiology (ACR) Standard for Communication: Diagnostic Radiology. After that, I express some of my own "pet peeves" about radiology reporting.

STANDARDS OF PRACTICE FOR RADIOLOGY REPORTING

The ACR publishes standards of practice that serve as national benchmarks for the performance of radiology-related professional tasks. Trial lawyers often refer to these standards in malpractice cases, both for and against radiologists. The ACR standards delineate the minimum requirements for diagnostic examinations such as chest CT and chest radiography. These standards also outline some of the professional obligations of radiologists, including (by way of example) the standard that describes the responsibilities for covering imaging services in emergency departments. The ACR Standard for Communication sets requirements for the elements of the radiology report and for the communication of the results. I now describe some of the points contained in the communication standard, emphasizing issues I believe have the most impact on the way we practice. Examples of case law will be cited as illustrations. These cases are abstracted from an article published by Cascade and Berlin (2), with permission from the *American Journal of Roentgenology*. I encourage the readers to become familiar with the ACR communication standard in its entirety. The publication can be obtained directly from the ACR (3).

The report should, when appropriate, identify factors that may limit the sensitivity and specificity of the examination. Standard Item II.C. 3

A patient fell from a truck and ended up in an emergency department complaining of neck pain. A cervical spine series was done that did not clearly show the junction of the cervical and thoracic spine. The examination was reported as normal, but the limitation of the study was not mentioned. Follow-up spine radiographs were obtained later because the neck pain persisted. A diagnosis of a fracture dislocation was made at C7-T1, and a lawsuit was filed.

The initial jury verdict found in favor of the radiologist. However, the verdict was reversed on appeal, specifying that the radiologist had the obligation to mention limitations of a study when there could be an impact on patient care.

Comparison with previous examinations and reports should be part of the radiologic consultation and report when appropriate and available. Standard Item II.C.5

A radiologist reported the presence of "questionable indeterminate calcifications" in the left breast of a 60-year-old woman. A prior mammogram was not available, although the typed report was. The prior report described the presence of benign-appearing calcifications, and for this reason the radiologist stated that the calcifications on the new study were probably benign. A subsequent screening mammogram 1 year later revealed changes in the calcifications that on biopsy showed carcinoma *in situ*.

At trial, an expert witness criticized the radiologist for not attempting to obtain the earlier mammogram for a comparison and to evaluate for interval change in the calcifications. The jury found in favor of the plaintiff, awarding her more than $100,000.

The timeliness of reporting any radiologic examinations varies with the nature and urgency of the clinical problem. The final report should be made available in a clinically appropriate timely manner. Standard Item III.A.

A venous hyperalimentation catheter was introduced into a young woman who suffered from chronic Crohn disease. A radiologist reported a concern that the catheter was positioned more medially in the mediastinum than usually seen. The radiologist tried unsuccessfully by phone to reach the surgeon who had placed the catheter. The radiologist did reach a nurse caring for the patient. She assured the radiologist that the catheter had free backflow and that the patient was asymptomatic after hyperalimentation. Hours later, the patient went into shock and died. Autopsy revealed that the catheter had perforated the superior vena cava with extravasation of hyperalimentation fluid into the thorax.

The family of the deceased sued, claiming that it was the responsibility of the radiologist to communicate directly with the surgeon in a timely fashion so that steps could be taken to remedy the problem. A radiologist expert witness testified that the defendant had breached the standard of practice by abandoning attempts to contact the surgeon directly and immediately when perforation was suspected. The case was settled before trial.

The final report should be proofread to minimize typographical errors, deleted words, and confusing or conflicting statements. Standard Item III.B.

A 32-year-old woman had chest radiography to evaluate for pneumonia. A radiologist reported the study as being within normal limits. Follow-up chest radiographs 18 months later revealed a right apical mass that turned out to be a neurofibroma. In retrospect, the mass had been present but missed on the initial chest radiographs.

A lawsuit was filed for missing the lesion on the initial chest examination. The radiologist named in the suit claimed that the report was not his and that the transcriptionist was in error when she put his name on the report as the dictating radiologist. The defendant did testify that it was his signature that was on the report but he had signed the report by mistake. It was his routine to sign all of his reports before going home in the evening, but he did not read the reports very carefully. The associate radiologist denied that he had dictated the report. The case was considered indefensible because both radiologists had accused each other of interpreting the study. The case was settled for $37,600.

In summary, the standards of practice for radiologists as developed by the ACR can be, and are, used by trial lawyers. All radiologists should be familiar with the standards that apply to radiology reporting. Sound risk management mandates close adherence to these standards for medical–legal reasons and, even more importantly, for good patient care.

MORE PET PEEVES

As Mark Twain once wrote, "It were not best that we should all think alike; it is difference of opinion that makes horse races" (from *Tragedy of Pudd'nhead Wilson*). In my experience, I found that reporting is one of the most controversial and passionate subjects that radiologists argue about. It seems as though each of us has his or her own style of dictating cases, a style thought (by each individual) to be the best. In the following section I point out examples of errors of composition and use of language and make recommendations for improvement. You can reject the thoughts, or adopt them if you are wise.

Do you remember your English composition classes in elementary school? From what I have seen, most radiologists have forgotten everything they learned. Basic principles of composition such as 1) use the active voice, 2) omit needless words, and 3) put statements in a positive form come to mind.

A typical chest radiographic report might read as follows:

> Findings: The lungs are well inflated. There is a calcified nodule in the right lower lobe that is compatible with a granuloma. The lungs are somewhat overexposed and nodules cannot be excluded. The heart is normal in size. There is no evidence of heart failure. There is no pleural effusion. The ribs and spine are normal for a patient of this age. There is a 5 mm osteoma in the proximal humeral metaphysis on the right. Impression: There are no significant findings on this somewhat limited examination (see paragraph above).

How boring and difficult to read! For some reason, radiologists continue to dictate in the passive voice, put in unnecessary words, and on occasion put sentences in a negative form. Hedging is common. I say, use the active voice, do not be verbose, be confident in your observations, and do not use the negative form. To ask the clinician "see paragraph above" or "correlate clinically" is unnecessary and insulting. Reading the body of the report is usually superfluous, and of course the clinician will correlate the report with his or her clinical knowledge.

Another way to write the report could be as follows:

> Findings: Fully inflated lungs. Benign calcified nodule in the right lower lobe. Overexposed images. Neoplasms could be present and obscured. Normal heart size, and no failure. Conclusion: Negative except for right lower lobe granuloma.

This report shows brevity, confidence, and clarity. I removed unnecessary words such as the description of the bones and insignificant findings such as a tiny osteoma, and I use phrases rather than full sentences to make the report more succinct. I took out hedges such as "there is no evidence of" I changed the double negative "cannot be excluded," replacing it with the positive statement "could be present." I also took the liberty of ending the report with "Conclusion" rather than "Impression." Conclusion portrays confidence.

An even better report, in my opinion follows:

> Conclusion: Negative except for right lower lobe granuloma.

This is my favorite type of report. There is no need to dictate *findings*; just a conclusion will suffice unless the findings are so complex that a full description is warranted. My expression is "few words, clear message."

In addition to poor grammar, radiologists often misuse terminology when reporting. The Fleischner Society, dedicated to excellence in chest radiology, has made comprehensive recommendations on appropriate and inappropriate terminology in chest radiology (4,5). Following is a list of terms related to chest radiography that should be banished, in my opinion, from radiology interpretive reports:

Diaphragms: Humans have one muscular diaphragm, not more. The singular form *diaphragm* should be used.

Adenopathy: Adeno comes from the Greek word meaning *gland*. There are no glands in lymph nodes! Use *lymph node enlargement* instead.

Density: Many reports contain the term *density* as a descriptor of an abnormal finding in the lung. In fact, *density* refers to the degree of darkening of the chest radiograph. Abnormalities in the lung such as nodules are relatively white on radiographs, not dark. Use *opacity* instead.

Bony: Radiologists often use the adjective *bony* when describing features related to the thoracic skeleton. For example, I have read reports of *bony* destruction of ribs. Would these same radiologists speak about *footy* pain instead of *foot* pain if they drop something on their foot or *lungy* congestion instead of *lung* congestion if they have an upper respiratory infection? Of course not. Therefore, use *bone* or *osseous* when describing abnormalities of bone (*bone destruction* not *bony destruction*).

Prominent: A frequent and classic hedge word used by many radiologists. For example, *prominent aortic arch* comes to mind. What is meant is that the aorta is, or might be, somewhat dilated or enlarged. In general, if you believe a structure is abnormal, say so. If you are not sure, do something to find out. In this example, call the aorta enlarged or recommend further imaging.

Nonspecific: The term *nonspecific* often appears in reports describing a bowel gas pattern. I have also seen the same term used to describe the interstitium of the lungs. When used, the term usually means that the radiologist believes the study is probably normal but is hedging his or her bets. Earn your paycheck. Do not dodge the decision by leaving the findings as *nonspecific*. Call the lungs normal, abnormal, or possibly abnormal with a recommendation of further imaging to find out.

Mainstem: Mainstem is an archaic term that should be replaced by *main* as in *right main bronchus*.

Poor Inspiration: Do not blame the patient. It could be that the technologist took the image during expiration.

Low Lung Volumes: Use lung volumes to refer to abnormal lungs. For example, patients with emphysema have large lung volumes and patients with pulmonary fibrosis can have small lung volumes. It is preferable to use degrees of inflation to describe the degree of aeration of the lungs, for example, *poor inflation* or *hyperinflation*.

REFERENCES

1. Chapman WW, Fiszman M, Frederick PR, et al. Quantifying the characteristics of unambiguous chest radiography reports in the context of pneumonia. *Acad Radiol* 2001;8:57–66.
2. Cascade PN, Berlin L. American College of Radiology standard for communication. *AJR Am J Roentgenol* 1999;173:1439–1442.
3. American College of Radiology. ACR standard for communication: diagnostic radiology. In: *Standards*. Reston, VA: American College of Radiology, 2000:1–3.
4. Tuddingham WJ. Glossary of terms for thoracic radiology: recommendations of the nomenclature committee of the Fleischner Society. *AJR Am J Roentgenol* 1984;143:509–517.
5. Austin JHM, Muller NL, Friedman PJ, et al. Glossary of terms for CT of the lungs: recommendations of the nomenclature committee of the Fleischner Society. *Radiology* 1996;200:327–331.

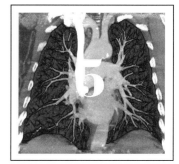

PNEUMONIA IN THE IMMUNOCOMPETENT HOST

- Clinical Clues to the Cause of Pneumonia
- Imaging Modalities
- Radiologic Signs of Pneumonia
- Radiologic Classification of Pneumonia
- Differential Diagnosis of Pneumonia
- Radiologic Clues to the Cause of Pneumonia
- Complications
- Bacterial Pneumonia
- Fungal Infections
- Viral Infections
- Parasitic Infections

Despite advances in medicine, pneumonia remains a major cause of morbidity and mortality. It affects six million American adults each year. With a mortality rate of 13.4 per 100,000, it is the sixth most common cause of death in the United States (1). Community-acquired pneumonia (CAP) in previously healthy individuals is caused by bacteria in 25% of patients, atypical pathogens (including mycoplasma) in 25%, and viruses in 20%. A few percent more feature multiple causative organisms, but many patients are treated without conclusive evidence.

In hospitalized adults with pneumonia, 60% to 80% are due to *Streptococcus pneumoniae*, up to 20% are caused by gram-negative bacteria, a few percent result from *Staphylococcus aureus*, and the remainder are due to viruses and *Mycoplasma*. For nosocomial or hospital-acquired pneumonia, gram-negative organisms are responsible for 35% to 40%, *S. pneumoniae* for 10%, *S. aureus* for 3%, and no agent is identified in approximately 40%.

The diagnosis of pneumonia is based on a combination of clinical history and examination, serologic tests, and diagnostic imaging (2–6) (Boxes 5.1 and 5.2). It is usually not possible to identify the etiology based on clinical or radiologic findings alone. Serologic tests require a few days. It is therefore important that the clinician and radiologist work together, pooling information and resources to narrow the differential diagnosis. The radiologist's role is to detect abnormality, define its location and extent, evaluate for compli-

---

Box 5.1: *Common Features of Bacterial Pneumonias*

- Respiratory symptoms predominate
- Acute onset of symptoms
- Focal signs on clinical examination
- Correlation between clinical and radiologic findings
- Pathologic changes in a focal area or areas of lung parenchyma

---

Box 5.2: Features of Atypical and Viral Pneumonia

- Systemic symptoms predominate over respiratory symptoms
- No response to usual antibiotic therapy
- Discrepancy between the severity and location of clinical signs and radiologic findings
- Pathologic changes mainly in the bronchial tree and interstitial parenchyma

---

cations, and monitor response to therapy. As in most clinical settings, the radiologist is significantly aided by having relevant clinical information.

CLINICAL CLUES TO THE CAUSE OF PNEUMONIA

Accurate early treatment is important in many of the bacterial pneumonias if complications (and even death) are to be avoided. The choice of an appropriate antibiotic rests on the radiologic and clinical findings. Several factors help to narrow the diagnostic possibilities. Patient age is one such factor. Viruses are the usual cause of pneumonia in children. Mycoplasma occurs mainly in children and young adults. Bacteria most commonly cause adult pneumonias.

Clinical symptoms can also be useful. An acute history of productive cough, pleuritic chest pain, and chills is characteristic of bacterial pneumonia (7). On physical examination, focal signs are often present, and there is a high incidence of radiologic findings. In atypical pneumonias systemic symptoms such as fatigue, malaise, arthralgias, and low-grade fever predominate, with a more gradual onset (8). There is often a discrepancy between the clinical and radiologic findings.

Predisposing factors may point to specific organisms. Alcoholism, dementia, neuro-muscular disease, swallowing disorders, and general anesthesia predispose to aspiration pneumonia. Anaerobic organisms, gram-negative bacteria, and *S. aureus* are most often isolated. Chronic obstructive pulmonary disease (COPD) exacerbations are often caused by *Hemophilus influenzae* or *Branhamella catarrhalis*. Pneumonia complicating influenza is often caused by *S. aureus*. *S. pneumoniae* is common in sickle cell disease and in patients who have previously undergone splenectomy. *Pseudomonas aeruginosa* and *S. aureus* are commonly responsible agents in cystic fibrosis. Immunocompromised patients are considered separately in Chapter 6.

IMAGING MODALITIES

Chest radiographs (CXR) are the first line of defense and the mainstay for imaging suspected pneumonia. If pneumonia is confirmed clinically and radiologically, therapy is generally begun. In elderly patients and heavy cigarette smokers, follow-up CXR is advised to complete resolution of disease, thereby excluding postobstructive pneumonia. Radiologic resolution may lag behind clinical improvement by as much as 6 to 8 weeks (and even longer in elderly and COPD patients). Ultrasound can be used to evaluate pleural opacity seen on CXR. The largest areas of pleural fluid can be marked radiologically for aspiration.

Chest computed tomography (CT) can be helpful in patients with pneumonia that resolves too slowly or fails to resolve. A small mass may be obscured by obstructive atelectasis on CXR. CT is better at detecting small calcifications and enlarged intrathoracic nodes. CT with contrast enhancement helps to differentiate lung abscess from empyema when CXR is equivocal.

Radiologic resolution of bacterial pneumonia often takes 6 to 8 weeks.

RADIOLOGIC SIGNS OF PNEUMONIA

OPACIFICATION

Focal opacity may be visible, especially when comparing one lung with the other on the frontal projection. On the lateral projection attention should be directed over the thoracic spine, the cardiac silhouette, and the retrosternal and retrocardiac regions, where faint opacity may otherwise escape detection (Figs. 5.1 and 5.2).

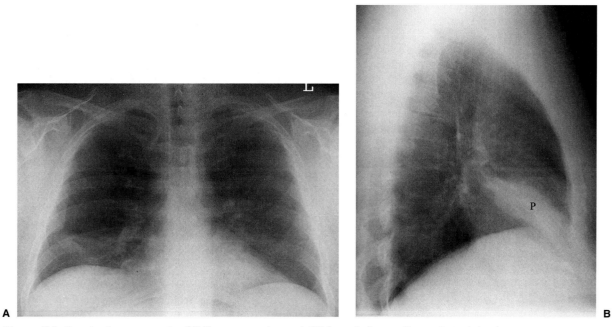

Figure 5.1 Opacity in pneumonia. *(A)* Posteroanterior and *(B)* lateral chest radiographs: minimal right basilar opacity, much better seen on the lateral view overlying the heart (P).

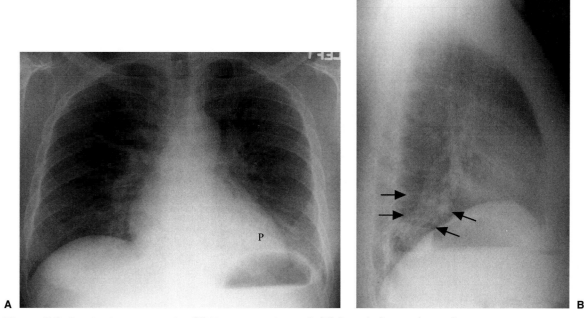

Figure 5.2 Opacity in pneumonia. *(A)* Posteroanterior and *(B)* lateral chest radiographs: vague retrocardiac abnormality (P) with corresponding increased opacity over the lower thoracic spine on the lateral view *(arrows)*.

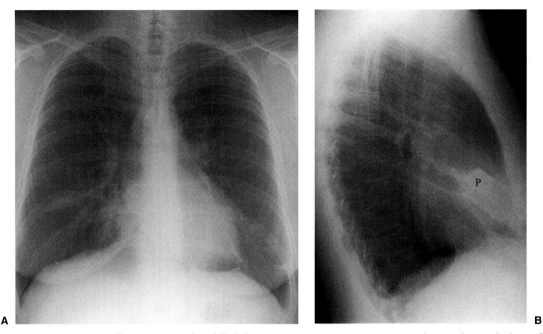

Figure 5.3 Silhouette sign of middle lobe pneumonia. *A.* Posteroanterior chest radiograph: loss of visualization of right heart border. *B.* Lateral chest radiograph: corresponding middle lobe pneumonia (P).

SILHOUETTE SIGN

Lung opacity contacting a mediastinal or diaphragmatic border will obliterate or silhouette that border ("silhouette sign"). Right middle lobe opacity can be subtle on the frontal CXR, necessitating careful scrutiny of the right heart border (Fig. 5.3). Lingular disease obliterates the left heart border (Fig. 5.4), whereas lower lobe opacity may obscure a hemidiaphragm.

AIRSPACE DISEASE

This describes replacement of the airspaces with fluid or exudate without gross destruction or displacement of lung morphology. Signs of airspace disease (Chapter 14) (Fig. 5.5)

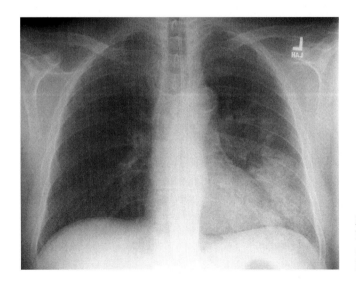

Figure 5.4 Silhouette sign of lingular pneumonia. Partial loss of visualization of lower left heart border.

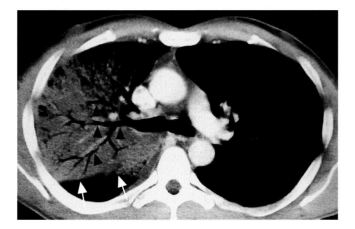

Figure 5.5 Airspace disease at computed tomography. Pneumonia shows air bronchograms (*arrowheads*), lobar distribution (*arrows* denote major fissure), and ill-definition anteriorly.

occur. At CT early airspace disease may manifest as ground glass opacity, with increased attenuation but with pulmonary vessels still visible.

PERIBRONCHIAL THICKENING

Perceptible thickening of a bronchus is most commonly seen in viral infections. It can often be discerned by comparing the bronchus diameter with its accompanying pulmonary artery.

ATELECTASIS

This describes loss of lung volume (Fig. 5.6), and the term collapse is used when a whole lobe or lung is involved. Mild atelectasis occurs in many patients, especially those with interstitial pneumonia. It usually manifests as linear or discoid atelectasis.

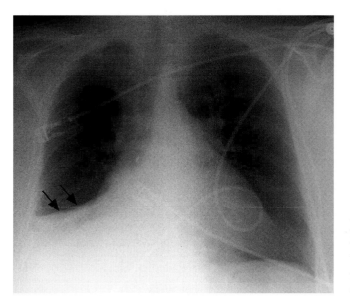

Figure 5.6 Atelectasis with pneumonia. Depression of major fissure (*arrows*) and silhouetting of right heart border indicate combined right middle and lower lobe atelectasis.

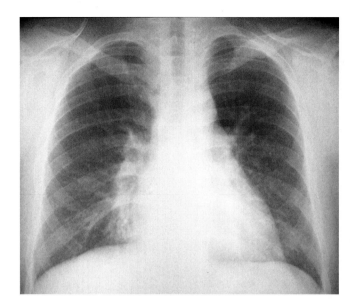

Figure ***5.7*** Bronchopneumonia. Multifocal central linear and patchy opacities.

RADIOLOGIC CLASSIFICATION OF PNEUMONIA

Pneumonia is recognized to have different radiologic appearances. These generally have no bearing on the final diagnosis, because the same organism may produce several patterns. In addition, the early use of antibiotics alters the evolution of these patterns. The patterns are as follows:

Bronchopneumonia: This is the most common pattern. Here, the inflammatory exudates are mainly related to the central bronchovascular structures and may be multifocal (Fig. 5.7). Some acini may be spared, resulting in a patchy distribution of opacity. There is often associated volume loss.

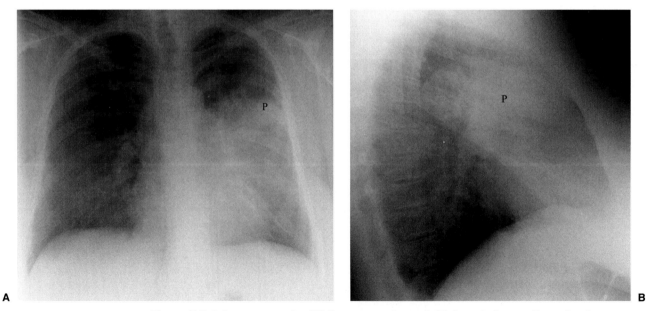

Figure 5.8 Lobar pneumonia. *(A)* Posteroanterior and *(B)* lateral chest radiographs demonstrate airspace opacity filling much of the left upper lobe (P).

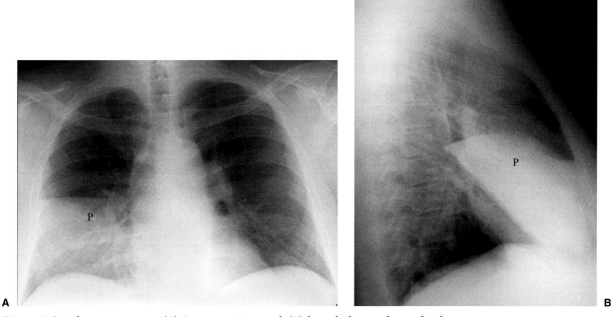

Figure 5.9 Lobar pneumonia. *(A)* Posteroanterior and *(B)* lateral chest radiographs demonstrate opacification of virtually the entire middle lobe (P).

Lobar pneumonia: The exudate begins distally and spreads circumferentially, giving rise to more homogeneous opacity (Figs. 5.8 and 5.9). It may eventually involve the whole lobe. The airways are not principally involved, so there is little volume loss, and air bronchograms are generally present.

Interstitial pneumonia: This consists of peribronchial thickening and ill-defined reticulonodular opacities (Fig. 5.10). This pattern is typical of *Mycoplasma* and viruses. Patchy distribution of atelectasis is often seen.

Round pneumonia: Some pneumonias have this configuration initially. There is usually an ill-defined border (Fig. 5.11). Air bronchograms are frequently present.

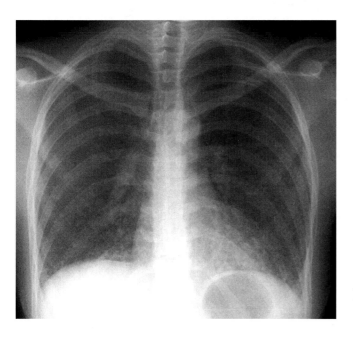

Figure 5.10 Interstitial pneumonia. Bilateral widespread ill-defined opacities.

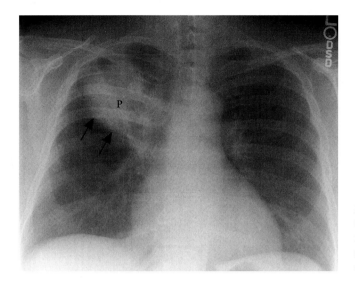

Figure 5.11 Round pneumonia (P), demonstrating a sharp margin inferiorly *(arrows)* and an ill-defined border superomedially.

DIFFERENTIAL DIAGNOSIS OF PNEUMONIA

Acute airspace disease has a reasonably brief differential diagnosis. Pneumonia generally differs from pulmonary edema in its more focal distribution. There is generally not associated cardiac enlargement in pneumonia. At CT pneumonia demonstrates nondependent opacity (as opposed to the dependent pattern of pulmonary edema). Pulmonary edema also improves or worsens in hours as opposed to days in the case of pneumonia.

Adult respiratory distress syndrome (ARDS) is often indistinguishable from pneumonia on a single radiographic study. Over time changes will occur more slowly in ARDS, and it is often more widespread than pneumonia. CT will show dependent changes in ARDS.

Subsegmental atelectasis may be indistinguishable from early pneumonia. The more linear the radiographic abnormality, the less likely it represents pneumonia. Associated clinical signs and symptoms may be helpful; transmitted breath sounds are often amplified in pneumonia but not in atelectasis.

The radiographic appearance of pulmonary infarct may be quite similar to pneumonia. Enlargement of a pulmonary artery or attenuated peripheral vessels may suggest a vascular etiology. Infarct is more likely to be well marginated at its borders and typically evolves more rapidly than pneumonia.

The appearance of pulmonary hemorrhage is very similar to pneumonia. There is often a history of frank hemoptysis. Clearance of opacity usually occurs more quickly than in pneumonia.

Some neoplasms, such as lymphoma and bronchoalveolar carcinoma, produce airspace opacification indistinguishable from pneumonia. Serial studies show more chronic abnormality with gradual change. Lymph node enlargement at CXR would be more typical of lymphoma than pneumonia.

RADIOLOGIC CLUES TO THE CAUSE OF PNEUMONIA

Lobar consolidation is often due to bacteria. Postobstructive pneumonia needs to be considered in patients at risk for lung carcinoma. Expansive consolidation occurs in *Klebsiella* pneumonia ("Friedlander pneumonia") (Fig. 5.12) but can also be seen with *S. pneumoniae*.

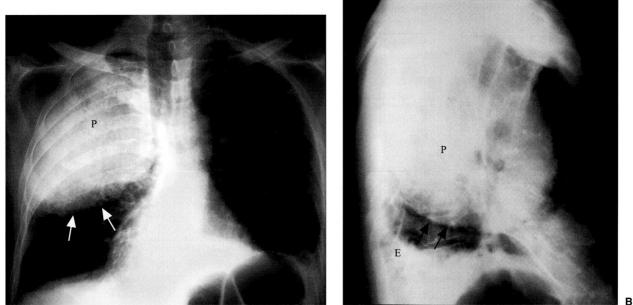

Figure 5.12 Pneumonia (P) enlarging the right upper lobe, suggesting the correct diagnosis of *Klebsiella* pneumonia. *(A)* Posteroanterior and *(B)* lateral chest radiographs: note bowing of major fissure *(arrows)*. There is an associated pleural effusion (E).

Cavitating consolidation (Figs. 5.13 and 5.14) suggests bacteria or fungi. *S. aureus, Klebsiella,* anaerobes, and *Mycobacterium tuberculosis* commonly cause cavitation. Pneumatoceles may result in a similar appearance (Fig. 5.15) and suggest *S. aureus* or *S. pneumoniae.* Emphysematous bullae within consolidated lung may mimic cavities.

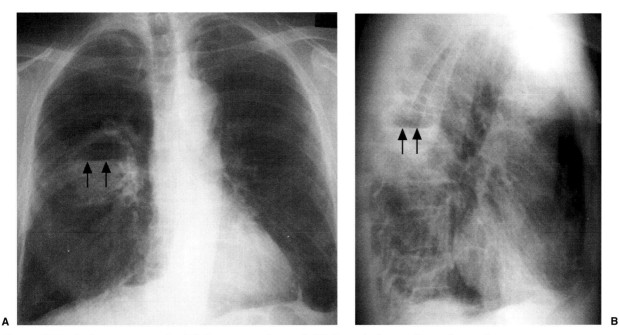

Figure 5.13 Cavitary pneumonia. *(A)* Posteroanterior, and *(B)* Lateral chest radiographs: cavity with a gas-fluid level *(arrows)* in the superior segment of the right lower lobe.

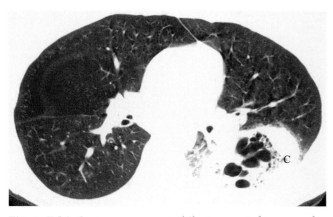

Figure 5.14 Cavitary pneumonia (C) at computed tomography.

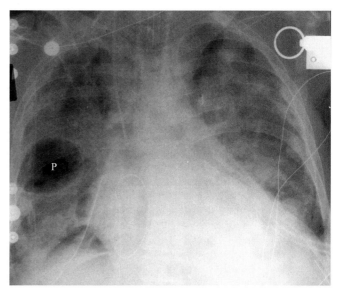

Figure 5.15 Diffuse pneumonia with pneumatocele formation (P).

Dependent pneumonia suggests aspiration, whereas cavitary upper lobe disease raises the possibility of TB.

Nodular or spherical pneumonia is usually due to pneumococcal, *Legionella*, Q fever, or fungal pneumonia. Hematogenous dissemination of *S. aureus* can cause spherical pneumonia or septic emboli. Reticulonodular opacity and peribronchial thickening are typical of viruses and *Mycoplasma*.

Patchy consolidation with a dependent distribution occurs with aspiration pneumonia. This is usually bilateral. Patchy upper lobe disease is suggestive of tuberculosis (TB) or histoplasmosis, especially if there is associated cavitation. Miliary opacities occur with overwhelming tuberculous or fungal infection.

Pleural effusions may develop with anaerobic bacteria, gram-negative bacteria, *S. aureus*, and *S. pyogenes*. Empyema should be suspected when pleural effusion is large or loculated or develops late in the course of disease.

COMPLICATIONS

Pleural effusions/empyema: these are indistinguishable radiographically.

Cavitation: if enlarging or greater than 4 cm in diameter, an indication for intervention.

Pneumatoceles: usually self-limiting and resolve within 4 weeks. They resemble bullae and blebs.

Pneumothorax: seen in *Pneumocystis carinii* pneumonia (Chapter 6).

Lymph node enlargement: seen with fungal and mycobacterial infections. In patients at risk, also consider bronchogenic carcinoma.

Bone destruction: may occur in actinomycosis, nocardiosis, fungal infections, and TB.

Abscess: may be difficult to distinguish from empyema. CT sometimes helpful to differentiate these two entities

Bronchiectasis: any chronic or severe infection may cause bronchiectasis, and in cystic fibrosis patients, upper lung bronchiectasis tends to occur.

Expansive consolidation:
  Klebsiella
  Haemophilus influenzae
  Pneumococcal pneumonia
  Plague pneumonia

TB
Lung abscess: *S. aureus, Klebsiella*
Lung mass
Cavitating pneumonia:
    S. aureus
    Klebsiella
    TB
    Aspiration
    Actinomycosis
    Nocardiosis
    Histoplasmosis
    Aspergillosis
    Coccidioidomycosis
    Echinococcosis
    Amoebiasis
Pneumatoceles:
    S. aureus
    S. pneumoniae
    Escherichia coli
    Klebsiella
    H. influenzae
    P. carinii
    Legionella pneumophila

BACTERIAL PNEUMONIA

STREPTOCOCCUS PNEUMONIAE (PNEUMOCOCCUS)

This gram-positive coccus is responsible for anywhere from 10% to 80% of cases of CAP (9,10). It is the most frequent organism resulting in hospitalization for pneumonia. It is common in healthy young adults, typically presenting with chills, fever, and cough productive of rust-colored blood-tinged sputum. Spread is by the airborne route. Diagnosis can be made by sputum or blood culture, although pneumococci are found in the sputum of 10% to 40% of normal patients. Sputum cultures are negative in nearly half of patients with positive blood cultures. Most patients are diagnosed presumptively, based on clinical and radiographic presentation, without the need for cultures.

Homogeneous airspace disease confined to a single lobe with an irregular margin (Fig. 5.16) is the most common radiographic pattern, seen in about one-third of patients. Pneumococcal pneumonia is one of the causes of expansive consolidation with bowing of fissures. More widespread patchy bronchopneumonia is seen in another one-third, usually confined to a single lobe. Interstitial opacification simulating viral or atypical pneumonia occurs in one-fourth of patients. The remainder show a mixed patchy and interstitial pattern. There is a predilection for the lower lobes. Pleural effusions are seen in one-third. Consolidation in pneumococcal pneumonia is said to clear by central "lysis." Patients with shorter clinical histories tend to show more rapid radiographic resolution. As in all pneumonias there is a lag period between clinical resolution and radiologic resolution, which can be several weeks.

Pneumococcus is the organism most frequently resulting in hospitalization for pneumonia.

STAPHYLOCOCCUS AUREUS

This gram-positive coccus is an uncommon but serious cause of CAP (11–13). It has a fulminant course with fever, cough, dyspnea, purulent sputum, hemoptysis, and chest pain. Spread occurs by the airborne or hematogenous route. When acquired via inhalation, *S. aureus* pneumonia is often a complication of influenza during epidemics. Airborne spread

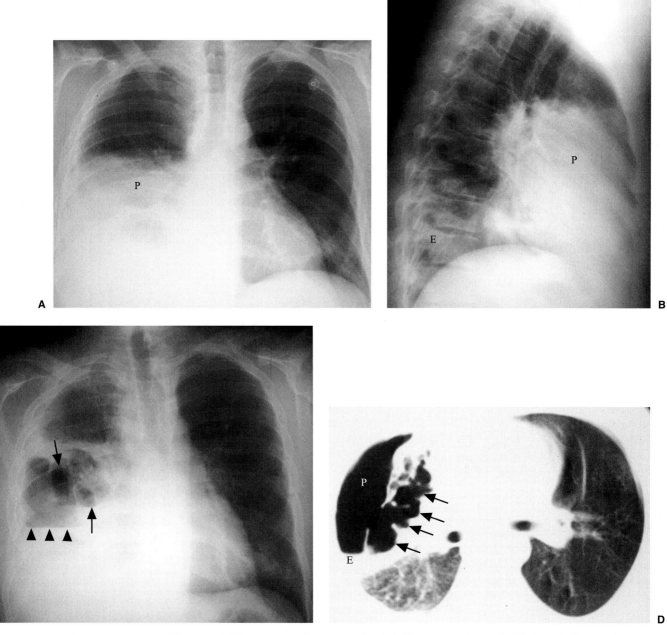

Figure 5.16 Pneumococcal pneumonia. *(A)* Posteroanterior and *(B)* lateral chest radiographs: homogeneous middle lobe pneumonia (P), possibly with slight expansion of the lobe, with associated right pleural effusion (E). *(C)* Later posteroanterior chest radiograph and *(D)* computed tomography: subsequent development of pneumatoceles *(arrows)* resulting in bronchopleural fistula with hydropneumothorax. P, pneumothorax; E, pleural effusion. *Arrowheads* mark gas–fluid level.

is also implicated in debilitated patients. Hematogenous spread occurs secondary to soft tissue infections, valve prostheses, hemodialysis, and intravenous drug use. Morbidity is high, with a reported mortality rate of 7% to 19%.

Initially, radiographs most commonly (75%) show multilobar homogeneous airspace disease (Fig. 5.17). Subsequent radiographic deterioration is often seen. Bilateral changes are noted in 35%. Cavitation or abscess formation (25%), pneumatoceles (40%), pleural

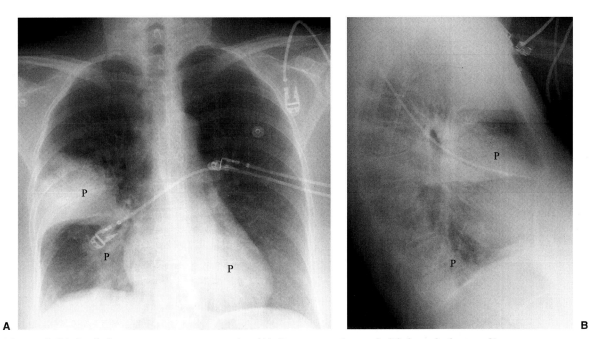

Figure 5.17 *Staphylococcus aureus* pneumonia. *(A)* Posteroanterior and *(B)* lateral chest radiographs demonstrate airspace disease in the right upper lobe and both lower lobes (P).

effusions (33%), and pneumothorax (20%, often associated with pleural effusion or empyema) are other common findings. Pneumonia with pneumatocele or pneumothorax should suggest *S. aureus* as the cause.

BACILLUS ANTHRACIS

This is a gram-positive sporulating nonmotile organism. It is endemic in the soil of Texas, Oklahoma, and the lower Mississippi valley (14). Cutaneous disease accounts for over 90% of cases, with gastrointestinal and inhalational disease causing 5% each. Inhalational disease results from industrial or agricultural exposure to animal hides, hair, wool, or bone meal of contaminated livestock. The disease is most prevalent among herbivores such as cattle, sheep, horses, and goats. Prior radiation exposure, alcoholism, and underlying pulmonary disease are thought to be risk factors. Spores of 2 to 5 μm reach the alveoli. Macrophages engulf the spores and transfer them to mediastinal and hilar nodes. Germination occurs with production of large amounts of anthrax toxin. This spills over into the systemic circulation with resultant edema, hemorrhage, necrosis, and septic shock. Massive hemorrhagic mediastinitis occurs. Inhalational anthrax manifests as an initial flu-like illness followed by rapidly progressive respiratory failure and death.

CXRs show widening of the mediastinum due to hemorrhagic mediastinitis and lymphadenitis (15,16). Pleural effusions also occur. Focal hemorrhagic pneumonia is only seen in one-fourth of patients. CT better demonstrates hemorrhagic mediastinitis and necrosis. It also excludes other etiologies of widened mediastinum.

KLEBSIELLA

This gram-negative bacillus is also known as Friedlander bacillus (17). It is found in the upper respiratory tract of 2% to 25% of healthy persons. It is an uncommon cause of pneumonia and a well-known cause of biliary and urinary tract sepsis. Middle-aged men are most commonly affected, and many patients have predisposing conditions such as alcoholism, malnutrition, and diabetes. Chronic pulmonary diseases such as asthma and bronchiectasis may also predispose to *Klebsiella* infections. The incubation period is short. Cough, pleuritic pain, and fever are frequent initial symptoms, with malaise, chills, and shortness of breath also occurring. The mortality rate is high, estimated at 70% to 80%. Of the remainder, a few recover slowly, whereas others suffer chronic disease with a clinical course similar to TB.

Klebsiella should be considered with opaque, extensive, expansive airspace disease.

Radiographs most commonly show scattered lobular foci of airspace disease that may coalesce to form larger opacities (18,19). Typically, opacity has a sharp advancing border. This pattern is indistinguishable from other bacterial pneumonias. The upper lobes are involved in two-thirds of cases. Healing generally leaves residual scarring and distortion of lung. Radiographs may show expansion of a lobe (Fig. 5.12) due to "drowned lung." Shift of the mediastinum to the opposite side may occur with whole lung involvement. Small pleural effusions are thought to occur because pleural thickening often remains after resolution of acute changes. Empyema occurs in about 6%. These patients have the worst clinical course. *Klebsiella* deserves consideration whenever opaque, extensive, expansive airspace disease is seen.

PSEUDOMONAS AERUGINOSA

Pseudomonas is implicated in 25% of ventilator-associated pneumonias, with 80% to 100% mortality.

This gram-negative organism is a rare cause of CAP in healthy persons (20,21). *Pseudomonas* colonizes bronchiectatic airways, especially in cystic fibrosis. It is sometimes present on normal skin and is also a secondary contaminant in wounds. Prematurity, chemotherapy, antibiotics, steroids, immunosuppressants, old age, and debility increase the risk of *Pseudomonas*. Neutropenia increases the risk of severe disease. Most cases occur in hospitalized patients, especially those on ventilators. Organisms have been cultured from sinks, catheters, receptacles, ventilator equipment, and staff. *Pseudomonas* is the most common pathogen isolated from the lower respiratory tract of ventilated patients and is implicated in 25% of ventilator-associated pneumonias. Mortality in these patients is in

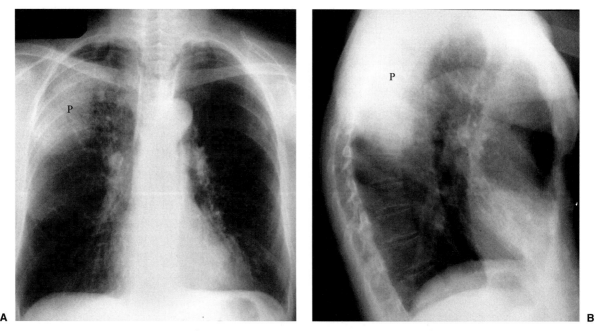

Figure 5.18 *Pseudomonas* pneumonia. (A) Posteroanterior and (B) lateral chest radiographs demonstrate airspace disease (P) predominantly in the posterior segment of the right upper lobe.

the 80% to 100% range. Pneumonia is usually secondary to aspiration of oropharyngeal contents in intensive care unit patients. Sedation, endotracheal intubation, and intermittent positive pressure ventilation predispose to infection. Person-to-person contact has been implicated in hospitals.

Radiographs most commonly demonstrate segmental or lobar disease (22) (Fig. 5.18). Abnormality is multilobar in 80% and bilateral in 65%. The lower lobes predominate. Pleural effusions are seen in 25%. Lucencies are seen in up to 20%, representing cavities or abscesses in necrotizing pneumonia, interspersed normal areas of lung, or pneumatoceles. Cavitation in a ventilated patient suggests *Pseudomonas*.

LEGIONELLA PNEUMOPHILA

This gram-negative organism is responsible for sporadic cases and outbreaks of pneumonia (23). The first reported outbreak of 182 cases occurred at an American Legion convention in 1977, after which the organism is named. It is thought to be an airborne infection with bacterial growth detected in cooling towers and air conditioning systems. *L. pneumophila* accounts for over 90% of cases of legionellosis. Diagnosis is based on sputum culture, urinary antigen detection, and rising antibody levels on paired serologic tests. Legionellosis has been classified as an atypical pneumonia due to the clinical prodrome of malaise and headache, the radiologic findings, and the poor correlation between these findings and clinical signs. It runs a long clinical course, taking even longer to resolve in debilitated patients. Death has been reported in a few cases.

Chest radiographic findings lag behind the clinical findings by a few weeks and cannot be used to differentiate legionellosis from other causes of pneumonia. Over 80% of patients have patchy airspace disease initially. In two-thirds of cases this is unilobar (Fig. 5.19). The lower lobes are involved in 75% of cases. The apices are rarely involved. Small pleural effusions are ultimately seen in over 60% of patients. Cavitation is very rare and occurs predominantly in immunocompromised patients. Enlarged lymph nodes have not been reported. Radiologic resolution is slow, and initial worsening of findings is often seen.

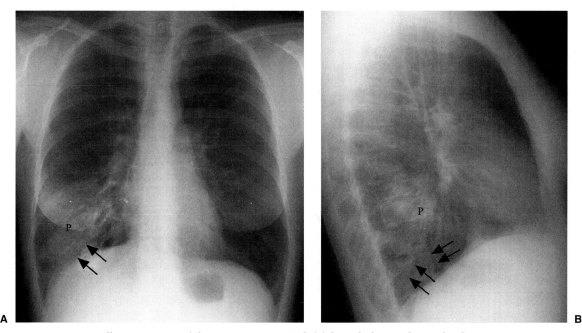

A   B

Figure 5.19 *Legionella* pneumonia. (A) Posteroanterior and (B) lateral chest radiographs demonstrate unilobar involvement of the right lower lobe (P) with prominent air bronchograms (*arrows*).

ASPIRATION PNEUMONIA

This may occur subsequent to the intake of solid or liquid materials into the lungs. Predisposing factors include impaired consciousness, alcoholism, general anesthesia, dementia, neuromuscular disorders, tracheoesophageal fistula, pharyngeal diverticulum, gastroesophageal reflux, achalasia, and hiatal hernia. Clinical and radiologic manifestations vary from asymptomatic to life-threatening disease (24). The most commonly involved lung sites are the posterior segments of the upper lobes and superior segments of the lower lobes in the recumbent position. The basal segments of the lower lobes, especially in the right lung, are most commonly involved when aspiration occurs in the upright position (Fig. 5.20). Chemical pneumonitis may occur, varying from mild bronchiolitis to pulmonary edema.

Aspiration of infected contents in hospitalized patients or those with poor oral hygiene may cause necrotizing pneumonia due to anaerobic organisms. *P. aeruginosa* is most commonly implicated. Complications include cavitation and empyema.

ACTINOMYCES

Actinomycosis does not respect anatomic barriers.

These slow-growing, filamentous, gram-positive bacteria are found normally in the oropharynx, especially in patients with poor dental hygiene (25). They form mycelium-like colonies that resemble fungi. Three disease patterns are described: cervicofacial, abdominopelvic, and thoracic. The latter accounts for 15% to 45% of cases. Men are affected three to four times more often than women. Thoracic infections may occur in the setting of trauma, surgery, alcoholism, COPD, or after aspiration. The primary lesion is based in the peribronchial tissues and spreads from lung to pleura, mediastinum, and chest wall with no regard for anatomic barriers. Direct spread relates to bacterial proteolytic activity. The organism can also disseminate hematogenously. Thoracic disease may also result from direct spread of disease in the neck or below the diaphragm. Diagnosis is difficult and often relies on demonstration of characteristic sulfur granules in sputum smears, consisting of conglomerate masses of mineralized organisms.

In acute infections, nonsegmental airspace disease (Fig. 5.21) is the usual CXR pattern, with peripheral and lower lobe predominance in over 75%. This may be multifocal

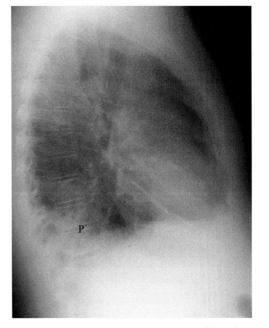

Figure 5.20 Aspiration pneumonia. Lower lobe distribution with increased opacity over the lower thoracic spine (P), silhouetting the posterior hemidiaphragms.

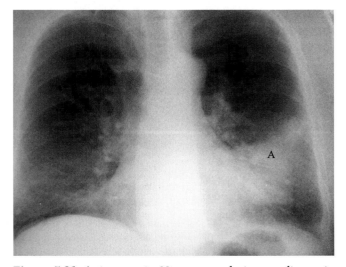

Figure 5.21 *Actinomycosis.* Nonsegmental airspace disease in the left upper lobe (A), silhouetting the left heart border.

and may cross fissures. Pleural thickening or small pleural effusions are found in most patients. Hilar and mediastinal lymph node enlargement is seen in one-third of patients. In chronic disease, spread to chest wall soft tissues can be well seen by CT.

NOCARDIA

This is a gram-positive filamentous bacterium with some similarity to *Actinomycetes*. It is present in soil and decaying organic matter and is acquired in humans by inhalation (26). *Nocardia asteroides* is responsible for 80% to 90% of all cases of nocardiosis. Pulmonary infection is the main clinical manifestation. About half of those affected are immunocompetent. The clinical syndrome is subacute, with productive cough, fever, weight loss, and malaise. Half of those infected develop disseminated disease. The central nervous system is affected in 25% of cases, and skin and subcutaneous tissues are commonly involved. Disseminated disease should be considered when the triad of pneumonia, central nervous system disease, and subcutaneus nodules occurs. With disseminated disease, the mortality rate is 80% to 90%, and death is especially likely when there is central nervous system involvement. Mortality is 38% without dissemination.

Radiographic manifestations are varied, including solitary and multiple nodules, airspace disease, and interstitial reticular opacities. Cavitation may occur. Pleural effusion and enlarged hilar and mediastinal lymph nodes may be seen.

CHLAMYDIA PNEUMONIAE

This organism has recently been identified as the cause of 6% to 12% of adult CAP (27). Before the advent of specific serologic tests, these infections were classified as "atypical" pneumonia or erroneously attributed to ornithosis. Two types of acute disease occur, primary (first exposure) and recurrent (in a previously exposed individual). Chronic lung disease is more common in those patients with the recurrent form. Transmission is by droplet spread. Symptoms include cough, fever, sore throat, hoarseness, and sinusitis.

Radiographs in the acute form show airspace disease, usually confined to one lung (Fig. 5.22) and in a single lobe in 75%. Interstitial opacities or mixed interstitial and air-

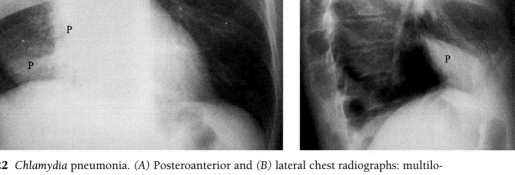

Figure 5.22 *Chlamydia* pneumonia. (A) Posteroanterior and (B) lateral chest radiographs: multilobar pneumonia (P) confined to one lung.

space opacities are less common. Pleural effusions are seen in over half of patients as disease progresses. In patients with recurrent disease findings are more variable, with bilateral disease in 63% and pleural effusions more likely. Hilar and mediastinal lymph node enlargement is uncommon.

MYCOPLASMA PNEUMONIAE

Mycoplasma is thought to cause up to 50% of atypical pneumonias.

This is a common cause of CAP, responsible for 10% to 30% of cases (9,28,29). It belongs to the group of organisms responsible for atypical pneumonia and is thought to cause up to 50% of such cases. Transmission is via the respiratory route, with most cases occurring in the fall and winter. Localized outbreaks in military camps, schools, families, and community groups have been described, cycling every 4 to 5 years. *Mycoplasma* is typically a disease of children and young adults and carries a good prognosis. The clinical course is often insidious, with malaise, fever, chills, headache, anorexia, and nonproductive cough. Complications include large pleural effusions, pleuropericarditis, myocarditis, ARDS, Guillain-Barré syndrome, lymph node enlargement, cold agglutinin-induced hemolytic anemia, and aseptic meningitis. Diagnosis is made by detecting a significant rise in serum cold hemagglutinins.

A common chest radiographic feature is segmental airspace disease (Fig. 5.23), occurring in 30% to 50% of patients. This may be dense or patchy in appearance. Involvement is unilateral in half to two-thirds, with lower lobe predominance in 77%. Reticulonodular opacities are said to occur just as often. Less commonly, perihilar bronchovascular thickening is seen. Pleural effusions are present in less than 10% of patients in most studies. Hilar lymph node enlargement is uncommon at CXR.

MYCOBACTERIUM TUBERCULOSIS

This bacillus, an obligate aerobe, is related to nocardia (30). It has a cell wall that resists staining by the usual Gram stain method. After accepting fuscin dyes it resists decolorization by acid-alcohol, hence the term acid-fast. Prevalence is highest in developing nations. Annual incidence is 200 to 250 cases per 100,000 in sub-Saharan Africa and Southeast

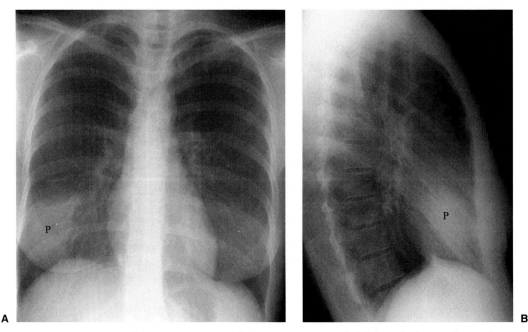

Figure 5.23 *Mycoplasma* pneumonia. (A) Posteroanterior and (B) lateral chest radiographs: segmental airspace disease (P) in the lateral segment of middle lobe.

Asia. Annual incidence in industrialized nations averages 23 per 100,000. In developing nations, 80% of cases affect adults in their productive years. In industrialized nations, most cases result from endogenous reactivation of remote infection, with rates highest in the elderly. Incidence is higher in non-white racial and ethnic groups and in immigrants.

Primary TB is transmitted by the airborne route. Particles measuring 1 to 5 mm can remain airborne for prolonged periods of time. Implantation of particles occurs preferentially in the middle and lower lung zones. Alveolar macrophages ingest and kill mycobacteria with variable success depending on host resistance and organism virulence. Macrophages may be overwhelmed and may burst, with released bacilli spreading via lymphatics and the bloodstream. Bacillary growth is usually arrested by the development of cell-mediated immunity and delayed hypersensitivity. Ninety percent of persons develop immunity and are asymptomatic. In 5% immunity is inadequate and active TB infection develops within a year (**progressive primary disease**). This is similar in morphology and course to postprimary disease. Another 5% will develop latent reactivation at a later stage. Progression to clinical disease is more likely with defects in T-cell or macrophage function, including acquired immunodeficiency syndrome, malnutrition, drug abuse, alcoholism, diabetes, immunosuppressive therapy, steroids, and silicosis.

Postprimary TB results from endogenous reactivation of previously acquired disease or, less commonly, exogenous reinfection. There is a predilection for the upper lung zones in postprimary TB, thought to relate to higher oxygen tensions and impaired lymphatic drainage. Cell-mediated immunity attacks TB via macrophage ingestion of particles. Delayed hypersensitivity causes caseous necrosis of TB-laden macrophages with local tissue destruction. Healing occurs with resorption of caseous material and accompanying fibrosis. Dystrophic calcification occurs in both primary and postprimary TB but does not necessarily indicate complete sterilization of infection. Endobronchial TB occurs along with pulmonary involvement and is believed to result from infected sputum, spread from adjacent parenchyma, eroded lymph nodes, and/or infected cavities. **Miliary TB** occurs when tubercle bacilli discharge into the bloodstream with distal organ dissemination. This can occur at the primary or postprimary stage. Symptoms of active TB include low-grade fever, anorexia, fatigue, cough, hemoptysis, chest pain, night sweats, and weight loss.

The CXR in primary TB commonly reveals lymph node enlargement (Fig. 5.24), especially involving the right paratracheal and hilar lymph nodes. The prevalence of lymph

> Miliary TB occurs both with primary and postprimary infections.

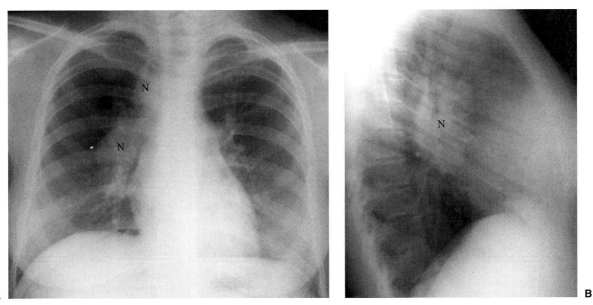

Figure 5.24 Primary tuberculosis. (*A*) Posteroanterior and (*B*) lateral chest radiographs demonstrate right hilar and paratracheal lymph node enlargement (N).

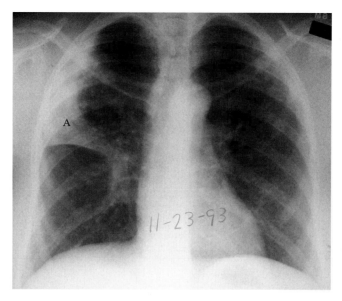

Figure 5.25 Primary tuberculosis. Right upper lobe airspace disease (A).

node enlargement decreases with age, from 40% of young adults to 10% of the elderly. Homogeneous consolidation in a segmental or lobar distribution is the most common parenchymal abnormality (Fig. 5.25). Patchy, linear, or nodular disease occurs less commonly. There is said to be a slight right lung predominance, but no zonal predominance. In contrast to lymph nodes, parenchymal disease increases in frequency with age. The initial site of parenchymal involvement at the time of first infection is known as the Ghon focus. The Ghon focus and enlarged regional lymph node together are known as the Ranke complex. Simon foci are apical nodules, frequently calcified, that result from hematogenous seeding at the time of initial infection. Prevalence of pleural effusion increases with age. Effusion is seen in one-third of adults, often on the side of parenchymal abnormality. Effusions are usually unilateral, with bilaterality in 15% of cases. In 5% effusion is the sole abnormality.

Contrast-enhanced CT may show a characteristic appearance in mediastinal tuberculous lymphadenitis, with central nodal low attenuation (Fig. 5.26) and peripheral

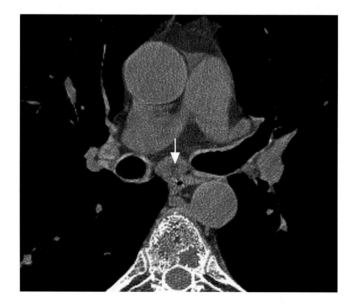

Figure 5.26 Primary tuberculosis. Computed tomography demonstrates low attenuation of a subcarinal lymph node (*arrow*).

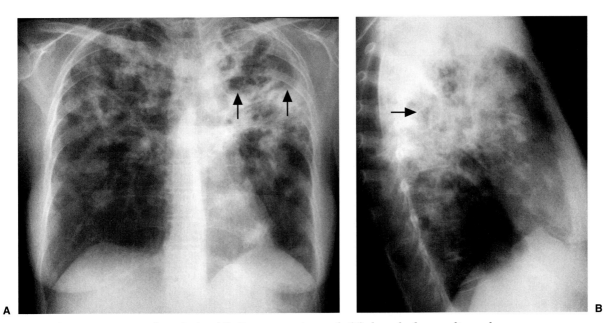

Figure 5.27 Postprimary tuberculosis. *(A)* Posteroanterior and *(B)* lateral chest radiographs demonstrate extensive bilateral upper lobe airspace disease, primarily posteriorly, with areas of cavitation *(arrows).*

enhancement. This appearance also occurs with atypical mycobacterial infections, lymphoma, metastases, and Whipple disease. CT is more sensitive for detection of calcification.

Radiographs in postprimary TB show parenchymal opacities in the apical and posterior segments of the upper lobes (Fig. 5.27) in over 80% and in the superior segments of the lower lobes in 10% to 15%. These opacities are most commonly heterogeneous, and cavitation (Fig. 5.28) is observed in 40% to 45%. Wall thickness is variable, and gas–fluid

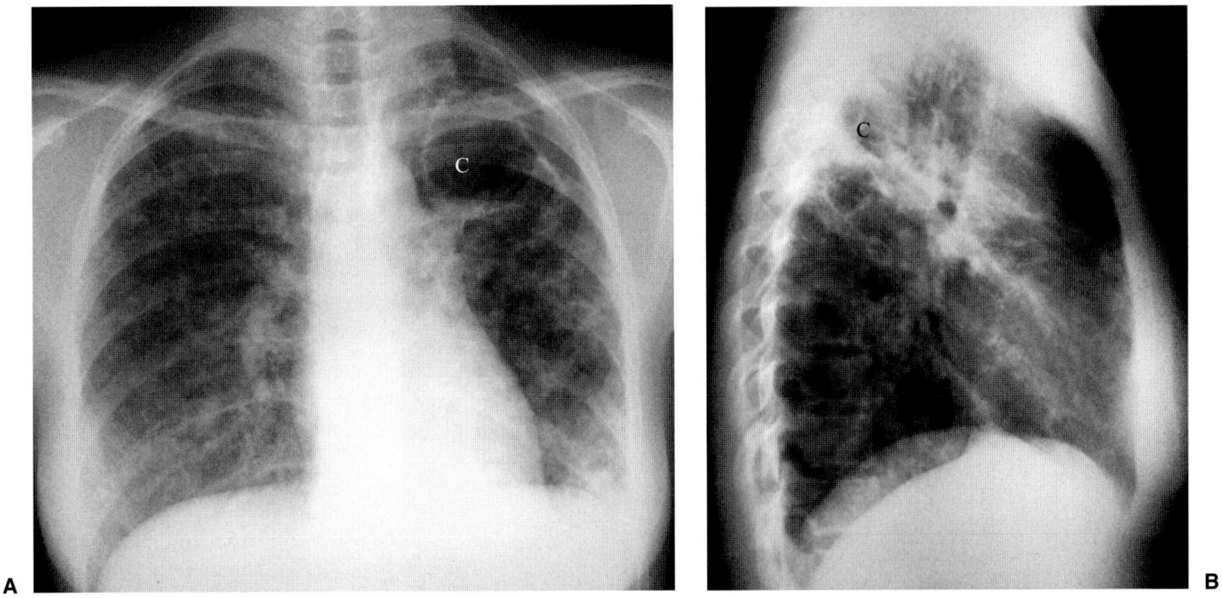

Figure 5.28 Postprimary tuberculosis. *(A)* Posteroanterior and *(B)* lateral chest radiographs demonstrate a large cavity *(C)* in the apicoposterior segment of the left upper lobe.

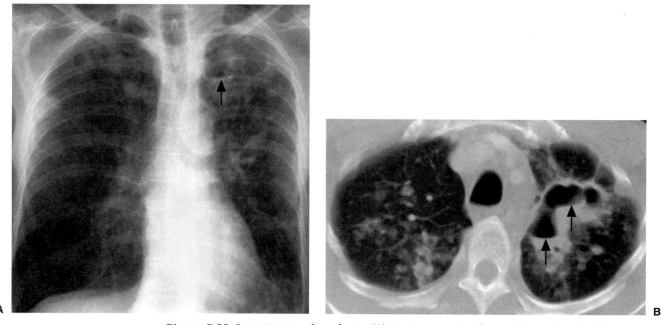

Figure 5.29 Postprimary tuberculosis. *(A)* Posteroanterior chest radiograph and *(B)* computed tomography with left upper lobe gas–fluid levels *(arrows)* and bilateral upper lobe disease.

levels are sometimes seen (Fig. 5.29). Bronchogenic spread may occur with resulting ill-defined nodules, typically involving the lower zones ("upstairs–downstairs" pattern). In 3% to 6% of patients tuberculomas subsequently develop (Fig. 5.30), often with calcification and generally ranging from 0.5 to 4 cm. Lymph node enlargement is uncommon in postprimary TB, seen in only 5%. Pleural effusion is present in 16% to 18% of cases and is usually unilateral. Radiographic evidence of the original primary infection, including calcified lymph nodes and granulomas, is seen in 20% to 40%. Upper lobe fibrotic changes

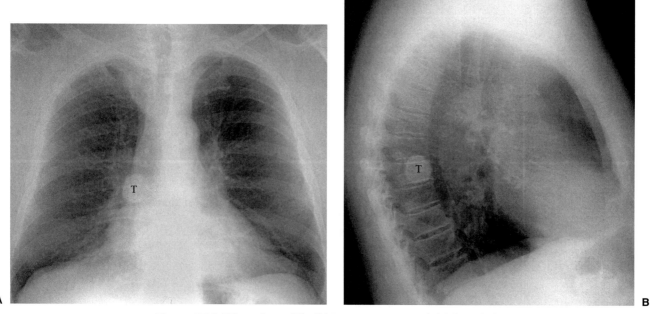

Figure 5.30 Tuberculoma (T). *(A)* Posteroanterior and *(B)* lateral chest radiographs demonstrate a solitary calcified right lower lobe nodule.

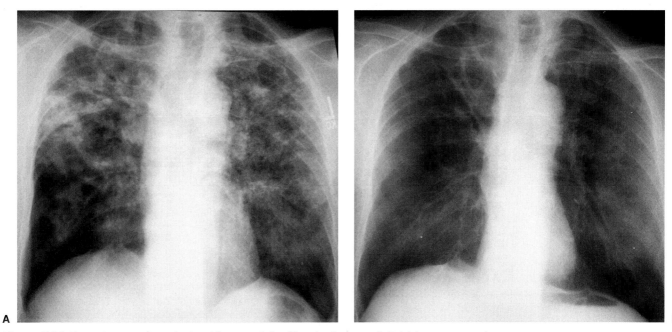

A   B

Figure 5.31 Postprimary tuberculosis with upper lobe fibrotic changes. *A.* Initial posteroanterior chest radiograph: exudative and cavitary upper lobe airspace disease, similar to Fig. 5.27. *B.* Posteroanterior chest radiograph 1 year later: marked resolution of exudative and cavitary disease, with residual linear, retractile abnormality.

(Fig. 5.31) are seen in a similar percentage of patients. Noncalcified miliary nodules are the hallmark of miliary TB (Fig. 5.32).

CT demonstrates internal details of cavities better than CXR. Bronchogenic spread, evidenced by centrilobular nodules and a tree-in-bud pattern (Fig. 5.33), is shown in 95% of cases of postprimary TB. Other findings on CT include lobular airspace disease and

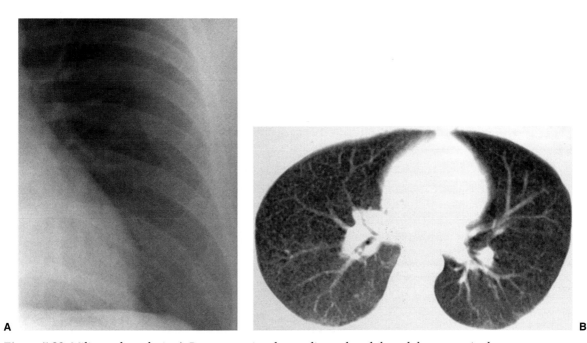

A   B

Figure 5.32 Miliary tuberculosis. *A.* Posteroanterior chest radiograph: subtle nodular pattern in the lower lungs. *B.* Computed tomography: innumerable tiny miliary bilateral nodules.

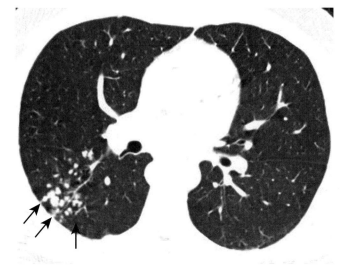

Figure 5.33 Bronchogenic spread of tuberculosis. Computed tomography demonstrates tree-in-bud pattern (*arrows*).

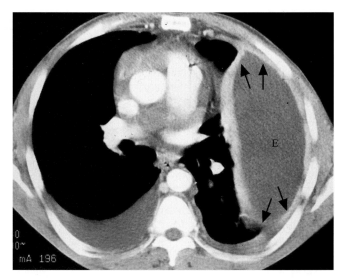

Figure 5.34 Tuberculous empyema (E) with split pleura sign (*arrows*).

interlobular septal thickening. Postprimary tuberculous effusions may show the "split pleura" sign on contrast-enhanced CT (Fig. 5.34). Miliary disease may be seen at high resolution CT before it is apparent on the CXR.

Complications of TB such as bronchiectasis are well demonstrated by CT. Dilated bronchi or cavities may be colonized by aspergillus species, resulting in aspergilloma(s) (Fig. 5.35). Rasmussen aneurysms are pulmonary artery pseudoaneurysms caused by erosion from an adjacent cavity. These are uncommon but may be shown on helical contrast-enhanced CT. Broncholiths occur when calcified lymph nodes erode into or obstruct bronchi (Fig. 5.36). Distal atelectasis and bronchoceles may ensue. A normal CXR cannot

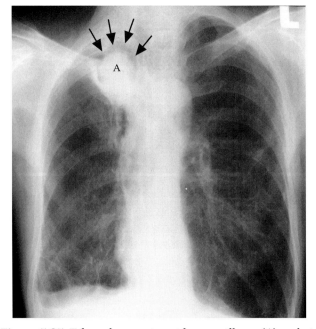

Figure 5.35 Tuberculous cavity with aspergilloma (A) and air crescent sign (*arrows*).

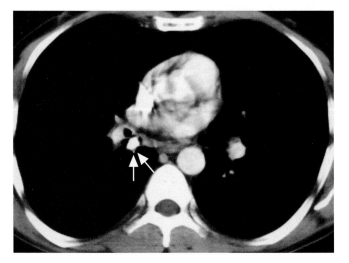

Figure 5.36 Broncholith (*arrows*) in tuberculosis.

exclude TB, nor can imaging studies differentiate active from inactive disease. Stability on follow-up studies generally indicates, but does not prove, inactivity.

NONTUBERCULOUS MYCOBACTERIA

Multiple species of nontuberculous mycobacteria (NTMB) exist. These are ubiquitous organisms that constitute part of the normal environmental flora. They have been isolated from lakes, streams, other natural waters, soil, milk and other foodstuffs, and domestic animals. Unlike TB, NTMB are not acquired by person-to-person spread (31). Rather, they are acquired from the environment by inhalation of aerosolized water droplets. *Mycobacterium avium* intracellulare and *Mycobacterium kansasii* account for the bulk of NTMB pulmonary infections. *M. avium* intracellulare is responsible for 61% of cases of NTMB infections alone. *M. avium* intracellulare is most prevalent in the southeastern United States, whereas *M. kansasii* is most prevalent in the midwestern and southwestern United States. Unlike *M. avium* intracellulare, *M. kansasii* responds favorably to antituberculous therapy. Clinical and radiographic findings in NTMB infections vary widely (32). The findings fall into two main groups, with three other discrete entities.

Classic Form of Infection

This form of infection is seen predominantly in middle-aged white men with predisposing illnesses. These include COPD, previous TB, lung fibrosis, silicosis, and asbestosis. Other risks are smoking, alcoholism, cardiac disease, and chronic liver disease. Symptoms are insidious and include cough (60% to 100%), hemoptysis (15% to 20%), weight loss, and weakness. Fever (10% to 13%) is notably uncommon as it is in all NTMB pulmonary infections. Radiographs reveal fibrotic and nodular opacities indistinguishable from postprimary TB (Fig. 5.37) Cavitation occurs in the majority (80% to 95%), and adjacent pleural thickening is frequent (37% to 56%). Bronchogenic spread to the lower lobes may occur, with patchy and nodular alveolar opacities. Pleural effusion is uncommon (5% to 20%), and enlarged lymph nodes (Fig. 5.38)are even less common (<4%). Bronchopleural fistula may occur.

Nontuberculous mycobacterial infections are often radiologically indistinguishable from postprimary TB.

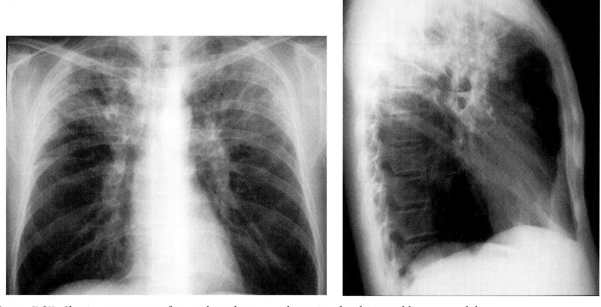

Figure 5.37 Classic appearance of nontuberculous mycobacteria, closely resembling upper lobe postprimary tuberculosis. (*A*) Posteroanterior and (*B*) lateral chest radiographs.

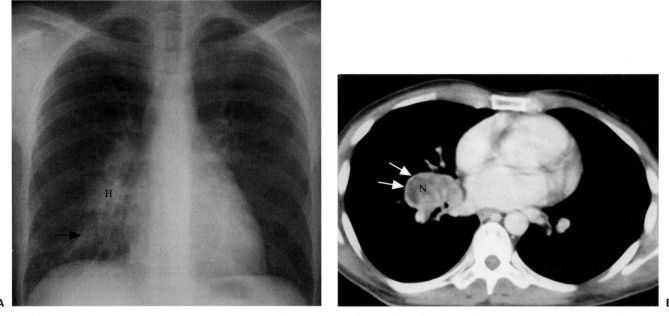

Figure 5.38 Atypical appearance of nontuberculous mycobacteria. *A.* Posteroanterior chest x-ray: large right hilum (H) with adjacent right lower lung airspace disease *(arrow)*. *(B)* Computed tomography: enlarged low attenuation right hilar lymph node (N) with enhancing rim *(arrows)*.

Nonclassic Form of Infection
This accounts for 20% to 30% of NTMB pulmonary infections in immunocompetent adults. Unlike the classic form, it is seen predominantly in elderly white women without predisposing illnesses. Clinical symptoms are similar, with chronic cough and hemoptysis. Fever is rare, and other constitutional symptoms are uncommon.

Radiographically, multiple bilateral nodular and interstitial opacities are randomly distributed. Bronchiectasis is sometimes seen. CT demonstrates linear opacities and clusters of opaque nodules predominantly in the lower zones, particularly in the lingula and middle lobe. Bronchiectasis is predominantly seen in the lingula and middle lobe. Volume loss is occasionally present. The high attenuation nodules likely represent peribronchial granulomas or mucous plugs in small airways. Branching centrilobular opacities (tree-in-bud) can be seen on high resolution CT. Patchy airspace disease or ground glass opacities may also be seen. Pleural thickening may develop adjacent to areas of bronchiectasis. Mediastinal lymph node enlargement is occasionally present.

Asymptomatic Nodules
Solitary or multiple granulomas may occur, as in granulomatous infections such as TB and histoplasmosis. When multiple, they may be in clusters. This helps to differentiate them from metastases, which usually have a more random distribution. Patients are usually asymptomatic and stability is shown on follow-up radiographic studies.

Achalasia Patients
The mechanism of infection in these patients is thought to be chronic aspiration. *M. fortuitum-chelonei* complex is almost always implicated. Radiographically, patchy alveolar airspace opacities are seen with a basal distribution, resembling aspiration pneumonia.

Immunocompromised Patients
The features of NTMB infection in patients with acquired immunodeficiency syndrome are discussed in Chapter 6.

Table 5.1: Summary of Radiographic Features in Fungal Infections

Lymph node enlargement—CO,H,N
Calcification—CO, H
Cavitation—A, B, CO, H, N, Z
Pleural disease—A, B, CO, N
CNS involvement—B, CO, CR, N, Z
Skin lesions—B, CO, CR, N

A, actinomycosis; B, blastomycosis; CNS, central nervous system; CO, coccidioidomycosis; CR, cryptococcosis; H, histoplasmosis; N, nocardiosis; Z, zygomycosis.

FUNGAL INFECTIONS

Table 5.1 lists the various radiographic features of fungal infections.

HISTOPLASMA

Histoplasmosis is a common granulomatous infection in parts of the United States (33). *Histoplasma capsulatum* is a fungus that exists as a mold in the soil. Soil rich in bird droppings encourages growth of this organism. Birds do not harbor the organism, but mammals such as bats may. Infection is acquired by inhalation of windborne spores blown from sources such as bird roosts or bat haunts. It is epidemic in the central United States in a triangular area extending from Ohio to Nebraska to Louisiana and encompassing the Mississippi, Missouri, and Ohio River valleys. Virtually all inhabitants of this area will acquire the infection.

Most infections are asymptomatic, with clinical pneumonia occurring in those exposed to a large number of infecting spores. Illness is mild with cough, fever, headache, and chest pain. At body temperature, inhaled spores germinate into yeast forms that are phagocytized by macrophages. The yeasts multiply in the macrophages, resulting in bronchopneumonia with granulomatous inflammation. The parasitized macrophages migrate to regional nodes and disseminate hematogenously to the reticuloendothelial system, especially the spleen. Within 1 to 2 weeks hypersensitivity develops with involution, encapsulation, and eventual calcification. Immunity to histoplasmosis is gradually lost over the next few years. However, in endemic areas the infection will be acquired again and again during a life span.

In symptomatic patients, radiographs demonstrate bilateral extensive nonsegmental areas of lobular airspace disease (Fig. 5.39). Hilar lymph node enlargement may also be

Virtually all inhabitants of the triangular region from Ohio to Nebraska to Louisiana will be infected by *Histoplasma capsulatum*.

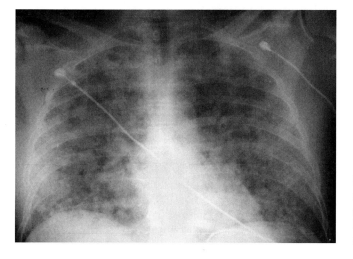

Figure 5.39 Acute histoplasmosis. Extensive bilateral airspace disease resulting from a large inhaled inoculum during caving.

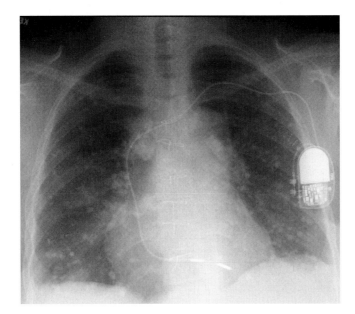

Figure 5.40 Histoplasmosis. Numerous small calcified lung nodules.

seen. After the findings resolve there are generally pulmonary and hilar calcifications (Fig. 5.40). Calcifications tend to be larger and more numerous than in TB.

Disseminated disease is rare and usually occurs in immunocompromised individuals. The very young and elderly are at increased risk for disseminated disease. This ranges from an acute rapidly fatal infection to a chronic intermittent illness. Radiographs are often normal. Multiple diffuse small nodular opacities are the most common abnormality (Fig. 5.41). Limited or diffuse linear or irregular opacities also occur. Airspace disease is less commonly seen.

Chronic histoplasmosis is rare and usually occurs in middle-aged white men. Disease is self-limiting and nonfatal. Most patients have a history of cigarette smoking and emphysema. Symptoms are similar to postprimary TB with malaise, cough, and night sweats. Like TB the apical and posterior segments of the upper lobes are most commonly affected (Fig. 5.42). However, true cavitation rarely occurs. Infection begins adjacent to blebs and bullae with lucencies due to emphysematous spaces in an area of disease. Lymph node

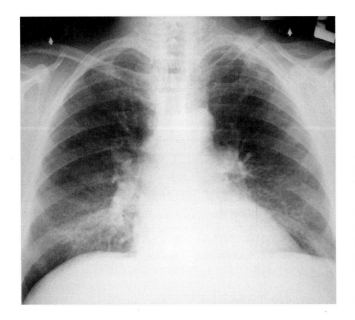

Figure 5.41 Miliary histoplasmosis. Miliary nodules are best visualized in the lower lungs. They were new from a chest x-ray 2 months earlier and resolved without therapy 4 months later. At that time, the patient died of Addison disease, and autopsy confirmed disseminated histoplasmosis as the cause.

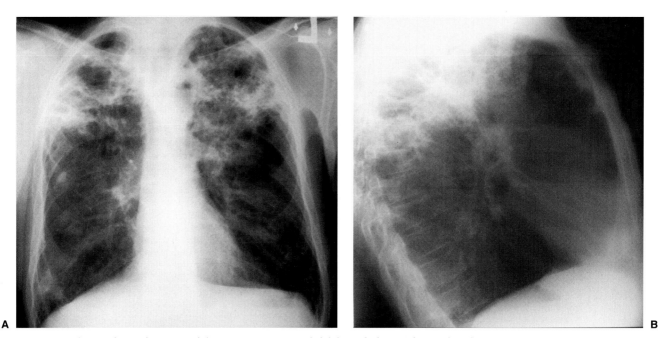

Figure 5.42 Chronic histoplasmosis. *(A)* Posteroanterior and *(B)* lateral chest radiographs: abnormality indistinguishable from postprimary tuberculosis and classic nontuberculous mycobacteria.

enlargement does not occur. Bronchogenic spread of cavitary contents from the upper lobes may occur, resulting in airspace disease in the lower lobes.

Delayed manifestations of histoplasmosis occur in a small number of patients for unknown reasons. These include histoplasmomas, broncholithiasis, and fibrosing mediastinitis.

In some individuals the calcified nodule of previous histoplasmosis continues to enlarge, termed a histoplasmoma. These are most common in the posterior lower lobes, peripheral and adjacent to the pleura. Growth is slow, with diameter increases of 0.5 to 3 mm per year (Fig. 5.43). Laminated calcific rings occur, with lack of peripheral calcifica-

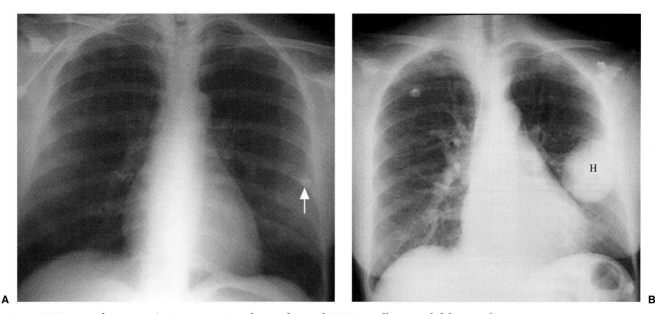

Figure 5.43 Histoplasmoma. *A.* Posteroanterior chest radiograph 1975: small opaque left lung nodule *(arrow)*. *B.* Posteroanterior chest radiograph 1984: same nodule (H) has enlarged considerably.

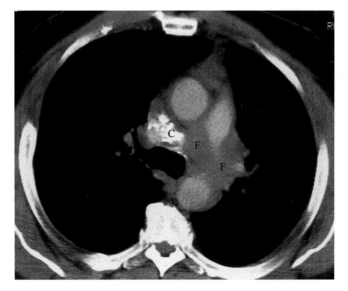

Figure 5.44 Fibrosing mediastinitis. Computed tomography reveals calcified lymph nodes (C) and noncalcified infiltrating soft tissue (F).

tion indicating further growth potential. In 20% of cases, histoplasmomas are associated with fibrosing mediastinitis.

Broncholithiasis occurs when peribronchial calcific nodal disease produces bronchial obstruction. A calcified node may erode into the bronchus and directly obstruct it, or associated inflammation may cause obstruction. Clinically, hemoptysis, fever, chills, and productive cough occur. Broncholiths are more common on the right because of airway anatomy and lymph node distribution. Distal atelectasis, air trapping, and mucus-filled bronchi may occur. Calcified nodes will be seen on radiographs, with atelectasis and dilated branching structures representing fluid-filled bronchi. Chest CT may show the relationship between the calcified lymph node and the dilated bronchus. Bronchiectasis may also be shown.

Fibrosing mediastinitis occurs when nonmalignant fibrous tissue encroaches on and obliterates vasculature and airways of the mediastinum. This process may be focal or generalized, with the former more common. Pathogenesis is unknown. Pathologically, enlarged lymph nodes surrounded by a fibrous capsule are found. Subcarinal and right paratracheal nodes are most commonly involved. Bilateral extension from the subcarinal region carries the worst prognosis. Radiographs show a widened mediastinum from fibrosis or enlarged collateral veins, with lung opacities due to atelectasis or infarcts. Calcification of nodes is usual at CT (Fig. 5.44). The nodes also demonstrate septa that enhance with contrast, separated by low attenuation areas.

COCCIDIOIDES IMMITIS

This infection is endemic to the southwestern United States, including southern California, Arizona, New Mexico, southern Utah and Nevada, and western Texas. Thousands of military personnel and their families as well as millions of tourists are exposed to the disease annually. Coccidioidomycosis is acquired by inhalation of arthrospores. The primary target for infection is the lung, and in about 60% of cases the patient is asymptomatic. Symptoms include fever, malaise, substernal or pleuritic chest pain, and cough. Skin rashes occur in two-thirds, including toxic erythema, erythema nodosum, and erythema multiforme.

Chest radiographs may be normal. The most common abnormal radiographic finding is segmental airspace disease (Fig. 5.45) extending out from the hilum (34). This is indistinguishable from other atypical or viral pneumonias. Progression of acute findings to a nodule may be seen over an extended time period. Nodules are usually noncalcified (Fig. 5.46). Hilar lymph node enlargement (Fig. 5.47) is found in 20%, with small unilateral

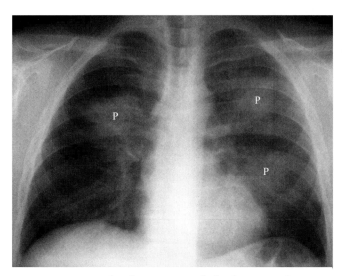

Figure 5.45 Coccidioidomycosis. Multifocal segmental airspace disease, extending out from the hila (P).

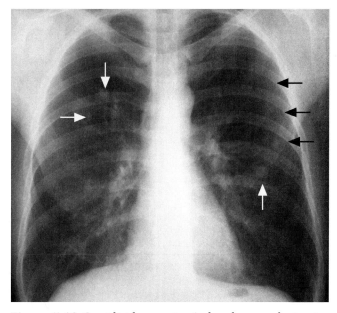

Figure 5.46 Coccidioidomycosis. Archaeology graduate student returned to the University of Michigan from a summer excavation in Arizona with multiple bilateral nodules (*arrows*).

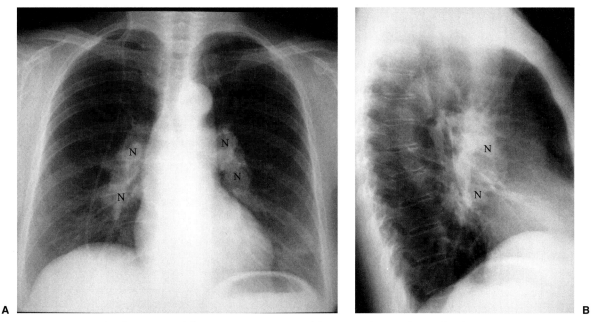

A

B

Figure 5.47 Coccidioidomycosis. (A) Posteroanterior and (B) lateral chest radiographs demonstrate bilateral hilar lymph node enlargement (N).

pleural effusions also seen in 20%. Cavitation is seen in 15%, with thin-walled cavities slightly more common than thick-walled ones.

ASPERGILLUS

Aspergillosis results in a spectrum of disease dependent on the virulence and number of organisms and the patient's immune and pulmonary status (35). Aspergillosis is caused by a ubiquitous soil fungus, usually *Aspergillus fumigatus*.

Noninvasive aspergillosis occurs when *Aspergillus* colonizes a preexisting cavity without tissue invasion (Figs. 5.35 and 5.48). Intertwined fungal hyphae mixed with mucus and cellular debris form an aspergilloma or fungus ball. Predisposing causes include TB and sarcoidosis as well as bronchogenic cysts, sequestrations, and pneumatoceles. Patients are usually asymptomatic, with hemoptysis being the most common symptom. Life-threatening hemoptysis is an indication for surgical resection or bronchial artery embolization.

A solid round or oval mass is seen at radiography (35,36). An air crescent is usually visible between the aspergilloma and wall of the cavity. Aspergillomas are usually single. CT shows the relatively high attenuation aspergilloma within the cavity. Change in position of the aspergilloma is usually seen with change in patient position.

Semiinvasive aspergillosis occurs in subjects debilitated by chronic illness, diabetes, malnutrition, alcoholism, advanced age, corticosteroids, or COPD. Clinical symptoms include chronic cough, sputum production, fever, and hemoptysis. The radiographic presentation is unilateral or bilateral segmental airspace disease with or without cavitation and adjacent pleural thickening (35,36). Pleural thickening may be the earliest sign of infection. Multiple nodules may also be seen.

Invasive aspergillosis occurs most commonly in immunocompromised patients and is discussed in Chapter 6.

Allergic bronchopulmonary aspergillosis occurs in patients with longstanding asthma (35). It is an allergic response to inhaled spores, with types I and III hypersensitivity reactions. *Aspergillus* organisms proliferate in the airway lumen, providing a supply of antigen. Immediate hypersensitivity reaction mediated by IgE occurs. IgG is also produced, and antigen–antibody immune complexes are deposited in the bronchial mucosa. Bronchial wall necrosis and dilation occur with eosinophilic infiltrates. Excess mucous production and abnormal ciliary function lead to mucous impaction. Expectoration of mucous plugs containing aspergillus organisms and eosinophils occurs. Symptoms include wheeze, cough, sputum production, chest pain, and low-grade fever.

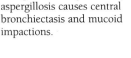

Allergic bronchopulmonary aspergillosis causes central bronchiectasis and mucoid impactions.

Radiographically, the characteristic appearance is of central mucoid impactions with tubular often branching structures in a bronchial distribution ("finger-in-glove" appearance) (Fig. 5.49). These represent bronchi plugged with mucus, organisms, and eosinophils. Lobar or segmental atelectasis may be seen. Central bronchiectasis is usually

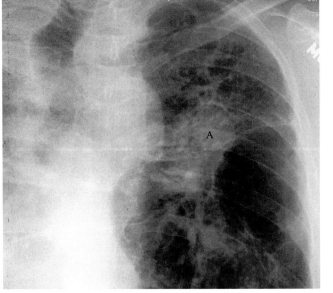

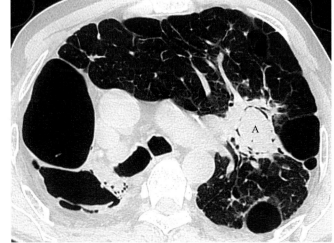

Figure 5.48 Aspergilloma (A) in a preexisting cavity on (A) chest radiograph and (B) computed tomography.

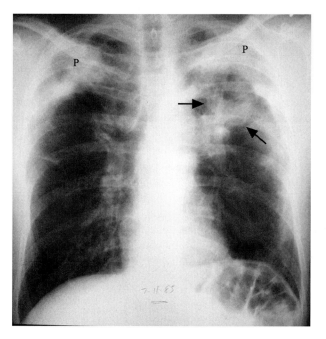

Figure 5.49 Allergic bronchopulmonary aspergillosis. Finger-in-glove appearance of mucoid impactions (*arrows*) and peripheral airspace disease from eosinophilic pneumonia (P).

present from previously expectorated mucous plugs. Patchy peripheral consolidations may be seen if there is concurrent eosinophilic pneumonia (Fig. 5.49). CT demonstrates dilated mucous-filled bronchi, often with high attenuation or calcified contents. Upper lobe central bronchiectasis is also well shown.

VIRAL INFECTIONS

INFLUENZA

Influenza A virus still causes significant morbidity and mortality despite major efforts at prevention and treatment (37,38). Although only a small percentage of infected patients develop pneumonia, those who do have a mortality rate of about 30%. Pneumonia occurs more commonly in the elderly and in those with chronic pulmonary disease. Comorbid illnesses such as diabetes, renal disease, heart disease, and immunosuppression are common. Dyspnea occurs along with the well-known influenza symptoms of fever, chills, myalgias, and cough. Superimposed bacterial infections occur in up to 50%, with *S. pneumoniae* and *S. aureus* most commonly isolated. Radiographs generally show bilateral diffuse alveolar (Fig. 5.50) or interstitial opacities. Lobar disease also occurs.

RUBEOLA (MEASLES)

Measles is rare in adulthood, and pneumonia is even rarer. Lymph node enlargement occurs before appearance of the rash and regresses shortly after. Pulmonary disease appears at the same time or just before the skin rash and regresses more slowly. Giant cell pneumonia with degeneration and hyperplasia of endothelial cells lining bronchi and bronchioles occurs.

CXR shows increased interstitial opacities with lower lobe predominance (39,40). Marked mediastinal and hilar lymph node enlargement occurs in over two-thirds of cases. Pleural effusions are seen in one-third.

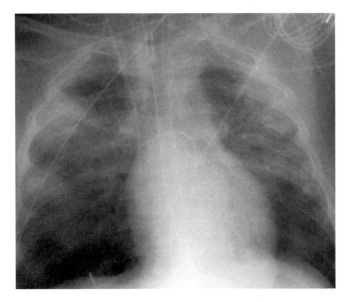

Figure 5.50 Influenza pneumonia. Diffuse bilateral airspace disease.

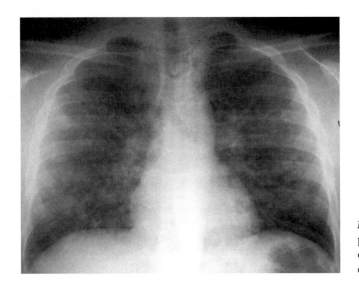

Figure 5.51 Chickenpox pneumonia. Typical appearance of widespread bilateral ill-defined nodules.

VARICELLA-ZOSTER

Pneumonia due to varicella infection in children is rare. In contrast, 10% to 30% of adults infected with chickenpox develop varicella-zoster interstitial pneumonitis. Affected patients are usually very ill, with dyspnea and cough. Diffuse, ill-defined, nodular, airspace opacities (Fig. 5.51) occur throughout the lungs (41). With coalescence, patchy segmental disease is seen. Pleural effusions and lymph node enlargement are not generally demonstrated. Clearing is slow, taking several months. Tiny punctate calcifications may develop in some patients.

PARASITIC INFECTIONS

ECHINOCOCCUS (HYDATID)

This parasitic infection is caused by the larval stage of the tapeworm *Echinococcus*. There are two main forms of disease, the most common being cystic unilocular disease caused by *Echinococcus granulosis.* This organism is widespread throughout the world and prevalent in most sheep- and cattle-raising countries. The parasitic life cycle involves two hosts, the definitive host (a canine, usually a dog) and an intermediate host (usually a grazing animal such as sheep or cattle). The mature adult tapeworm lives in the intestine of the definitive host. Ova are laid and pass to pastures where the intermediate hosts graze. This is the step where humans may be accidentally infected. After ova are ingested, digestive enzymes dissolve the coat, freeing the embryo, which burrows through the duodenal mucosa to enter veins and lymphatics. Most embryos are filtered by the liver, the lungs filter some of the remainder, and a small proportion reach distant organs.

If the host tissues do not destroy the embryos, they transform into tiny cysts. Most (65% to 75%) occur in the liver, with 10% to 25% in the lungs and 10% to 15% in other body tissues. In the thorax, most cysts are intrapulmonary, with only 2% to 5% occurring in the mediastinum, pleura, or diaphragm. Hydatid cysts have three "layers." The outer pericyst is composed of vascularized connective tissue formed by the host's response. The ectocyst is the laminated outer layer of the parasite. The innermost layer is the endocyst, consisting of germinating membrane from which daughter cysts and cyst fluid arise.

Most patients are asymptomatic, with incidental discovery of lesions. If cysts rupture, there is abrupt onset of cough, fever, expectoration, and acute hypersensitivity. Occasionally, anaphylaxis occurs. With rupture, viable scolices may be discharged into the peritoneum, mesentery, lung parenchyma, pleura, liver, and/or spleen, causing secondary hydatidosis.

Growth rate of hydatid cysts varies, with sizes more than 20 cm reported. In 60% they are solitary, and in 40% multiple. The lower lobes and posterior lungs are the most frequent sites. In 20% of patients, cysts are bilateral. Calcification of lung cysts is very rare.

Radiographs of an intact "simple" cyst demonstrate a smooth, homogeneous, round or oval well-demarcated nodule or mass (42) (Fig. 5.52). On contrast-enhanced CT and magnetic resonance imaging, the pericyst may enhance. If infarction, hemorrhage, or infection occurs, the clear demarcation with adjacent parenchyma is lost and the hydatid cyst may simulate pneumonia or carcinoma. In these cases a dense or hyperintense halo is

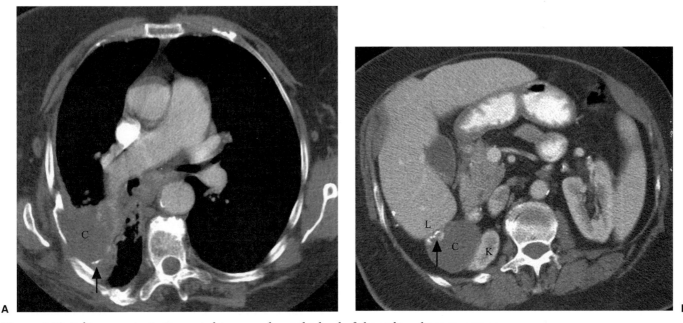

A   B

Figure 5.52 *Echinococcosis. A.* Computed tomography at the level of the right pulmonary artery: cyst (C) apparently involving right lower lobe and pleura, with calcification *(arrow). B.* Computed tomography of upper abdomen: additional cyst (C) between tip of liver (L) and right kidney (K), also calcified *(arrow).*

seen on CT and magnetic resonance imaging, representing surrounding inflammatory change (43).

If air enters a cyst after invasion of an airway, a lucent "air crescent" occurs between the pericyst and ectocyst (42). This is a sign of impending cyst rupture. As more air enters a cyst, the parasite shrinks and ruptures with expulsion of cyst contents and entry of air between ectocyst and endocyst. Two air crescents may then be visible with the ectocyst in between, known as the Cumbo sign. CT shows small air lucencies to advantage.

With further collapse, the endocyst membrane may be seen floating on top of any remaining fluid, simulating a water lily (the Camalote sign) (42). On CT and magnetic resonance imaging, the crumpled membranes are seen as curvilinear structures within the pericyst wall, variously called the "serpent sign," "spin sign," or "whirl sign" (43).

REFERENCES

1. Mandell LA. Community-acquired pneumonia: etiology, epidemiology and treatment. *Chest* 1995;108:35S–42S.
2. Armstrong P, Wilson AG, Dee P, et al. *Imaging of diseases of the chest.* St. Louis: Mosby, 2000: 163–253.
3. Katz DS, Leung AN. Radiology of pneumonia. *Clin Chest Med* 1999;20:549–562.
4. Franquet T. Imaging of pneumonia: trends and algorithms. *Eur Respir J* 2001;18:196–208.
5. Tanaka N, Matsumoto T, Kutamitsu, et al. High resolution CT findings in community acquired pneumonia. *J Comput Assist Tomogr* 1996;20:600–608.
6. Tomiyama N, Müller NL, Johkoh T, et al. Acute parenchymal lung disease in immunocompetent patients: diagnostic accuracy of high resolution CT. *AJR Am J Roentgenol* 2000;174:1745–1750.
7. Genereux GP, Stilwell GA. The acute bacterial pneumonias. *Semin Roentgenol* 1980: 15:9–16.
8. Berkmen YM. Uncommon acute bacterial pneumonias. *Semin Roentgenol* 1980;15:17–24.
9. MacFarlane JT, Miller AC, Roderick Smith WH, et al. Comparative radiographic features of community acquired legionnaires disease, pneumococcal pneumonia, mycoplasma pneumonia, and psittacosis. *Thorax* 1984;39:28–33.
10. Kantor HG. The many radiologic facies of pneumococcal pneumonia. *AJR Am J Roentgenol* 1981; 137:1213–1220.
11. Musher DM, Franco M. Staphylococcal pneumonia. *Chest* 1981;79:172–173.
12. Naraqi S, McDonnell G. Hematogenous staphylococcal pneumonia secondary to soft tissue infection. *Chest* 1981;79:173–175.
13. Macfarlane J, Rose D. Radiographic features of staphylococcal pneumonia in adults and children. *Thorax* 1996;51:539–540.
14. Shafazand S, Doyle R, Ruoss S, et al. Inhalational anthrax: epidemiology, diagnosis and management. *Chest* 1999;116:1369–1376.
15. Penn C, Klotz SA. Anthrax pneumonia. *Semin Respir Infect* 1997;12:28–30.
16. Earls JP, Cerva D, Berman E, et al. Inhalational anthrax after bioterrorism exposure: spectrum of imaging findings in two surviving patients. *Radiology* 2002;222:305–312.
17. Ritvo M, Martin F. The clinical and roentgen manifestations of pneumonia due to bacillus mucosus capsulatus (primary Friedlander pneumonia). *AJR Am J Roentgenol* 1949;62:211–225.
18. Holmes RB. Friedländer's pneumonia. *Radiology* 1956;75:728–743.
19. Moon WK, Im JG, Yeon M, et al. Complications of *Klebsiella* pneumonia: CT evaluation. *J Comput Assist Tomogr* 1995;19:176–181.
20. Lipchik RJ, Kuzo RS. Nosocomial pneumonia. *Radiol Clin North Am* 1996;34:47–57.
21. Winer-Muram HT, Jennings SG, Wunderink RG, et al. Ventilator-associated *Pseudomonas aeruginosa* pneumonia: radiographic findings. *Radiology* 1995;195:247–252.
22. Shah RM, Wechsler R, Salazar AM, et al. Spectrum of CT findings in nosocomial *Pseudomonas aeruginosa* pneumonia. *J Thorac Imag* 2002;17:53–57.
23. Tan MJ, Tan JS, Hamor RH, et al. The radiologic manifestations of Legionnaires disease. *Chest* 2000;116:398–403.
24. Franquet T, Gimenez A, Roson N, et al. Aspiration diseases: findings, pitfalls, and differential diagnosis. *Radiographics* 2000;20:673–685.
25. Kwong S, Muller NL, Goodwin JD, et al. Thoracic actinomycosis: CT findings in eight patients. *Radiology* 1992;183:189–192.

26. Marrie TJ. Pneumonia caused by *Nocardia* species. *Semin Respir Infect* 1994;9:207–213.
27. McConnell CT, Plouffe JF, File TM, et al. Radiographic appearance of *Chlamydia pneumoniae* (TWAR strain) respiratory infections. *Radiology* 1994;192:819–824.
28. Cameron DC, Borthwick RN, Philp T. The radiographic patterns of acute *Mycoplasma* pneumonitis. *Clin Radiol* 1977;28:173–180.
29. Reittner P, Muller NL, Heyneman L, et al. *Mycoplasma pneumoniae* pneumonia: radiographic and high-resolution CT features in 28 patients. *AJR Am J Roentgenol* 2000;174:37–41.
30. Leung AN. Pulmonary tuberculosis: the essentials. *Radiology* 1999;210:307–322.
31. Miller WT. Spectrum of pulmonary nontuberculous mycobacterial infection. *Radiology* 1994; 191:343–350.
32. Rosenzweig DY. Nontuberculous mycobacterial disease in the immunocompetent adult. *Semin Respir Infect* 1996;11:252–261.
33. Gurney JW, Conces DJ. Pulmonary histoplasmosis. *Radiology* 1996;199:297–306.
34. Greendyke WH, Resnick DL, Harvey WC. The varied roentgen manifestations of primary coccidioidomycosis. *AJR Am J Roentgenol* 1970;109:491–499.
35. Franquet T, Muller NL, Gimenez A, et al. Spectrum of pulmonary aspergillosis: histologic, clinical, and radiologic findings. *Radiographics* 2001;21:825–837.
36. Aquino SL, Kee ST, Warnock ML, et al. Pulmonary aspergillosis: imaging findings with pathologic correlation. *AJR Am J Roentgenol* 1994;163:811–815.
37. Olivera EC, Marik PE, Colice G. Influenza pneumonia. A descriptive study. *Chest* 2001;119: 1717–1723.
38. Janower ML, Weiss EB. Mycoplasmal, viral and rickettsial pneumonias. *Semin Roentgenol* 1980; 15:25–32.
39. Quinn JL. Measles pneumonia in an adult. *AJR Am J Roentgenol* 1964;91:560–563.
40. Margolin FR, Gandy TK. Pneumonia of atypical measles. *Radiology* 1978;131:653–655.
41. Sargent EN, Carson MJ, Reilly ED. Roentgenographic manifestations of varicella pneumonia with postmortem correlation. *AJR Am J Roentgenol* 1966;98:305–317.
42. Balikian JP, Mudarris FF. Hydatid disease of the lungs. A roentgenologic study of 50 cases. *AJR Am J Roentgenol* 1974;122:692–706.
43. Von Sinner WN. New diagnostic signs in hydatid disease: radiography, ultrasound, CT and MRI correlated to pathology. *Eur J Radiol* 1991;12:150–159.

INFEC

IMMU

HOST

Immunocompromis
humoral, and are pr
an important catego
all human immuno
tory illness over the
other forms of imn
plant recipients (2)

The radiologist
infections. This inc
(CXR), generating ;
sion, response to tre
evaluation with co
needed and should
choscopy, open lun
related to acquired
compromise are the

PULMONAR
IMMUNODE

APPROACH

HIV-infected patien
tors are crucial in m
immune status and
(Table 6.1). For exa

Table 6.1. CD4 Counts in AIDS—Correlation with Associated Diseases

Disease	CD4 Count (cells/mm³)	Demographic Data
Bacterial infection		
Bacterial pneumonia	Any	i.v. drug users—*S. aureus, S. epidermidis,* gram negatives
Nocardia	<200	
M. tuberculosis	Any	PPD+, i.v. drug users, African Americans, exposure to *Mycobacteria*
	<350	Reactivation of dormant bacteria; similar appearance to reactivation TB in immunocompetent hosts
	<200	Similar appearance to primary TB in immunocompetent hosts
MAC	<50	
Fungal infection		
Histoplasma	<100	Endemic area
Aspergillus	<50	
PCP	<200	
CMV	<20	Infection with HIV through sexual contact
Neoplasms		
Kaposi sarcoma	<200	Male homosexual/bisexual
Lymphoma	<200	
Lung cancer	Any	Smoker, male

PPD+, tuberculin purified protein derivation; MAC, mycobacterium arium complex; TB, tuberculosis; PCP, pneumocystis carinii pneumonia; CMV, cytomegalovirus; HIV, human immunodeficiency virus.

with CD4 counts under 20 cells/mm³, whereas *Nocardia* pneumonia and Kaposi sarcoma are encountered when the count is less than 200 cells/mm³ (4).

Patient demographics also help to determine likely pulmonary manifestations (Table 6.1). Intravenous drug abusers are more likely to suffer infections such as *Staphylococcus aureus* pneumonia, septic emboli, and tuberculosis (5), whereas CMV infections are more frequent in patients infected by HIV through sexual contact (6).

Prophylactic antimicrobial therapy decreases the likelihood of infection with drug-susceptible organisms (4) but may delay diagnosis by interfering with blood and sputum culture results (7). Integration of the radiographic appearance with demographic data, laboratory results, and clinical presentation is necessary to reach a reasonable differential diagnosis (8).

BACTERIAL INFECTIONS

AIDS patients have altered B-cell function and are therefore susceptible to severe infections by encapsulated bacteria, such as *Streptococcus pneumoniae* and *Hemophilus influenza*, with any CD4 count (9). As the CD4 count falls, the susceptibility to bacterial infection increases (10). The introduction of *Pneumocystis carinii* pneumonia (PCP) prophylaxis has increased the incidence of bacterial pneumonia relative to that of PCP (10). Intravenous drug abusers are at greater risk to develop *S. aureus* pneumonia, septic emboli, and empyema (5).

Bacterial pneumonia typically presents with segmental or lobar airspace disease. In patients with AIDS there is a higher incidence of multilobar pneumonia (4) and of rapid progression and cavitation (7) (Fig. 6.1) than in non-immunocompromised hosts. Pyogenic airway disease with bronchitis, bronchiolitis, and bronchiectasis is common in HIV-

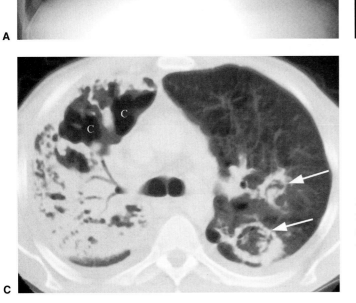

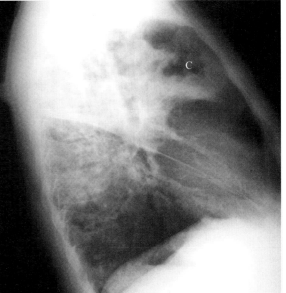

Figure 6.1 Cavitary *Nocardia* pneumonia in acquired immunodeficiency syndrome (AIDS). *(A)* Posteroanterior and *(B)* lateral chest radiographs: multifocal airspace disease with cavitation (C). *C.* Computed tomography 11 days later: extensive right upper lobe pneumonia with cavitation (C). Cavitary disease also present in the left upper lobe *(arrows)*. (Courtesy of Dr. Rosita Shah, Philadelphia, Pennsylvania.)

infected patients with normal CD4 counts. The radiographic findings are subtle and include bronchial wall thickening on the CXR and tree-in-bud opacities, bronchiectasis, bronchial wall thickening, and mucoid impactions on HRCT (11).

MYCOBACTERIAL INFECTIONS

Tuberculosis

The estimated infection rate with *Mycobacterium tuberculosis* among HIV-infected patients is 5%. The rate is higher among specific groups such as Latinos, African Americans, and intravenous drug abusers (12). Because tuberculosis is a highly contagious and treatable disease, it needs to be recognized promptly (13).

The clinical presentation and radiographic appearance are influenced by immune status and CD4 level. With CD4 counts below 350 cells/mm^3, reactivation of dormant *M. tuberculosis* may occur (8). Findings will be similar to reactivation tuberculosis in immune competent hosts, with upper lobe predominant exudative and cavitary disease. Pleural effusions in AIDS patients are more prevalent and tend to be bigger, with a higher inoculum of bacteria (14). When the CD4 counts drop below 200 cells/mm^3, the

A typical finding of tuberculosis in AIDS patients is low attenuation lymph nodes with enhancing rims.

radiographic appearance is more like primary tuberculosis, with randomly distributed focal airspace disease, diffuse infiltrates, miliary nodules, and/or multiple pulmonary nodules. Cavitation is rare in this setting (15). Bulky hilar and mediastinal lymph node enlargement are typical in HIV patients (Fig. 6.2), unlike in non-AIDS patients. On enhanced CTs lymph nodes may demonstrate low attenuation centers with enhancing rims (16) (Fig. 6.3).

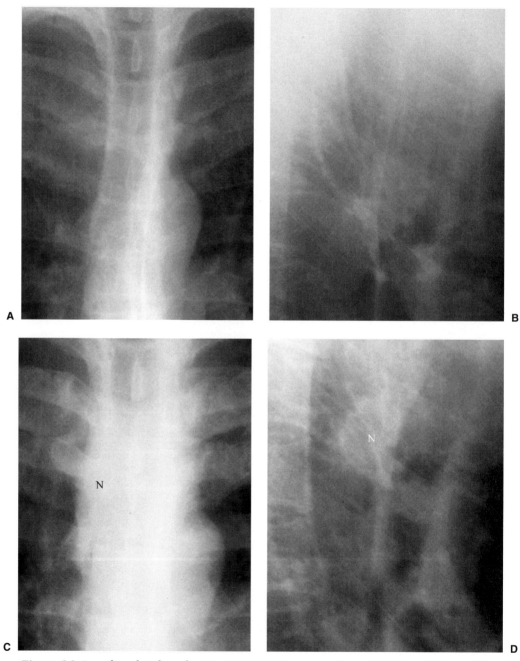

Figure 6.2 Lymph node tuberculosis in AIDS. (*A*) Posteroanterior and (*B*) lateral chest radiograph 11-84: normal. (*C*) Posteroanterior and (*D*) lateral chest radiograph 5-85: interval development of mediastinal lymph node enlargement (N). (Courtesy of Dr. David Spizarny, Detroit, Michigan.)

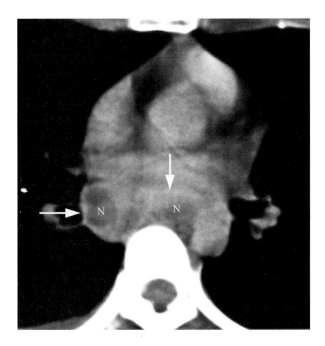

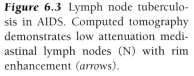

Figure 6.3 Lymph node tuberculosis in AIDS. Computed tomography demonstrates low attenuation mediastinal lymph nodes (N) with rim enhancement (*arrows*).

Atypical Mycobacteria

Mycobacterium avium complex infection occurs in severely immunocompromised patients, with CD4 counts less than 50 cells/mm³. Disease is disseminated throughout the reticuloendothelial system and may involve the lungs as well. Disease tends to be subacute, with constitutional symptoms (4). The radiographic appearance ranges from a normal CXR to large pulmonary nodules that may cavitate, often with lymph node enlargement (17,18). On HRCT there is a tendency for bilateral lower lobe distribution and ground glass opacities (GGOs) (19). Other forms of atypical mycobacteria are rare (Fig. 6.4).

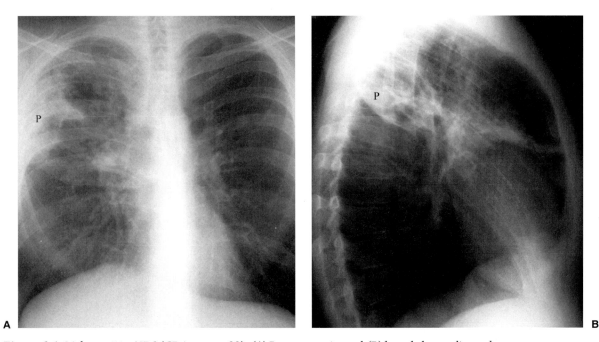

Figure 6.4 *M. kansasii* in AIDS (CD4 count = 23). (*A*) Posteroanterior and (*B*) lateral chest radiograph: cavitary upper lobe pneumonia (P), especially involving the right upper lobe.

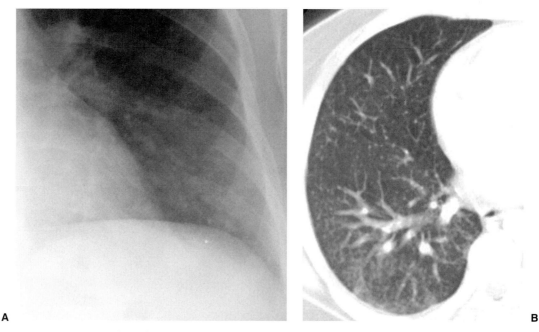

A   B

Figure 6.5 Miliary histoplasmosis in AIDS (CD4 count = 160). *(A)* Posteroanterior chest radiograph and *(B)* computed tomography: miliary nodules.

FUNGAL INFECTION

Fungal pneumonia is uncommon in AIDS patients because neutrophil activity is preserved. Patients receiving antiviral therapy that induces granulocytopenia are susceptible to fungal infections (7) (Fig. 6.5). The common pathogens causing fungal pneumonia are *Cryptococcus* and *Aspergillus. Cryptococcus* is a fungus that commonly causes meningitis. The radiographic features of *Cryptococcus* pneumonia include nodular interstitial infiltrates, solitary or multiple pulmonary nodules or masses that may cavitate, pleural effusions, and lymph node enlargement (20). The radiographic appearance of *Aspergillus* is discussed later in this chapter (Fig. 6.6).

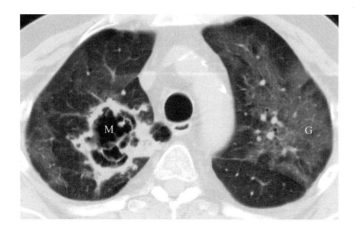

Figure 6.6 Two diagnoses in a patient with AIDS. Computed tomography shows ground glass opacity bilaterally (G) and a cavitary right upper lobe mass (M). Percutaneous aspiration of the right upper lobe mass revealed *Aspergillus*. Because of continued fevers, bronchoscopy was subsequently performed and revealed *Pneumocystis*.

PNEUMOCYSTIS CARINII PNEUMONIA

P. carinii is a unicellular organism that behaves like a protozoan but is classified as a fungus (21). The organism cannot be grown in cultures, and therefore the diagnosis is based on visualizing the organism (or its cyst) in special stains preformed on sputum or bronchoalveolar lavage fluid. PCP can occur at any level of immunosuppression, but it becomes common when CD4 counts are at or below 200 cells/mm^3. Despite the use of effective prophylactic therapy and the resultant decline in PCP, it remains the most common opportunistic pulmonary infection in AIDS. Approximately 70% of AIDS patients will suffer at least one PCP infection during the course of their disease. It is more common in homosexual and male patients (21,22). PCP in AIDS patients is insidious and presents with nonproductive cough, dyspnea, low-grade fever, and malaise (8).

Pneumocystis remains the most common opportunistic pneumonia in AIDS, ultimately affecting roughly 70% of AIDS patients.

The radiologic manifestations of PCP are varied. In most cases it presents as bilateral, diffuse, symmetric parenchymal abnormality with a perihilar and basilar predominance (Fig. 6.7). Early findings are often subtle, and the CXR is normal or nearly normal in anywhere from 10% to as many as 39% of patients (8). Infection may appear as interstitial granular or reticular opacities or as airspace disease. Without treatment PCP often progresses to confluent airspace disease (22,23). Upper lobe disease is classically seen in patients receiving aerosolized prophylactic pentamidine therapy (23). Radiographic improvement is expected within 10 days of appropriate treatment, although there is usually initial radiographic worsening due to capillary leak. Atypical manifestations are encountered in approximately 5% and include isolated lobar disease, focal parenchymal opacities, nodules and masses, a miliary pattern, endobronchial lesions, and pleural effusions (23).

AIDS patients may present with cystic lesions (Fig. 6.8), thin or thick walled, regular or irregular in shape, that may be surrounded by GGOs (Fig. 6.9), indicating inflammatory pneumonitis. This form of disease is termed cystic PCP and is rare in non-AIDS patients (21,23). The cystic lesions show a predilection for the lung apices and subpleural

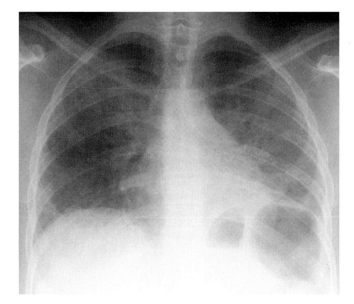

Figure 6.7 *Pneumocystis* pneumonia in AIDS (CD4 count = 27). Widespread bilateral parenchymal abnormality with perihilar confluent airspace disease, left greater than right.

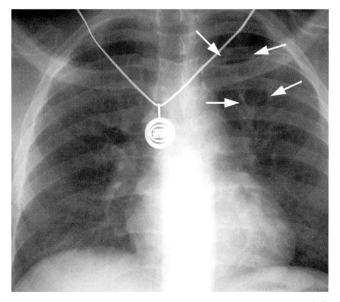

Figure 6.8 *Pneumocystis* pneumonia in AIDS. Two cysts in left upper lobe (*arrows*).

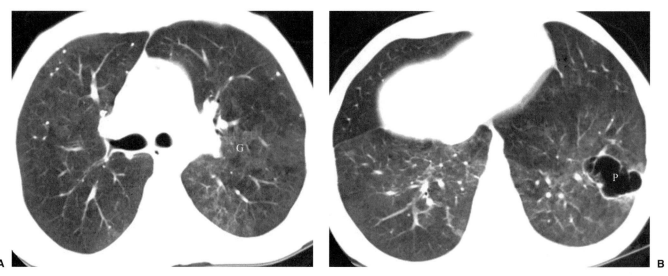

Figure 6.9 *Pneumocystis* pneumonia in AIDS (CD4 count = 169). *A.* Computed tomography at the level of the carina: ground glass opacity, especially in the left perihilar lung (G) and smaller cysts. *B.* Computed tomography more caudal than (*A*): left lower lobe pneumatocele (P).

areas, and patients present with spontaneous pneumothorax in 6% to 7% of cases (Fig. 6.10). The pneumothoraces are frequently bilateral, associated with a higher mortality rate of 33% to 57%, and not always responsive to standard chest tube placement (21).

Chest CT and HRCT are helpful for the patient with a nonspecific clinical presentation and normal or near normal CXR or when PCP relapse is suspected in the presence of an abnormal CXR from a previous episode of infection (21). At HRCT, PCP manifests as GGOs that may be diffuse and homogeneous or patchy and geographic in distribution, often in the perihilar lungs (7,21). GGO is attributed to accumulation of fluid, organisms, and debris within the alveoli and is considered highly suggestive of *P. carinii* infection in the setting of HIV infection (Figs. 6.6, 6.9, and 6.10). HRCT may show thickening of interlobular septa secondary to edema and cellular infiltration and may delineate the extent and distribution of cyst formation and changes of interstitial fibrosis secondary to chronic PCP. CT findings may suggest an alternative diagnosis, an additional diagnosis along with PCP (Fig. 6.6), or another pathogen and may help to direct a biopsy.

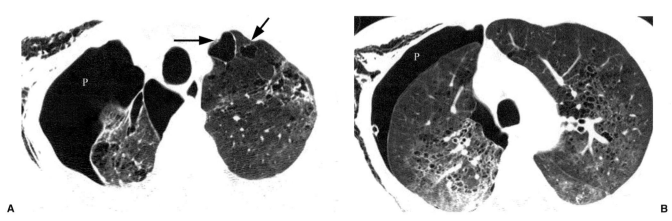

Figure 6.10 Chronic *Pneumocystis* pneumonia in AIDS (CD4 count = 24). Computed tomography at two different levels (*A and B*) reveals numerous small cysts, larger cysts in the left lung anteriorly (*arrows*), ground glass opacity, and a large right pneumothorax (P).

VIRAL INFECTIONS

CMV is a common pathogen in AIDS patients with CD4 counts below 100 cells/mm³. It is more prevalent in patients who contracted AIDS through sexual contact (6). The lungs are infected with CMV in 50% to 90% of patients (4,8). The exact role of CMV as a pulmonary pathogen is not clear, and it is often not the cause of death. Chronic CMV pneumonitis is thought to be related to extrathoracic manifestations of CMV, including retinitis, colitis, esophagitis, and encephalitis.

The classic radiographic appearance includes diffuse GGO, patchy airspace disease, and pulmonary nodules (24). Airway disease such as bronchiectasis and bronchial wall thickening is commonly seen and may be the sole manifestation (25). Other viruses such as herpes simplex, varicella-zoster, and Epstein-Barr virus seldom cause pulmonary infection in AIDS patients (8).

NONINFECTIOUS PULMONARY MANIFESTATIONS OF ACQUIRED IMMUNODEFICIENCY SYNDROME

AIDS patients are continuously exposed to viruses associated with malignancy, such as Epstein-Barr virus and human papilloma virus. AIDS patients are thus predisposed to neoplasms, including Kaposi sarcoma, lymphoma, lung cancer, and pulmonary metastases.

KAPOSI SARCOMA

Among AIDS patients, Kaposi sarcoma almost exclusively affects homosexual or bisexual men and is thought to be related to human papilloma virus-8 (4). It initially manifests as purplish skin lesions, but as CD4 counts drop below 100 cells/mm³, disease often disseminates to abdominal organs and to the larynx, tracheobronchial tree, and lungs (26).

The radiographic findings are typical, often enabling the radiologist to reach a diagnosis without the need for invasive procedures. In fact, CT is reported to be more then 90% accurate (8). Kaposi sarcoma is characterized by nodularity along the bronchovascular bundles that spreads to the perihilar regions (Fig. 6.11). As disease progresses, lung

CT is reported to be more than 90% accurate for the diagnosis of Kaposi sarcoma.

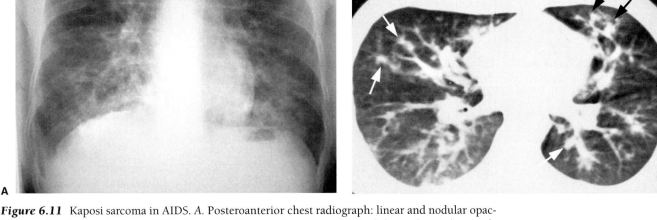

Figure 6.11 Kaposi sarcoma in AIDS. *A.* Posteroanterior chest radiograph: linear and nodular opacities, predominantly in the perihilar lungs. *B.* Computed tomography: nodularity (*arrows*) extends along the bronchovascular bundles.

nodules and septal lines develop. The nodules tend to be ill-defined and may obstruct airways, thereby causing postobstructive pneumonia. In advanced disease, pleural effusions and enlarged lymph nodes may appear. The lymph nodes are not markedly enlarged but typically are high in attenuation as a result of contrast enhancement (7,27).

Lymphoma

The most common lymphoma in AIDS patients is B-cell non-Hodgkin lymphoma. It is termed AIDS-related lymphoma and is thought to result from Epstein-Barr virus (28). AIDS-related lymphoma is an extranodal disease that primarily involves the central nervous system and gastrointestinal tract and occurs when CD4 counts are less than 55 cells/mm^3. The chest is involved in only 10% to 50% of patients (4), either via spread from extrathoracic foci or rarely as primary pulmonary lymphoma.

Unilateral pleural effusion is the most common thoracic manifestation of extrapulmonary AIDS-related lymphoma (Fig. 6.12) and may be the only manifestation. Other findings include parenchymal nodules (Fig. 6.13), masses, and airspace disease. Enlarged mediastinal lymph nodes occur but are not the hallmark of disease (29).

There are few reports of primary pulmonary AIDS-related lymphoma. The disease is characterized by pulmonary nodules, often bilateral and basilar, sometimes with air bronchograms or cavitation. Enlarged thoracic lymph nodes are less typical, and pleural effusions are rare (30).

Lung Cancer

Lung cancer is known to be associated with HIV infection, and because its manifestations overlap with AIDS-related infections, diagnosis is frequently delayed and prognosis is grim.

There is a known association between HIV infection and lung cancer. There is controversy about whether HIV infection is a risk factor for lung cancer or a coincidental disease (31). However, lung cancer deserves consideration in AIDS patients. HIV-infected patients with lung cancer are typically younger than the general population of lung cancer patients. There is a strong male predilection, and there is usually a history of smoking (32), identifying a subpopulation that is at particular risk. There is no correlation with CD4 counts. Adenocarcinoma is the usual cell type, but other cell types are reported as well. The diagnosis is typically only made late in the course of disease, and prognosis is grim. This is

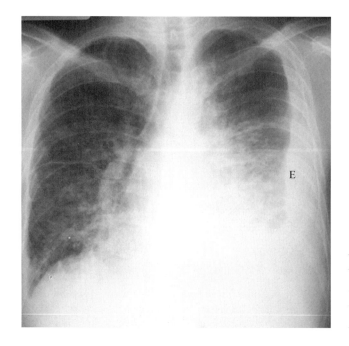

Figure 6.12 Two diagnoses in AIDS. Loculated left pleural effusion (E) results from large cell lymphoma. Underlying nodular lung disease represents Kaposi sarcoma.

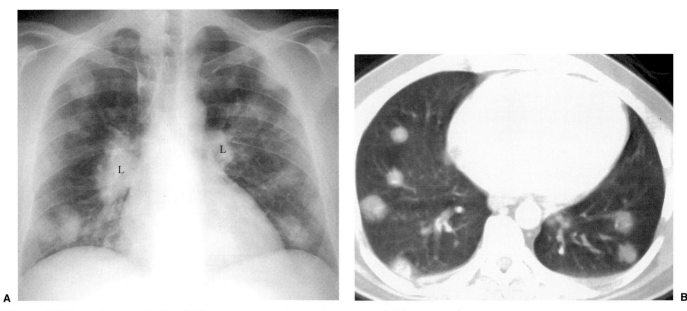

Figure 6.13 Lymphoma in AIDS. *(A)* Posteroanterior chest radiograph and *(B)* computed tomography: enlarged hilar lymph nodes (L) and multiple lung nodules.

because the more common infections and neoplasms that AIDS patients develop are considered long before lung cancer, and the younger than expected age and sometimes confusing radiographic presentation in lung cancer patients with AIDS can be misleading. It is therefore suggested that transbronchial or percutaneous biopsy should be obtained whenever abnormality persists despite antibiotic therapy.

The typical radiographic presentation is of a lung nodule or mass, peripheral or central, predominantly in the upper lobes (Fig. 6.14). Postobstructive airspace disease is also frequently seen. Lymph node enlargement and pleural effusion are common but are not

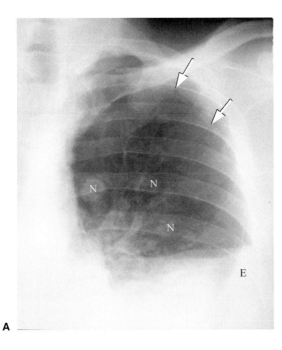

Figure 6.14 Small cell carcinoma of lung in AIDS. *A.* Posteroanterior chest radiograph: nodules (N) and hydropneumothorax. *Arrows* mark lung edge. E, effusion.

(continued on next page)

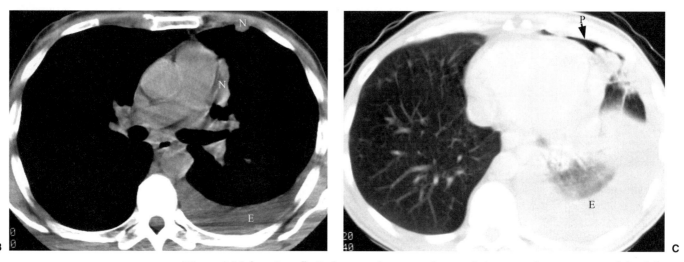

Figure 6.14 (continued) *B.* Computed tomography at soft tissue window settings: nodules (N) are pleural. *C.* Computed tomography at lung window settings: left lung volume loss despite left hydropneumothorax. E, effusion; P, pneumothorax. (Courtesy of Dr. Rosita Shah, Philadelphia, Pennsylvania.)

specific and may be caused by many other AIDS-related diseases (32). Diffuse pleural thickening has been reported as a rare manifestation of lung cancer in AIDS. This situation presents particular diagnostic difficulty, because bacterial and mycobacterial infections, lymphoma, and Kaposi sarcoma may present in this exact way. CT demonstration of underlying pleural and lung masses and metastases may be helpful.

PULMONARY MANIFESTATIONS IN NON–ACQUIRED IMMUNODEFICIENCY SYNDROME IMMUNOCOMPROMISED PATIENTS

APPROACH

In the last several decades there has been a steady increase in the number of patients with immune compromise as a result of advances in cancer therapy, more frequent organ transplantation, and aggressive immunosuppressive therapy for collagen vascular disorders and autoimmune diseases (33). There are four main categories of lung defense against infection: mechanical barriers, phagocytic defense, cell-mediated defense, and humoral immunity (34). Impairment of one or more defense mechanisms results in different forms of immune compromise and predisposes affected patients to specific organisms.

Defining the nature of immune defect and its severity helps to determine the organisms to which the patient is susceptible (33). For example, lymphoma patients or patients receiving corticosteroids have altered cell-mediated immunity and are susceptible to fungal infections such as *Cryptococcus*, *Histoplasma*, and *Candida* and to bacterial infections such as *Legionella* and *Nocardia*. Patients receiving chemotherapy or patients with myeloproliferative disorders have granulocyte dysfunction and are susceptible to infections with gram-negative bacteria, *Staphylococcus*, *Aspergillus*, and *Candida* (33,34).

Duration of immune compromise also influences the organisms that are likely to infect a patient. Cancer patients treated with cytotoxic drugs are prone to develop bacterial pneumonia with typical pathogens such as *S. aureus* in the first few days after therapy. Patients with severe neutropenia over a prolonged period of time are at greater risk of developing *Aspergillus* infections (35). After organ transplantation, patients are susceptible to infection with different organisms depending on the time interval since transplantation. From 1 to 4 months after kidney transplantation, T-cell-mediated immunity is severely impaired, rendering patients at risk for infection with *Aspergillus*, *Cryptococcus*, *Mucorales*, *Nocardia*, PCP, CMV, and *Mycobacteria*. Later, as immunosuppression is tapered, the immune system recovers. Patients in this stage are more likely to develop community-acquired pneumonias, although the risk of PCP and *Cryptococcus* persists (36).

After heart transplantation, in addition to the effects of potent immunosuppressive therapy, there is increased susceptibility to pulmonary infection as a result of prolonged intubation, pulmonary edema, and effects of thoracic surgery on lung mechanics. After lung transplantation there is added lung liability due to impaired mucociliary clearance, organ injury during transplantation, and the presence of recipient alveolar macrophages in transplanted lungs. Patients are therefore at risk for nosocomial pneumonias with gram-negative bacteria and *Staphylococcus* in the immediate postoperative period and later are susceptible to viral, PCP, and fungal infections (37).

Pre–bone marrow transplantation (BMT) induction includes high dose chemotherapy and whole body radiation, which cause severe neutropenia (38). Similarly, after BMT patients suffer from severe neutropenia and are at increased risk for lung infections by gram-negative bacteria, *Staphylococcus*, *Streptococcus*, and *Aspergillus*. In the subacute phase (30 to 100 days after transplantation) granulocytes recover, but cell-mediated immunity and antibody production are impaired, leading to infection with CMV and PCP. From that point on, graft-versus-host disease may involve the lungs. In the chronic post-BMT phase, patients suffer from combined immunodeficiency as a result of immunosuppressive therapy, reduced antibody production, and graft-versus-host disease. At this stage there is increased susceptibility to infections with encapsulated organisms such as *Streptococcus*.

Radiographic Patterns

Radiographic features of opportunistic infections are nonspecific. However, there is some correlation between the radiologic pattern and the responsible pathogen. Some organisms have typical radiographic patterns of presentation. Correlating the radiographic pattern with clinical data helps to narrow the differential diagnosis (39,40).

The main radiographic patterns encountered in non-AIDS immunocompromised patients include airspace disease, nodules, and diffuse lung disease. The role of chest CT and HRCT is discussed later.

Normal Chest Radiograph

Chest radiography plays a major role in evaluating febrile immunocompromised patients. The CXR has limited sensitivity for detection of early infection, especially in neutropenic patients. A normal CXR does not exclude lung infection (Fig. 6.15). Neutropenic patients have an altered inflammatory response, with subtle and delayed radiographic findings (40). The CXR is normal in up to 78% of such patients with initial febrile episodes, recurrent fevers, or persistent fevers (41). HRCT may increase sensitivity for subtle abnormality in neutropenic patients, suggest the causative pathogen, help to guide diagnostic procedures, and allow early initiation of therapy to improve survival (42,43). In a febrile immunocompromised patient with a normal CXR or questionable findings, HRCT deserves serious consideration (41,42).

> A febrile immunocompromised patient with a normal CXR may benefit from HRCT.

Airspace Disease

Bacteria are the most common organisms to cause pulmonary infections in the non-AIDS immunocompromised host. In a neutropenic patient, bacterial pneumonia typically develops in the acute neutropenic stage, whereas fungal pneumonia will develop in the subacute neutropenic phase (about 2 weeks later). The clinical presentation of bacterial pneumonia is of an acute rapidly progressive febrile illness. *S. aureus* is a frequent pathogen.

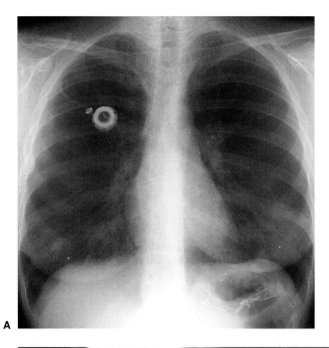

A

Figure 6.15 Infection with nearly normal chest radiograph in patient with acute myelogenous leukemia and bone marrow transplant. *A.* Posteroanterior chest radiograph: questionable nodularity in lower lungs, left greater than right. *B and C.* Computed tomography 1 day after *A:* multiple bilateral lung nodules with a computed tomography halo sign *(arrows)* and several cavities *(arrowheads)* result from invasive pulmonary aspergillosis. P, pneumomediastinum.

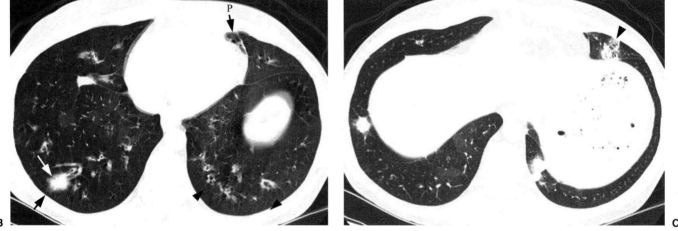

B   C

Gram-negative bacteria are common pathogens, because the organisms colonizing the oropharynx are altered in debilitated patients. Altered phagocytosis in neutropenic patients also increases the susceptibility to gram-negative infections. *Legionella* and *Pseudomonas* may develop in moist ventilation tubing (40).

The typical radiographic pattern caused by bacteria is airspace disease resulting from filling of alveoli with inflammatory exudate. It may occur in a lobar, segmental, subsegmental, or patchy distribution. Disease is characteristically confluent, and air bronchograms are common. Cavitation is also common, either solitary or in the form of multiple microabscesses. Large pleural effusions and empyemas are infrequent (39).

Airspace disease most commonly reflects bacterial infection, but infection with other organisms may manifest similarly. Fungi such as *Aspergillus, Histoplasma,* and *Coccidioides* and other species of bacteria such as *Nocardia* may manifest as indolent pneumonia clinically and may cause airspace disease, with or without cavitation (33). *M. tuberculosis* and *M. avium* complex infections are generally uncommon in non-AIDS immunocompromised hosts but are relatively more prevalent in patients after organ transplantation or in patients with lymphoproliferative diseases and primary neoplasms of lung, head, and neck. The most common radiographic picture is typical reactivation tuberculosis, with consolidation of the apical or posterior segments of the upper lobes, often with cavitation (33).

Nodules

Rapidly growing nodules are the hallmark of fungal infection. Nodules may be single or multiple, and cavitation is frequent. Several fungi cause nodules in the immunocompromised host. *Aspergillus* is the most frequent pathogen. Invasive pulmonary aspergillosis (IPA) is a form of *Aspergillus* infection in severely immunocompromised hosts, most frequently encountered in patients with acute leukemia who are receiving cytotoxic therapy. These patients typically have prolonged neutropenic fevers treated with broad-spectrum antibiotics (43). *Aspergillus* is also encountered in patients on prolonged corticosteroid therapy or other immunosuppressive therapy for collagen vascular disease and in AIDS. Definitive diagnosis of IPA is difficult, because the organism is seldom isolated in sputum and is isolated in bronchoalveolar lavage or transbronchial biopsy specimens in only 50% of patients (43). Therefore, the diagnosis is generally empirical, based on the presence of typical radiographic findings in immunocompromised patients not responding to broad-spectrum antibiotics. HRCT demonstrates increased sensitivity for early detection of disease and plays a major role in the diagnosis of IPA (42). Radiographic features of IPA vary. Classically there are multiple ill-defined nodules. A rim of GGO around nodules, termed the "CT halo sign," provides a significant HRCT clue for early diagnosis (Fig. 6.15). The "halo sign" reflects areas of hemorrhagic infarction and/or edema (33), likely resulting from the angioinvasive nature of the infection (Fig. 6.16).

Cavitation occurs relatively late in the course of disease, usually as the white blood cell count recovers (Figs. 6.17 and 6.18). At this stage crescentic lucency may appear, termed the "air crescent sign." This should not be confused with a mycetoma in an immune competent host (43). A mycetoma is usually single; IPA typically results in multiple cavities. A mycetoma arises in the setting of an old pulmonary cavity; IPA usually arises in previously normal lung. A mycetoma is typically freely mobile in its cavity; the central opacity in an IPA cavity is usually fixed, a finding that has been called "the mural nodule" (Figs. 6.19 and 6.20). Aspergillosis may even involve the tracheobronchial tree (Fig. 6.21).

> Rapidly growing nodules are the hallmark of fungal infection.

> A rim of ground glass around nodules ("CT halo sign") at HRCT suggests invasive pulmonary aspergillosis.

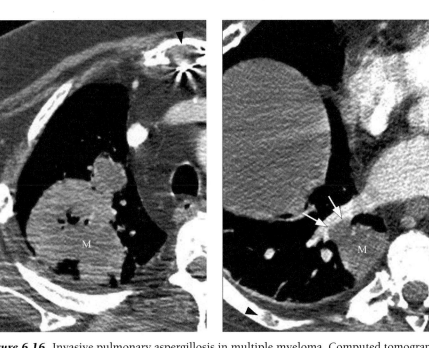

Figure 6.16 Invasive pulmonary aspergillosis in multiple myeloma. Computed tomography at two different levels (*A and B*) reveals cavitary lung masses (M), one of which directly invades the right inferior pulmonary vein (*arrows*). Lytic skeletal lesions of multiple myeloma are also seen (*arrowheads*).

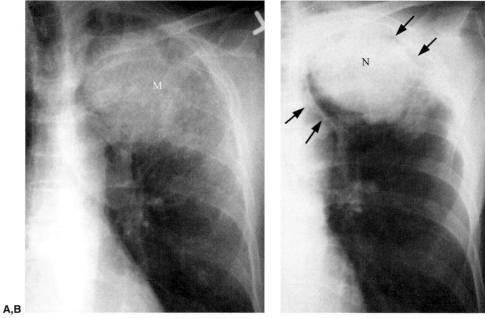

Figure 6.17 Invasive pulmonary aspergillosis in acute myelogenous leukemia. *A.* Posteroanterior chest radiograph May 1st: mass-like left upper lobe opacity (M). *B.* Posteroanterior chest radiograph May 23rd: interval cavitation *(arrows)* with a large suspended mural nodule (N).

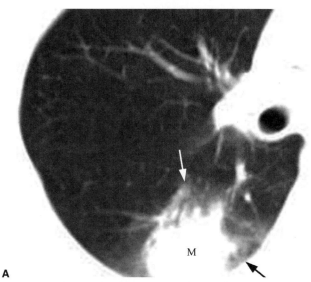

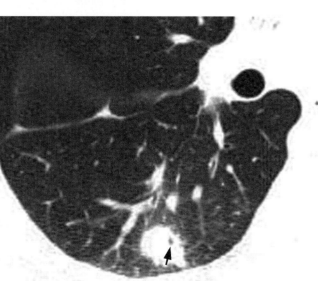

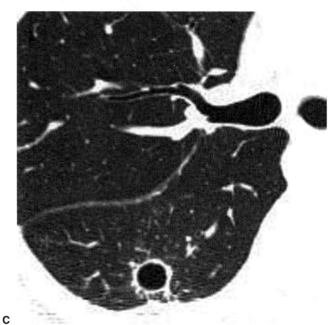

Figure 6.18 Invasive pulmonary aspergillosis in acute lymphocytic leukemia. *A.* Computed tomography January 25th: right lower lobe mass (M) with computed tomography halo sign *(arrows)*. *B.* Computed tomography March 4th: smaller nodule with early cavitation (arrow). *C.* Computed tomography March 26th: nodule is almost entirely cavitary.

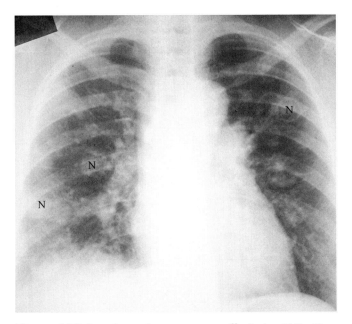

Figure 6.19 Invasive pulmonary aspergillosis in AML. Posteroanterior radiograph demonstrates multiple cavitary nodules, many with central suspended mural nodules (N).

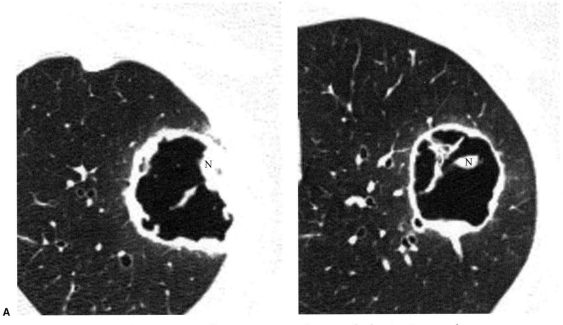

Figure 6.20 Invasive pulmonary aspergillosis in acute myelogenous leukemia. Computed tomography at two different levels (*A and B*) demonstrates nondependent mural nodules (N).

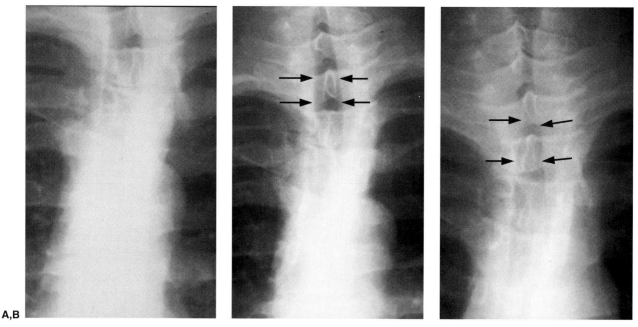
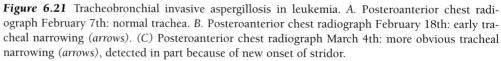

Figure 6.21 Tracheobronchial invasive aspergillosis in leukemia. *A.* Posteroanterior chest radiograph February 7th: normal trachea. *B.* Posteroanterior chest radiograph February 18th: early tracheal narrowing *(arrows)*. *(C)* Posteroanterior chest radiograph March 4th: more obvious tracheal narrowing *(arrows)*, detected in part because of new onset of stridor.

Other fungi manifesting with nodules include *Mucorales, Candida, Coccidioides, Blastomyces,* and *Cryptococcus.* Zygomycosis, now the preferred term for the clinical manifestations of *Mucorales* infection, is quite similar, clinically and radiologically (Figs. 6.22 and 6.23), to IPA (39). *Cryptococcus* pneumonia is rare and often presents with associated meningitis. Radiographic features are of single or multiple nodules, sometimes with cavi-

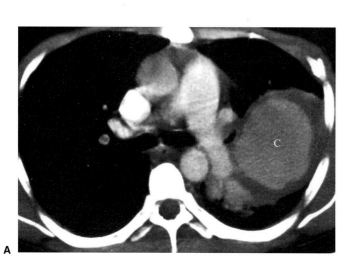
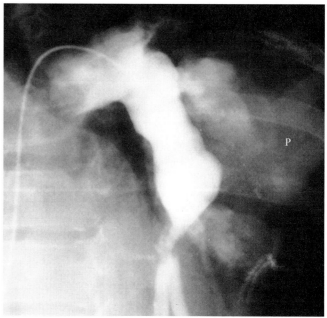

Figure 6.22 Zygomycosis in systemic lupus erythematosus treated with steroids, with vascular invasion. *A.* Computed tomography: large low attenuation left lung lesion with amorphous central contrast (C). *B.* Left pulmonary arteriogram: lesion is a large pseudoaneurysm (P).

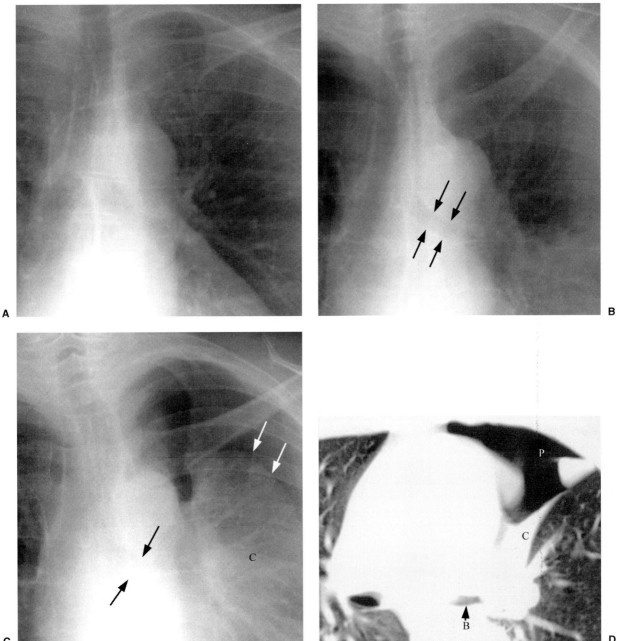

Figure 6.23 Tracheobronchial zygomycosis in diabetic with renal transplant on immunosuppressive therapy. *A.* Posteroanterior chest radiograph in 1993 is normal. *B.* Posteroanterior chest radiograph 1-2-95: mild narrowing of the left main bronchus *(arrows)*. *C.* Posteroanterior chest radiograph 2-1-95: marked narrowing of the left main bronchus *(arrows)* with development of left upper lobe collapse (C) and pneumothorax *(arrows* mark lung edge). *D.* Computed tomography 2-2-95: confirmation of abnormality of left main bronchus (B), left upper lobe collapse (C), and pneumothorax (P).

tation. *Candida* is a common oropharyngeal commensal organism and may easily contaminate sputum cultures. A lung biopsy is therefore required for the diagnosis of *Candida* pneumonia.

Patients with decreased cellular immunity, especially patients on prolonged corticosteroid therapy, are susceptible to *Nocardia* pneumonia. Radiographically, there are single or multiple nodules that may cavitate (Fig. 6.24). Extension to the pleural cavity and chest wall invasion are suggestive of *Nocardia*.

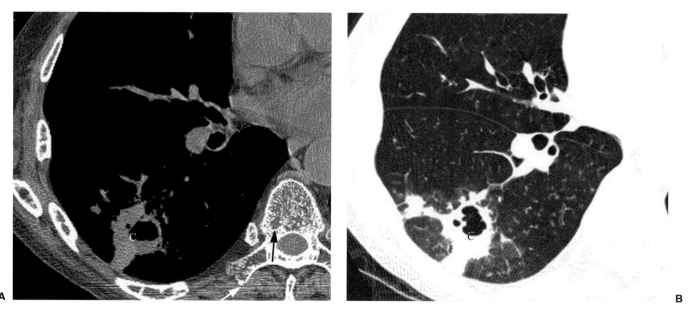

Figure 6.24 Cavitary nocardiosis in multiple myeloma. Computed tomography at *(A)* soft tissue and *(B)* lung window settings: cavitary right lower lobe pneumonia (C) (*arrows* mark lesions of multiple myeloma).

Septic emboli are a nodular complication of indwelling catheters, commonly used in immunocompromised patients. *S. aureus* and *Staphylococcus epidermidis* are the most common pathogens. Radiographic features include multiple nodules (Fig. 6.25), often with indistinct margins, and frequent cavitation (Fig. 6.26).

Diffuse Lung Disease

CMV is an important pathogen in organ transplant recipients.

Viral lung infections may result in diffuse bilateral lung disease. CMV is the most common such pathogen. Organ recipients are susceptible to CMV pneumonia, particularly through seropositive organ donors or blood transfusions (33). Infection is often asymptomatic.

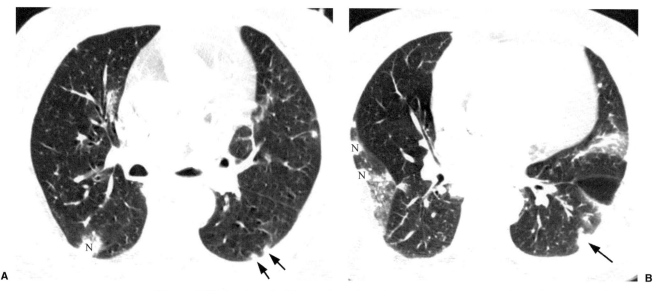

Figure 6.25 Septic emboli in esophageal carcinoma patient receiving chemotherapy. *A and B.* Computed tomography at lung window settings: multiple peripheral lung nodules (N), several recognizably wedge-shaped (*arrows*).

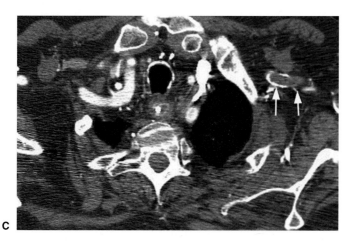

C

Figure 6.25 (continued) C. Computed tomography at soft tissue window settings: thrombus *(arrows)* in left axillary vein.

Symptomatic disease is usually self-limited, but rapid deterioration may occur, typically in BMT recipients. Symptomatic CMV pneumonia may manifest with a normal chest radiograph or may produce diffuse bilateral linear, small nodular, ground glass, or airspace opacities (Fig. 6.27). A single nodule or lobar airspace disease occurs infrequently. Other viral causes of diffuse lung disease include herpes zoster, herpes simplex, and respiratory syncytial virus. Again, organ recipients are at risk. Viral pneumonias characteristically result in diffuse interstitial opacity, GGO, or a reticular or reticulonodular pattern and may progress to diffuse airspace disease.

PCP is the most common protozoan to cause diffuse lung disease. Although it is closely linked to AIDS, PCP infection also occurs after corticosteroid withdrawal or completion of chemotherapy. The clinical presentation is often fulminant, with rapidly progressive tachypnea and hypoxemia. Diffuse lung disease is often seen (Fig. 6.28), as detailed in the section on AIDS.

Diffuse small nodular disease, the so-called miliary pattern, may be a manifestation of overwhelming *M. tuberculosis* infection (Figs. 6.29 and 6.30). It is not commonly seen in atypical mycobacterial infections. Disseminated fungal infections, including histoplasmosis, coccidioidomycosis, and blastomycosis, may all present radiographically with miliary nodules (33).

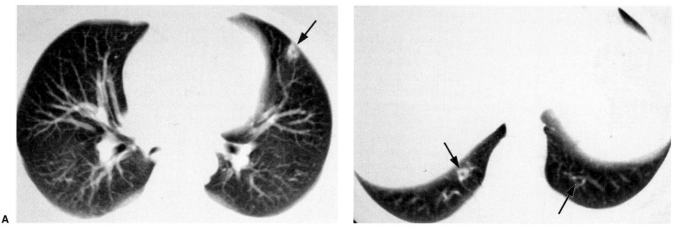

A   B

Figure 6.26 Septic emboli in systemic lupus erythematosus patient on steroids with indwelling catheter. *A and B.* Computed tomography at two different levels: bilateral cavitary nodules *(arrows).*

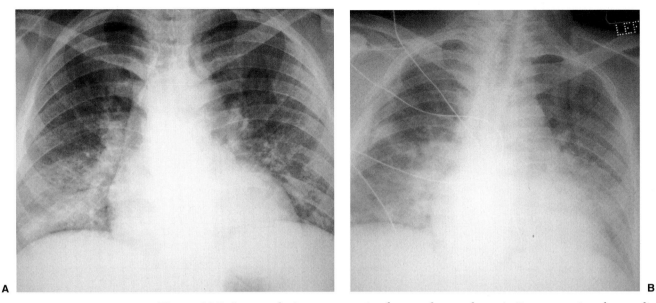

Figure 6.27 Cytomegalovirus pneumonia after renal transplant. *A*. Posteroanterior chest radiograph September 14th: early diffuse parenchymal abnormality with septal lines, nodularity, and ground glass opacity. *B*. Posteroanterior chest radiograph September 17th: diffuse bilateral airspace disease.

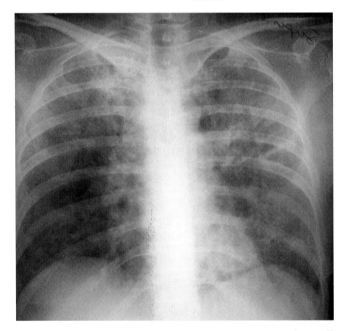

Figure 6.28 *Pneumocystis* pneumonia in patient with T-cell defect. Bilateral airspace disease, predominantly in the central upper lungs.

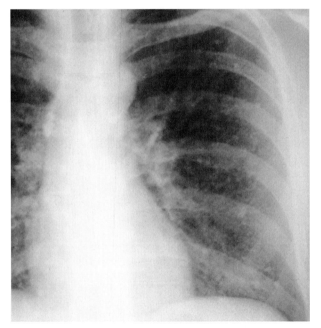

Figure 6.29 Miliary tuberculosis in patient receiving steroids. Chest radiograph reveals miliary nodules.

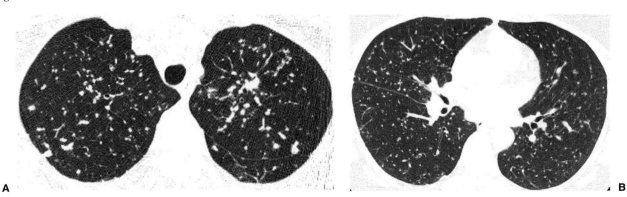

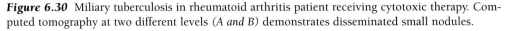

Figure 6.30 Miliary tuberculosis in rheumatoid arthritis patient receiving cytotoxic therapy. Computed tomography at two different levels (*A and B*) demonstrates disseminated small nodules.

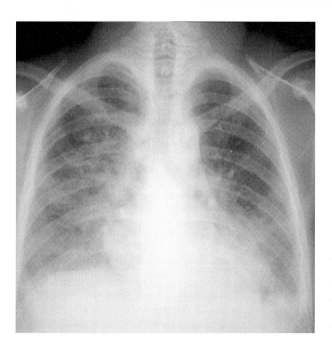

Figure 6.31 Leukemic infiltration of lung in acute myelogenous leukemia. Posteroanterior chest radiograph shows bilateral airspace disease, greatest in the right perihilar lung and left lower lobe.

NONINFECTIOUS LUNG DISEASE

Many noninfectious processes occur in the non-AIDS immunocompromised host. The radiologist should be aware of these diseases and should suggest them in the appropriate clinical and radiographic setting. For example, the lungs may be infiltrated with the patient's primary disease, such as leukemic (Fig. 6.31) or lymphomatous infiltration, creating airspace disease, nodules, and, rarely, diffuse lung disease. Metastatic carcinoma usually presents with lung nodules, but lymphangitic carcinomatosis presents with small irregular opacities (reticulonodular pattern), in some patients resembling miliary nodules or other interstitial patterns.

Intrathoracic lymphoproliferative disorders are more common in AIDS patients but are also well documented in organ transplant recipients. Radiographic findings vary and include multiple nodules, diffuse GGO, and airspace disease. Pleural effusions and lymph node enlargement may or may not occur (42,44) (Fig. 6.32). Posttransplant lymphopro-

Intrathoracic lymphoproliferative disease deserves special consideration in AIDS patients and in organ transplant recipients.

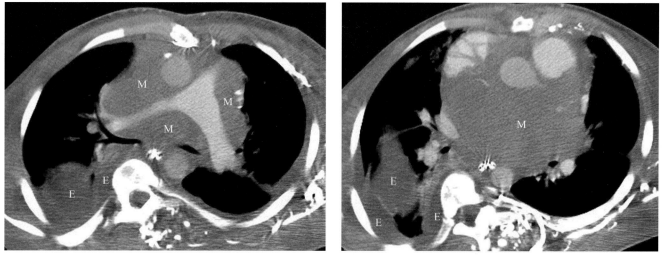

Figure 6.32 Posttransplant lymphoproliferative disorder 12 years after heart transplant for transposition of the great vessels with a single ventricle. *A and B.* Computed tomography at two different levels: extensive lymph node mass (M) throughout the mediastinum with loculated right pleural effusion (E). Patient presented with 2- to 3-day history of dry cough on October 7th and died on October 21st.

liferative disorder may regress as immunosuppression is withdrawn. Immunocompromised patients also develop complications of therapy.

Pulmonary hemorrhage may complicate chemotherapy-induced thrombocytopenia and usually manifests as airspace disease. Cytotoxic therapy, especially with Adriamycin (Doxorubicin), is potentially cardiotoxic. It may cause heart failure and resultant pulmonary edema. Pulmonary edema may also develop after excessive hydration. Other chemotherapeutic agents such as bleomycin and busulfan are known to cause pulmonary fibrosis. Radiation pneumonitis may follow radiation therapy, usually conforming to the radiation port. Rejection of transplanted lung and pulmonary graft-versus-host disease in BMT patients both result in bronchiolitis obliterans. HRCT features of bronchiolitis obliterans include air trapping, centrilobular nodules, and bronchiectasis.

REFERENCES

1. Miller R. HIV associated respiratory disease. *Lancet* 1996;348:307–312.
2. Neiman PE, Thomas ED, Reeves WC, et al. Opportunistic infection and interstitial pneumonia following marrow transplantation for aplastic anemia and hematologic malignancy. *Transplant Protoc* 1976;8:663.
3. Bodey GP, Powell RD, Hersh EM, et al. Pulmonary complications of acute leukemia. *Cancer* 1966;19:781.
4. Haramati LB, Jenny-Avital ER. Approach to the diagnosis of pulmonary disease in patients infected with the human immunodeficiency virus. *J Thorac Imag* 1998;13:247–260.
5. White DA, Zaman MK. Pulmonary disease. Medical management of AIDS patients. *Med Clin North Am* 1992;76:19–44.
6. Markowitz GS, Conception L, Factor SM, et al. Autopsy patterns of disease among subgroups of an inner-city Bronx AIDS population. *J Acquir Immune Defic Syndr Hum Retrovirol* 1996;13: 48–54.
7. McGuiness G. Pulmonary complications of acquired immunodeficiency syndrome. In: Naidich DP, Webb WR, Muller NL, et al., eds. *Computed tomography and magnetic resonance of the thorax*, 3rd ed. Philadelphia: Lippincott-Raven, 1999:465–503.
8. Maki DD. Pulmonary infections in HIV/AIDS. *Semin Roentgenol* 2000;35:124–139.
9. Noskin GA, Glassroth J. Bacterial pneumonia associated with HIV-1 infection. *Clin Chest Med* 1996;17:713–723.
10. Hirschtick RE, Glassroth J, Jordan MC, et al. Bacterial pneumonia in persons infected with the immunodeficiency virus. *N Engl J Med* 1995;333:845–851.
11. McGuiness G, Gurden JF, Bhalla M, et al. AIDS related airway disease. *AJR Am J Roentgenol* 1997; 168:67–77.
12. Kuhlman JE. Pulmonary manifestations of acquired immunodeficiency syndrome. *Semin Roentgenol* 1994;29:242–274.
13. Barnes PF, Bloch AB, Davidson PT, et al. Tuberculosis in patients with human immunodeficiency virus infection. *N Engl J Med* 1991;324:1644–1650.
14. Jones BE, Young SMM, Antoniskis D, et al. Relationship of the manifestations of tuberculosis to CD4 cell counts in patients with human immunodeficiency virus infection. *Am Rev Respir Dis* 1993;148:1292–1297.
15. Haramati LB, Jenny-Avital ER, Alterman DD. Effect of HIV status on chest radiographic and CT findings in patients with tuberculosis. *Clin Radiol* 1997;52:31–35.
16. Pastores SM, Naidich DP, Aranda CP, et al. Intrathoracic adenopathy associated with pulmonary tuberculosis in patients with human immunodeficiency virus infection. *Chest* 1993;103: 1433–1437.
17. Aronchick JM, Miller WT Jr. Disseminated nontuberculous mycobacterial infections in immunosuppressed patients. *Semin Roentgenol* 1993;28:150–157.
18. Kalayjilan RC, Toossi Z, Tomashefski JF Jr, et al. Pulmonary disease due to infection by mycobacterium avium complex in patients with AIDS. *Clin Infect Dis* 1995;20:1186–1194.
19. Laissy JP, Cadi M, Cinqualbre A, et al. Mycobacterium tuberculosis versus nontuberculous mycobacterial infection of the lungs in AIDS patients: CT and HRCT patterns. *J Comput Assist Tomogr* 1997;21:312–317.
20. Miller WT Jr, Edelmann JM, Miller WT. Cryptococcal pulmonary infection in patients with AIDS. *Chest* 1990;92:725–728.

21. Kuhlman JE. Pneumocystic infections: The radiologist perspective. *Radiology* 1996;198: 623–635.
22. Goodman PC. *Pneumocystis carinii* pneumonia. *J Thorac Imag* 1991;6:16–21.
23. Kennedy CA, Goetz MB. Atypical roentgenographic manifestations of *Pneumocystis carinii* pneumonia. *Arch Intern Med* 1992;152:1390–1398.
24. McGuinness G, Scholes JV, Garay SM, et al. Cytomegalovirus pneumonitis: spectrum of CT parenchymal findings in 21 AIDS patients. *Radiology* 1994;192:451–459.
25. Waxman AB, Goldie SJ, Brett-Smith H, et al. Cytomegalovirus as primary pulmonary pathogen in AIDS. *Chest* 1997;111:128–134.
26. Garden JF, Huang L, Webb WR, et al. AIDS-related Kaposi sarcoma of the lung: radiographic findings and staging system with bronchoscopic correlation. *Radiology* 1995;195:545–552.
27. Herts BR, Megibow AJ, Birnbaum BA, et al. High attenuation lymphadenopathy in AIDS patients: significance of findings at CT. *Radiology* 1992;185:777–781.
28. Joachim HL, Cooper MC, Hellman GC. Lymphomas in men at high risk for acquired immune deficiency syndrome (AIDS). *Cancer* 1985;56:2831–2842.
29. Seider L, Weiss AJ, Smith MD, et al. Varied appearance of AIDS-related lymphoma in the chest. *Radiology* 1989;171:629–632.
30. Bazot M, Cadranel J, Benayoun S, et al. Primary pulmonary AIDS-related lymphoma. *Chest* 1999;116:1282–1286.
31. Bazot M, Cadranel J, Khalil A, et al. Computed tomographic diagnosis of bronchogenic carcinoma in HIV-infected patients. *Lung Cancer* 2000;28:203–209.
32. Fishman JE, Schwartz DS, Sais GJ, et al. Bronchogenic carcinoma in HIV-infected patients: findings on chest radiographs and CT scans. *AJR Am J Roentgenol* 1995;164:57–61.
33. Conces DJ. Immunocompromised patients who do not have acquired immunodeficiency syndrome: a systematic approach. *J Thorac Imag* 1998;13:247–260.
34. Toews GB. Pulmonary defense mechanisms. *Semin Respir Infect* 1993;8:160–167.
35. Bodey GP, Buckley M, Sathe YS, et al. Quantitative relationships between circulating leukocytes and infection in patients with acute leukemia. *Ann Intern Med* 1966;64:328–340.
36. Peterson PK, Balfour HH, Marker SC, et al. Cytomegalovirus disease in renal allograft recipients: a prospective study of the clinical features, risk factors and impact on renal transplantation. *Medicine* 1989;59:283–300.
37. Dummer SJ, Mentero CG, Griffith BP, et al. Infections in heart-lung transplant recipients. *Transplantation* 1986;41:725–729.
38. Soubani AO, Miller KB, Hassoun PM. Pulmonary complications of bone marrow transplantation. *Chest* 1996;109:1066–1077.
39. McLoud TC. Pulmonary infections in the immunocompromised host. *Radiol Clin North Am* 1989;27:1059–1066.
40. Oh YW, Effmann EL, Godwin JD. Pulmonary infections in immunocompromised host: the importance of correlating the conventional radiologic appearance with the clinical setting. *Radiology* 2000;217:647–656.
41. Donowitz GR, Harman C, Pope T, et al. The role of chest roentgenogram in febrile neutropenic patients. *Arch Intern Med* 1991;151:701–704.
42. Heussel CP, Hans-Ulrich K, Heussel GE, et al. Pneumonia in febrile neutropenic patients and in bone marrow and blood stem-cell transplant recipients: use of high resolution computed tomography. *J Clin Oncol* 1999;17:796–805.
43. Miller WT. Aspergillosis: a disease with many faces. *Semin Roentgenol* 1996;31:52–66.
44. Carigan S, Staples CA, Muller NL. Intrathoracic lymphoproliferative disorders in the immunocompromised patient: CT findings. *Radiology* 1995;197:53–58.

LUNG CANCER

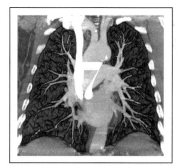

- Detection
- Diagnosis
- Staging

Lung cancer is the most common fatal malignancy in humans. It is strongly associated with cigarette smoking and asbestos exposure; viral infections, pulmonary fibrosis, and radiation exposure play a less defined and/or less frequent role (1–7). Imaging plays a crucial role in detection, diagnosis, and staging.

DETECTION

Although history and physical examination may suggest a pulmonary process, they seldom result in a specific diagnosis of carcinoma of the lung. Sputum cytology is somewhat better in that it may reveal malignant cells. However, radiology alone allows direct noninvasive visualization of the pulmonary parenchyma and mediastinum.

The chest x-ray (CXR) is the cheapest, easiest, most convenient method for this examination. On the CXR, lesions are often detected when they are in the 1-cm size range, and smaller lesions may be detected. Unfortunately, smaller lesions are most likely to be seen if they are calcified, in which case they are probably benign. Frontal and lateral radiographs increase the likelihood of detecting important small lesions, and comparison with prior radiographs can also improve diagnostic accuracy and assessment of the lesion's malignant potential. A nodule that has been present for more than 2 years or less than 2 months is unlikely to be malignant, depending on its size and growth rate.

Interpretation of the CXR requires great care and awareness of locations that are more difficult to evaluate (and therefore require more scrutiny). Lesions that may be missed may occur in the lung apices, where overlapping ribs, clavicles, neck soft tissues, and variable pleural and parenchymal scarring from old granulomatous infections result in significant camouflage (Fig. 7.1). "Pseudo-lesions" also occur in this location, because calcification and/or ossification at the first costochondral junctions may simulate lung nodules. Apical lordotic chest radiography, with the patient leaning back and the x-ray beam angled upward, projects anterior structures cephalad, allowing better visualization of the lung apices.

The hila, with branching arteries and superimposed veins, may conceal an enlarged lymph node or obscure a nearby lung nodule. Hilar masses are sometimes better appreciated on the lateral radiograph (Fig. 7.2). The mediastinum may conceal an especially large mass, and lung lesions close to the mediastinum are also harder to detect because of overlap with the heart, aorta and its branches, and superior vena cava. Nodules in any part of the lung may be rendered invisible by surrounding parenchymal abnormality (Fig. 7.3). In

The CXR is the cheapest, easiest, most convenient method for detecting lung cancer.

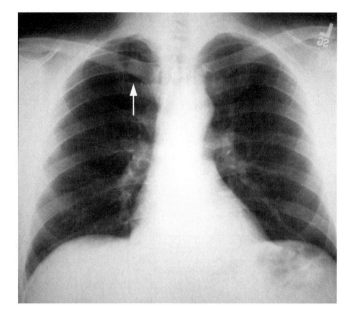

Figure 7.1 A nodule behind the medial right clavicle that could potentially be missed *(arrow)*.

addition, small nodules anywhere at the periphery of the lungs may be overlooked. Shallow oblique radiographs may be a very helpful first step in evaluating a suspicious opacity.

A particularly dangerous nodule location is in the posterior costophrenic sulci of the lungs, below the domes of the diaphragm (Fig. 7.4). In some patients a central endobronchial lesion will clearly be undetectable based on size alone, but careful assessment of secondary signs (such as postobstructive atelectasis, pneumonia, or air trapping) may still allow diagnosis (Fig. 7.5).

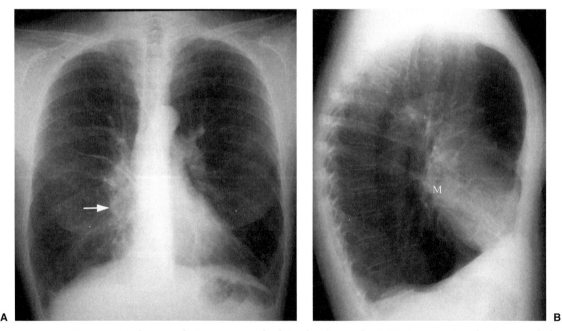

Figure 7.2 Hilar mass better seen on the lateral radiograph. *A.* Posteroanterior chest x-ray: slight enlargement of right lower hilum *(arrow)*. *B.* Lateral chest x-ray: mass (M) more easily appreciated.

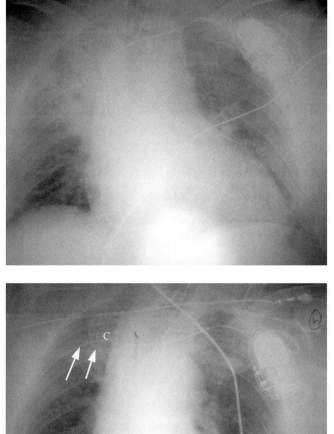

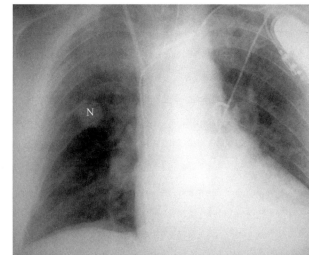

Figure 7.3 The case of the missing lung nodule. *A.* Anteroposterior chest x-ray 3-6: pulmonary edema but no obvious nodule. *B.* Anteroposterior chest x-ray 3-8: right upper lobe collapse (C), with elevation of the minor fissure *(arrows)*, but no obvious nodule. *C.* Anteroposterior chest x-ray 3-9: the nodule (N) is finally visible.

To broach the topic of malpractice, a discussion of missed lung cancer (as the flip side of lung cancer detection) is in order. Malpractice has well-defined legal elements (such as duty, breach of duty, negligence, and injury), but jurors are not legal scholars. Jurors may sympathize with young attractive plaintiffs who have obviously suffered from illness; the suffering may not be related to the radiologist in any way. The radiologist is particularly at risk because the images that reveal the radiologist's "mistake" (important note: mistake does *not* equal malpractice) are generally available for review, and abnormalities seem to grow before your very eyes in retrospect.

I offer the following ideas for defense of alleged radiologic malpractice in missed lung cancer:

1. Small lesions: It could not be diagnosed prospectively (usually easy to get supportive expert witness testimony, although it is also easy for the plaintiff to hire someone to testify that they could see this lesion).
2. Larger lesions: It did not affect the outcome (especially worth consideration with bad cell types like small cell and large cell carcinoma).
3. The "Mayo Clinic" defense: In a study (8) of CXR screening for lung cancer at 4-month intervals, two or three experts in pulmonary disease (at least one a radiologist)

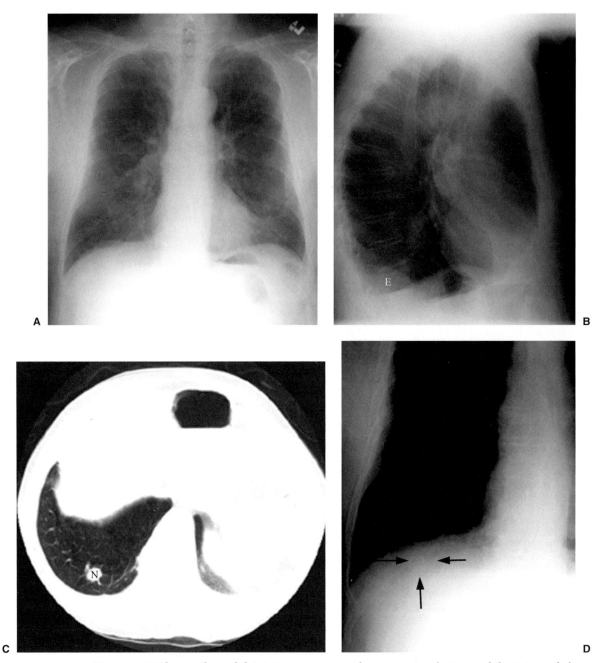

Figure 7.4 Where is the nodule? *A.* Posteroanterior chest x-ray: no obvious nodule. *B.* Lateral chest x-ray: posterior right hemidiaphragmatic eventration (E), but no nodule. *C.* Computed tomography: right lower lobe nodule (N) below dome of right hemidiaphragm not seen on chest x-ray. *D.* Close-up of right lung base in *A* with adjusted viewing parameters: with hindsight and ample imagination, the nodule is possibly visible *(arrows).*

reviewed radiographs specifically for evidence of lung cancer in high-risk patients (older males who were heavy smokers). When cancer was detected, in 45 of 50 peripheral lung cancers and in 30 of 42 central lung cancers the lesion could also be seen in retrospect on at least one earlier CXR; four were visible on radiographs dating back at least 2 years. Their conclusion: "Our results suggest that failure to detect a small pulmonary nodule on a single CXR should not constitute negligence or be the basis for malpractice litigation."

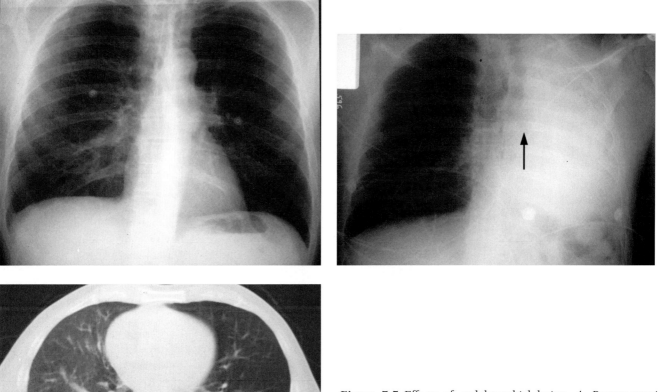

Figure 7.5 Effects of endobronchial lesion. *A.* Posteroanterior chest x-ray: slightly increased lucency of left lung compared with right, with fewer vessels per unit area in that lung, compatible with air trapping distal to an endobronchial mass. *B.* Computed tomography of lower lungs: lucency of left lung and sparsity of left lung vessels more clearly revealed. *C.* Anteroposterior chest x-ray 2 weeks after *A*: left lung collapse with bronchial cutoff *(arrow).*

4. The "Where's Waldo?" defense: In an elegant letter to the editor of the journal *Radiology* (9), Dr. Ronald Hendrix pointed out the need for an analogy to explain to members of a lay audience how a well-qualified careful radiologist could ever miss a lesion that they now easily see on a radiograph. He likened this to the search for Waldo in the series of "Where's Waldo?" books. As Dr. Hendrix pointed out, everyone understands how hard it can be to locate Waldo in a given illustration. However, once he has been found, Waldo is incredibly obvious when the same illustration is reviewed. Dr. Hendrix added that it is even harder to look for lung cancer (or any other radiographic finding) because, whereas Waldo is definitely present on every page of a "Where's Waldo" book, a radiograph may be normal (in other words, it may contain no radiographic findings *or* Waldos).

I offer the following advice to potential radiologists: If you cannot stand to make mistakes (or more to the point, if you do not want proof of your errors to be part of the permanent medical record), choose another specialty.

Compared with the CXR, computed tomography (CT) is more sensitive for identifying lung nodules; unfortunately, this is accompanied by decreased specificity. Many small nodules detected only at CT are scars, intrapulmonary lymph nodes, or other nonspecific benign lesions. Unfortunately, some are early lung cancers. This is the crux of the issue currently being addressed by trials of CT for lung cancer screening.

Cancer screening would certainly seem to make sense for the leading cause of cancer-related deaths in the United States. However, the biological characteristics of a neoplasm influence the utility of screening for that neoplasm in an at-risk population. Screening evaluates individuals who manifest no signs of disease; in lung cancer, the at-risk population consists of heavy smokers. For effective screening, the following must apply:

1. Disease must be identifiable before symptoms develop.
2. Earlier treatment of the disease must be shown to have more effect than later treatment.
3. Benefits to the few treated for disease must outweigh the expense and harm to the screened population caused by the screening process.
4. To be considered effective, screening needs to demonstrate a decrease in the mortality of a given disease.

Certain biases need to be considered when evaluating the effectiveness of screening. *Lead time bias* refers to the fact that earlier detection of disease in a screened population compared with a control group makes it seem that patients live longer in the screened group, even if they die at the same age as control group patients with the same disease. *Length time bias* means that slowly growing tumors have a longer detectable preclinical phase than rapidly growing tumors and are therefore more likely to be identified at screening. *Overdiagnosis bias* is the failure to correct for preclinical disease that would not have produced signs or symptoms before the subject would have died of other causes. In general, a large number of subjects (more than 500) and a long observation time (usually more than 5 years) are required to validate the utility of screening.

Four large randomized trials (10–13) of lung cancer screening in the past 30 years (before the advent of CT screening) failed to detect a statistically significant decrease in lung cancer mortality. This subject is currently being reassessed with the addition of chest CT. CT screening for lung cancer certainly allows identification of disease before symptoms are present. However, it is not yet certain that this can be done cost-effectively, particularly because so many detected nodules turn out to be benign (14,15). In fact, the possibility that screening can even prove harmful has also been raised (16). It is probably best to describe lung cancer screening as a technique that is unproven but not yet discredited.

> Lung cancer screening is currently best described as unproven but not yet discredited.

DIAGNOSIS

Lung cancer often manifests as a single nodule or mass. Diagnosis or exclusion of lung cancer starts with an assessment of the radiographic features of the detected nodule or mass. A lesion is generally considered benign if it remains stable for at least 2 years. Thus, the single best test of a lesion's malignant potential is comparison with old films. This simple fact is so often ignored that it must need more emphasis. Apart from its greater diagnostic accuracy, comparison with old films also results in lower expense (subject to the next rate increase from the U.S. Postal Service) and *much* less radiation than alternative imaging strategies for assessing a demonstrated lung nodule.

When old films are unavailable, the lesion can be assessed for benign radiographic features. Calcification may be helpful if there is a benign pattern of calcification (diffuse, central, "popcorn," or concentric) (Fig. 7.6); other patterns of calcification are unrevealing as to a lesion's malignant potential (Fig. 7.7). Another suggestive finding of benign disease is "rabbit ears" (a feeding artery and draining vein) in a pulmonary arteriovenous malformation (Fig. 7.8). Thin-section CT may be more helpful in this setting, because it may demonstrate calcification that escapes CXR detection (Fig. 7.9), and it can also reveal fat within a lesion (diagnostic of hamartoma) (Fig. 7.10). There has been some enthusiasm for CT assessment of nodule enhancement, with lung cancers enhancing more than benign nodules. Early CT follow-up of a lesion (sometimes in just a few weeks) has also been applied to this issue.

Most of these approaches (apart from comparison with old films) have been superseded by positron emission tomography (PET). PET is the imaging equivalent of compar-

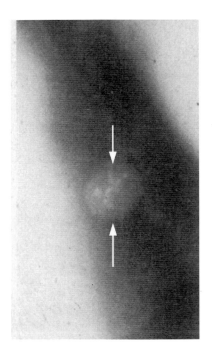

Figure 7.6 Hamartoma with popcorn calcification (*arrows*).

ison with old films, in that it allows assessment of the activity of a lesion, not just its morphology (Fig. 7.11). We still generally attempt thin-section CT in the assessment of a nodule, but if there is any remaining doubt, PET is generally the next step. We use it increasingly frequently in the assessment of lung nodules, with three caveats:

Assessment of a lesion's activity (via PET or comparison with old films) is the crux of imaging a lung nodule or mass.

1. A lesion must be 7 mm or greater in size for accurate PET assessment.
2. Bronchoalveolar carcinoma may be PET negative.
3. PET has false positives (inflammatory lesions, a particular problem in some parts of the country with abundant fungi such as histoplasmosis or coccidioidomycosis) and false negatives (well-differentiated carcinomas, particularly adenocarcinoma).

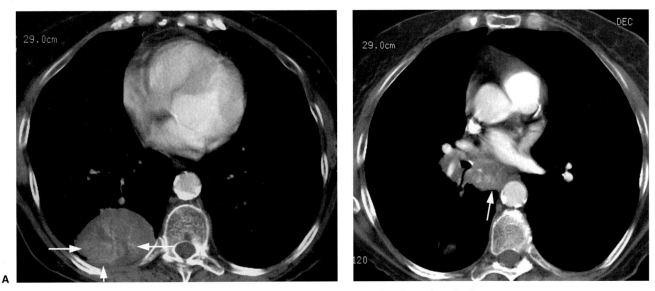

Figure 7.7 Calcified non–small cell lung cancer. *A.* Computed tomography through right lower lobe mass: irregular calcifications throughout (*arrows*). *B.* Computed tomography through subcarinal lymph node metastases: similar calcifications (*arrow*).

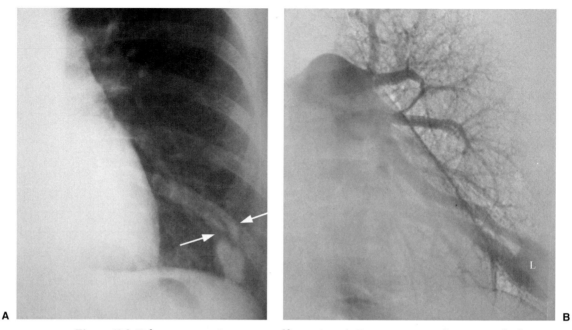

Figure 7.8 Pulmonary arteriovenous malformation. *A.* Posteroanterior chest x-ray: feeding artery and draining vein *(arrows)* resemble "rabbit ears." *B.* Digital subtraction angiography: vascular nature of lesion (L) confirmed.

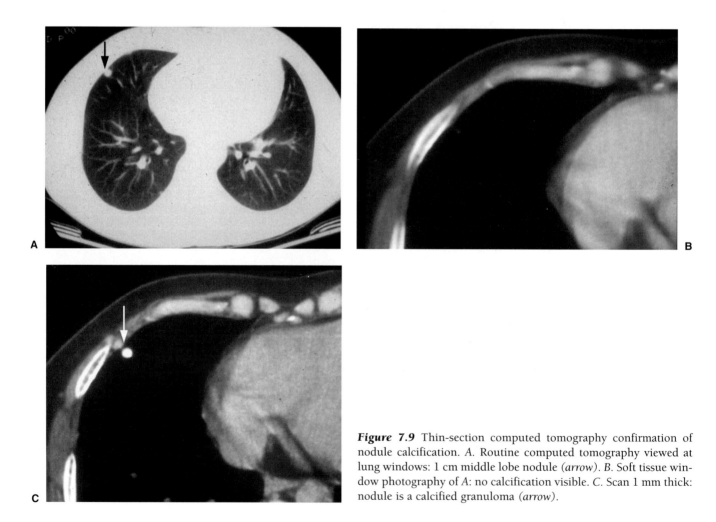

Figure 7.9 Thin-section computed tomography confirmation of nodule calcification. *A.* Routine computed tomography viewed at lung windows: 1 cm middle lobe nodule *(arrow)*. *B.* Soft tissue window photography of *A:* no calcification visible. *C.* Scan 1 mm thick: nodule is a calcified granuloma *(arrow)*.

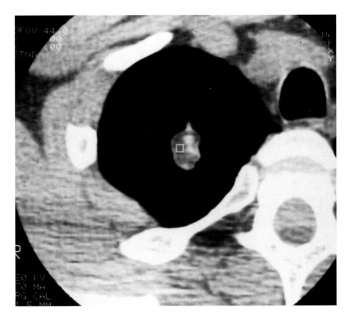

Figure 7.10 Hamartoma. Thin-section computed tomography demonstrates fat within the lesion (marked by *cursor*).

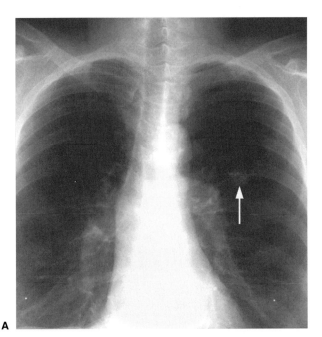

A

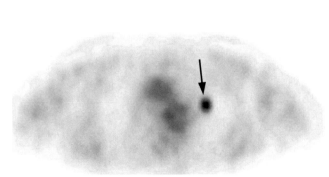

Figure 7.11 Adenocarcinoma of lung. *A*. Posteroanterior chest x-ray: poorly visible left lung nodule *(arrow)*. *B*. Projection and *(C)* axial positron emission tomography images: easily visible focus of uptake *(arrows)*. (Courtesy of Dr. Chuong Bui, Ann Arbor, MI.)

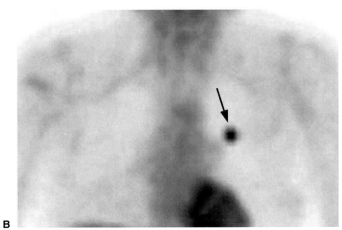

B

C

An important aspect of lung cancer diagnosis is a consideration of the typical CXR appearances of different cell types. The radiographic presentations are emphasized, along with a discussion of the demographics and other features of the various cell types. This is an approach whose merits have been championed by Dr. Michael McCarthy.

SOLITARY PULMONARY NODULE

Solitary pulmonary nodule (SPN) refers to a single nodular lesion in the lung, but the literature is inconsistent with regard to the upper size limit that is included. Most authors use 4 cm as a cutoff, above which the abnormality is considered a mass. Lung cancers and granulomas account for at least 80% of SPNs in most series. In Siegelman et al.'s classic article (17) on CT of the SPN, the literature review indicated that 54% of SPNs were granulomas and 28% were bronchogenic carcinomas or other primary malignancies. Combining two large recent series, 49% of 955 SPNs were malignant. In six of nine series from the early 1960s, more than 40% of SPNs were malignant.

In lung cancer, the model for this radiographic presentation is adenocarcinoma; other cell types that may manifest this pattern are squamous cell carcinoma and bronchoalveolar carcinoma. Adenocarcinoma is now the most common cell type of lung cancer, accounting for 30% to 35% of such cancers. It is associated with cigarette smoking but less strongly than squamous cell and small cell carcinoma. It is the typical cell type when cancer develops at the site of a previous scar ("scar carcinoma") and may also occur in the setting of pulmonary fibrosis.

> Most malignant solitary pulmonary nodules are adenocarcinoma, and adenocarcinoma usually presents as a solitary pulmonary nodule.

Most malignant SPNs are adenocarcinoma, and more than half of adenocarcinomas present as SPNs. Adenocarcinoma has an upper lobe predilection, occurring there in almost 70% of cases (Fig. 7.12). Early lymphogenous and hematogenous spread is typical of adenocarcinoma, although not invariably seen (Fig. 7.13), but cavitation is uncommon.

Lung cancer is generally morphologically distinct from pulmonary metastatic disease because the latter usually manifests as multiple nodules. In the setting of a previous extrapulmonary primary neoplasm, the relative likelihood that a new SPN is a solitary metas-

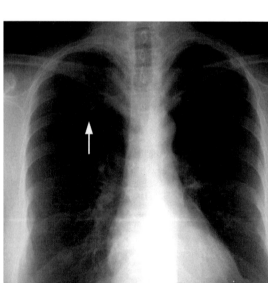

Figure 7.12 Adenocarcinoma as right upper lobe single pulmonary nodule *(arrow)*.

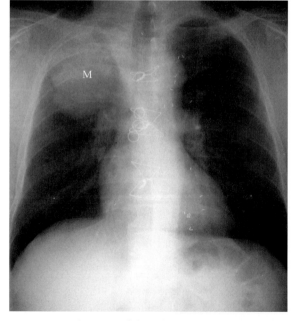

Figure 7.13 Right upper lobe adenocarcinoma. Mass (M) is 10.2 cm in size, but clinically and pathologically there was no evidence of spread (T2N0M0). In contrast, the 1.5-cm nodule in Fig. 7.12 presented with a brain metastasis (T1N0M1).

tasis or a new lung cancer depends on the previous primary (Box 7.1). In a CXR-based series from the 1970s (18), the odds sometimes favored a new lung primary. This was true of head and neck carcinoma (15.8:1), bladder carcinoma (8.3:1), and cervical carcinoma (6:1). In fact, with some primaries all malignant SPNs were lung cancers (prostate, 26 patients; stomach, 7 patients; esophagus, 4 patients; pancreas, 3 patients). With other primaries a solitary metastasis was more likely. This applied to soft tissue sarcoma (17.5:1), osteosarcoma (6.7:1), melanoma (4.1:1), and testicular carcinoma (2:1). With many common primaries the odds were far from definitive but favored lung cancer slightly, such as with breast carcinoma (1.7:1), colon carcinoma (1.4:1), renal cell carcinoma (1.2:1), and endometrial carcinoma (1.1:1). A more recent study addressed this issue in patients with SPNs demonstrated at CT (19). In this series breast carcinoma moved more definitively into the lung cancer camp, but the other observations were reconfirmed.

LARGE CENTRAL MASS

The models for this appearance are squamous cell carcinoma and small cell carcinoma, but large cell carcinoma and adenocarcinoma sometimes manifest this way. Squamous cell carcinoma, formerly the most common cell type of lung cancer, still accounts for 30% of cases. It is the cell type most likely to produce a parathormone-like hormone. Squamous cell carcinoma typically arises endobronchially. It is known for relentless local growth and is relatively locally invasive. Hematogenous dissemination tends to occur late in the course of disease.

Radiographically, squamous cell carcinoma most often presents with postobstructive findings of atelectasis or pneumonia (Fig. 7.14). Exophytic growth with or without (or else +/−) ipsilateral hilar lymph node metastases can result in the large central mass that we are discussing here, which is the second most common pattern of presentation (Fig. 7.15). Squamous cell carcinoma has significant heterogeneity of its radiographic appearance, with more than 25% presenting as a SPN. In fact, cavitation occurs in up to 20%, and

> Squamous cell carcinoma often arises endobronchially and is known for relentless local growth.

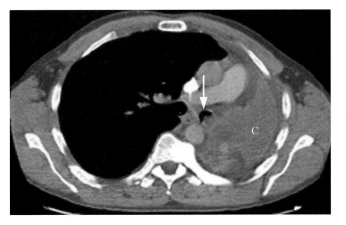

Figure 7.14 Endobronchial squamous cell carcinoma (*arrow*) presenting with collapse of the left upper lobe (C).

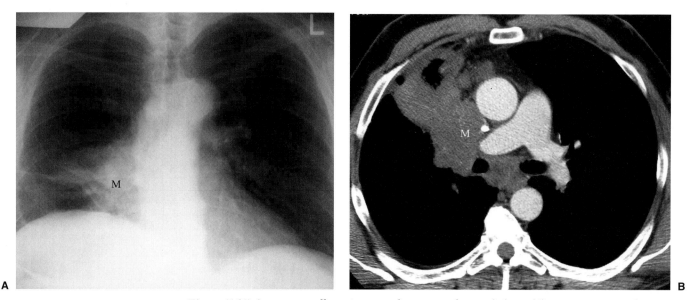

Figure 7.15 Squamous cell carcinoma as large central mass (M) on (*A*) posteroanterior chest x-ray and (*B*) computed tomography.

squamous is by far the most common cell type in the presence of a cavitary lesion (Fig. 7.16). An important simulator of lower lobe cavitary neoplasm is illustrated in Fig. 7.17.

Small cell carcinoma accounts for 20% to 25% of lung cancers. It is the cell type most likely to be associated with paraneoplastic syndromes. This includes hormonal syndromes in 14% of small cell patients, especially syndrome of inappropriate antidiuretic hormone (Fig. 7.18), Cushing syndrome, and other syndromes of less certain origin like Eaton-Lambert syndrome, a sort of reverse myasthenia gravis (at least at electromyography).

The large central mass of small cell carcinoma is often bigger, more multifocal, and more mediastinal than the large central mass of squamous cell carcinoma (which tends to

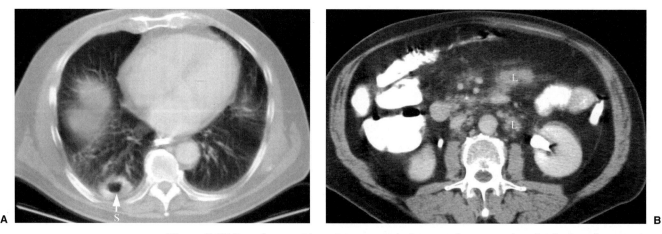

Figure 7.16 Lymphoma with cavitary mass. *A.* Computed tomography of right lung base: cavitary right lower lobe nodule is squamous cell carcinoma (S). *B.* Abdominal computed tomography: mesenteric and left paraaortic lymphoma (L).

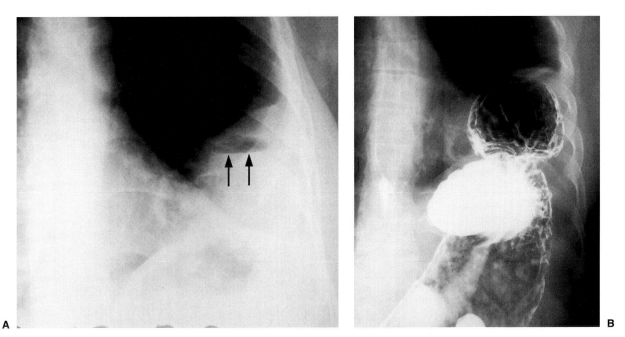

A   B

Figure 7.17 Apparent left basilar cavity. *A.* Posteroanterior chest x-ray: air–fluid level *(arrows)* in left basilar abnormality. Any "cavity" not clearly separable from the diaphragm should be considered a bowel loop until proven otherwise. *B.* Barium swallow: diaphragmatic hernia containing a portion of stomach.

be centered in a hilum). Although 15% of small cell carcinomas are thought to arise peripherally, even in those patients hilar and mediastinal lymph node metastases often grow much more quickly than the lung lesion (Fig. 7.19). Tumor necrosis is common, but cavitation is rare. Because small cell carcinoma is often quite responsive to radiation and chemotherapy, the result can be disappearance of a mass in a relatively short period of time (Fig. 7.20).

Small cell carcinoma generally manifests predominantly in hilar and mediastinal lymph nodes.

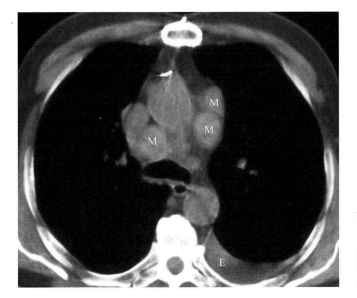

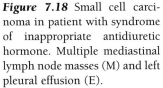

Figure 7.18 Small cell carcinoma in patient with syndrome of inappropriate antidiuretic hormone. Multiple mediastinal lymph node masses (M) and left pleural effusion (E).

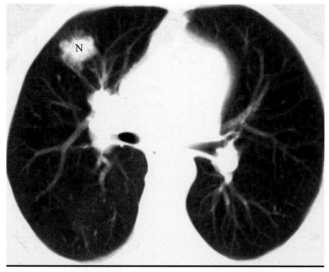

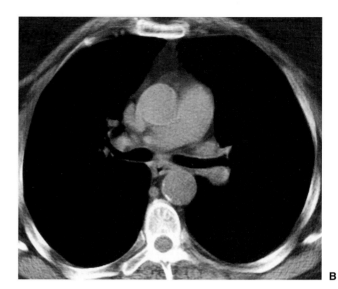

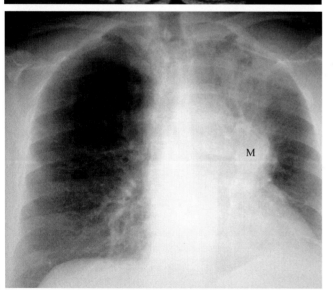

Figure 7.19 Small cell carcinoma with rapid growth of lymph node metastases. *A.* Computed tomography 1-13: lung nodule (N) is small cell carcinoma. *B.* Computed tomography 1-13: no abnormal thoracic lymph nodes. *C.* Computed tomography 3-26: marked interval enlargement of right hilar, paratracheal, and subcarinal lymph nodes (N).

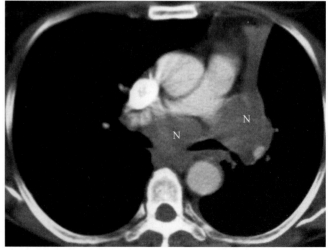

Figure 7.20 Small cell carcinoma with rapid response. *A.* Posteroanterior chest x-ray 12-22: central left lung mass (M) with left upper lobe collapse. *B.* Computed tomography confirms small cell carcinoma involving left hilar and subcarinal lymph nodes (N).

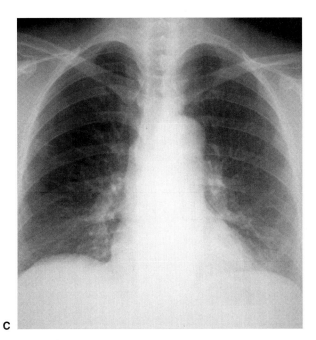

C

Figure 7.20 (continued) C. Posteroanterior chest x-ray 1-16: after radiation and chemotherapy, 25-day follow-up chest x-ray is normal.

LARGE PERIPHERAL MASS

The model for a large peripheral mass is large cell carcinoma. It is sometimes a presentation of squamous cell carcinoma and adenocarcinoma. Large cell carcinoma accounts for 10% to 15% of lung cancers. This rapidly growing neoplasm tends to early lymphogenous and hematogenous spread, with resultant poor 5-year survival rates. It is the most common cause of a malignant peripheral mass larger than 6 cm in size.

Slightly more than half of large cell carcinomas appear as a peripheral mass (Fig. 7.21). Most of the remainder are large central masses. As with small cell carcinoma, necrosis is common, but cavitation is rare.

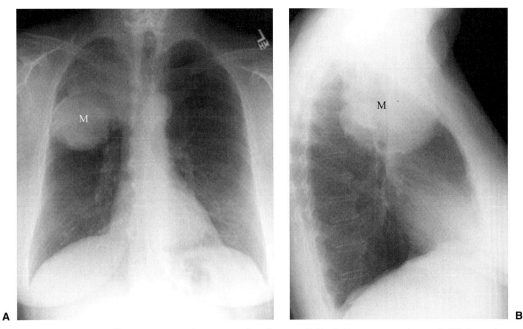

A   B

Figure 7.21 Large cell carcinoma as large peripheral mass (M). *A.* Posteroanterior and *(B)* lateral chest x-ray.

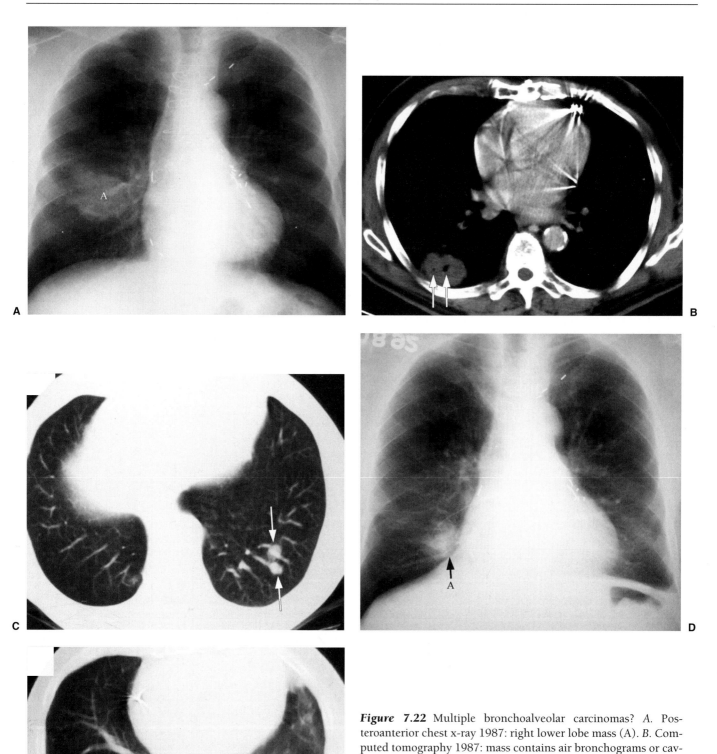

***Figure* 7.22** Multiple bronchoalveolar carcinomas? *A.* Posteroanterior chest x-ray 1987: right lower lobe mass (A). *B.* Computed tomography 1987: mass contains air bronchograms or cavitation *(arrows)*. *C.* Computed tomography 1989: two left lower lobe nodules *(arrows)*. *D.* Posteroanterior chest x-ray and *(E)* computed tomography 1992: chronic right lower lung airspace disease (A). These are all manifestations of bronchoalveolar carcinoma in the same patient, a common pitfall that sometimes causes radiologists to overestimate the frequency of disease "in their own experience."

PERIPHERAL INFILTRATE

The model for this mode of presentation is bronchoalveolar carcinoma. Adenocarcinoma may instead manifest this way, which is not surprising given that bronchoalveolar carcinoma is a subtype of adenocarcinoma (but with distinctive pathologic and radiographic findings). Bronchoalveolar carcinoma is responsible for 2% to 5% of lung cancers, although recent articles suggest that it is increasing in incidence. My own experience at Multidisciplinary Thoracic Oncology Conference emphatically corroborates the trend of rising incidence (Fig. 7.22). Bronchoalveolar carcinoma arises from bronchiolar epithelium and type 2 alveolar cells. This cell type has no relationship to cigarette smoking, but there is a relationship to pulmonary fibrosis in general and scleroderma lung in particular.

Bronchoalveolar carcinoma has a variable growth rate, but it is sometimes quite indolent. SPN is the most common presentation of bronchoalveolar carcinoma, and disease has been documented to progress from SPN to focal or diffuse alveolar disease. Peripheral infiltrate is the second most common manifestation of bronchoalveolar carcinoma. Air bronchograms are typically a prominent finding, as opposed to postobstructive alveolar disease distal to a central obstructing lesion. When infiltrate is present the patient may demonstrate bronchorrhea, a symptom suggestive of this diagnosis. Indolent growth results in a relatively good prognosis when SPNs are bronchoalveolar carcinoma; once disease spreads in the lungs (a typical pattern of dissemination), the prognosis is grim.

> Bronchoalveolar carcinoma accounts for 2% to 5% of lung cancers and appears to be increasing in incidence.

MULTIPLE PULMONARY NODULES

This pattern, more typical of metastatic disease from an extrathoracic primary, is also seen with bronchoalveolar carcinoma. Less frequently, adenocarcinoma may present in this fashion. Multiple nodules are the presenting radiographic appearance in up to 10% of patients with bronchoalveolar carcinoma. This pattern was initially thought to reflect multifocal origin of disease, but it is now believed to be secondary to aerogenous and/or hematogenous spread from one focus (Fig. 7.23). Disease is occasionally cavitary. Although it can be difficult to distinguish between prominent air bronchograms and cavitation in some patients (Fig. 7.22B), in others there is no such difficulty (Fig. 7.24). Bronchoalveolar carcinoma is the second most likely cell type to explain a cavitary mass (after squamous cell carcinoma) (Box 7.2).

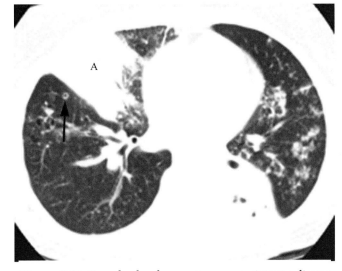

Figure 7.23 Bronchoalveolar carcinoma as airspace disease (A) and multiple nodules, some cavitary (*arrow*).

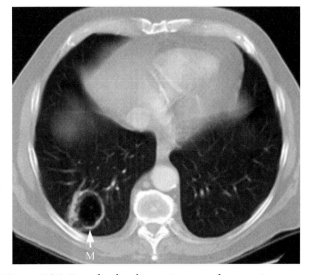

Figure 7.24 Bronchoalveolar carcinoma as large cavitary mass (M).

Box 7.2: Summary: Morphology of Lung Cancer

Solitary pulmonary nodule
    Model: adenocarcinoma
    Others: squamous, bronchoalveolar
Large central mass
    Model: squamous, small cell
    Others: large cell, adenocarcinoma
Large peripheral mass
    Model: large cell
    Others: squamous, adenocarcinoma
Peripheral infiltrate
    Model: bronchoalveolar

Others: adenocarcinoma
Multiple pulmonary nodules
    Model: bronchoalveolar
    Others: adenocarcinoma
Cavity
    Model: squamous
    Others: bronchoalveolar
Postobstructive volume loss
    Model: squamous
    Others: small cell

STAGING

Patients with limited small cell lung cancer receive radiation and chemotherapy, whereas those with extensive disease receive only chemotherapy.

Staging differs significantly between small cell carcinoma and non–small cell lung cancer. Small cell carcinoma is generally considered inoperable, because more than 70% have metastasized at the time of diagnosis. It is staged as limited or extensive, depending on whether disease is confined to a single radiation port (limited) or not (extensive). In some patients with rather widespread disease confined to one radiation port, the resultant morbidity from the amount of lung that would have to be radiated leads to treatment of the patient as if disease had been extensive. The differentiation of limited versus extensive disease is mirrored in a difference in therapy (which is after all the intent of a staging scheme); patients with limited disease receive radiation and chemotherapy, whereas patients with extensive disease receive only chemotherapy. Patients with limited disease have a higher rate of disease remission and a higher cure rate, but overall this is still a terrible disease to have.

In non–small cell lung cancer, the primary goal of staging is to determine resectability. Although advances in radiation and chemotherapy have resulted in significant improvements in response to therapy and even sometimes cure, surgical resection remains the best chance for cure. The staging scheme that is most widely used is the TNM system of the American Joint Committee on Cancer, revised in 1997 (20). This scheme is detailed in Table 7.1. In staging, the break between resectable and unresectable disease generally occurs between stages IIIA and IIIB. Thus, it is critical to detail the extent of mediastinal spread (differentiating ipsilateral mediastinal disease, stage IIIA, from contralateral mediastinal spread, stage IIIB) and to exclude more distant metastases (stage IV).

CXR evaluation is of limited utility in staging lung cancer. The problem is very low sensitivity. CXR evaluation is probably most helpful in the setting of thoracic skeletal metastases; CXR is sometimes better at demonstrating such lesions than CT. Mediastinal lymph node enlargement and contralateral lung nodules or hilar lymph nodes may also be suspected from the CXR, but CT evaluation will virtually always be far better.

The perceived value of CT staging has gone up and down over the past 20 years—not figuratively, but literally. In the 1970s CT was considered a poor staging tool, an apt reflection of the quality of scanners then available, the limited options for vascular enhancement, variable scanning techniques, and the more rudimentary knowledge of thoracic lymph node anatomy of that era. In the 1980s a number of studies (21,22) with better CT equipment, bolus administration of intravenous contrast, standardized contiguous scanning, and improved appreciation of nodal anatomy demonstrated that CT staging of mediastinal lymph nodes was highly sensitive (in the 90% range) but not specific (in the 65% range). Interestingly, CT at this time was not being uniformly applied to lung cancer

Table 7.1: American Joint Committee Staging Scheme

Primary tumor (T)

Tx — Primary tumor cannot be assessed or tumor proven by presence of malignant cells in the sputum or bronchial washings but not visualized by bronchoscopy or CT.

T0 — No evidence of primary tumor.

Tis — Carcinoma *in situ.*

T1 — Tumor 3 cm or less in greatest dimension, surrounded by lung or visceral pleura, without bronchoscopic evidence of invasion more proximal than the lobar bronchus[a] (i.e., not in main bronchus).

T2 — Tumor with *any* of the following features of size or extent: a) More than 3 cm in greatest dimension. b) Involves main bronchus, 2 cm or more distal to the carina. c) Invades the visceral pleura. d) Associated with atelectasis or obstructive pneumonitis that extends to the hilar region but does not involve the entire lung.

T3 — Tumor of any size that directly invades any of the following: chest wall (including superior sulcus tumor), diaphragm, mediastinal pleura, parietal pericardium; or tumor in the main bronchus less than 2 cm distal to the carina but without involvement of the carina; or associated atelectasis or obstructive pneumonitis of the entire lung.

T4 — Tumor of any size that invades any of the following: mediastinum, heart, great vessels, trachea, esophagus, vertebral body, carina; separate tumor nodule(s) in the same lobe; or tumor with a malignant pleural effusion.[b]

Regional lymph nodes (N)

NX — Regional lymph nodes cannot be assessed.

N0 — No regional lymph node metastases.

N1 — Metastases to ipsilateral peribronchial and/or ipsilateral hilar lymph nodes and intrapulmonary nodes involved by direct extension of the primary tumor.

N2 — Metastases to ipsilateral mediastinal and/or subcarinal lymph node(s).

N3 — Metastasis in contralateral mediastinal, contralateral hilar, ipsilateral or contralateral scalene or supraclavicular lymph nodes.

Metastases (M)

MX — Distant metastases cannot be assessed.

M0 — No distant metastases.

M1 — Distant metastases present (includes synchronous separate nodule(s) in a different lobe).

Stage grouping

Occult	TX	N0	M0
Stage 0	Tis	N0	M0
Stage IA	T1	N0	M0
Stage IB	T2	N0	M0
Stage IIA	T1	N1	M0
Stage IIB	T2	N1	M0
	T3	N0	M0
Stage IIIA	T3	N1	M0
	T1	N2	M0
	T2	N2	M0
	T3	N2	M0
Stage IIIB	Any T	N3	M0
	T4	Any N	M0
Stage V	Any T	Any N	M1

[a]The uncommon superficial tumor of any size with its invasive component limited to the bronchial wall, which may extend proximal to the main bronchus, is also classified as T1.

[b]Most pleural effusions associated with lung cancer are due to tumor. However, there are a few patients in whom multiple cytopathologic examinations of pleural fluid are negative for tumor. In these cases, fluid is nonbloody and is not an exudate. When these elements and clinical judgment dictate that the effusion is not related to the tumor, the effusion should be excluded as a staging element and the patient should be staged T1, T2, or T3.

CT, computed tomography.

From Mountain CF. Revision in the international staging system for staging lung cancer. *Chest* 1997;111:1710–1717, with permission.

patients for the purposes of staging. By the 1990s, several large studies (23,24) indicated that CT staging was not actually sensitive or specific (in the 50% range for both). Surprisingly, with CT's reputation in shambles, virtually every patient diagnosed with lung cancer now undergoes CT staging.

The fact is that CT remains the workhorse of lung cancer staging. Although it is not clear why CT sensitivity and specificity are no better than flipping a coin, most decisions regarding surgery, radiation, and chemotherapy are based on CT data. It may be that CT misses (such as metastases to normal-size lymph nodes) (25) would not change the therapeutic approach, even if they were appreciated beforehand. CT has the important advantage of evaluating numerous potential sites of metastatic disease throughout the lower neck, chest, and upper abdomen, and a few words about some of them follows:

- Thoracic lymph nodes: 1 cm in short axis should be used as the threshold.
- Lungs: CT is very sensitive for detecting small nodules but is not at all specific.
- Adrenals: Many detected nodules are non-hyperfunctioning adenomas; dedicated adrenal CT can be helpful for distinguishing benign from malignant (26,27).
- Liver: CT again is sensitive and somewhat able to characterize lesions (such as cysts and hemangiomas); small lesions may still be problematic, and hepatic magnetic resonance imaging can be helpful as a problem-solving tool.
- Bones: CT is generally not very good at detecting or characterizing skeletal lesions, although careful attention to the bones sometimes yields critical information. Radionuclide bone scan is far preferable.

CT is the workhorse for lung cancer staging, but more and more patients are also undergoing PET.

When CT detects a single questionable finding of potential importance for subsequent therapy, a variety of imaging tools may be called upon for more definitive diagnosis, as noted above (e.g., adrenal CT, hepatic magnetic resonance imaging, radionuclide bone scan). However, more and more the next step turns out to be PET (28). This is particularly helpful in a patient with several questionable findings or for further characterization of borderline or mildly enlarged thoracic lymph nodes. Currently, it seems that almost one-fourth of our lung cancer patients have PET as part of the staging process. However, a patient with no evidence of distant spread at CT will generally go directly to surgery without PET. The need for other imaging tests (such as head CT or magnetic resonance imaging) will depend on the cell type and the presence or absence of symptoms.

The best measure of the final product of staging is probably the satisfaction of the thoracic surgeon. Surgeons in general do not like to operate on patients only to discover that the extent of disease is far greater than previously appreciated, necessitating surgical closure without cancer resection (apparently, only attorneys truly appreciate "open and shut cases"). Surgeons in general are not shy about expressing their opinions, and we have seldom encountered surgeons who were in particular shy about telling us when our radiographic interpretations were problematic. It probably bespeaks their satisfaction with the current imaging approach to diagnosis and staging of lung cancer that our surgeons have not complained of an increasing number of so-called staging thoracotomies.

With the current approach some limitations should be acknowledged. We are generally poor at detecting local extension of disease, such as chest wall or mediastinal invasion. Chest wall invasion generally does not change resectability, although it changes the extent of the surgical procedure. It is therefore probably best to suggest the possibility of pleural or chest wall involvement whenever there is extensive contact between tumor and pleura, localized pleural thickening, or gross abnormality of adjacent chest wall structures. As for mediastinal involvement, some patients with minimal contact between tumor and mediastinum cannot be resected (Fig. 7.25); in others, tumor that appears to invade mediastinum at imaging is easily peeled off the mediastinal pleura at surgery (Fig. 7.26). Not all examples of mediastinal invasion are so equiv-

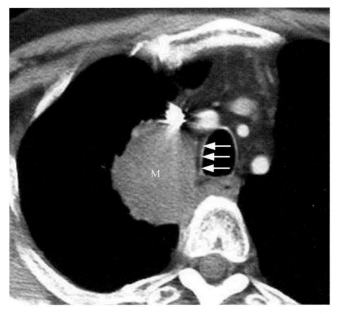

Figure 7.25 Unresectable lung cancer because of mediastinal invasion. Despite an apparent fat plane *(arrows)*, mass (M) could not be separated from mediastinum.

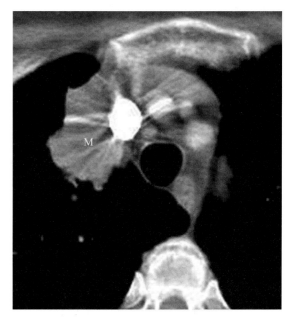

Figure 7.26 Resectable lung cancer. Despite apparent mediastinal involvement, mass (M) readily peeled away from mediastinum at surgery.

ocal (Fig. 7.27). CT after introduction of pleural air (artificial pneumothorax) has been suggested to solve this vexing problem. However, pleural adhesions can simulate mediastinal invasion by neoplasm. Because surgical resection provides the best hope for cure of disease, it is probably best to give the patient the benefit of the doubt whenever uncertainty remains.

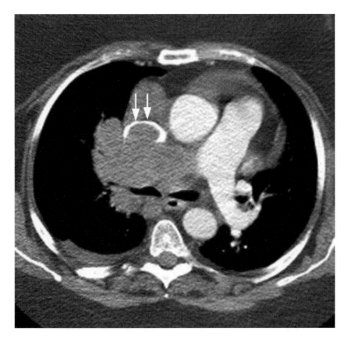

Figure 7.27 Gross mediastinal invasion, with involvement of superior vena cava *(arrows)*.

REFERENCES

1. Boucot KR, Cooper DA, Weiss W, et al. Cigarettes, cough and cancer of the lung. *JAMA* 1966;196:985–990.
2. Janerich DT, Thompson WD, Varela LR, et al. Lung cancer and exposure to tobacco smoke in the household. *N Engl J Med* 1990;323:632–636.
3. Finkelstein MM. Mortality among employees of an Ontario asbestos cement factory. *Am Rev Respir Dis* 1984;129:754–761.
4. Bejui-Thivolet F, Liagre N, Chignol MC, et al. Detection of human papilloma virus DNA in squamous bronchial metaplasia and squamous cell carcinoma of the lung by in situ hybridization using biotinylated probes in paraffin-embedded specimens. *Hum Pathol* 1990;21:111–116.
5. Butler AE, Colby TV, Weiss L, et al. Lymphoepithelioma-like carcinoma of the lung. *Am J Surg Pathol* 1989;13:632–639.
6. Roumm AD, Medsger TA Jr. Cancer and systemic sclerosis: an epidemiologic study. *Arthritis Rheum* 1985;28:1336–1340.
7. Neuberger JS. Residential radon exposure and lung cancer: an overview of published series. *Cancer Detect Prev* 1991;15:435–443.
8. Muhm JR, Miller WE, Fontana RS, et al. Lung cancer detected during a screening program using four-month chest radiographs. *Radiology* 1983;148:609–615.
9. Hendrix RW. In defense of a missed lesion. *Radiology* 1995;195:578–579.
10. Frost JK, Ball WC, Levin ML, et al. Early lung cancer detection: results of the initial (prevalence) radiologic and cytologic screening in the Johns Hopkins Study. *Am Rev Respir Dis* 1984;130: 549–554.
11. Flehinger BJ, Melamed MR, Zama MB, et al. Early lung cancer detection: results of the initial (prevalence) radiologic and cytologic screening in the Memorial Sloan-Kettering study. *Am Rev Respir Dis* 1984;130:555–560.
12. Fontana RS, Sanderson DR, Taylor WF, et al. Early lung cancer detection: results of the initial (prevalence) radiologic and cytologic screening in the Mayo Clinic study. *Am Rev Respir Dis* 1984;130:561–565.
13. Kubik A, Polak J. Lung cancer detection: results of a randomized prospective study in Czechoslovakia. *Cancer* 1986;57:2427–2437.
14. Patz EF Jr, Black WC, Goodman PC. CT screening for lung cancer: not ready for routine practice. *Radiology* 2001;221:587–591.
15. Miettinen OS, Henschke CI. CT screening for lung cancer: coping with nihilistic recommendations. *Radiology* 2001;221:592–596.
16. Reich J. Hazards of lung cancer screening. *Chest* 2001;119:659–660.
17. Siegelman SS, Zerhouni EA, Leo FP, et al. CT of the solitary pulmonary nodule. *AJR Am J Roentgenol* 1980;135:1–13.
18. Cahan WG, Shah HP, Castro EB. Benign solitary lung lesions in patients with cancer. *Ann Surg* 1978;187:241–244.
19. Quint LE, Park CH, Iannettoni MD. Solitary pulmonary nodules in patients with extrapulmonary neoplasms. *Radiology* 2000;217:257–261.
20. Mountain CF. Revision in the international staging system for staging lung cancer. *Chest* 1997; 111:1710–1717.
21. Glazer GM, Orringer MB, Gross BH, et al. The mediastinum in non-small cell lung cancer: CT-surgical correlation. *AJR Am J Roentgenol* 1984;142:1101–1105.
22. Lewis JW Jr, Pearlberg JL, Beute GH, et al. Can computed tomography of the chest stage lung cancer? Yes and no. *Ann Thorac Surg* 1990;49:591–596.
23. Webb WR, Gatsonis C, Zerhouni EA, et al. CT and MR imaging in staging non-small cell carcinoma: report of the Radiologic Diagnostic Oncology group. *Radiology* 1991;178:705–713.
24. McLoud TC, Bourgouin PM, Greenberg RW, et al. Bronchogenic carcinoma: analysis of staging in the mediastinum with CT by correlative lymph node mapping and sampling. *Radiology* 1992; 182:319–323.
25. Gross BH, Glazer GM, Orringer MB, et al. Bronchogenic carcinoma metastatic to normal-sized lymph nodes: frequency and significance. *Radiology* 1988;166:71–74.
26. Korobkin M, Brodeur FJ, Yutzy GY, et al. Differentiation of adrenal adenomas from nonadenomas using CT attenuation values. *AJR Am J Roentgenol* 1996;166:531–536.
27. Korobkin M, Brodeur FJ, Francis IR, et al. Delayed enhanced CT for differentiation of benign from malignant adrenal masses. *Radiology* 1996;200:737–742.
28. Pieterman RM, van Putten JWG, Meuzelaar JJ, et al. Preoperative staging of non-small-cell lung cancer with positron-emission tomography. *N Engl J Med* 2000;343:254–261.

OTHER THORACIC NEOPLASMS

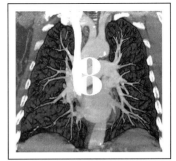

- Tracheobronchial Neoplasms
- Benign Tracheobronchial Neoplasms
- Malignant Tracheobronchial Neoplasms
- Benign Pulmonary Neoplasms
- Malignant Pulmonary Neoplasms
- Lymphoma and Lymphoproliferative Diseases
- Metastatic Disease
- Esophageal Carcinoma

This chapter covers a variety of benign and malignant thoracic neoplasms, arising with the airway, lung parenchyma, esophagus, and the lymphatic system, as well as metastases to the thorax. Lung cancer was discussed in Chapter 7, pleural neoplasms are discussed in Chapter 17, and the rare tumors of the vascular system are discussed briefly in Chapters 18, 20, and 21. A full discussion of all these neoplasms could easily be the topic of an entire text unto itself. What you will read here is a discussion of the more common of these entities and, when possible, specific imaging features that can be helpful in distinguishing one from another.

TRACHEOBRONCHIAL NEOPLASMS

Benign and malignant tracheobronchial neoplasms are rare and vary widely histologically. When they occur in the trachea, they may present with a nonproductive cough due to irritation, hemoptysis if they bleed, or wheezing and/or dyspnea due to airway obstruction. When they occur in the bronchi, they may also cause postobstructive pulmonary infection. Recurrent infection, especially within the same lobe or segment, is suggestive of an endobronchial lesion.

Tracheobronchial neoplasms often present with stridor and wheezing.

On chest radiographs, lobar or segmental airspace disease, obstructive pneumonitis, or atelectasis may be seen. Abscess or bronchiectasis may also develop when the obstruction is longstanding. Endobronchial lesions may create a ball–valve phenomenon, with an open airway at inspiration and a closed airway in early expiration, creating hyperinflation and obstructive emphysema distal to the occlusion. Although sometimes visible on an inspiratory radiograph, this phenomenon is best recognized on expiratory or ipsilateral decubitus radiographs. The tumor itself is uncommonly identified on the chest radiograph; however, the tumor, extent of tumor spread, and associated findings are readily identified on computed tomography (CT). Characteristically, the recognition of malignant lesions is based on the following triad:

1. Abnormal or obstructed airways;
2. A central mass, causing distinct bulging of the proximal contour of the collapsed lobe or segment;
3. Differential enhancement of tumor versus collapsed peripheral lung after administration of intravenous contrast (1).

CT with multiplanar reconstructions is the preferred imaging modality for evaluating airway lesions (Chapter 16). Inspiratory and expiratory CT examinations are usually performed to evaluate the impact of the lesion on the airway during the respiratory cycle. Intravenous contrast is usually administered for better evaluation of the neoplasm with

Table 8.1: Benign Tracheobronchial Neoplasms

Epithelial tumors	Smooth muscle tumors
Papilloma	Leiomyoma
Squamous cell papilloma	Skeletal muscle tumors
Adenoma	Cartilaginous tumors
Soft tissue	Chondroma
Vascular tumors	Osteogenic tumors
Hemangiomas	Neurogenic tumors
Hemangioendothelioma	Neurilemmoma
Fatty tumors	Neurofibroma
Lipoma	Miscellaneous tumors
Fibrous tumors	Granular cell tumor (myoblastoma)
Fibroma	Tumor-like lesions

Adapted from *Histological typing of lung tumors*, 2nd ed. Vol. 1. International Histological Classification of Tumors No. 1. Geneva: World Health Organization, 1981.

Table 8.2: Benign Pulmonary Neoplasms

Epithelial tumors	Neurogenic tumors
Papilloma	Neurilemmoma
Squamous cell papilloma	Neurofibroma
Soft tissue	Miscellaneous tumors
Vascular tumors	Clear cell tumor
Hemangioma	Benign germ cell tumor
Fatty tumors	Teratoma
Lipoma	Chemodectoma
Fibrous tumors	Sclerosing hemangioma
Fibroma	Tumor-like lesions
Smooth muscle tumors	Hamartoma
Leiomyoma	Amyloidoma
Skeletal muscle tumors	Endometriosis
Cartilaginous tumors	
Chondroma	
Osteogenic tumors	

Adapted from *Histological typing of lung tumors*, 2nd ed. Vol. 1. International Histological Classification of Tumors No. 1. Geneva: World Health Organization, 1981.

Table 8.3: Malignant Tracheobronchial Neoplasms

Epithelial tumors	Fibrous tumors
Squamous cell carcinoma	Smooth muscle tumors
Adenocarcinoma	Skeletal muscle tumors
Adenosquamous carcinoma	Cartilaginous tumors
Large cell carcinoma	Chondrosarcoma
Small cell carcinoma	Osteogenic tumors
Carcinoid	Neurogenic tumors
Bronchial gland carcinomas	Miscellaneous tumors
Soft tissue	Malignant lymphoma
Vascular tumors	Tumor-like lesions
Fatty tumors	Metastases

Adapted from *Histological typing of lung tumors*, 2nd ed. Vol. 1. International Histological Classification of Tumors No. 1. Geneva: World Health Organization, 1981.

Table 8.4: Malignant Pulmonary Neoplasms

Epithelial tumors	Skeletal muscle tumors
Bronchial gland carcinomas	Rhabdomyosarcoma
Adenocystic carcinoma	Cartilaginous tumors
Mucoepidermoid carcinoma	Chondrosarcoma
Soft tissue	Osteogenic tumors
Vascular tumors	Osteosarcoma
Hemangiopericytoma	Neurogenic tumors
Epithelioid hemangioendothelioma	Neurofibrosarcoma
Kaposi sarcoma	Miscellaneous tumors
Pulmonary angiosarcoma	Carcinosarcoma
Fatty tumors	Pulmonary blastoma
Fibrosarcoma	Askin tumor
Fibrous tumors	Malignant lymphoma
Fibrosarcoma	Plasmacytoma
Malignant fibrous histiocytoma	Lymphoma and lymphoproliferative
Smooth muscle tumors	disorders
Leiomyosarcoma	Metastases

Adapted from *Histological typing of lung tumors*, 2nd ed. Vol. 1. International Histological Classification of Tumors No. 1. Geneva: World Health Organization, 1981.

respect to adjacent mediastinal structures, particularly when there is extension outside the airway (2–4). Many of the benign and malignant tracheobronchial neoplasms can also arise within the small bronchi of lung parenchyma, and some tumors of the same cell type may arise from pleura, as can be seen from the overlap in Tables 8.1 to 8.4.

BENIGN TRACHEOBRONCHIAL NEOPLASMS

PAPILLOMA

Squamous papillomas are the most common laryngeal tumor in childhood. In 2% to 17% of patients they involve the tracheobronchial tree (Fig. 16.17). More rarely they involve the lung parenchyma. Lesions may be single or multiple, and the laryngeal disease may be present for up to 10 years before tracheobronchial disease occurs. Malignant transformation has been described and is extremely rare. Papillomas are much rarer in adults than children, usually presenting between the ages of 50 and 70 years. In adults, laryngeal papillomatosis is usually absent. As of 1991 only 59 adult cases were documented in the literature (3,5).

> Squamous cell papilloma is the most common laryngeal tumor in children.

The chest radiograph and CT findings of papilloma include pneumonia, bronchiectasis or abscess formation secondary to obstruction. When the lungs are involved, multiple, small, well-defined, scattered pulmonary nodules are found, which may cavitate.

LIPOMA

This is a benign tumor of adipose tissue or lipocytes. It has a mean age at onset in the fifth decade. They are more common in smokers than nonsmokers and more common in males than females, with a ratio of 5:1. Approximately 80% of lesions arise in the tracheobronchial tree and 20% within the lung parenchyma; 109 cases have been reported. Lesions are usually solitary, may be pedunculated, and have been reported up to 3 cm in size. Lipomas can also arise from the pleura (Fig. 17.25). Radiologically, findings are related to airway obstruction or the mass itself. On CT they demonstrate characteristic homogeneous fat attenuation. Liposarcoma is the malignant equivalent. It is very rare, with less than 10 cases reported. It usually occurs in the lung parenchyma and occurs equally in men and women. At CT, liposarcoma should be suspected when the fat attenuation mass also contains areas of soft tissue nodularity (5–7).

FIBROMA

Fibromas occur equally in males and females. They arise from within the bronchial wall, but may also arise within the lung parenchyma. They may grow to be very large. The endobronchial lesions may cause lobar or segmental atelectasis due to obstruction. They may also present as a solitary pulmonary nodule, often incidentally detected in asymptomatic individuals. Fibrosarcoma is the malignant equivalent of fibroma. Similarly, lesions may be endobronchial or lung parenchymal in location. The mean age at onset is 49 years. At CT, both fibroma and fibrosarcoma appear as soft tissue masses; the latter may have features of invasion and spread outside the airway, into or around other mediastinal structures (8,9).

CHONDROMA

Carney syndrome: bronchial chondromas, gastric leiomyoma, and extraadrenal paragangliomas.

Chondromas usually arise from the cartilage in the walls of large bronchi and are usually 1 to 2 cm in size. When multiple, they should raise suspicion of Carney syndrome, a triad of bronchial chondroma, gastric leiomyoma, and extraadrenal functional paragangliomas. Less commonly, chondromas arise within the lung parenchyma and appear as a solitary pulmonary nodule, usually detected incidentally in asymptomatic individuals. The malignant equivalent is a chondrosarcoma. It is very rare. It occurs equally within the endobronchial tree and lung parenchyma, is slightly more common in women, and has a mean age at onset of 55 years. Like fibromas, the radiologic and clinical features depend on the presence or absence of airway obstruction. In addition to a soft tissue mass, they may also contain areas of calcification (5,7,9).

GRANULAR CELL TUMOR (MYOBLASTOMA)

Granular cell tumors, otherwise known as myoblastomas, may arise within the skin, breast, tongue, or esophagus. Approximately 6% are endobronchial in location, of which approximately 100 cases have been reported. They appear as either polypoid or sessile soft tissue masses in the large bronchi or in the trachea near the carina, ranging in size from 5 to 60 mm (Fig. 8.1). Rarely, they arise in the lung parenchyma. The imaging features are similar to fibroma (5,9,10).

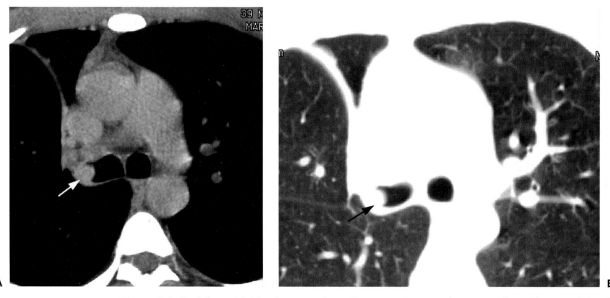

Figure 8.1 Endobronchial benign granular cell tumor. Computed tomography of lung at (A) soft tissue and (B) lung window settings demonstrate a right main bronchus soft tissue mass (arrow).

MALIGNANT TRACHEOBRONCHIAL NEOPLASMS

The most common epithelial neoplasms are bronchogenic carcinomas (Chapter 7). Carcinoid tumors and bronchial gland tumors are discussed here. The most common malignant neoplasms of the trachea are squamous cell carcinoma and adenocarcinoma. CT is the preferred imaging modality for evaluation of malignant tracheal neoplasms.

CARCINOID

Carcinoid tumors represent 5% of pulmonary tumors and are usually seen in either young adults when benign or in adults older than 50 years when more aggressive. Low and intermediate grade tumors occur equally in males and females, whereas the high grade tumors are two to four times more common in men. Carcinoid tumors are also up to 25 times more common in Caucasians than in African Americans. Carcinoid tumors are a spectrum of benign, invasive, and malignant lesions, representing a histopathologic spectrum of neuroendocrine neoplasms that originate from neurosecretory cells (Kulchitsky cells) of the bronchial mucosa. These slow-growing malignant neuroendocrine tumors are part of the amine precursor uptake and decarboxylation system and may secrete a number of hormones, including calcitonin, bradykinin, norepinephrine, antidiuretic hormone, and adrenocorticotrophic hormone. Histologically, they are divided into three groups (Table 8.5).

> Carcinoid tumors are neuroendocrine in origin and are on a histopathologic spectrum that ranges from benign carcinoids to small cell carcinoma.

Approximately 80% of carcinoid tumors are endobronchial in location, and the remaining 20% arise in the lung parenchyma as a solitary pulmonary nodule. The latter arise from small bronchi, a feature seen at pathologic examination but usually not recognizable with imaging. Given the histopathologic spectrum, the clinical presentation and radiologic findings are variable, ranging from locally confined and usually low grade tumors to locally invasive tumors. The intermediate and high grade tumors have a tendency to recur and metastasize to extrathoracic sites; the incidence of metastases depends on tumor grade (11–14).

Classic carcinoid is the least aggressive and has a mean age at onset of 50 years. These tumors are usually centrally located in the airway and are less than 2.5 cm in size. They infrequently metastasize to lymph nodes and have a good prognosis. They occur more frequently in the right middle lobe than other lobes of the lung and have a 5-year survival of 87%. Atypical carcinoid tumors are usually greater than 2.5 cm in size, with a mean age at onset of 57 years. Although they have well-defined margins, lymph node metastases occur in 50% of patients and other organ metastases in 30% of patients. The prognosis is therefore less favorable, with a 5-year survival rate of 56% (12,13,14).

Small cell carcinoma has a mean age at onset of 62 years and is twice as common in males than females. It is the most aggressive form of carcinoid tumor and has the worst prognosis. It is usually an ill-defined lesion (Fig. 8.2), with extensive mediastinal lymph node involvement at the time of diagnosis. Similarly, large cell neuroendocrine carcinoma has a mean age at onset of 62 years and is four times more common in males than females. The 27% 5-year survival of large cell neuroendocrine carcinoma is better than the 9% 5-year survival for small cell carcinoma; however, the 10-year survival rate for both is poor, at just over 5% (12–14).

With carcinoid tumors, 90% of the chest radiographs are abnormal. Abnormalities include lobar or segmental atelectasis or hyperinflation, obstructive pneumonitis, bronchiectasis or lung abscess. They can also appear as a solitary nodule (Figs. 8.2 and 8.3)

Table 8.5: Histopathologic Spectrum of Carcinoid Tumors

I	Low grade	Classic carcinoid
II	Intermediate grade	Atypical carcinoid
III	High grade	Small cell carcinoma
		Large cell neuroendocrine carcinoma

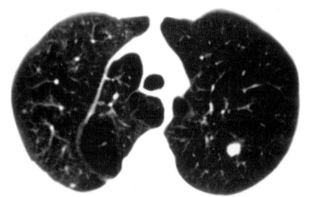

Figure 8.2 Limited stage small cell carcinoma presenting as a left upper lobe solitary pulmonary nodule on computed tomography.

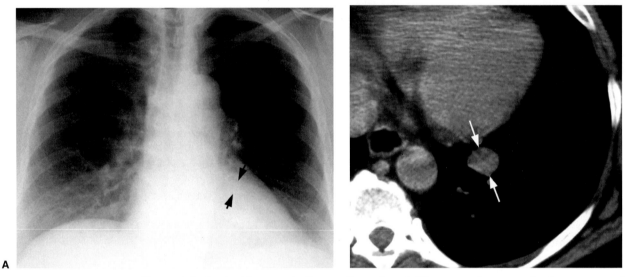

Figure 8.3 Carcinoid tumor. A. Chest radiograph and (B) computed tomography demonstrate a left lower lobe solitary pulmonary nodule of soft tissue attenuation (*arrows*).

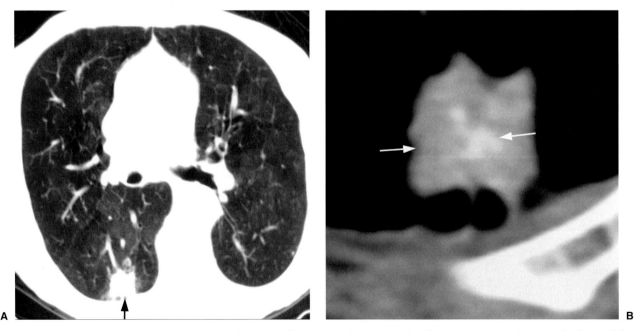

Figure 8.4 Atypical carcinoid. Computed tomography demonstrates a solitary right lower lobe nodule on (A) lung and (B) soft tissue window settings (*arrow*). Note calcification seen as central high attenuation, which represents ossification histologically.

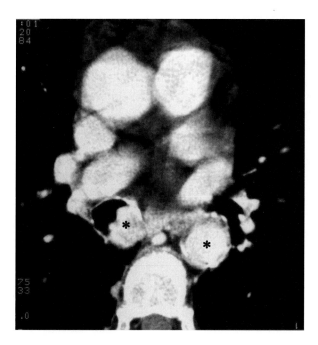

Figure 8.5 Carcinoid tumor. Computed tomography with intravenous contrast. Carcinoids are vascular tumors. The tumor (*left asterisk*) and aorta (*right asterisk*) have similar enhancement.

or as a pedunculated mass. Occasionally, they contain areas of apparent calcification (Fig. 8.4), which represents ossification histologically. CT is excellent at demonstrating both the intraluminal and extraluminal component of these tumors. Up to 25% of classic and atypical carcinoid tumors have calcification on CT. Intravenous contrast enhancement of the lesions is classically intense (Fig. 8.5), not surprising given what is often referred to at bronchoscopy as a "cherry red" lesion that commonly has visible vessels on its surface. Carcinoid tumors can also be demonstrated with radiolabeled octreotide scans or with magnetic resonance imaging (MRI) (Fig. 8.6) due to high signal from the tumor and the low background signal from normal lung and flowing blood (2,15).

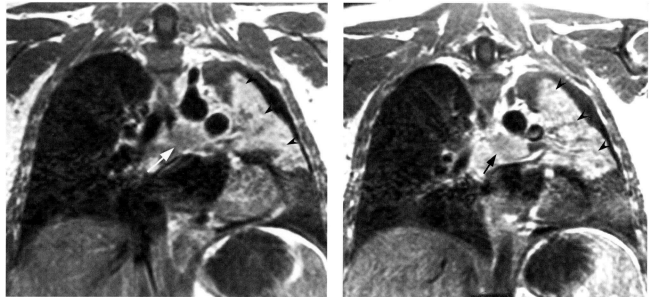

Figure 8.6 Carcinoid tumor. T1-weighted coronal magnetic resonance imaging before (*A*) and after (*B*) gadolinium. Left main and upper lobe bronchus tumor (*arrow*), which enhances postcontrast (*arrow*), and causes upper lobe post-obstruction consolidation (*arrowheads*).

(continued on next page)

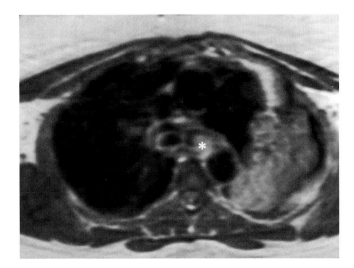

Figure 8.6 (continued) T1-weighted axial magnetic resonance. The endobronchial component is better appreciated (*asterisk*).

BRONCHIAL GLAND CARCINOMAS

Bronchial gland tumors include adenoid cystic carcinoma, also known as cylindroma, and mucoepidermoid carcinoma. The term "bronchial adenoma" was used in the past to include these tumors as well as carcinoid tumor. Inclusion of the latter group is incorrect, because they have a different cell of origin.

Adenoid cystic carcinoma arises from mixed serous and mucinous glands located in the posterolateral wall of the trachea and major bronchi. They occur in middle age, are more aggressive than carcinoid tumors, and have a greater propensity for both local invasion and metastases. They usually arise in the lower trachea, main or lobar bronchi. Chest radiograph abnormalities are usually due to chronic bronchial obstruction and may be present for a number of years before diagnosis. Adenoid cystic carcinoma has a tendency to grow along the length of the airway in a submucosal manner, so that the length of the airway involved is usually greater than is appreciated with CT examination (Fig. 16.20). The length of the airways excised is usually greater that what is visible with imaging. The tumor can locally recur, often many years after initial resection. In a series from the Mayo Clinic, 55% of patients were alive at 10 years (13,16).

Mucoepidermoid carcinoma is a mixture of mucous-secreting, squamous, and intermediate cells. It usually affects the trachea as a locally invasive sessile or polypoid tumor. It is rare. Half of patients are less than 30 years of age. Low-grade tumors rarely are locally invasive or metastasize; local resection (such as sleeve resection) has an excellent prognosis. High grade lesions are treated with surgery and postsurgical radiotherapy (13,16).

BENIGN PULMONARY NEOPLASMS

There is a wide spectrum of benign pulmonary neoplasms that may arise from the many cellular elements present in the lung. In general, they appear on imaging as indeterminate solitary pulmonary nodules. The most common are the pulmonary hamartomas, and they are discussed first. Where possible, specific imaging findings that can lead one to a specific diagnosis are indicated. Others neoplasms that also occur within the tracheobronchial tree have already been discussed.

HAMARTOMA

A hamartoma represents an abnormal quantity of cellular elements normally present in the organ in which they are found.

Hamartomas are an abnormal quantity, mixture, or arrangement of the normal constituents of the organ in which they are found. They usually occur in patients between 40 and 70 years of age and are two to four times more common in males than females. Most

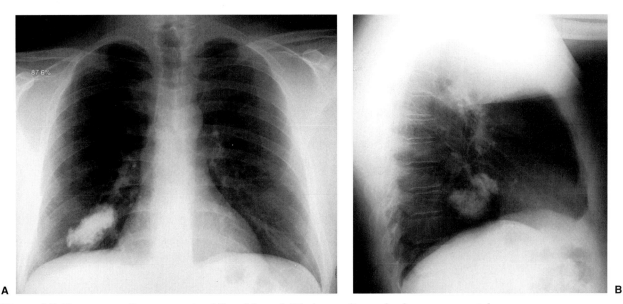

A   B

Figure 8.7 Hamartoma. Posteroanterior *(A)* and lateral *(B)* chest radiographs demonstrate a right lower lobe lobulated calcified mass.

arise within the lung periphery; however, 10% to 20% have an endobronchial origin. Rarely, they may be multiple.

On chest radiograph or CT lesions are seen as well-defined round or ovoid nodules that can be lobulated or notched (Fig. 8.7). They are usually 2 to 5 cm in diameter, with most less than 4 cm in diameter. Calcification is common, being more common the larger the diameter of the hamartoma (Figs. 8.7 and 8.8). On chest radiography and CT, hamartomas are most commonly seen as homogeneously soft tissue opacity and attenuation, respectively (Fig. 8.9). At chest radiography or CT, the presence of "popcorn calcification" is classic and nearly pathognomonic (Fig. 8.10). Fat attenuation with the nodule on CT is demonstrated in approximately one-third of hamartomas and is pathognomonic (Fig. 8.8).

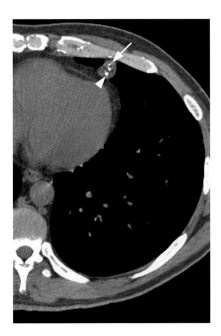

Figure 8.8 Calcified hamartoma. Computed tomography demonstrates a hamartoma within the lingula *(arrow)* with central calcifications *(arrowhead)* and adjacent low attenuation representing fat.

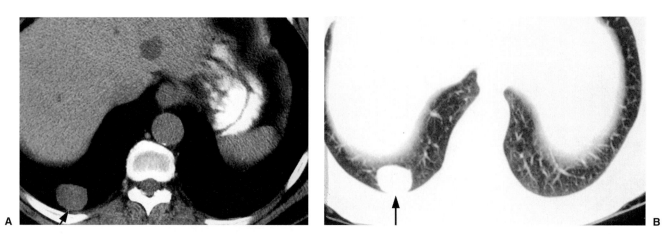

Figure 8.9 Hamartoma. Computed tomography at (A) soft tissue window settings and (B) lung window settings demonstrates a solitary right lower lobe lung nodule of soft tissue attenuation (*arrow*).

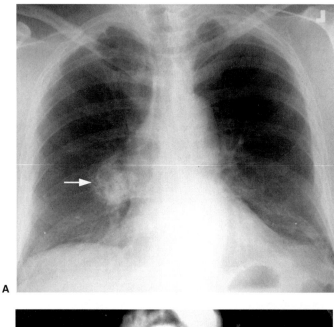

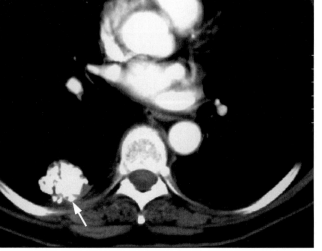

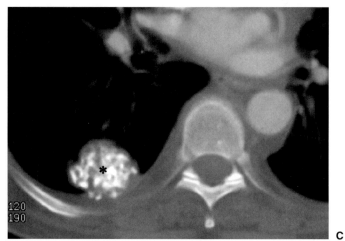

Figure 8.10 Calcified hamartoma on (A) chest radiograph and (B) computed tomography. Soft tissue settings demonstrates a lobulated and calcified right lower lobe mass (*arrow*). Computed tomography on bone window settings (C) more clearly demonstrates the morphology of the internal calcification (*asterisk*).

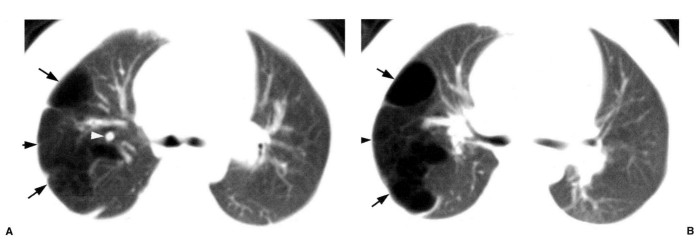

Figure 8.11 Cystic adenomatoid malformation. Computed tomography images (*A and B*) demonstrate a multicystic right upper lobe mass (*arrows*) with a small nodular soft tissue component (*white arrowhead*).

Cavitation is extremely rare. At MRI, hamartomas have intermediate signal on T1-weighted images and high signal on T2-weighted images. Septa may be demonstrated dividing the lesion into lobules within the nodule, and these septa may enhance intensely after intravenous gadolinium. Endobronchial lesions cause radiologic signs of obstruction (5,17).

Infantile hamartoma or congenital cystic adenomatoid malformation is composed of increased structures resembling terminal bronchioles, epithelium, stroma, and smooth muscle. They are slightly more common in males, occur equally on both sides, and usually affect only one lobe. They are prone to recurrent infection and treatment is surgical resection. On chest radiograph and CT, a solid mass with cystic or radiolucent foci is seen, and air–fluid levels may be present (Fig. 8.11) (18).

> One-fourth to one-third of hamartomas can be specifically diagnosed by the presence of fat or fat and calcium in a nodule on CT.

> Cystic adenomatoid malformation is an infantile form of hamartoma.

HEMANGIOMA

Hemangiomas arise from benign proliferations of blood vessels with little surrounding stroma. Histologically, cavernous and capillary types are described. The usual age at diagnosis is 30 to 40 years, and they are more common in females than males. They most commonly arise in the peripheral pulmonary parenchyma in a subpleural location, and rarely may be endobronchial in location. Hemoptysis is a common presenting symptom.

On the chest radiograph and CT, hemangiomas are usually solitary, round, well-marginated nodules or masses, with an average diameter of 3 cm in the lung periphery. Uncommonly, they may be multiple. They are usually soft tissue in attenuation on CT. Discrete round calcifications, representing phleboliths, may be seen on CT, less commonly appreciated on chest radiographs. Hemangiomas may present with obstructive signs when endobronchial (3,7,9).

LEIOMYOMA

A leiomyoma arises from smooth muscle, either within the lung parenchyma peripherally or walls of the tracheobronchial tree, in 55% and 45% of cases, respectively. They are 1.5 times more common in females than males, and usually present between 30 and 40 years of age. A leiomyoma is usually a solitary pulmonary nodule or mass ranging in size from 2 to 8 cm. Although usually soft tissue in attenuation on CT, they may calcify. They may also appear as multiple small pulmonary nodules, usually 5 to 10 mm in diameter. With central lesions (Fig. 8.12), patients may have wheezing as a presenting symptom, with

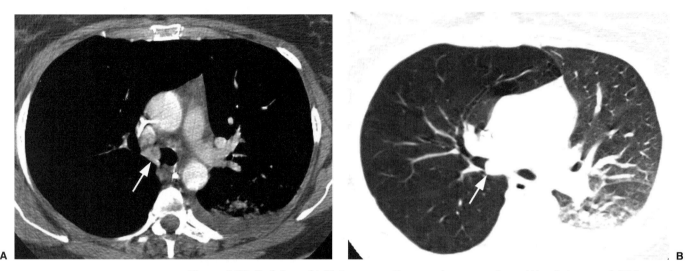

Figure 8.12 Endobronchial leiomyoma. Computed tomography at (*A*) soft tissue and (*B*) lung window settings demonstrates a right main bronchus soft tissue nodule (*arrow*).

radiologic findings of obstruction (5,7,9). Leiomyosarcoma is the very rare malignant equivalent.

NEUROGENIC TUMORS

Although relatively common in the mediastinum (Figs. 9.15 and 9.17), the neural tissue tumors, such as neurofibroma and neurilemmoma, are exceedingly rare in the lung. They usually occur as a peripheral solitary pulmonary nodule. Even more rarely they may be endobronchial in location and cause signs of obstruction. Neurofibromas are three times more common than neurilemmomas. Neurofibromas are more common in men, whereas neurilemmomas are more common in women. Malignant equivalents of these tumors also occur (5,7).

BENIGN CLEAR CELL TUMOR

These are very rare tumors of the lung parenchyma that are benign, although histologically they resemble clear cell renal carcinoma. They are slightly more common in women, with a mean age at onset of 51 years (9,10).

TERATOMA

Typically thought of as an anterior mediastinal mass (Fig. 9.19), rarely teratomas arise in the lung, with only 33 pulmonary teratomas reported. They are slightly more common in females than males and usually occur in young adults. Most are benign, but a malignant form is described. Expectoration of hair is pathognomonic clinically. On chest radiograph or CT they appear as lobulated masses with calcification that tend to occur in the left upper lobe. Fat has been described on chest radiograph, but not yet on CT; only a few have been reported with CT so far. They may cavitate (10).

Tricholithoptysis may be seen with pulmonary teratomas.

CHEMODECTOMA

Chemodectomas are nonchromaffin paragangliomas with no hormonal activity. They are more frequent in females than males, occurring with a ratio of 4:1.5. The mean age at onset is 58 years. Chemodectomas occur much more frequently in the mediastinum than the lung. Within the lung they appear as a round solitary pulmonary nodule, 1 cm or greater in size, with a 17 cm mass reported (10).

PULMONARY ENDOMETRIOSIS

Intrathoracic endometriosis is very rare. It occurs in two forms: pleurodiaphragmatic and bronchopulmonary. Pleurodiaphragmatic is the most common form and may be a source of recurrent pneumothorax that occurs during menstruation (catamenial) (Fig. 17.19). Less commonly it may involve the lung parenchyma or airway and manifests as catamenial hemoptysis. Radiologically, it appears as single or multiple nodules that may cavitate and may be associated with bronchiectasis (3).

MALIGNANT PULMONARY NEOPLASMS

Unlike bronchogenic carcinoma, the other malignant pulmonary neoplasms are rare. Like the benign pulmonary neoplasms, malignant pulmonary neoplasms may arise from a variety of cells, giving rise to a list of tumors of varying histopathology and radiologic manifestations (Table 8.4). Lymphoma and lymphoproliferative disease processes are discussed after malignant pulmonary neoplasms in their own section.

HEMANGIOPERICYTOMA

Hemangiopericytoma usually occurs in patients between 40 and 60 years of age and affects males and females equally. It may be benign or malignant, and this distinction usually depends on lesion size. The larger the lesion, the more likely it is to be malignant. An endobronchial component may occur. Patients may present with hemoptysis, but frequently it is first discovered as an incidental "solitary pulmonary nodule" on a chest radiograph (7,9).

EPITHELIOID HEMANGIOENDOTHELIOMA

Epithelioid hemangioendothelioma is four times more common in females than males. Patients present between 12 and 60 years of age, with a mean onset of 35 years. Half of cases occur in individuals below the age of 40 years. Survival may be up to 15 years in the less aggressive form of the disease; however, there is a more aggressive form of the tumor with a survival of approximately 1 year. At initial presentation, epithelioid hemangioendothelioma often effects multiple organs, including the lung, liver, bones, and soft tissues simultaneously or sequentially. When this occurs it may be difficult to know if the tumor arose initially as a multicentric process, similar to lymphoma, or as a primary lesion with metastases to other tissues, though metastases are uncommon.

The most characteristic feature of epithelioid hemangioendothelioma on chest radiograph or CT is the presence of multiple bilateral lung perivascular nodules with well-defined or ill-defined margins in both lungs (Fig. 8.13). The nodules range in size up to 2 cm, but most are less than 1 cm in size and redundant to calcify. They are usually found in relation to small and medium-sized vessels and bronchi. The lung nodules uncommonly calcify (19–21).

PRIMARY PULMONARY SARCOMA

Primary pulmonary sarcomas are usually fibrosarcomas or leiomyosarcomas, although chondrosarcoma (Fig. 8.14), osteosarcoma, malignant fibrous histiocytoma, rhabdomyosarcoma and neurofibrosarcoma also occur. Overall, most pulmonary sarcomas are secondary metastases from extrathoracic primary sites. On imaging they appear as a solitary pulmonary nodule or mass. Rarely, they may be endobronchial and cause atelectasis.

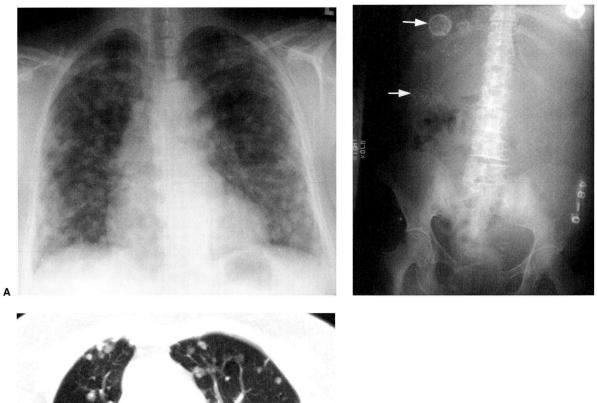

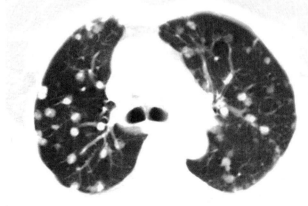

Figure 8.13 Epithelial hemangioendothelioma. Chest radiograph (A) and computed tomography (B) demonstrate multiple pulmonary nodules. Abdominal radiograph (C) demonstrates multiple calcified hepatic tumors (*arrows*).

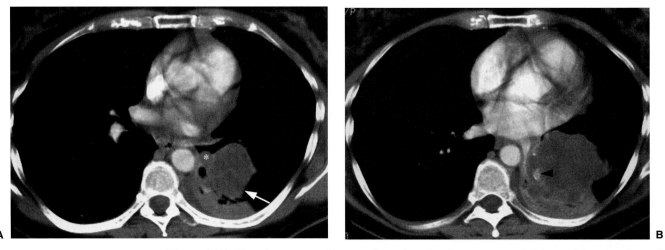

Figure 8.14 Chondrosarcoma. Computed tomography demonstrates a left lower lobe mass (*arrow*) with endobronchial component (*asterisk*) (A) and matrix calcification seen as eccentric high attenuation (*arrowhead*) (B).

CARCINOSARCOMA AND PULMONARY BLASTOMA

Carcinosarcoma usually occurs in patients over the age of 50 years, with 90% of patients between 50 and 80 years of age. It is much more common in males than females and has an increased incidence in smokers. They usually manifest as a solitary large peripheral mass in the upper lobes. Occasionally, it may be an endobronchial lesion and present with clinical and radiologic signs of obstruction (9,13,22).

Pulmonary blastoma is now believed to be a form of carcinosarcoma. It occurs in a younger age group than carcinosarcoma. On chest radiograph or CT it appears as a large, solitary, well-defined, peripheral nodule or mass, ranging from 2 cm upward but usually about 10 cm; they may have cystic structures. Occasionally they can be multiple. At least one case of cavitation and calcification is described (9,13,22).

LYMPHOMA AND LYMPHOPROLIFERATIVE DISEASES

A variety of malignancies may be found in the thorax arising from the lymphatic system, as listed in Table 8.6. Lymphoma, Castleman disease, and plasma cell granuloma are discussed here. The other lymphoproliferative diseases, leukemias, multiple myeloma, and amyloid are discussed in Chapter 13.

LYMPHOMA

Lymphomas are tumors of the immune system, divided into Hodgkin lymphoma and non-Hodgkin lymphomas. Lymphoma is the seventh leading cause of death from cancer in the United States. The incidence of Hodgkin lymphoma is 2.5 per 100,000. It has a bimodal age distribution, with a large peak in the second and third decade and a smaller peak in the sixth and seventh decade. It occurs more often in males than females, with a ratio of 1.7:1. Non-Hodgkin lymphoma is more common than Hodgkin lymphoma and occurs in an older age group. In the thorax, lymphoma can affect almost any structure, including the intrathoracic and axillary lymph nodes and thymus, as well as extranodal involvement of the pulmonary parenchyma, airway, pleura, pericardium, chest wall and spine (3,11).

Thoracic lymph node enlargement is the most common manifestation of both Hodgkin and non-Hodgkin lymphoma (Fig. 9.9). Whereas Hodgkin lymphoma predictably spreads in a contiguous fashion, non-Hodgkin lymphoma is often noncontiguous and asymmetric. Lymph node enlargement is present on the chest radiographs in 67% of Hodgkin lymphoma, versus 43% of non-Hodgkin lymphoma. These figures are much higher for CT in both forms of lymphoma. The incidence of visible lymph node enlargement on chest radiography is lower in younger patients. Most patients with Hodgkin lymphoma have involvement of two or more nodal groups; hilar involvement is rare in the absence of mediastinal involvement. In non-Hodgkin lymphoma, half of cases may have only one nodal group involved. The paracardiac nodes are rarely involved at presentation, but are an important site for relapse.

Lymphoma is the seventh leading cause of cancer death in the United States.

Table 8.6: Lymphoproliferative Disease within the Thorax

Plasma cell granuloma (inflammatory pseudotumor)
Posttransplant lymphoproliferative disorder
Lymphoid interstitial pneumonitis
Lymphomatoid granulomatosis
Lymphoma
Pseudolymphoma
Angioimmunoblastic lymphadenopathy
Castleman disease

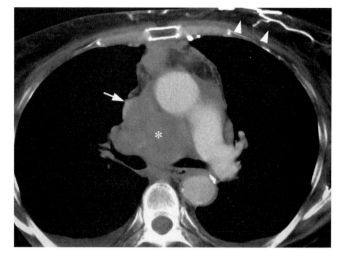

Figure 8.15 Lymphoma. Computed tomography demonstrates massive mediastinal lymph node enlargement (*asterisk*). The superior vena cava is compressed to a thin slit (*arrow*). Note the collateral vessels within the left anterior chest wall (*arrowheads*).

Lymph nodes in lymphoma may calcify after treatment.

Hodgkin lymphoma is the most common lymphoma to involve the lungs. Non-Hodgkin lymphoma is the most common primary pulmonary lymphoma.

Nodules with air bronchograms or consolidation are the classic findings of pulmonary lymphoma.

Lymph node calcification is rare at presentation but may occur after radiation therapy or chemotherapy. Superior vena cava obstruction may occur as a presenting symptom or later in the course of the disease (Fig. 8.15). Thymic enlargement is commonly seen and lymphoma may arise solely within the thymus.

Pulmonary parenchymal involvement associated with nodal disease occurs in 10% to 15% of patients with lymphoma at presentation and is three times more common in Hodgkin lymphoma than in non-Hodgkin lymphoma (Fig. 8.16). The most common presentation is one or more discrete nodules (Fig. 8.17), which are typically ill defined or contain air bronchograms (Fig. 8.18) and uncommonly cavitate. Lung parenchymal involvement without nodal involvement is rare. Primary pulmonary Hodgkin lymphoma is very rare. Primary pulmonary non-Hodgkin lymphoma is a low grade B-cell lymphoma that arises from mucosa-associated lymphoid tissue and is known specifically as bronchus-associated lymphoid tumor (Fig. 8.19). Because of the widespread pulmonary lymphatic tissue there can be enlarged peribronchovascular lymph nodes and thickening of the interlobular septa. High resolution CT is particularly useful in the evaluation of the interstitium. Lymph node enlargement can extend to involve the adjacent pulmonary parenchyma with resultant chronic airspace disease and air bronchograms. Infectious complications can occur secondary to immunosuppressive therapy due to bacterial, fungal, viral, or mycobacterial infections. CT is particularly useful in early detection of these findings, with high resolution CT being especially useful in the detection of invasive pulmonary aspergillosis. A "CT halo sign," though not specific, is highly suggestive of invasive aspergillosis in immunocompromised patients (13,23–27).

Pleural effusion can occur secondary to lymphatic obstruction or pleural invasion and can be unilateral or bilateral. They are usually small to moderate in size. More commonly

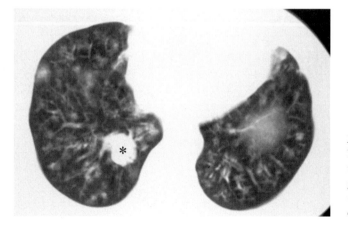

Figure 8.16 Low-grade non-Hodgkin lymphoma. Computed tomography demonstrates a single large right lower lobe mass (*asterisk*) and innumerable ill-defined bilateral lung nodules.

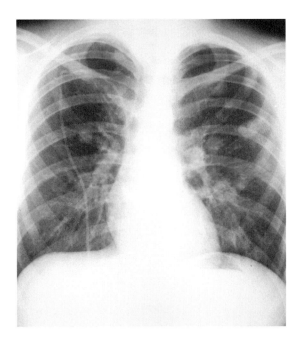

Figure 8.17 Metastatic lymphoma. Chest radiograph shows multiple bilateral pulmonary nodules of varying size.

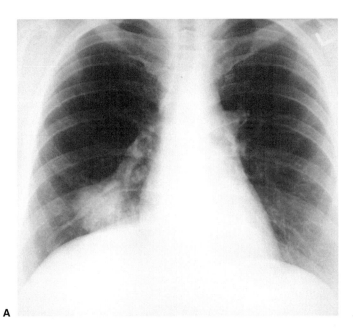

A

Figure 8.18 Pseudolymphoma. Chest radiograph (*A*), and computed tomography on (*B*) soft tissue and (*C*) lung window settings demonstrate a well-defined right lower lobe mass containing air bronchograms (*arrow*).

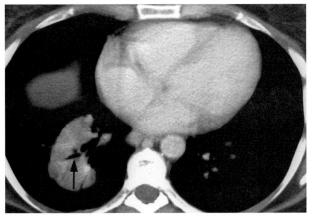

B

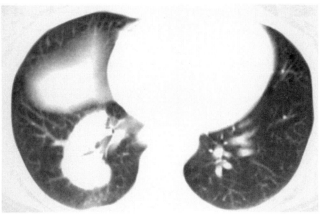

C

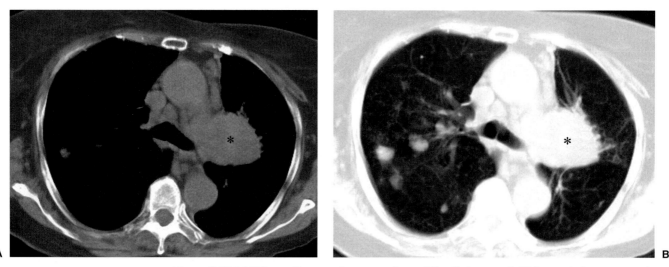

Figure 8.19 MALToma. Computed tomography at (*A*) soft tissue and (*B*) lung window settings demonstrates a large central mass (*asterisk*) extending into the lingula and multiple pulmonary nodules.

Pleural effusions in lymphoma patients are more commonly due to heart failure or infection than to lymphoma.

pleural effusions in patients with lymphoma are secondary to cardiac failure or infection. Chest wall involvement can also occur. Lymphomatous involvement of the pericardium and myocardium, often due to direct invasion, is seen in a small number of patients (3).

CASTLEMAN DISEASE

Castleman disease is a form of lymphoma with localized and generalized (systemic) forms.

Castleman disease is also known as angiofollicular hyperplasia or giant lymph node hyperplasia. It occurs in two forms: a localized form known as unicentric angiofollicular hyperplasia and a generalized form known as multicentric angiofollicular hyperplasia. There are also two histologic forms, the hyaline-vascular type and the plasma cell type. Patients may be asymptomatic. Fever, weight loss, and lassitude are common symptoms with the localized form, especially with the plasma cell type. Elevated erythrocyte sedimentation rate, an IgG, IgA, or IgM hypergammaglobulinemia, and chronic anemia also occur. The generalized form presents with skin lesions, papilledema, or a monoclonal gammopathy. There may also be a symmetric sensorimotor peripheral neuropathy. Current thinking is that this disease is a form of lymphoma (3,11).

The hyaline vascular type of Castleman disease enhances intensely with intravenous contrast on CT or MRI. The plasma cell type does not.

Localized or unicentric angiofollicular hyperplasia is usually of the hyaline-vascular type in up to 96% of cases. Hyaline-vascular localized Castleman disease usually occurs between 30 and 40 years of age and occurs equally in males and females; it may have a slight female predominance. Radiologically, there is usually a solitary, well-circumscribed, encapsulated mass, with or without cervical or mediastinal lymph node enlargement. This form of Castleman disease characteristically enhances intensely with intravenous contrast administration on either CT or MRI (Fig. 9.22). Plasma cell type localized Castleman disease usually occurs in young adults, equally in males and females. Lymph node enlargement usually is more often disseminated. Treatment is with surgical resection, radiotherapy, and steroids; this can achieve a cure rate of up to 100% (3,28).

Generalized Castleman disease is usually the plasma cell type, occurs in patients over the age of 40 and is twice as common in males than females. It occurs in two forms, hyperplasia without neuropathy and hyperplasia with neuropathy. Both are treated as described above; however, the prognosis is poor, with a mean life expectancy of approximately 30 months. Radiologically, there is disseminated lymph node involvement, with adjacent soft tissue infiltration at multiple sites (3,28).

PLASMA CELL GRANULOMA (INFLAMMATORY PSEUDOTUMOR)

Plasma cell granuloma is a benign tumor, which may originate as an organizing pneumonia. Sixty percent of patients are under the age of 40, and it is the most common benign lung

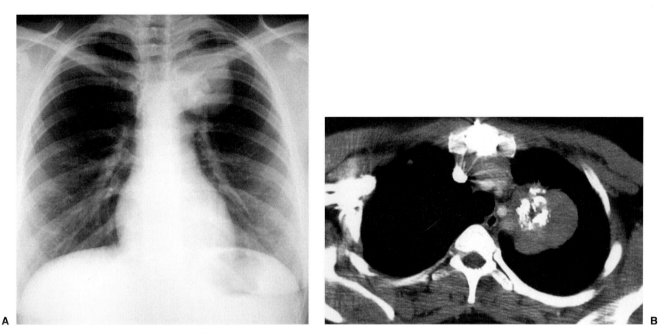

A   B

Figure 8.20 Plasma cell granuloma (inflammatory pseudotumor). Chest radiograph *(A)* and computed tomography *(B)* demonstrate a 6 cm left upper lobe mass with central calcification.

tumor in children. It occurs equally in males and females. Most patients are asymptomatic, and it is usually diagnosed as an incidental mass on a chest radiograph. When symptomatic, patients present with fever, cough, chest pain, wheezing or hemoptysis. The chest radiograph and CT demonstrate a solitary well-defined nodule in 70% of cases. In the remainder there may be an ill-defined or spiculated nodule, a large mass or multiple (up to three) lesions. Calcification may be extensive (Fig. 8.20), and cavitation is described. Occasionally, plasma cell granuloma may arise in a bronchus, with consolidation or atelectasis distally (Fig. 8.21). A pleural origin is also described. Plasma cell granuloma may or may not enhance with intravenous contrast on CT or MRI. They are hyperintense to muscle on T1-weighted sequences and high signal on T2-weighted sequences (3,28).

Plasma cell granuloma (a.k.a. inflammatory pseudotumor) is the most common benign primary lung tumor in children.

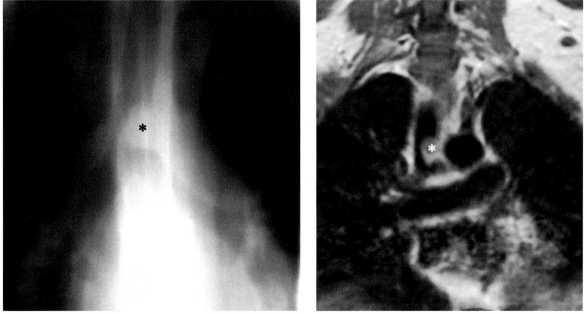

A   B

Figure 8.21 Plasma cell granuloma (inflammatory pseudotumor). Tomogram *(A)* and T1-weighted coronal magnetic resonance postgadolinium *(B)* demonstrate a sessile tracheal nodule *(asterisk)*.

METASTATIC DISEASE

Metastases to the thorax may deposit in many structures, most commonly the lungs, lymph nodes, pleura, ribs, and spine. Metastases to the pericardium are common at autopsy but are uncommonly diagnosed antemortem. Metastases to the airway and esophagus are unusual. The incidence of thoracic metastases varies with the primary tumor and with the stage of the disease.

LUNG METASTASES

The lung is a very common site for metastases. The tumors most likely to metastasize to the lung are renal cell carcinoma, sarcoma, thyroid cancer, breast cancer, and melanoma (3,11). Tumor may spread by a number of routes, as listed in Table 8.7.

Hematogenous spread is the most common form of dissemination of metastases to the lung. The main radiologic features are multiple bilateral round or ovoid nodules of varying size. They occur in the lower lungs more than the upper lungs due to the greater distribution of blood flow to the lower lobes. Lung metastases are usually in the peripheral one-third of the lung and range in size from 1 to 2 mm to several centimeters (Figs. 8.22 and 8.23). Although these features are seen on both the chest radiograph and CT, CT is more sensitive for the detection of smaller nodules and nodules obscured by the heart and mediastinum. Lung metastases are usually well defined but may have irregular margins if

> Hematogenous lung metastases are found in the portion of the lungs with the greatest blood flow, namely the lower lobes.

Table 8.7. Routes of Metastatic Dissemination within the Thorax

Endobronchial
Hematogenous
Lymphatic
Pleural
Direct

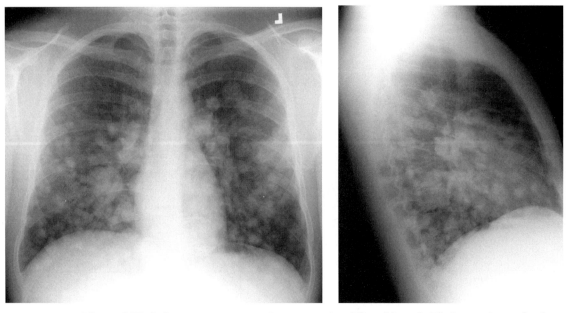

A   **B**

Figure 8.22 Pulmonary metastases. Posteroanterior (*A*) and lateral (*B*) chest radiographs demonstrate multiple bilateral pulmonary nodules of varying size.

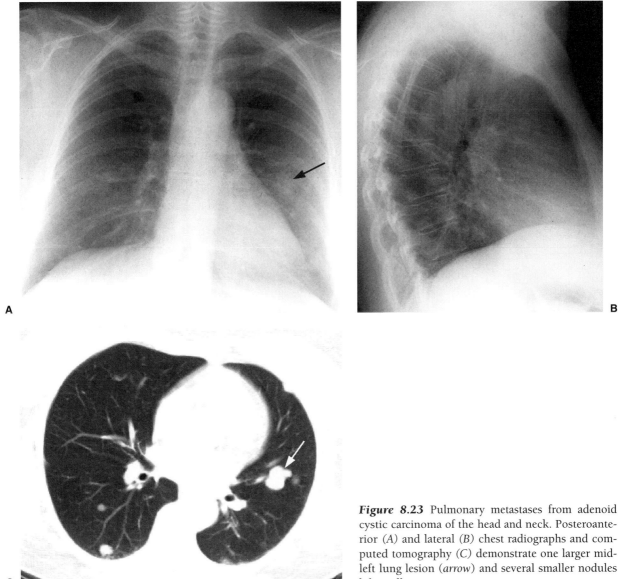

Figure 8.23 Pulmonary metastases from adenoid cystic carcinoma of the head and neck. Posteroanterior (*A*) and lateral (*B*) chest radiographs and computed tomography (*C*) demonstrate one larger mid-left lung lesion (*arrow*) and several smaller nodules bilaterally.

they bleed into the adjacent lung. The latter may be seen with adenocarcinoma, choriocarcinoma, and with metastases after treatment. Uncommonly, metastases appear as innumerable 3- to 5-mm miliary nodules, similar to the miliary pattern seen with miliary tuberculosis. This pattern is most commonly seen with thyroid cancer, renal cell carcinoma, and melanoma. Very rarely metastases present as areas of pulmonary consolidation; this occurs with melanoma and breast cancer (3,13,29).

Cavitation is not common and occurs most frequently with squamous cell carcinoma, sarcoma, melanoma, transitional cell carcinoma, colon, uterine, and cervix cancers and after chemotherapy. Metastases can cavitate while still small, and usually cavitary and noncavitary nodules coexist. Cavitation with sarcoma metastases causing spontaneous pneumothorax occurs relatively frequently (Fig. 8.24) (Fig. 17.18) (3,13,29).

Calcification is very uncommon but does occur in breast, thyroid (papillary), testicular, and ovarian cancers and in mucinous adenocarcinoma. More frequently, calcification occurs in sarcomas of osteoid or chondroid origin, where calcification occurs as matrix mineralization as in the primary tumor (Fig. 8.25). They may simulate calcified granulomas on chest radiographs and CT. Dystrophic calcification can be seen in treated metastases (3,13,29).

Miliary hematogenous metastases are most commonly seen with very vascular tumors that shower thousands of tumor cells and then grow slowly, namely thyroid and renal cancers.

Metastatic osteosarcoma to lung may appear as multiple calcified nodules, mimicking granulomas.

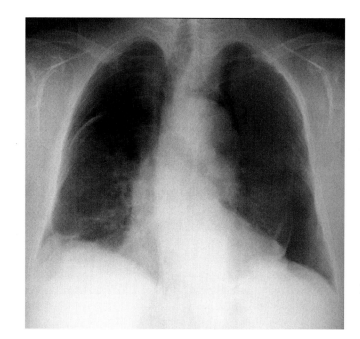

Figure 8.24 Spontaneous bilateral pneumothoraces secondary to metastatic sarcoma on chest radiograph.

Occasionally, metastatic disease can present as a single nodule, occurring in less than 10% of patients. In patients with known extrathoracic malignancy it can be difficult to know if this represents a primary bronchogenic carcinoma or solitary metastasis. If the extrathoracic primary is from carcinoma of the head and neck, bladder, breast, cervix, bile ducts, esophagus, ovary, prostate, or stomach, then this was more likely to be primary bronchogenic carcinoma than lung metastasis. This is also true of squamous cell carcinoma. In patients with carcinomas of the salivary glands, adrenal gland, colon, parotid gland, kidney, thyroid gland, thymus, or uterus, the likelihood of the nodule in the lung representing a solitary metastasis equals the incidence of a secondary primary tumor. This is also true of ade-

A new solitary pulmonary nodule in a patient with head and neck, bladder, or cervical cancer is more likely to be a new lung cancer than a metastases; all share cigarette smoking as a risk factor.

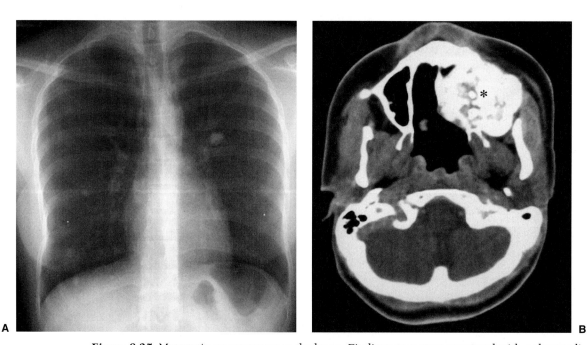

Figure 8.25 Metastatic osteosarcoma to the lungs. Findings were new compared with a chest radiograph 7 months earlier. Appearance on a chest radiograph simulates multiple calcified granulomas. *A.* Chest radiograph demonstrates multiple ossified bilateral lung nodules. *B.* Computed tomography of the head demonstrates the primary osteosarcoma of the left maxilla (*asterisk*).

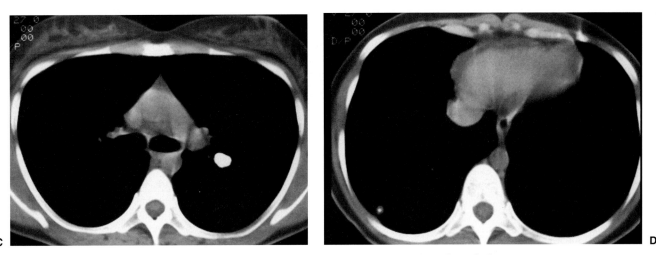

C   D

Figure 8.25 (continued) *C* and *D*. Computed tomography images demonstrate bilateral ossified lung nodules.

nocarcinomas. Patients with melanoma, sarcoma, or testicular carcinoma are more likely to have a solitary metastasis than a bronchogenic carcinoma (3,13,29,30).

Lymphatic spread of tumor may occur secondary to direct invasion of lymphatic vessels, by tumor embolization to blood vessels with spread through blood vessel walls and subsequent invasion of lymphatic vessels, and by retrograde spread through the pulmonary lymphatics from involved mediastinal lymph nodes. The most common tumors to spread this way are bronchogenic carcinoma, melanoma, breast, kidney, stomach, pancreas, colon, thyroid, larynx, and cervical cancers. The chest radiograph may be normal; when abnormal there is usually a mixed picture of reticulonodular opacities with thickening of the interlobular septa (Kerley B lines). There may also be pleural effusion. The main differential diagnosis is intersitial pulmonary edema secondary to cardiac failure, and distinguishing the two can be difficult. A normal sized heart or the presence of enlarged mediastinal lymph nodes favors the diagnosis of lymphangitic carcinomatosis, but often progression on repeat radiographs or failure to improve after diuretic or other therapy makes the diagnosis. CT is more sensitive than chest radiography, particularly high resolution CT, which demonstrates irregular or nodular thickening of the interlobular septa (Fig. 8.26). Nodular or patchy airspace shadowing can also occur. Either localized areas of interlobular thickening or diffuse thickening not lower lobe predominant help distinguish from cardiac failure, as does irregular septal thickening. Nodular septal thickening is very specific for lymphangitic carcinomatosis and is termed the "beaded septum sign" (3,13,29).

There are two forms of lymphangitic tumor spread: central hilar mass causing lymphatic obstruction and hematogenous dissemination with lymphatic invasion.

Nodular septal thickening and polygons are the typical features of lymphangitic tumor spread on high resolution CT.

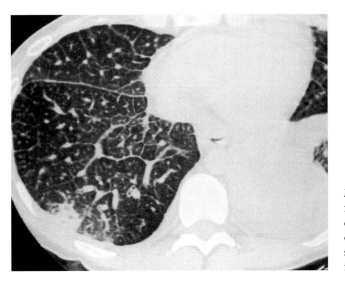

Figure 8.26 Lymphangitic carcinomatosis from bronchoalveolar cell carcinoma. High resolution computed tomography demonstrates nodular thickening of the interlobular septa and fissure.

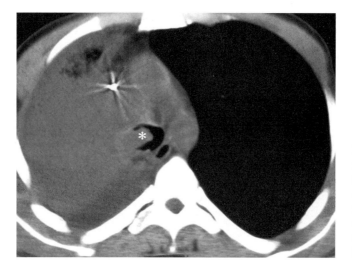

Figure 8.27 Endobronchial metastasis from teratocarcinoma. Computed tomography demonstrates a bronchus intermedius nodule *(asterisk)* with obstructive consolidation of the middle and right lower lobes.

AIRWAY METASTASES

The most common tumors to manifest clinically with endobronchial metastases are lung, renal, colon and thyroid cancer, melanoma, and lymphoma.

Endobronchial metastases are not common but are found in 18% to 51% of autopsied patients with extrathoracic malignancy if other intrathoracic metastases are present. Metastases to the bronchus alone occur in less than 5% of patients at autopsy. Usually, endobronchial metastases occur late in the clinical course. The most common primary sites are bronchogenic carcinoma, lymphoma, renal cell carcinoma, colorectal carcinoma, breast cancer, melanoma, and thyroid cancer. Metastases may spread from tumor in the local lung parenchyma, via lymph nodes or from an extrathoracic primary. Occasionally, metastases may produce a clinical and radiologic appearance similar to primary bronchogenic tumor, with either focal bronchial narrowing or mass or obstructive signs (Figs. 8.27 and 8.28) (3,11,13,29).

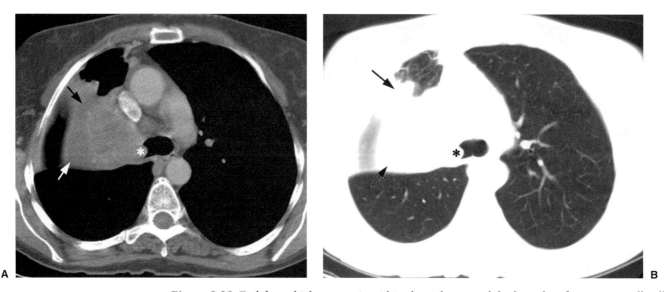

Figure 8.28 Endobronchial metastasis within the right upper lobe bronchus from non–small cell lung cancer. Computed tomography at *(A)* soft tissue and *(B)* lung window settings demonstrates a right main bronchus nodule *(asterisk)* and consolidation of the right upper lobe *(arrows)*.

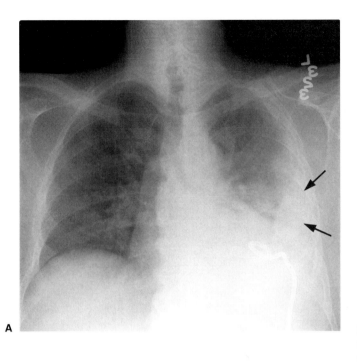

A

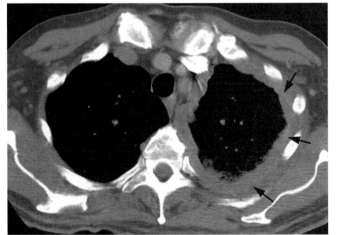

B

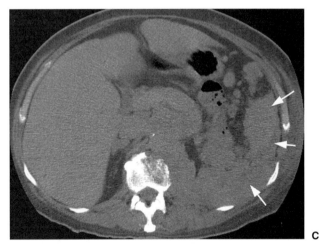

C

Figure 8.29 Pleural metastases. Chest radiograph *(A)* and computed tomography *(B and C)* demonstrate left pleural thickening *(arrows)*.

PLEURAL METASTASES

Pleural spread of tumor occurs most commonly with lung and breast cancers and lymphoma but also occurs with cancer of the pancreas, stomach, and ovary. The visceral pleura is usually involved, but parietal pleura may also be involved if the visceral pleura is affected. On chest radiography, CT, and ultrasound, pleural nodules may be identified (Fig. 8.29). However, the usual finding is a pleural effusion. This occurs in up to 60% of patients with pleural metastases. The pleural fluid has high protein and lactate dehydrogenase levels and low glucose level and low pH. Pleural effusions do not always occur in the presence of pleural metastases, and even when pleural metastases are present the effusion may be due to lymphatic obstruction (3,11,13,29).

The most common manifestation of ovarian carcinoma in the thorax is a pleural effusion.

ESOPHAGEAL CARCINOMA

There are approximately 11,000 deaths a year in the United States due to esophageal cancer. It is rare under the age of 40, and the incidence increases with each subsequent

Table 8.8: Rare Esophageal Malignancies

Mucoepidermoid carcinoma
Adenoid cystic carcinoma
Small cell carcinoma
Carcinosarcoma (spindle cell carcinoma)
Sarcoma (leiomyosarcoma, rhabdomyosarcoma, fibrosarcoma)
Kaposi sarcoma
Primary melanoma

decade. It is two to four times more common in males than females and twice as common among African Americans than whites. In the last two decades the incidence of adenocarcinoma has increased, and this now represents one-third to one-half of cases. In contrast, up to 20 years ago squamous cell carcinoma accounted for greater than 90% of cases. The reason for this is not fully known, but it is due to an increase in cases of adenocarcinoma rather than a relative reduction in numbers of squamous carcinoma. Adenocarcinoma is found to arise on a background of Barrett's mucosa, which is due to longstanding gastroesophageal reflux and reflux esophagitis. A variety of other histologic esophageal tumors are listed in Table 8.8; all are very rare (31).

> A normal esophagus on CT does not exclude esophageal carcinoma.

Early esophageal cancers can manifest as irregularities, plaque-like lesions, and sessile or polypoid masses with or without ulceration on double-contrast esophograms. The presence of stricturing may suggest Barrett's esophagitis, a premalignant condition associated with an increased risk of adenocarcinoma (Fig. 8.30). Advanced esophageal cancer may manifest on chest radiography as a dilated or obstructed esophagus, as mediastinal widening, or as thickening of the retrotracheal stripe. CT typically reveals circumferential esophageal thickening; squamous cell carcinoma tends to be located in the upper and middle thirds of the esophagus and adenocarcinoma in the lower third and are therefore more likely to invade the gastric cardia and fundus (Fig. 8.30) (32).

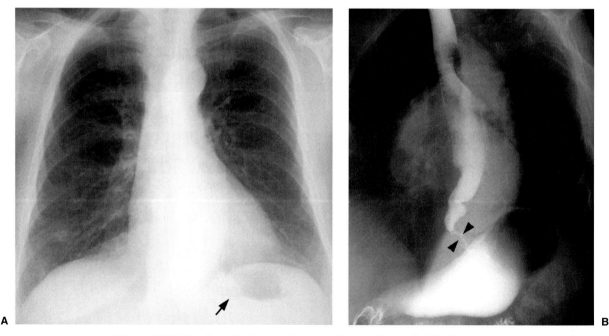

Figure 8.30 Esophageal adenocarcinoma. Chest radiograph (A) demonstrates tumor at the gastroesophageal junction indenting the gastric fundus (*arrow*). Double-contrast esophogram swallow (B) demonstrates tight stricture of the lower esophagus (*arrowheads*).

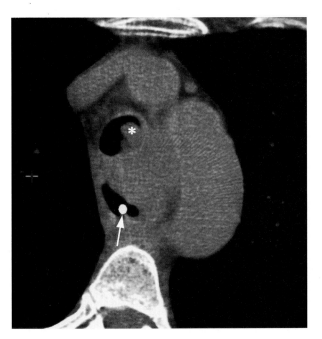

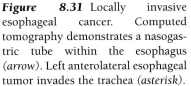

Figure 8.31 Locally invasive esophageal cancer. Computed tomography demonstrates a nasogastric tube within the esophagus (*arrow*). Left anterolateral esophageal tumor invades the trachea (*asterisk*).

CT is used to stage esophageal carcinoma by the detection of mediastinal, cervical, and abdominal lymph node enlargement, as well as the detection of distant metastases to lung, liver, kidneys, adrenals, and occasionally bone. CT is also important to evaluate for invasion of adjacent mediastinal structures, such as the airway (Figs. 8.31 and 8.32), aorta, and pericardium. CT has moderate to good accuracy at detecting extraluminal spread and tracheobronchial or aortic involvement. Esophageal cancers typically spread to regional lymph nodes, with upper and middle third of the esophagus tumors spreading to mediastinal lymph nodes and lower third tumors spreading to upper

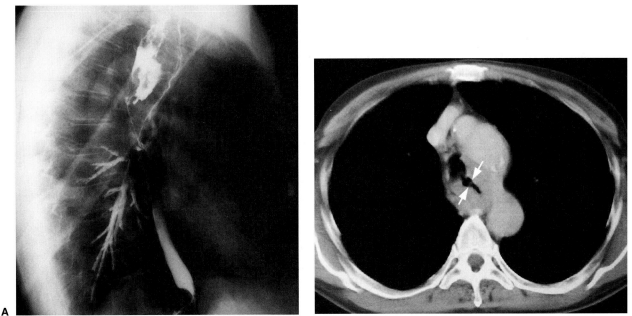

A   B

Figure 8.32 Esophageal carcinoma with tracheoesophageal fistula. This is demonstrated on esophogram (*A*), with contrast spilling into the tracheobronchial tree and bronchi. The fistula is also demonstrated on computed tomography (*arrows*) (*B*).

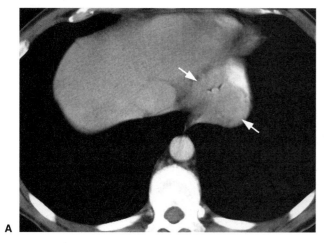

Figure 8.33 Metastatic esophageal carcinoma at the time of diagnosis. Computed tomography demonstrates the primary esophageal tumor at the gastroesophageal junction with extension into the cardia (*arrows*) (*A*), gastrohepatic ligament lymph node metastases (*arrowheads*) (*B*), and liver metastases (*asterisks*) (*C*).

For a distal esophageal adenocarcinoma, lymph node metastases to paraesophageal and gastrohepatic nodes are considered to be resectable; celiac axis and more caudal nodes in the abdomen and supraclavicular nodes are considered to be unresectable.

abdominal (lymph nodes, gastrohepatic ligament and left gastric nodal chains). CT is only moderately accurate because normal size lymph nodes may contain metastatic disease, lymph node enlargement may be due to benign disease, and it can be difficult to distinguish enlarged nodes from esophageal wall thickening. The prevalence of distant metastases at the time of diagnosis is low; however, CT is very accurate in detecting distant metastases (33,34).

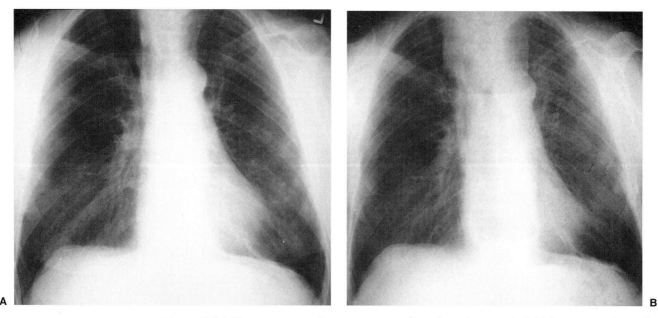

Figure 8.34 Upper anastomotic recurrent esophageal carcinoma. *A.* Initial postoperative radiograph and (*B*) later radiograph with widened mediastinum due to recurrent tumor.

The accuracy of MRI for staging esophageal cancer is comparable with CT at present. Endoscopic ultrasound can be used to assess the depth of tumor invasion in the esophageal wall and the presence, size, and morphology of lymph nodes. It has an accuracy of 85% to 90% for T staging, is more accurate at staging adenocarcinoma than squamous cell carcinoma, and with local disease is more accurate than CT. The main limitation of endoscopic ultrasound is tumor stenosis, preventing passage of the scope. At some institutions patients are preoperatively staged with CT and endoscopic ultrasound (33,35).

It is also important to assess for distant metastases at the time of diagnosis. Quint et al. (36) showed that 18% of patients had distant metastatis at the time of their newly diagnosed esophageal carcinoma (Fig. 8.33). CT is superb at detecting liver and adrenal metastases. Distant metastases are most commonly diagnosed in abdominal lymph nodes, liver, lung, cervical/supraclavicular lymph nodes, bone, adrenal glands, peritoneum, and brain (33,36).

Postoperatively, CT can be used to assess for disease recurrence. CT accuracy is moderate to good. Recurrent disease is usually at the resection site or anastomosis (Figs. 8.34 and 8.35) or a combination of local-regional disease and distant metastases with abdominal lymph node enlargement (37).

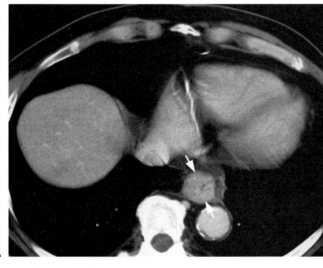

A

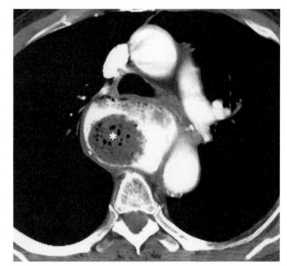

B

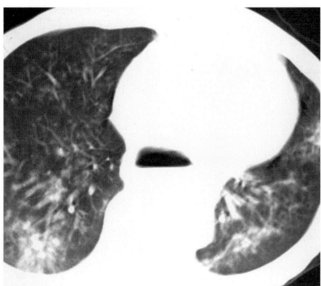

C

Figure 8.35 Recurrent esophageal tumor. Computed tomography demonstrates recurrent disease with abnormal concentric soft tissue within the distal gastric pull-through *(arrows)* *(A)*. This results in dilatation proximally with a bezoar *(asterisk)* present within the dilated gastric pull-through *(B)*. This also resulted in bilateral aspiration pneumonia *(C)*.

REFERENCES

1. *Histological typing of lung tumors*, 2nd ed. Vol 1. International Histological Classification of Tumors No. 1. Geneva: World Health Organization, 1981.
2. Naidich DP. CT/MR correlation in the evaluation of tracheobronchial neoplasia. *Radiol Clin North Am* 1990;28:555–571.
3. Armstrong P, Wilson AG, Dee P et al. *Imaging of diseases of the chest*, 3rd ed. Mosby, St. Louis, 2000.
4. Colletti PM. Computed tomography in endobronchial neoplasms. *Comput Med Imaging Graph* 1990;14:257–262.
5. Wilson RW, Kirejczyk W. Pathological and radiological correlation of endobronchial neoplasms. Part I. Benign tumors. *Ann Diagn Pathol* 1997;1:31–46.
6. Hirata T, Reshad K, Itoi K, et al. Lipomas of the peripheral lung-a case report and review of the literature. *Thorac Cardiovasc Surg* 1989;37:385–387.
7. Colby TV, Koss MN, Travis WD. Miscellaneous mesenchymal tumors. In: Colby TV, Koss MN, Travis WD, eds. *Atlas of tumor pathology, third series: tumors of the lower respiratory tract*. Washington, DC: Armed Forces Institute of Pathology, 1995.
8. Colby TV, Koss MN, Travis WD. Fibrous and fibrohistiocytic tumors and tumor-like conditions. In: Colby TV, Koss MN, Travis WD, eds. *Atlas of tumor pathology, third series: tumors of the lower respiratory tract*. Washington, DC: Armed Forces Institute of Pathology, 1995.
9. Sperber M. *Radiologic diagnosis of cheat disease*. Springer, London, England, 2001.
10. Colby TV, Koss MN, Travis WD. Miscellaneous tumors and tumors of uncertain histogenesis. In: Colby TV, Koss MN, Travis WD, eds. *Atlas of tumor pathology, third series: tumors of the lower respiratory tract*. Washington, DC: Armed Forces Institute of Pathology, 1995.
11. Dahnert W. *Radiology review manual*, 4th ed. Baltimore: Williams & Wilkins, 1999.
12. Colby TV, Koss MN, Travis WD. Carcinoid and other neuroendocrine tumors. In: Colby TV, Koss MN, Travis WD, eds. *Atlas of tumor pathology, third series: tumors of the lower respiratory tract*. Washington, DC: Armed Forces Institute of Pathology, 1995.
13. Wilson RW, Frazier AA. Pathological-radiological correlations: pathological and radiological correlation of endobronchial neoplasms. Part II. Malignant tumors. *Ann Diagn Pathol* 1998;2:31–34.
14. Flieder DB, Vazquez MF. Lung tumors with neuroendocrine morphology. A perspective for the new millennium. *Radiol Clin North Am* 2000;38:563–577.
15. Marom EM, Goodman PC, McAdams HP. Focal abnormalities of the trachea and main bronchi. *AJR Am J Roentgenol* 2001;176:707–711.
16. Colby TV, Koss MN, Travis WD. Tumors of salivary gland type. In: Colby TV, Koss MN, Travis WD, eds. *Atlas of tumor pathology, third series: tumors of the lower respiratory tract*. Washington, DC: Armed Forces Institute of Pathology, 1995.
17. Colby TV, Koss MN, Travis WD. Hamartoma. In: Colby TV, Koss MN, Travis WD, eds. *Atlas of tumor pathology, third series: tumors of the lower respiratory tract*. Washington, DC: Armed Forces Institute of Pathology, 1995.
18. Colby TV, Koss MN, Travis WD. Embryology, anatomy, and congenital, developmental, and related lesions. In: Colby TV, Koss MN, Travis WD, eds. *Atlas of tumor pathology, third series: tumors of the lower respiratory tract*. Washington, DC: Armed Forces Institute of Pathology, 1995.
19. Luburich P, Carmen Ayuso M, Picado C, et al. CT of pulmonary epithelioid hemangioendothelioma. *J Comp Assist Tomogr* 1994;18:562–565.
20. Ross GJ, Violi L, Friedman AC, et al. Intravascular bronchioloalveolar tumor: CT and pathologic correlation. *J Comp Assist Tomogr* 1989;13:240–243.
21. Dail DH, Liebow AA, Gmelich JT, et al. Intravascular, bronchiolar, and alveolar tumor of the lung (IVBAT). An analysis of twenty cases of a peculiar sclerosing endothelial tumor. *Cancer* 1983;51:452–464.
22. Colby TV, Koss MN, Travis WD. Mixed epithelial and mesenchymal tumors. In: Colby TV, Koss MN, Travis WD, eds. *Atlas of tumor pathology, third series: tumors of the lower respiratory tract*. Washington, DC: Armed Forces Institute of Pathology, 1995.
23. Castellino RA. Hodgkin disease: practical concepts for the diagnostic radiologist. *Radiology* 1986;159:305–310.
24. Edwards JR, Matthay KK. Hematologic disorders affecting the lungs. *Clin Chest Med* 1989;10:723–746.

25. Balikian JP, Herman PG. Non-Hodgkin lymphoma of the lungs. *Radiology* 1979;132:569–576.
26. Lee KS, Kim Y, Primack SL. Imaging of pulmonary lymphomas. *AJR Am J Roentgenol* 1997;168: 339–345.
27. North LB, Libshitz HI, Lorigan JG. Thoracic lymphoma. *Radiol Clin North Am* 1990;28:745–762.
28. Bragg DG, Chor PJ, Murray KA, et al. Lymphoproliferative disorders of the lung: histopathology, clinical manifestations, and imaging features. *AJR Am J Roentgenol* 1994;163:273–281.
29. Colby TV, Koss MN, Travis WD. Tumors metastatic to the lung. In: Colby TV, Koss MN, Travis WD, eds. *Atlas of tumor pathology, third series: tumors of the lower respiratory tract.* Washington, DC: Armed Forces Institute of Pathology, 1995.
30. Quint LE, Park CH, Iannettoni MD. Solitary pulmonary nodules in patients with extrapulmonary neoplasms. *Radiology* 2000;217:257–261.
31. Gore RM. Esophageal cancer. Clinical and pathologic features. *Radiol Clin North Am* 1997;35: 243–263.
32. Levine MS. Esophageal cancer. Radiologic diagnosis. *Radiol Clin North Am* 1997;35:265–279.
33. Saunders HS, Wolfman NT, Ott DJ. Esophageal cancer. Radiologic staging. *Radiol Clin North Am* 1997;35:281–294.
34. Quint LE, Francis IR, Glazer GM, et al. CT and MR staging of tumors of the esophagus and gastroesophageal junction and detection of postoperative recurrence. In: Freeney PC, Stevenson GW, et al. *Margulis & Burhenne's alimentary tract radiology*, 5th ed. St. Louis: Mosby Yearbook, 1994.
35. McLoughlin RF, Cooperberg PL, Mathieson JR, et al. High resolution endoluminal ultrasonography in the staging of esophageal carcinoma. *J Ultrasound Med* 1995;14:725–730.
36. Quint LE, Hepburn LM, Francis IR, et al. Incidence and distribution of distant metastases from newly diagnosed esophageal carcinoma. *Cancer* 1995;76:1120–1125.
37. Carlisle JG, Quint LE, Francis IR, et al. Recurrent esophageal carcinoma: CT evaluation after esophagectomy. *Radiology* 1993;189:271–275.

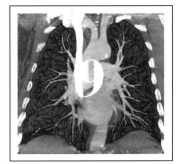

RADIOLOGY OF MEDIASTINAL MASSES

■ Localizing Mediastinal Masses
■ Differential Diagnosis
■ Computed Tomography of
   Mediastinal Masses
■ Current Role of Magnetic
   Resonance Imaging

Evaluation of the mediastinum is an important part of the interpretation of a chest x-ray (CXR). Saying that it is important is not the same as saying that it is well done. The mediastinum is the giant blind spot of the CXR. Mediastinal masses in particular represent a significant challenge to the diagnostic capabilities of the radiologist. Plain-film analysis of mediastinal masses is considered, with pointers for differential diagnosis. The roles of computed tomography (CT) and magnetic resonance imaging (MRI) are also addressed.

LOCALIZING MEDIASTINAL MASSES

Localization of mediastinal masses on CXR is a two-part job. The first part is to determine that a mass is actually mediastinal, and the second part is to place it in the anterior, middle, or posterior mediastinum. Several signs place a mass in the mediastinum. Configuration of the interface of the mass with adjacent lung is sometimes helpful. Parenchymal lung masses are generally almost completely surrounded by lung, forming an acute angle with the mediastinum. Mediastinal masses instead have the shape of extraparenchymal masses, pushing toward lung with resultant obtuse angles (Fig. 9.1). As with lateral extraparenchymal masses, it may be very difficult to distinguish a mediastinal mass from one in medial pleura. Bone destruction (involving spine, ribs, or sternum) resolves the issue, indicating that a medial mass is mediastinal. Bilaterality of abnormality also strongly suggests a mediastinal origin (Fig. 9.2). Conversely, air bronchograms in a lesion indicate that it arose in lung, not mediastinum.

Cardiopericardial abnormalities constitute an important pitfall in diagnosis of mediastinal masses. On the one hand, a soft anterior mediastinal mass such as a thymolipoma may droop down along the heart border (Fig. 9.3), resembling pericardial effusion or cyst (1). On the other hand, a pericardial cyst or neoplasm may extend cephalad into the pericardial recesses, simulating a mediastinal mass. CT may be very helpful in this regard.

The ability of radiologists to localize mediastinal masses via CXR has atrophied because of CT. Certain signs (silhouette sign, hilum overlay and convergence signs, and cervicothoracic and thoracoabdominal signs) (Chapter 3) can be enormously helpful in localizing mediastinal masses. Effect of a mass on adjacent mediastinal structures (trachea,

Bilaterality of abnormality in proximity to the thoracic midline suggests a mediastinal origin.

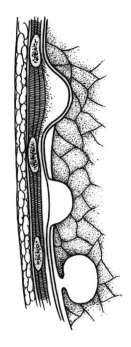

Figure 9.1 Drawing of different medial thoracic lesions, illustrating differences in shape and in configuration of margins. M, mediastinal; P, pleural; L, lung. The same applies to lateral lesions, where M is the configuration of an extrapleural mass.

paraspinal line, anterior and posterior junction lines, and ribs) should also be assessed. These observations, in combination, will often be more useful for localizing mediastinal masses than will lateral chest radiographs (Fig. 9.4). Although the advantage of having two right-angle radiographs for evaluating three-dimensional anatomy has previously been emphasized, lateral radiography is frequently not very helpful for mediastinal mass localization.

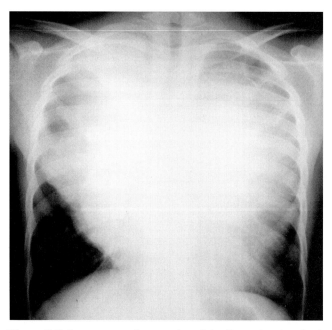

Figure 9.2 Large mass of uncertain origin. Extension into both hemithoraces is typical of a mediastinal mass, in this case Hodgkin disease.

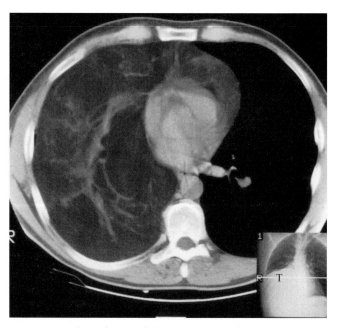

Figure 9.3 Thymolipoma fills the right hemithorax with fat and vessels. The computed tomography scout demonstrates that the mass (T) droops down toward the diaphragm.

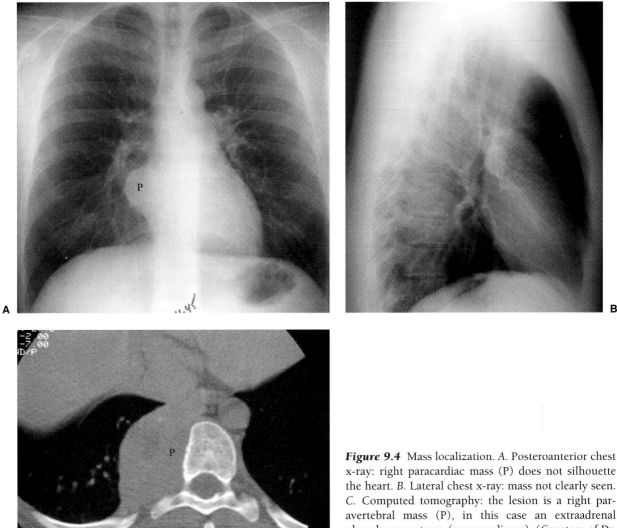

Figure 9.4 Mass localization. *A.* Posteroanterior chest x-ray: right paracardiac mass (P) does not silhouette the heart. *B.* Lateral chest x-ray: mass not clearly seen. *C.* Computed tomography: the lesion is a right paravertebral mass (P), in this case an extraadrenal pheochromocytoma (paraganglioma). (Courtesy of Dr. David Spizarny, Deroit, MI.)

DIFFERENTIAL DIAGNOSIS

Generating a differential diagnosis for a mediastinal mass starts with a classification scheme. The system used by Felson (2) (Fig. 9.5) divides the mediastinum into anterior, middle, and posterior compartments by drawing one line along the front of the trachea and the back of the heart and a second line 1 cm posterior to the anterior margin of the thoracic vertebrae. This system does not classify the superior mediastinum as a separate compartment.

For anterior mediastinal masses, the classic differential diagnosis is the "4 Ts": thymoma, thyroid, teratoma, and terrible lymphoma (Table 9.1). Further clues can be obtained from the radiographic appearance, the patient's age, and associated clinical manifestations. For example, mediastinal thyroid is rare if there is not demonstrable direct extension from the neck. Calcification, teeth, and/or fat in a lesion favor teratoma. Lymphoma is the likeliest diagnosis when there is a multilobular mass (Fig. 9.6). Thymoma often (although not always) overlies the aortopulmonary window (Fig. 9.7).

The "4 Ts" delineate the important entities in anterior mediastinal mass differential diagnosis—thymoma, thyroid, teratoma, and terrible lymphoma.

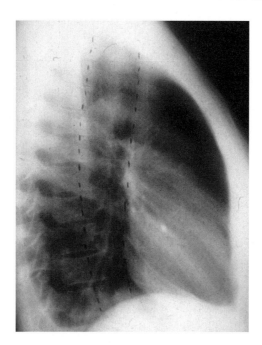

Figure 9.5 Compartments of the mediastinum. (From Felson B. *Chest roentgenology*. Philadelphia: WB Saunders, 1973:419, with permission.)

Table 9.1: Anterior Mediastinal Masses

The 4 Ts: Thymoma, teratoma, thyroid, terrible lymphoma
   Hemangioma
   Hemorrhage
   Metastases
   Parathyroid adenoma
   Vascular lesions

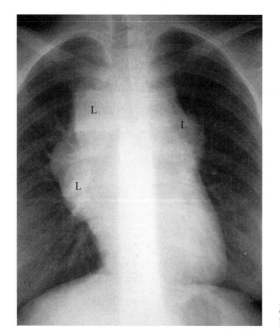

Figure 9.6 Multilobular mass (L) typical of lymphoma.

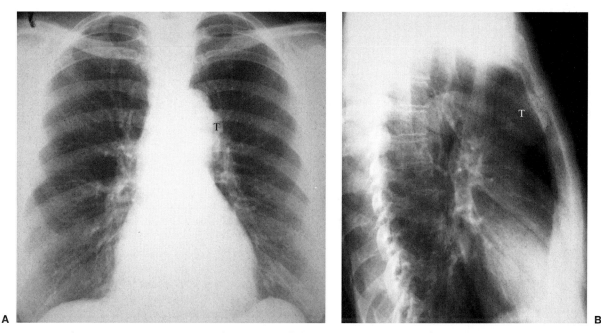

Figure 9.7 Thymoma. *A.* Posteroanterior chest x-ray: subtle mass overlying aortopulmonary window (T). *B.* Lateral chest x-ray: much more obvious mass (T).

Turning to clinical clues, teratoma is typically a disease of teenagers, whereas thymoma usually affects those aged 40 to 60 years. Hodgkin disease has a bimodal age distribution, particularly affecting patients in their teens or 20s and those over age 50. There are a number of clinical conditions associated with thymoma, including myasthenia gravis (MG), pure red cell aplasia, and hypogammaglobulinemia. MG is the most common of these, occurring in roughly 50% of patients with thymomas; among patients with MG, 10% to 15% have an underlying thymoma.

The classic mnemonic is not all inclusive. There are thymic lesions other than thymoma to consider, for example. Thymic carcinoid demonstrates some of the same features as bronchial carcinoid (Fig. 9.8). Metastatic disease and vascular lesions (such as aneurysms) can occur in any mediastinal compartment. Trauma or nontraumatic mediastinal hemorrhage probably affects the anterior mediastinum more than any other mediastinal compartment (Fig. 9.9). Finally, when parathyroid adenomas are not found in the neck, they usually occur in the anterior mediastinum (Fig. 9.10). Only a small percentage (less than 2%) of normal parathyroid glands are mediastinal, but in patients with previously unsuccessful neck exploratory surgery for primary hyperparathyroidism, the incidence of a mediastinal adenoma rises to 47% (3). Whereas most ectopic parathyroid glands are in the superior aspect of the mediastinum, readily accessible to a neck incision, the percentage of mediastinal glands requiring sternotomy rises to 17% in those being reexplored for hyperparathyroidism.

Turning to the middle mediastinum (Table 9.2), the key structure that traverses this compartment from top to bottom is the esophagus (Fig. 9.11). As a result, even in the twenty-first century CT is not the only alternative to the CXR for diagnosis and further characterization of middle mediastinal masses. Barium swallow actually is better than CT at delineation of esophageal lesions, which account for many middle mediastinal masses. In fact, it is surprising how many patients with documented esophageal carcinomas have normal or nearly normal chest CTs. Other esophageal masses (such as leiomyomas) are similarly better seen with barium swallow than with CXR or CT.

In patients with prior neck exploration and continued primary hyperparathyroidism, the incidence of mediastinal adenoma is 47%, and 17% of such glands cannot be reached from a neck incision.

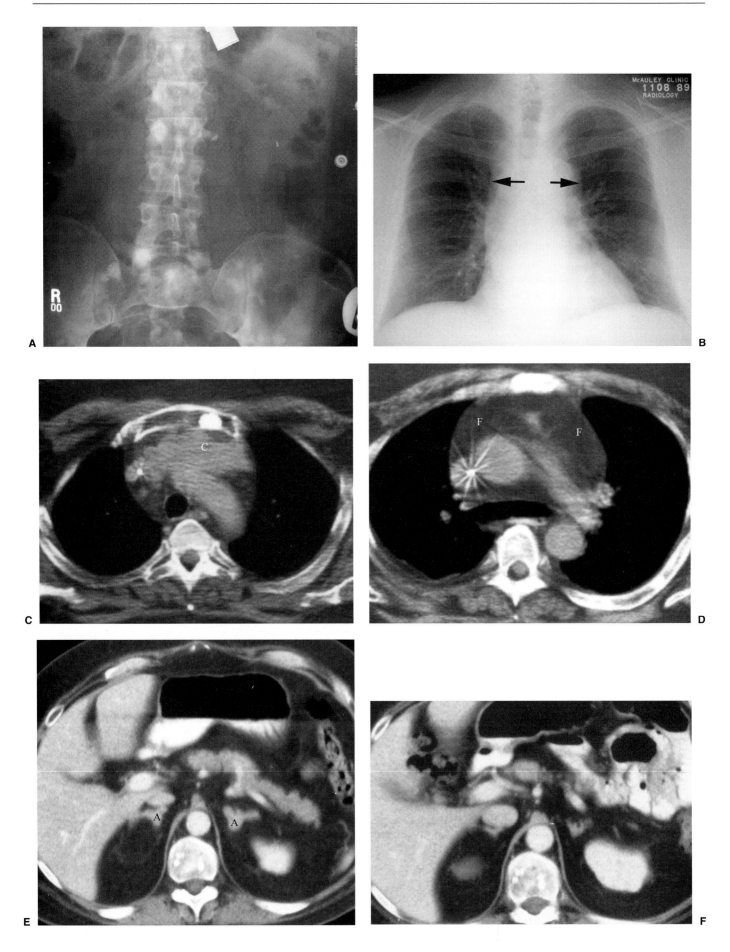

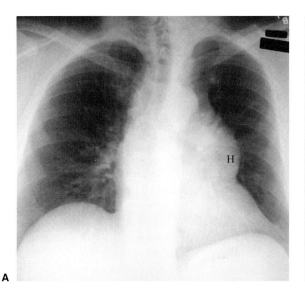

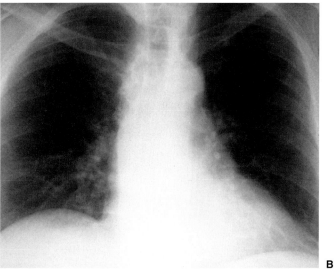

A

B

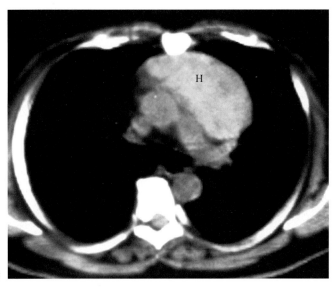

C

Figure 9.9 Disappearing anterior mediastinal mass. *A.* Posteroanterior chest x-ray 3-27: anterior mediastinal mass (H) blends with left heart border. Note the hilum overlay sign, with vessels converging medial to the mass border. *B.* Posteroanterior chest x-ray 4-1: mass no longer present. *C.* Noncontrast computed tomography 3-28: high attenuation of the mass (H) reveals that it is spontaneous mediastinal hemorrhage.

Figure 9.8 This book cannot omit one of the all-time great cases. *A.* Abdominal radiograph obtained because of pain after a motor vehicle accident: multiple sclerotic skeletal lesions. *B.* Posteroanterior chest x-ray: mild mediastinal widening *(arrows).* *C.* Computed tomography at the level of the aortic arch: anterior mediastinal soft tissue mass (C). *D.* Computed tomography several centimeters caudal to C: mediastinal widening is also partly due to mediastinal lipomatosis (F). *E.* Computed tomography of the upper abdomen: the adrenals (A) are incredibly thick. The diagnosis is thymic carcinoid, accounting for the mediastinal mass and the sclerotic skeletal metastases and causing Cushing syndrome, with mediastinal lipomatosis and adrenal hyperplasia. *F.* Computed tomography of the upper abdomen after resection of the thymic carcinoid: the adrenals have returned to normal. (Courtesy of Dr. David Baker, Ann Arbor, MI.)

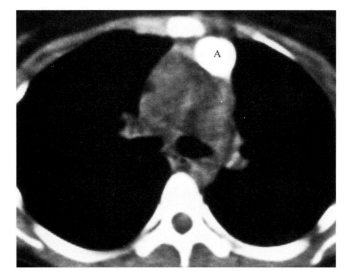

Figure 9.10 Parathyroid adenoma (A) after angiographic ablation, accounting for intense contrast enhancement. (Courtesy of Dr. Murray Rebner, Royal Oak, MI.)

Table 9.2: Middle Mediastinal Masses

Esophageal abnormality
Lymph node disease
   Lymphoma
   Metastases
   Sarcoidosis
   Infection
Bronchogenic cyst
Vascular lesions (aneurysms, pseudoaneurysms)

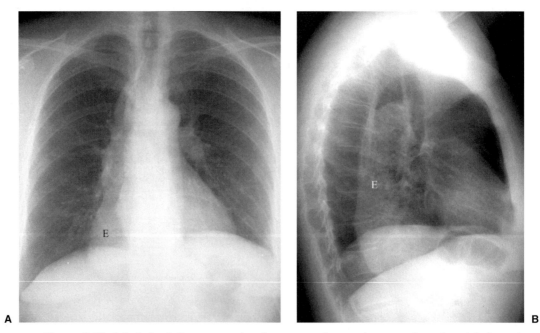

Figure 9.11 Achalasia. *A.* Posteroanterior chest x-ray: abnormal contour lateral to right heart border (E). *B.* Lateral chest x-ray: massively dilated esophagus (E) containing debris.

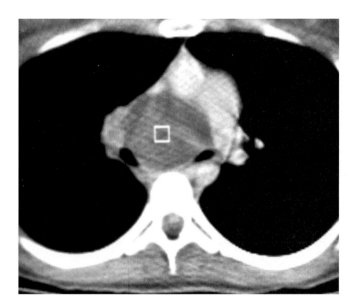

Figure 9.12 Bronchogenic cyst. Computed tomography reveals typical water attenuation mass (marked by *cursor*) in subcarinal middle mediastinum.

If a middle mediastinal mass is unrelated to the esophagus, the differential diagnosis includes bronchogenic cyst (Fig. 9.12), lymph node abnormalities (sarcoid, lymphoma, metastases), and vascular lesions (Fig. 9.13). Bronchogenic cyst most often occurs between the carina and the esophagus, but the right lower paratracheal region is not an uncommon alternative location (Fig. 9.14). Among lymph node diseases, tuberculous lymphadenitis has become a more important entity because it is common in patients with acquired immunodeficiency syndrome and frequently involves middle mediastinal lymph nodes. Metastatic disease usually affects lymph nodes in the anterior and/or middle mediastinum. Lung cancer is the most common primary neoplasm to involve mediastinal lymph nodes. Most extrathoracic neoplasms do not commonly metastasize to intratho-

Extrathoracic neoplasms that metastasize to intrathoracic lymph nodes include primaries of head and neck, breast, stomach, kidney, and testis, as well as melanoma.

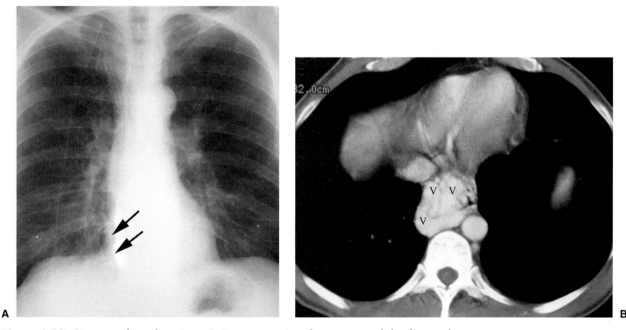

A

B

Figure 9.13 Giant esophageal varices. *A.* Posteroanterior chest x-ray: subtle abnormal contour (*arrows*) in right lower paravertebral region. *B.* Computed tomography: massive enhancing esophageal varices (V).

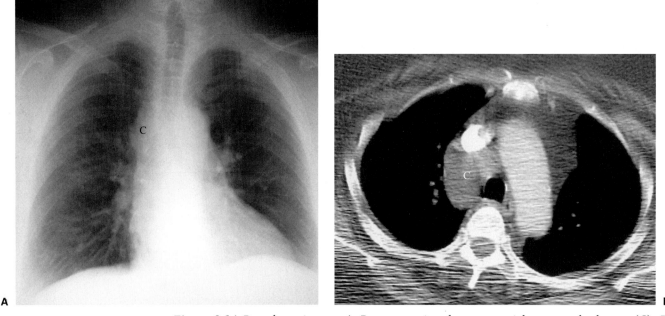

Figure 9.14 Bronchogenic cyst. *A.* Posteroanterior chest x-ray: right paratracheal mass (C). *B.* Computed tomography: uniform water attenuation mass (C) is typical of bronchogenic cyst.

racic lymph nodes, but there are exceptions. Head and neck tumors, genitourinary neoplasms (especially testicular and renal cell carcinomas), breast carcinoma, gastric carcinoma, and melanoma are extrathoracic primaries with a predilection for hilar and mediastinal lymph nodes.

Posterior mediastinal masses (Table 9.3) generally represent neurogenic tumors (neurofibroma, schwannoma, ganglioneuroma, and so on) (Fig. 9.15). Posterior mediastinal masses may grow to incredible sizes. (A thoracic surgeon in our institution notes that the largest intrathoracic masses he has encountered have almost always been posterior mediastinal masses.) Interestingly, in patients with neurofibromatosis, posterior mediastinal masses are nearly as often lateral meningoceles (Fig. 9.16) as they are neurogenic tumors. Experience teaches that masses near the medial lung apices are often posterior mediastinal in origin, even when the angle between lesion and mediastinum is not well assessed (Fig. 9.17). This applies to most medial lesions above the clavicles, at least if they are well outlined by lung (the cervicothoracic sign).

For posterior mediastinal masses in general, other diagnostic considerations include disc space or vertebral body infection, vascular lesions, and extramedullary hematopoiesis (Fig. 9.18). The latter condition usually produces bilateral lobulated paravertebral masses in the lower thoracic region and is commonly associated with hereditary spherocytosis, thalassemia, or other severe congenital anemias.

Table 9.3: Posterior Mediastinal Masses

Neurogenic tumors
Extramedullary hematopoiesis
Hemangioma
Infection
Vascular lesions

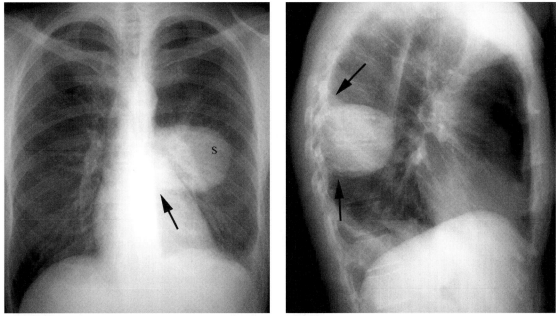

A

B

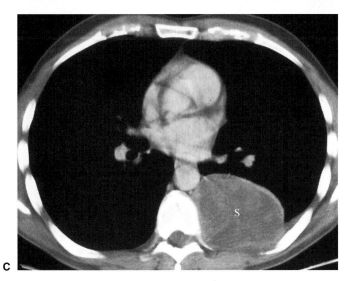

C

Figure 9.15 Large schwannoma. *A.* Posteroanterior chest x-ray: large left thoracic mass (S) with right angle margin medially *(arrow).* Note hilum overlay sign. *B.* Lateral chest x-ray: mass again demonstrates right angle margins *(arrows).* *C.* Computed tomography: reasonably uniform low attenuation (but not water attenuation) left paravertebral mass (S).

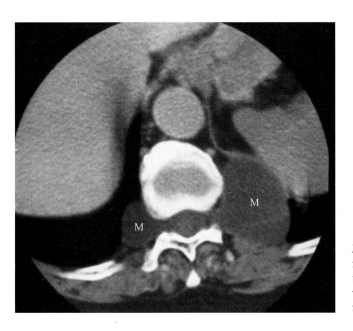

Figure 9.16 Bilateral lateral meningoceles (M). Computed tomography reveals water attenuation masses adjacent to the neural foramina.

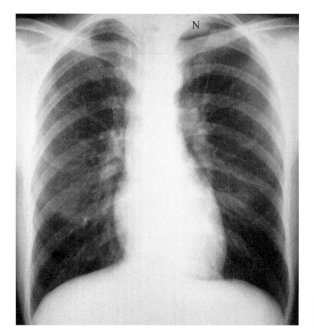

Figure 9.17 Apical neurofibroma (N) in a patient with neurofibromatosis.

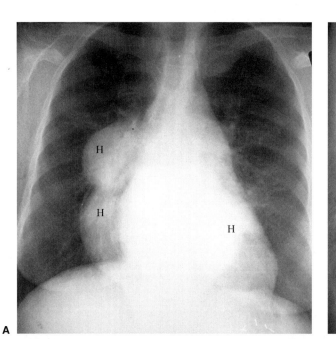

A

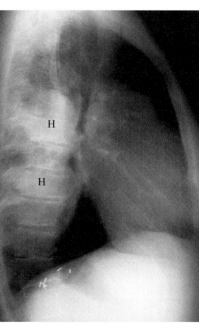

B

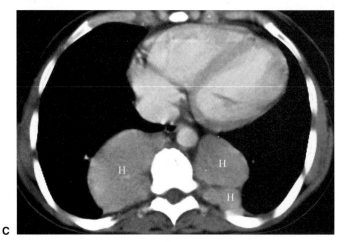

C

Figure 9.18 Extramedullary hematopoiesis. *A.* Posteroanterior chest x-ray: multilobular bilateral mediastinal masses (H) in lower hemithoraces. *B.* Lateral chest x-ray: masses (H) are posterior. *C.* Computed tomography: lobular bilateral soft tissue masses (H).

Computed Tomography of Mediastinal Masses

CT has revolutionized the imaging of mediastinal masses. Compared with CXR, CT has major advantages in detection and characterization of mediastinal masses. These advantages are considered in turn, and the ability of CT to arrive at a specific diagnosis is also addressed.

Detection

CT is considerably better than CXR in detecting mediastinal masses. This has been particularly well studied in patients with MG, where underlying thymoma is an important concern. In an early series of six patients with MG (4), CT detected a thymoma missed by CXR in one and accurately localized to the thymus a second calcified lesion whose CXR location was indeterminate. In a second series of 23 consecutive MG patients who underwent thymectomy regardless of neurologic status or imaging results (5), CT detected all four thymomas that were present; CXR was positive in three of four. At CT there were two false-positive examinations, but there were three false positives at CXR. In a larger series of 57 MG patients (6), 16 of whom had thymoma, CT detected 14 of 16. CXR in these patients was positive in nine, equivocal in two, and normal in five.

> CT is indicated to rule out thymoma in MG, even when CXR is normal.

Lesion detection was also addressed in a large series of proven mediastinal masses that had been demonstrated by CT (7). Of 90 patients with concurrent CXR, only 62 (69%) had mediastinal masses that could be detected by the chest radiograph. The rate of detection depended on the mediastinal compartment. Only 48% (10/21) of middle mediastinal masses were detected by CXR, with 67% (20/30) of anterior and 100% (4/4) of posterior mediastinal masses visualized. The smallest mass detected by CXR was a $2 \times 2 \times 2$-cm anterior mediastinal mass caused by sarcoidosis. The largest mass missed by CXR was a $6 \times 5 \times 7$ cm middle mediastinal mass in small cell carcinoma of lung.

> CXR detected only 69% of CT-demonstrated mediastinal masses in one series.

Confirmation of Location and Extent

The ability of CT to confirm location and extent of mediastinal abnormality has important consequences in differential diagnosis. It is obvious that when CT precisely localizes a mass that cannot be localized by CXR, this will improve differential diagnosis. It is less obvious (but also true) that the ability of CT to differentiate patients with a single mediastinal mass from those with multiple masses also has important diagnostic implications. Patients with multiple masses are very unlikely to have thymoma or teratoma and are much more likely to have lymphoma, metastatic disease, or sarcoidosis (7). On the other hand, a single middle mediastinal mass virtually excludes lymphoma (7). This does not apply to a single anterior mediastinal mass; lymphoblastic lymphoma presented this way in several patients. CT is much better at distinguishing single from multiple masses than CXR. Of 28 patients with multiple masses at CT and an abnormal CXR, 12 (43%) were thought to have a single mass based on the chest radiograph (7).

Identification of Fat, Water, and Calcium

The ability of CT to identify different tissues by their attenuation characteristics can be very important in diagnosing mediastinal masses. Tables 9.4, 9.5, and 9.6 list the masses that may be fat attenuation, fluid attenuation, or calcified, respectively, on CT. An anterior mediastinal mass containing fat, water, calcium, and/or teeth is a teratoma (8) (Fig. 9.19). Thymoma may have a rim of calcification (Fig. 9.20), whereas thymic cyst is a water attenuation lesion. In the middle mediastinum, bronchogenic cyst is often a water

Table 9.4: Fat Attenuation Mediastinal Masses

Lipomatosis
Lipoma
Thymolipoma
Teratoma
Diaphragmatic hernias
   Morgagni
   Bochdalek
   Hiatal
   Posttraumatic

Table 9.5: Fluid Attenuation Mediastinal Masses

Bronchopulmonary foregut duplication anomalies
   Bronchogenic cyst
   Esophageal duplication cyst or diverticulum
   Neuroenteric cyst
Thymic cyst
Pericardial cyst
Lateral thoracic meningocele
Teratoma
Hematoma / seroma / abscess
Abdominal source
   Pancreatic pseudocyst
   Ascites through diaphragmatic hiatus

Table 9.6: Calcified Mediastinal Masses

Goiter
Fibrosing mediastinitis
Lymph nodes
   Silicosis
   Sarcoidosis
   Tuberculosis
   Histoplasmosis
   Pneumocystis carinii infection
   Treated lymphoma
Teratoma

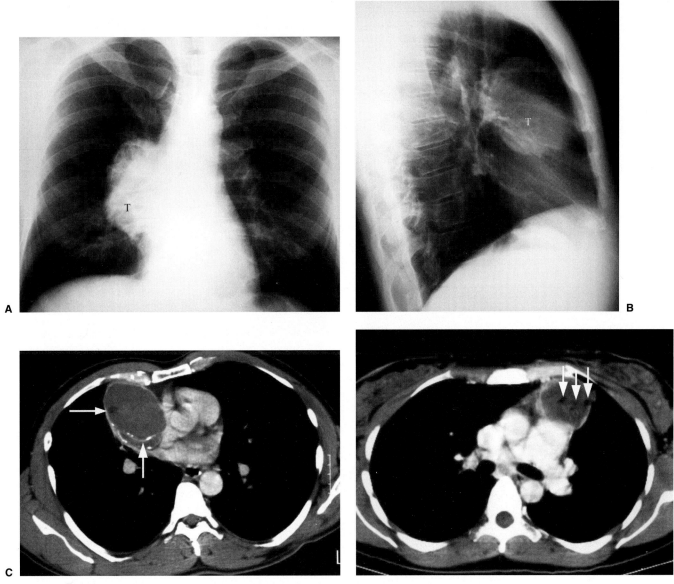

Figure 9.19 Anterior mediastinal teratomas. *A.* Posteroanterior chest x-ray: mass (T) overlying right hilum and blending with right heart border. *B.* Lateral chest x-ray: anterior location confirmed (T). *C.* Computed tomography: mass largely consists of fluid, with curvilinear calcification *(arrow)* and smaller low attenuation foci indicating fat *(left arrow). D.* Computed tomography in a different patient: similar mass with foci of fat *(arrows).*

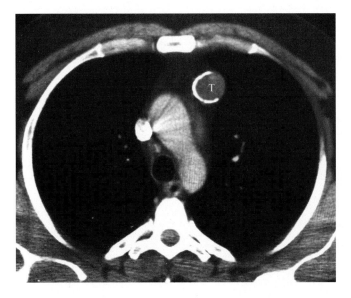

Figure 9.20 Thymoma with peripheral calcification. Note that computed tomography demonstrates a solid mass, not one of water attenuation as in Fig. 9.19.

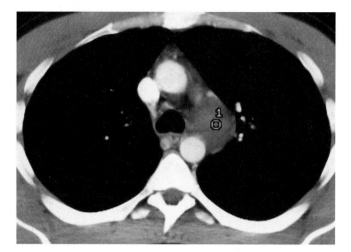

Figure 9.21 Bronchogenic cyst with uniform high attenuation contents. Computed tomography attenuation measured 36 Hounsfield units.

attenuation lesion, although uniform higher attenuation in a bronchogenic cyst is a well-known phenomenon (9) (Fig. 9.21). Low attenuation lymph nodes with enhancing rims are typical of tuberculous lymphadenitis (10). As for posterior mediastinal masses, many neurogenic tumors are relatively low in attenuation (Fig. 9.15C) but not of water attenuation. Calcification may be seen in neurogenic tumors, particularly those containing elements of neuroblastoma. Lateral meningoceles are water attenuation paravertebral masses (Fig. 9.16).

Enhancement Characteristics

Mediastinal thyroid and paraganglioma account for most enhancing mediastinal masses, whereas lymphoma and metastatic disease almost never enhance.

Bolus injection of intravenous contrast optimizes CT demonstration of enhancement of intrathoracic structures. This in turn facilitates differentiation of mediastinal from cardiac masses, the demonstration of mediastinal vascular abnormalities, and the recognition of enhancing mediastinal masses (Table 9.7). The demonstration of an enhancing mediastinal mass results in a more specific differential diagnosis (11). Mediastinal thyroid is the most common enhancing mediastinal mass. At the University of Michigan, a referral center for extraadrenal pheochromocytomas because the radionuclide ^{131}I MIBG was developed there (12), intrathoracic pheochromocytomas accounted for 4 of enhancing mediastinal masses and an aortic body tumor accounted for a fifth (11). These tumors can be lumped together because of their common origin from paraganglionic cells, and it has been suggested that all aortic and carotid body tumors, chemodectomas, glomus tumors, and extraadrenal pheochromocytomas should instead be called paragangliomas.

Other causes of enhancing mediastinal masses include Castleman disease (Fig. 9.22), parathyroid adenoma (Fig. 9.23), and carcinoid tumor. On rare occasions the pattern of contrast enhancement may suggest a specific diagnosis (13) (Fig. 9.24). Contrast enhancement virtually eliminates lymphoma and metastatic disease from consideration.

Table 9.7: Enhancing Mediastinal Masses

Aneurysm
Esophageal varices
Goiter
Castleman disease
Paraganglioma (extraadrenal pheochromoctyoma)
Ectopic parathyroid adenoma
Carcinoid tumor

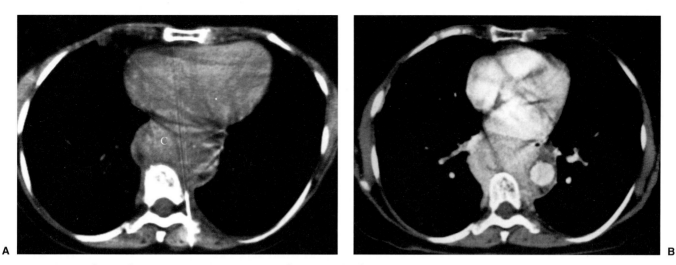

Figure 9.22 Castleman disease. *A*. Precontrast computed tomography during percutaneous biopsy: soft tissue attenuation middle mediastinal mass (C). *B*. Postcontrast computed tomography: marked enhancement of mass.

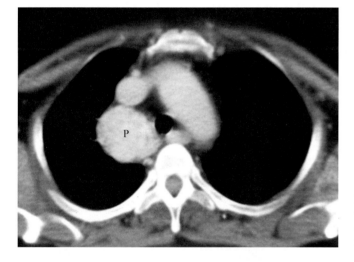

Figure 9.23 Mediastinal parathyroid adenoma. Computed tomography demonstrates contrast enhancement of mass (P).

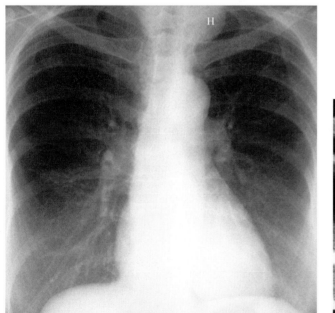

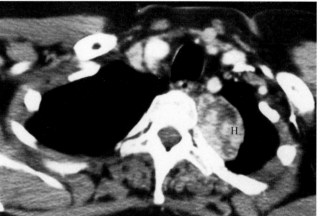

Figure 9.24 Characteristic enhancing pattern of mediastinal mass. *A*. Posteroanterior chest x-ray: left medial apical mass (H); lesions in this location are virtually always posterior mediastinal masses. *B*. Computed tomography reveals puddles of contrast enhancement in the mass (H), typical of cavernous hemangioma.

DETECTION OF CONCURRENT ABNORMALITIES

Associated abnormalities in the chest or upper abdomen are common in patients with mediastinal masses, and they definitely affect differential diagnosis. Concurrent axillary lymph node enlargement favors lymphoma, whereas a focal pulmonary mass, focal hepatic or adrenal lesions, or bone lesions suggest metastatic disease (7). A very important clue to the diagnosis of malignant thymoma is focal or multifocal, usually unilateral pleural implants. These can be in either hemithorax, although in our experience they are more common in the left pleural space. Amazingly, in some patients it may be more difficult to detect these implants with CT than with CXR. Various other concurrent abnormalities are demonstrable (e.g., pericardial disease, neck mass, abdominal lymph node enlargement), but they do not narrow the differential diagnosis significantly.

SPECIFIC COMPUTED TOMOGRAPHY DIAGNOSES

Certain mediastinal masses can be characterized with confidence at CT, but specific diagnosis generally remains an elusive goal.

With the advantages enumerated above it would be expected that CT would improve one's ability to reach a specific diagnosis in many patients with mediastinal masses. An elaborate algorithm has been developed that uses the capabilities of CT (14). However, in the previously cited series (7) of proven mediastinal masses demonstrated by CT, specific diagnosis was possible in only 16 of 132 patients. Most patients had metastatic disease or lymphoma. These common soft tissue attenuation masses could not reliably be distinguished from each other (or from sarcoidosis), and it was also generally impossible to distinguish Hodgkin disease from non-Hodgkin lymphoma or to distinguish metastatic lung cancer from other metastatic disease. CT may narrow the differential diagnosis, as previously noted, by demonstrating multiple masses or certain concurrent extramediastinal abnormalities, but specific CT attenuation characteristics were encountered infrequently. A more recent study (15) of anterior mediastinal masses concurred, noting "although CT is better than chest radiography in determining the pathologic diagnosis of an anterior mediastinal mass, CT is still poor at making that prediction with confidence."

CURRENT ROLE OF MAGNETIC RESONANCE IMAGING

Several series have shown that MRI can clearly display mediastinal masses in a manner comparable with CT (16,17). Although MRI has theoretical and real advantages (including multiplanar imaging capability, lack of ionizing radiation, avoidance of intravenous contrast agents or use of less toxic agents, and potential for tissue characterization), to date these are outweighed by considerations such as availability, cost, and, most important, examination time. As a result, CT remains the examination of choice for the mediastinum, with MRI assuming a secondary problem-solving role. This has been the state of affairs since the 1980s, and it is unlikely to change in the near future.

REFERENCES

1. Rosado-de-Christenson ML, Pugatch RD, Moran CA, et al. Thymolipoma: analysis of 27 cases. *Radiology* 1994;193:121–126.
2. Felson B. *Chest roentgenology*. Philadelphia: WB Saunders, 1973.
3. Krudy AG, Doppman JL, Brennan MF, et al. The detection of mediastinal parathyroid glands by computed tomography, selective arteriography, and venous sampling. *Radiology* 1981;140: 739–744.
4. Mink JH, Bein ME, Sukor R, et al. Computed tomography of the anterior mediastinum in patients with myasthenia gravis and suspected thymoma. *AJR Am J Roentgenol* 1978;130: 239–246.

5. Moore AV, Korobkin M, Powers B, et al. Thymoma detection by mediastinal CT: patients with myasthenia gravis. *AJR Am J Roentgenol* 1982;138:217–222.

6. Fon GT, Bein ME, Mancuso AA, et al. Computed tomography of the anterior mediastinum in myasthenia gravis. *Radiology* 1982;142:135–141.

7. Rebner M, Gross BH, Robertson JM, et al. CT evaluation of mediastinal masses. *Comput Radiol* 1987;11:103–110.

8. Moeller KH, Rosado-de-Christenson ML, Templeton PA. Mediastinal mature teratoma: imaging features. *AJR Am J Roentgenol* 1997;169:985–990.

9. Mendelson DS, Rose JS, Efremidis SC, et al. Bronchogenic cysts with high CT numbers. *AJR Am J Roentgenol* 1983;140:463–465.

10. Im J, Song KS, Kang HS, et al. Mediastinal tuberculous lymphadenitis: CT manifestations. *Radiology* 1987;164:115–119.

11. Spizarny DL, Rebner M, Gross BH. Enhancing mediastinal masses: CT evaluation. *J Comput Assist Tomogr* 1987;11:990–993.

12. Francis IR, Glazer GM, Shapiro B, et al. Complementary roles of CT and ^{131}I-MIBG scintigraphy in diagnosing pheochromocytoma. *AJR Am J Roentgenol* 1983;141:719–725.

13. McAdams HP, Rosado-de-Christenson ML, Moran CA. Mediastinal hemangioma: radiographic and CT features in 14 patients. *Radiology* 1994;193:399–402.

14. Feigin DS, Padua EM. Mediastinal masses: a system for diagnosis based on computed tomography. *J Comput Tomogr* 1986;10:11–21.

15. Ahn JM, Lee KS, Goo JM, et al. Predicting the histology of anterior mediastinal masses: comparison of chest radiography and CT. *J Thorac Imag* 1996;11:265–271.

16. Aronberg DJ, Glazer HS, Sagel SS. MRI and CT of the mediastinum: comparisons, controversies, and pitfalls. *Radiol Clin North Am* 1985;23:439–448.

17. Von Schulthess GK, McMurdo KC, Tscholakoff D, et al. Mediastinal masses: MR imaging. *Radiology* 1986;158:289–296.

THORACIC IMAGING IN THE CRITICALLY ILL

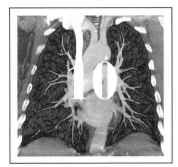

- ■ Radiologic Approach
- ■ Pulmonary Parenchymal Opacification
- ■ Evaluation of Cardiovascular Status
- ■ Cardiogenic Edema versus Noncardiogenic Edema versus Other Causes of Lung Opacity
- ■ Abnormal Air Collections

Imaging of the thorax in critically ill and/or intensive care unit (ICU) patients has an important role in successful patient management. Portable chest radiography is the mainstay for evaluation of the thorax in these patients. Chest radiographs are either performed as daily routine examinations or are performed as urgent or immediate examinations due to abrupt changes in clinical status or the manipulation of indwelling diagnostic, therapeutic or monitoring lines, tubes, and devices. The latter are covered in detail in Chapter 11. Performing daily routine portable chest radiographs on ICU patients has been shown to detect unexpected problems, with subsequent alterations in the diagnostic approach or treatment after nearly 40% of "routine" examinations and after nearly two-thirds of all portable chest radiographs on ICU patients (1–3). Although routine testing faces considerable scrutiny by health care facilities and third-party payers facing constant pressure to reduce costs, such imaging for critically ill intensive care unit patients may be justified as an effective method to discover unexpected problems that may be a source of morbidity or mortality. Guidelines for portable radiography can be developed successfully by multidisciplinary teams, so that imaging is appropriate (4,5).

Important elements of acute care radiology include not only the timely performance and accurate interpretation of examinations, but prompt communication of abnormalities to the ordering physician. Daily radiology rounds between radiologists and the ICU team, including physicians, nurses, and respiratory therapists, promotes quality patient care. Bitetti and Zimmerman (6) described the concepts of such a team, indicating the positive benefits of improved diagnostic information, facilitated sequencing of studies, and decreased hospital length of stay.

In the last decade, computed tomography (CT) has played a greater role in the imaging of critically ill ICU patients (7–11). Clinical indications for CT in this setting include distinguishing between pleural and parenchymal disease (Fig.10.1) and evaluating pleural fluid collections, including empyema (Chapter 17), lung abscess (Fig. 10.2), mediastinal abnormality, abnormal or unusual fluid or air collections (Fig.10.3), and pulmonary embolism (Chapter 21). CT may also be used for CT-guided percutaneous drainage and fluid aspiration (12). CT for ICU patients generally requires the transportation of ill and often medically unstable patients to the radiology department, with careful attention to the logistical difficulties of maintaining life support systems during transportation. Physiologic changes are common during transportation, as frequently occurs when these patients

Daily routine portable radiographs in ICU patients commonly reveals significant findings.

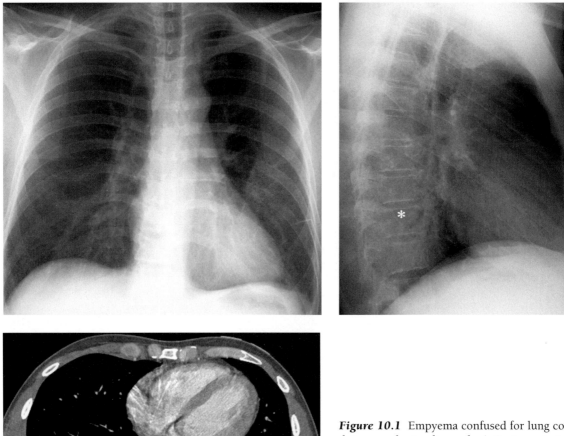

Figure 10.1 Empyema confused for lung consolidation on chest radiograph. *A.* Posteroanterior and *(B)* lateral chest radiographs demonstrate ill-defined opacity over the mid-lower left lung, seen over the spine on the lateral view *(asterisk)*, without sharp borders. *C.* Computed tomography demonstrates a loculated left pleura fluid collection, heterogeneous in attenuation, with pleural thickening and enhancement.

are in the ICU. In one study, 39% of all patients transported to radiology had a change in management within 48 hours of the diagnostic examination; for abdominal CT examinations, that number was even higher, at 51% (13). At our institution the transportation of adult ICU patients to radiology is done by a specialized team of six registered nurses with critical care training, called the SWAT team (Smiling, Willing, Able and Technical), a concept developed at the University of Missouri (14). Up to two SWAT nurses and a respiratory therapist usually transport the ICU patients, depending on their clinical status. Use of specially trained nursing staff has been shown to reduce adverse outcomes associated with intrahospital transportation of critically ill patients (14).

Mobile or portable CT scanners are also available to use in or adjacent to the ICU (15,16). In general, image quality is poorer than the modern fast helical CT scanners that are prevalent today. Portable CT scanners are not technically capable of performing fast CT angiographic examinations, as required to evaluate for suspected pulmonary embolism or vascular emergencies. They are capable of basic evaluation of the lungs, pleural spaces and mediastinum, abdomen, and intracranial structures. In one series, the physicians who ordered portable CTs cited that patient severity of illness, use of extracorporeal life support, and cardiovascular instability were the most common indications for the study; when faced with a situation in which the portable CT scanner was not available, 67% of physi-

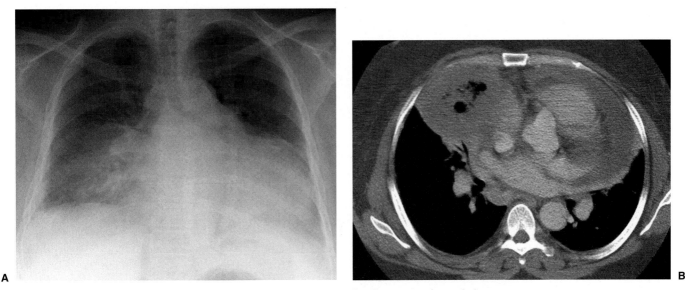

A   B

Figure 10.2 Right middle lobe lung abscess secondary to methicillin-resistant *Staphylococcus aureus* (MRSA) with pericardial effusion. *A.* Posteroanterior chest radiograph demonstrates a mass-like opacity in the right middle lobe and a large cardiac silhouette. *B.* Computed tomography demonstrates the mass to be a fluid and air-filled lung abscess with a moderately sized pericardial fluid collection that required a surgical pericardial window for drainage.

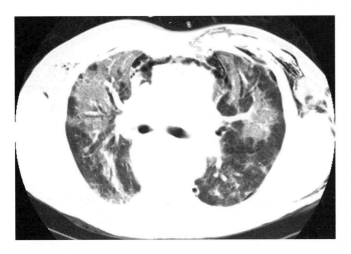

Figure 10.3 Negative pressure pulmonary edema. Computed tomography image after traumatic intubation for thoracoscopic thoracic duct ligation demonstrates ground glass opacities predominantly in the central and anterior aspect of the lungs.

cians ordered fixed helical CTs requiring transportation to the radiology department (15). In contrast to CT, ultrasound examinations may be performed at the bedside and are particularly useful for the evaluation of pleural fluid collections, both for diagnosis and percutaneous ultrasound-guided intervention (Chapter 22) (17,18).

RADIOLOGIC APPROACH

Comprehensive and systematic assessment of chest radiographs in critically ill patients includes evaluation of lung parenchymal abnormalities, pleural disease, mediastinum, cardiovascular structures, and physiologic parameters. The visualized portion of the abdomen should also be evaluated for signs of disease processes that are often silent clinically in intubated, sedated, and/or paralyzed patients. It is important to look at the musculoskeletal structures as well. The correct position of all diagnostic, therapeutic, and

Table 10.1: Lung Parenchymal Opacification in the ICU Setting

ARDS
Edema (cardiogenic and noncardiogenic)
Pneumonia
Aspiration
Hemorrhage
Underlying lung disease

ICU, intensive care unit; ARDS, acute respiratory distress syndrome.

monitoring devices should be confirmed, as detailed to a greater extent in Chapter 11. The use of computed radiography with soft-copy interpretation of images on workstations by radiologists improves the delivery of portable chest images and facilitates the initiation of clinical actions, without any reduction in diagnostic quality, when compared with conventional film-screen radiography (19,20). As a by-product, the use of computed radiography also reduces consultation with radiologists.

The interpretation of portable chest radiography is made more difficult by the limited power output of portable equipment and subsequent inconsistency of filming technique. The latter can be overcome in many cases by the use of computed radiography, which allows manipulation of image parameters at a computer workstation to optimize evaluation of the thorax. Patient factors also contribute to reduced image quality and include the inability to position patients fully upright, the inability to obtain images free of respiratory motion at full inspiration in intubated and often medically paralyzed patients, and the superimposition of the internal and external components of lines, tubes, and devices.

Causes of lung parenchymal abnormality are discussed here, including acute respiratory distress syndrome (ARDS), acute interstitial pneumonitis (AIP), infection (Chapters 5 and 6), atelectasis, aspiration, and both cardiogenic and noncardiogenic pulmonary edema (Table 10.1). Abnormal air collections are then discussed, including pneumomediastinum, pneumopericardium, pneumatoceles, and interstitial emphysema. Pneumothorax is discussed briefly here in the setting of barotrauma and in greater detail in Chapters 12 and 17.

PULMONARY PARENCHYMAL OPACIFICATION

ACUTE RESPIRATORY DISTRESS SYNDROME

Definition
Previously termed adult respiratory distress syndrome, the modern definition of acute respiratory distress syndrome (ARDS) was reported in 1967 by Ashbaugh et al. (21). Today, ARDS is defined as the onset of acute respiratory failure, accompanied by severe and persistent hypoxemia despite the administration of high concentrations of inspired oxygen (ratio of arterial partial pressure of oxygen-to-fraction of inspired oxygen less than 200 mm Hg), pulmonary capillary wedge pressure (PCWP) less than 18 mm Hg, and the absence of elevated left heart filling pressures, with consolidation in three or four quadrants of the lungs on the chest radiograph. This definition was reported by a joint American–European Consensus Conference on ARDS (22). The definition had previously included diffuse pulmonary opacity, shunt physiology, increased dead space, and decreased lung compliance in the absence of increased left-sided filling pressures (23). Systemic inflammatory response syndrome may be a precursor to or trigger acute lung injury, ARDS, and multiple organ system failure (24). Systemic inflammatory response syndrome is defined as a systemic inflammatory response to a variety of clinical insults and is manifested by two or more of the items

Table 10.2: Systemic Inflammatory Response Syndrome (Defined as Two or More of the Items Below)

Temperature >38°C or <36°C
Heart rate >90 beats/min
Respiratory rate >20 breaths/min
WBC count
>12,000/mm^3 or
<4,000/mm^3 or
>10% immature forms

WBC, white blood cell.

listed in Table 10.2 (24). There are many potential proinflammatory and antiinflammatory mediators of acute lung injury, and it is the balance between these factors that culminates in the clinical manifestations of acute lung injury and ARDS. The former includes platelets and white blood cells, cytokines, endorphins and histamine, endotoxins, and vasoactive neuropeptides. The latter includes interleukins, epinephrine, leukotriene B4 receptor antagonist, and lipopolysaccharide binding protein.

Clinical Presentation and Risk Factors

ARDS is a clinical syndrome and is diagnosed clinically not radiographically. Patients with ARDS usually present acutely with rapidly progressive dyspnea, tachypnea, and respiratory distress. The risk factors for ARDS are listed in Table 10.3, with sepsis accounting for up to 35% of cases (25). Risk factors are synergistic, with more risk factors further increasing the risk of ARDS. The mortality of ARDS remains high, between 40% and 60%, despite advances in treatment and understanding of the pathophysiology of ARDS. There has been a gradual reduction in mortality. In general, mortality from ARDS is lower in patients less than 60 years of age and in patients with ARDS secondary to sepsis (26).

ARDS is a clinical syndrome, not a radiographic diagnosis.

Radiography and Phases

Although the diagnosis of ARDS is based primarily on clinical findings, the chest radiograph may provide additional diagnostic information concerning the effectiveness of treatment, complications, and prognosis. Bachofen and Weibel (27) described the three pathologic phases of ARDS lung injury and response in 1977: the acute exudative phase/stage, a fibroproliferative phase, and a fibrotic phase or healing stage. The acute phase, represented pathologically by diffuse endothelial cell injury with alveolar capillary leak of proteinaceous fluid and neutrophils, manifests radiologically as diffuse ill-defined alveolar opacities predominantly in the lung periphery (Fig. 10.4A) (28). As capillary leak

Table 10.3. Risk Factors for Acute Respiratory Distress Syndrome

Sepsis
Systemic inflammatory response syndrome
Disseminated intravascular coagulation
Prolonged hypotension
Gastric acid aspiration
Near drowning
Trauma, lung contusion, fat embolism
Burn injury
Pancreatitis
Multiple emergency transfusions
Post-cardiopulmonary bypass

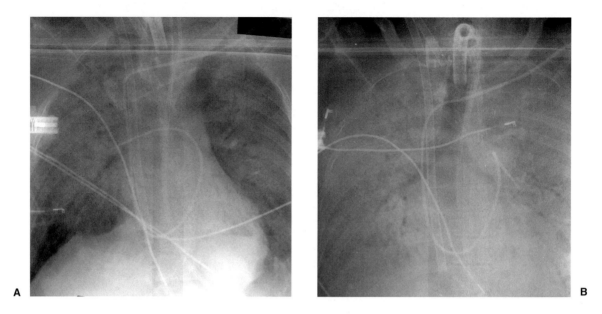

Figure 10.4 Progression of acute respiratory distress syndrome on serial chest radiographs in a patient on extracorporeal life support over 12 days. *A.* Diffuse alveolar opacity. *B.* Dense bilateral alveolar opacity with extensive air bronchograms. Little to no alveolar air filling, only air within the bronchial tree.

progresses, with greater extravasation of fluid from the intravascular space into the alveoli, widespread pulmonary opacification and complete "white-out" of the lungs occurs radiographically (Fig. 10.4B) (29). Grossly, the lungs are heavy and wet. Other microscopic pathologic features include platelet microthrombi and white blood cells in the capillary lumen, swelling of capillary endothelial cells, infiltration by polymorphonuclear leukocytes, and hyaline membrane formation within the alveoli. Injury to alveolar epithe-

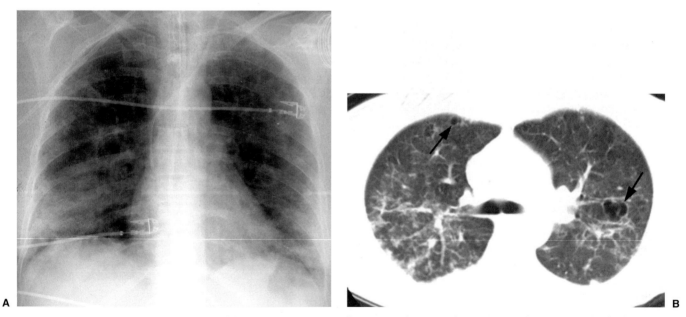

Figure 10.5 Acute respiratory distress syndrome with pneumatoceles in a patient with late-stage acute respiratory distress syndrome, day 19 after clinical diagnosis of acute respiratory distress syndrome. *A.* Chest radiograph and *(B)* computed tomography demonstrate bilateral thin walled lucencies *(arrows)* representing pneumatoceles on a background of ground glass and reticular lung opacities.

Table 10.4: Radiologic Manifestations of Barotrauma
Pneumothorax
Pneumomediastinum
Pneumopericardium
Pulmonary interstitial emphysema
Pneumoperitoneum
Pneumoretroperitoneum

lial cells results in decreased surfactant production and therefore decreased lung compliance, reflected on radiographs as small lung volume and atelectasis (27).

In general, during the acute exudative phase, the alveolar opacities of ARDS progress over several days on chest radiographs, until there is diffuse or near diffuse opacification of the lungs. Subsequently, the appearance changes very slowly from day to day. The alveolar edema of ARDS is not associated with widening of the vascular pedicle, cardiomegaly, or altered pulmonary blood flow distribution, which is in contrast to cardiogenic, uremic, and hypervolemic pulmonary edema. Because capillary leak occurs directly into the alveolar spaces, septal lines are usually absent on chest radiographs in ARDS. Although the pulmonary vessels are generally not visible through the alveolar opacities, when seen they may be vasoconstricted. In the subacute phase, which occurs over the next 5 to 10 days after the acute phase, the pathologic findings are proliferation of epithelial cells and fibroblasts, together with collagen deposition. This produces the radiographic findings of progressive lung destruction and a transition from alveolar to combined alveolar and interstitial opacities (Fig. 10.5). Findings of barotrauma (Table 10.4), including pneumothorax and pneumatocele formation, are frequent during this fibroproliferative phase, during which fibrosis has developed and the lungs become stiff and noncompliant (30,31). Although some patients recover from ARDS with no pulmonary function deficit, other patients eventually enter the chronic phase several weeks after the initial lung injury, manifested by fibrosis and focal emphysema on chest radiographs.

ARDS generally changes slowly on radiographs from day to day.

Early recognition of barotrauma in ARDS patients is important to minimize potentially serious complications, such as tension pneumothorax.

Computed Tomography

CT of ARDS was first reported in the early-to-mid 1980s and has been studied extensively since that time. Much of the work has been performed by Gattinoni and colleagues (32–34). What was once thought to be a disease process that homogeneously involved both lungs based on chest radiography is now recognized to be a more heterogeneous process based on CT investigations. The CT appearance varies with the etiology of ARDS, mechanical ventilation, patient position, and time. For example, in ARDS secondary to direct lung injury, such as pneumonia or aspiration, the radiologic appearance is more patchy and multifocal. In contrast, in ARDS with indirect lung injury, such as sepsis or sustained hypotension, lung injury is more diffuse (Fig. 10.6) (35). CT is clinically useful in patients with ARDS who are not improving or are deteriorating clinically, by identifying pleural effusions, lung abscess, lobar atelectasis, barotrauma, and malpositioned lines and tubes more accurately than chest radiographs (36,37).

Ground glass opacity, consolidation, and a reticular pattern are the hallmarks of ARDS on CT. The ground glass opacity is believed to represent active inflammation in lung interstitium and alveolar wall, coupled with incomplete alveolar filling by inflammatory cells, cellular debris, and edema. Consolidation is due to either complete filling of the alveolar spaces with fluid and debris, and/or atelectasis, referred to as the collapse of potentially recruitable lung units. If a patient were to be placed prone, the potentially recruitable lung units may reexpand and fill with air, thereby improving gas exchange. This has lead to the theory that patients with ARDS should be rotated regularly, with changes in the distribution of lung abnormality demonstrated on CT with changes in position (34,38). The reticular pattern may be seen both acutely, secondary to edema or inflammation, or in the chronic phase of ARDS, representing fibrosis. During the acute phase of ARDS, the ante-

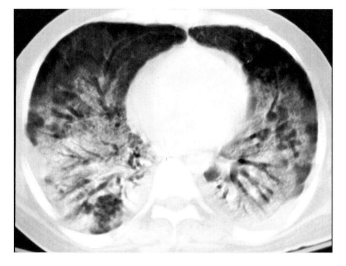

Figure 10.6 Computed tomography of acute respiratory distress syndrome demonstrates dense bilateral alveolar consolidation, more severe in the dependent (posterior) regions of the lungs than the nondependent (anterior) regions. Scattered small lucencies within the consolidation are pneumatoceles.

rior or most nondependent lung may be normal or near normal, whereas the mid-third of the lungs in the ventral to dorsal direction is ground glass in attenuation, with consolidation in the dorsal or most dependent lung, creating a ventral to dorsal gradient of lung attenuation. A cranial-to-caudal gradient is also noted, being more consolidated in the lower lungs than at the apices.

If ARDS resolves within 1 week, there are usually few if any radiologic sequelae. With a more protracted course of ARDS, the exudated fluid is reabsorbed from the lung and the fibroproliferative organizing phase sets in. Lung attenuation improves, whereas signs of fibrosis, including distortion of the normal bronchovascular architecture, may be found. Subpleural cysts, also known as pneumatoceles, varying in size from a few millimeters to a few centimeters, develop in both the dependent and nondependent lung.

Follow-up high resolution CT of the lungs after ARDS demonstrates fibrosis in most patients (39,40). The extent of fibrosis correlates with the severity of ARDS, the duration of mechanical ventilation using high peak inspiratory pressures, and a higher fraction of inspired oxygen. The location of the fibrosis is predominantly in the ventral or nondependent lung in the supine position, suggesting that it may be secondary to the high peak inspiratory pressures and oxygen therapy used to treat ARDS rather than to the ARDS itself. The collapsed dependent lung may be spared from this injury, protected by the fail-

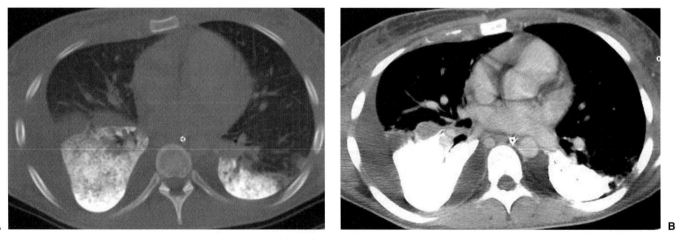

A   B

Figure 10.7 Partial liquid ventilation with perfluorocarbon. Computed tomography images photographed on (*A*) bone and (*B*) soft tissue windows settings demonstrate the gravity dependent distribution of the high attenuation perfluorocarbon.

ure to ventilate this region of the lung. Partial liquid ventilation is an experimental treatment for ARDS, in which perfluorocarbon is instilled into the airway with continuous gas ventilation through the endotracheal tube. Perfluorocarbon is a clear odorless liquid that is radiopaque (41). It distributes within the lungs in a gravity-dependent distribution, which matches the distribution of the most severely consolidated lung in ARDS, where it reduces alveolar surface tension and keeps the alveoli distended to facilitate gas exchange (Fig. 10.7).

ACUTE INTERSTITIAL PNEUMONITIS

AIP is an idiopathic form of acute lung injury, characterized by rapidly progressive cough and dyspnea leading to severe hypoxemia and respiratory failure over days. This short duration is in contrast to other chronic idiopathic interstitial pneumonias, such as usual and nonspecific interstitial pneumonitis that have a more insidious disease onset (Chapter 14). AIP was formerly referred to as Hamman-Rich syndrome. In 1935 Hamman and Rich (42) described five patients with acute lower respiratory tract illness, four of whom died after hospital stays of up to 6 months; one died within days. At autopsy, organizing diffuse alveolar damage and diffuse interstitial fibrosis was present in all cases (42). In 1986 Katzenstein and colleagues (43) coined the phrase "acute interstitial pneumonia" to reflect the acuity of the disease and distinguish it from other chronic interstitial pneumonias. Others later reviewed the autopsy material of the original 1935 cases and compared them with current cases of AIP, confirming that the pathologic lesion of AIP was identical to that described by Hamman and Rich (44).

AIP should be suspected in patients diagnosed initially with severe diffuse bilateral community-acquired pneumonia that does not respond to broad-spectrum antibiotics and from whom no infectious organism is isolated (45). It is distinguished from ARDS by the absence of a known cause of ARDS and the lack of systemic involvement or multisystem organ failure. Surgical lung biopsy in AIP demonstrates organizing diffuse alveolar damage, the same pathologic lesion seen in the fibroproliferative phase of ARDS (45). Similar to ARDS, the chest radiographic manifestations of AIP are bilateral, patchy, alveolar opacities that may progress to extensive diffuse consolidation. Reported survival in AIP ranges from 26% to 67%; however, the higher numbers likely reflect case series contaminated by ARDS and the lower figure is from a series of well-documented biopsy-proven cases. The number of pathologically confirmed AIP cases is small, and the impact of treatment, such as corticosteroids or cytotoxic drugs that are used for other forms of interstitial pneumonitis, is unclear.

AIP is acute diffuse alveolar damage of unknown etiology.

INFECTION

Pulmonary infections are covered extensively in Chapters 5 and 6. Aspects of infection as they relate to ICU patients are discussed here. The radiographic hallmark of pneumonia is airspace consolidation with air bronchograms, which may be segmental, lobar, or diffuse in distribution. New or progressing consolidation, together with two or more of the following, should raise suspicion for pneumonia: fever, hypothermia, peripheral leukocytosis or leukopenia, purulent respiratory secretions, and worsening respiratory failure (22). In critically ill patients the diagnosis of pneumonia may be delayed or unrecognized, because fever and leukocytosis may be absent. Fever may also be present in at least 50% of patients with atelectasis and no pneumonia, making it a poor clinical sign of infection (46,47). Pneumonia is difficult to diagnose in the setting of ARDS, with a high false-negative rate, as high as 29% (27). In a series by Mock et al. (48), the clinical variables and radiographic findings of 80 patients with positive sputum cultures were reviewed. One point each was given for the presence of new airspace "shadows," air bronchograms, segmental infiltrates, asymmetric infiltrates, infiltrates in nondependent lung, ipsilateral pleural effusion, and for the absence of volume loss, cardiomegaly, and hilar enlargement on chest radiographs. Clinical symptoms of fever, leukocytosis, respiratory failure, and

Clinical signs of pneumonia are often absent in critically ill patients.

Table 10.5: Risk Factors for Nosocomial Pneumonia in the Intensive Care Unit

Prolonged mechanical ventilation
Depressed consciousness
Massive gastric aspiration
Prophylactic antimicrobial therapy
Histamine 2 receptor blockers
Continuous enteral feeding
Corticosteroid use

mortality did not correlate with the radiographic findings. Patients with high radiographic scores, ranging from 4 to 10, were more likely to have positive blood and fluid cultures, polymicrobial cultures, multisystem organ failure, *Escherichia coli* or *Pseudomonas* infection, and improvement on antibiotics.

The risk of nosocomial pneumonia increases by 1% for each day intubated.

Nosocomial infections in the ICU setting are of particular concern, both in surgical and medical ICUs. They occur in 20% to 40% of patients, increasing morbidity, mortality, and costs (49–52). For example, in one series of trauma ICU patients, mortality was 43.5% in the patients with nosocomial pneumonia compared with 18% in the patients without nosocomial pneumonia (49). Risk factors for nosocomial infection are listed in Table 10.5. Prolonged mechanical ventilation is a major risk factor. Endotracheal tubes bypass natural host defenses, allow leakage of bacteria and secretions around the cuff into the airway, damage the ciliated tracheal epithelium, reduce bacterial clearance from the trachea, and direct bacteria into the lungs through tube manipulation and airway suctioning. It has been estimated that for each day of mechanical ventilation, the risk of nosocomial pneumonia increases by 1% (53). The organisms responsible for the infection and the rate of infection may vary from hospital to hospital and even from ICU to ICU within the same hospital (54). CT may be useful in ICU patients with sepsis of unknown origin, identifying the source of fever within the thorax or abdomen in nearly 20% of patients (55).

Patchy subpleural alveolar or nodular opacities should raise the suspicion of septic pulmonary emboli.

Another form of thoracic infection that should be considered in ICU patients is septic pulmonary emboli. ICU patients are at risk due to indwelling vascular catheters for combined underlying infection or nosocomial infection. When patchy bilateral lung parenchymal opacities or wedge-shaped nodularity develops, often subpleural in distribution, the possibility of septic pulmonary emboli should be raised (Figs. 21.24 and 21.25). Although the lung abnormality usually increases slowly, in some cases progression can be quite rapid. The nodules are usually less than 3 cm in size and may cavitate (56). CT is more sensitive than plain radiography for diagnosing septic emboli and may yield a diagnosis before it is clinically or radiographically suspected (56–58)

ASPIRATION AND ASPIRATION PNEUMONIA

Critically ill patients are at increased risk of aspiration and aspiration pneumonia. Predisposing reasons for this are given in Table 10.6. Aspiration should be suspected when chest radiographs demonstrate the sudden appearance of new focal alveolar opacities (Fig.

Table 10.6: Factors that Contribute to Aspiration in Intensive Care Unit Patients

Tracheal and esophageal intubation
Depressed cough reflex
Impaired mucociliary function
Increased secretions
Supine position
Cardiopulmonary resuscitation events

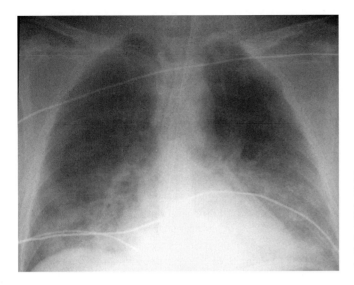

Figure 10.8 Aspiration in an intubated intensive care unit patient manifesting as new bibasilar consolidation. The chest radiograph was normal the previous day and returned to normal 5 days later.

10.8). Unless occurring acutely related to manipulation of airway or esophageal tubes, episodes of aspiration are often unrecognized by caretakers. Aspiration can be divided into three categories, according to the type of fluid aspirated and subsequent lung reaction: toxic, bland, and infectious (Table 10.7) (59).

Toxic aspiration occurs with the aspiration of acidic gastric contents with an acidic pH of less than 2.5 or water-soluble radiographic contrast material. In toxic aspiration, severe bronchospasm and chemical pneumonitis may develop within minutes of aspiration, manifesting radiographically as noncardiogenic pulmonary edema. When massive, toxic aspiration may result in immediate apnea, hypotension, and shock. Half of these patients will subsequently develop fever and leukocytosis, in the absence of infection, confounding the caretakers into diagnosing pneumonia. In milder forms, there may be mild bronchiolitis. The radiographs may also mimic pneumonia; however, unlike pneumonia, the alveolar opacities gradually improve over 1 to 2 days, which is faster than bacterial pneumonia.

When bland fluid, such as water, blood, or fluid, is aspirated, the radiograph may be normal unless a large volume of fluid is aspirated. Transient respiratory distress usually improves after airway suctioning, and there is usually no significant inflammatory lung response. If either toxic or bland fluid is aspirated in conjunction with solid foreign material such as food, the radiographs will demonstrate airway obstruction with distal atelectasis and frequently subsequent pneumonia.

The aspiration of infected material, such as pharyngeal or airway secretions colonized by multiple organisms, results in radiographic findings of pneumonia, with persistent alveolar consolidation. The location of the abnormality is related to patient position during the aspiration event. When supine, the superior segments of the lower lobes, particularly on the right, are most common, followed by the posterior segments of the upper lobes (60). When upright, the basilar segments of the lower lobes are usually involved (Fig. 5.20). If the patient is prone, as is common when using a rotational bed, the abnormality may be located in the anterior segments of the upper or lower lobes, the middle lobe, or lingula. Aspiration occurring when in a decubitus position may involve multiple or even all segments of the dependent lung and completely spare the nondependent lung. Aspira-

Acute focal or multifocal alveolar opacities, particularly at the lung bases or in superior segments of lower lobes, should raise the suspicion of aspiration, which is often clinically silent.

The location of opacities due to aspiration depends on patient position during the aspiration event.

Table 10.7: Categories of Aspiration

Toxic
Bland
Infectious

tion of infected contents in hospitalized patients or patients with poor oral hygiene may cause necrotizing pneumonia due to anaerobic organisms, often accompanied by cavitation and empyema. The most commonly implicated organism is *Pseudomonas aeruginosa*.

ATELECTASIS

In contrast to the hazy increased lung parenchymal opacity of pulmonary edema, diffuse atelectasis can often be recognized by secondary signs of volume loss, including low lung volumes and crowding of the bronchovascular structures and ribs. In intubated patients, chest radiographic exposure should be timed to peak inspiration of the ventilatory cycle after tidal volume has been delivered, because images at end-expiration will suffer from diffuse atelectasis and therefore be suboptimal for the evaluation of lung disease. Focal bibasilar subsegmental atelectasis is more common and often transient. After cardiac surgery, the left lower lobe is a common location for both atelectasis and pneumonia, secondary to stretching and cold-induced injury of the phrenic nerve (61). Angulation of the x-ray beam is important. With as little as 10 degrees of lordotic angulation the beam is no longer tangential to the apex of the hemidiaphragm, creating pseudo-opacity in the left retrocardiac region that may be interpreted as atelectasis or consolidation behind the heart (62).

Acute partial or complete lung collapse in an intubated patient is most commonly due to a mucous plug in the airway.

Intubated patients are at increased risk of mucous plugging of the airway due to decreased ciliary function, depressed cough reflex, and increased secretions. Mucous plugging may be a source of acute respiratory decompensation. Whenever acute lobar collapse or even whole lung collapse is identified radiographically, mucous plugging should be suspected. Suctioning of the airway usually results in radiographic and clinical improvement (Fig. 10.9). Atelectasis without air bronchograms is more responsive to suctioning than atelectasis with air bronchograms because of the presence of occlusive secretions within the airway that are amenable to removal (63).

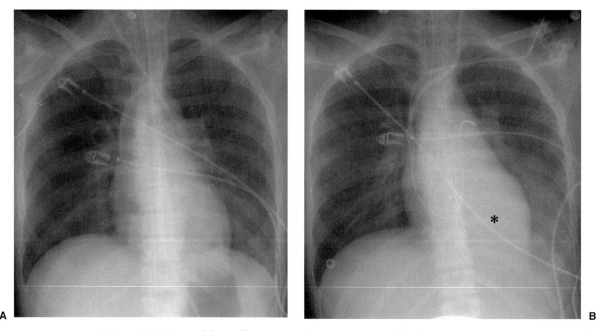

Figure 10.9 Acute lobar collapse secondary to a mucous plug in an intensive care unit patient. *A.* Initial radiograph demonstrates normal lungs. *B.* Radiograph a few hours later demonstrates acute left lower lobe collapse with retrocardiac and left lower lung opacity (*asterisk*) obscuring the left hemidiaphragm, slight shift of the heart toward the left, crowding together of the left posterior ribs compared with the right side, and leftward positioning of the esophagus compared with *A* as demonstrated by the esophageal tube.

EVALUATION OF CARDIOVASCULAR STATUS

Circulating blood volume (CBV), central venous pressure (CVP), pulmonary blood volume (PBV), pulmonary arterial pressure (PAP), capillary wedge pressure, and systemic extravascular water are indications of cardiovascular status that can be evaluated with chest radiographs (64–67). The radiographic findings of these cardiovascular status indicators are listed in Table 10.8 and have been shown to correlate with both clinical symptoms and physical examination findings.

CIRCULATING BLOOD VOLUME

CBV, also known as systemic blood volume, is defined as the total volume of blood within the systemic circulation, including the heart, arteries, veins, and capillaries and excluding the pulmonary circulation. The vascular pedicle width across the superior mediastinum can be used to evaluate CBV (64,66,68,69). The term vascular pedicle width was introduced in the 1970s by Eric Milne, to whom a great deal of our understanding of physiology as it relates to chest radiography interpretation is credited (64,68,70). The right margin of the vascular pedicle is formed by the lateral aspect of the right brachiocephalic vein and the superior vena cava. The left margin is formed by the lateral aspect of the left subclavian artery and the aortic arch. The thoracic vessels that make up the borders of the vascular pedicle are distensible and respond to changes in CBV. The right border of the vascular pedicle is made up entirely of venous structures that are more distensible than the arterial structures that make up the left border; therefore, the right border changes more readily in response to changes in systemic blood volume.

Changes in the vascular pedicle width on radiographs obtained with consistent positioning indicate changes in CBV and fluid status (66,69,71). Changes in the vascular pedicle width are more important than an absolute measurement and have been shown to have a greater correlation with CBV. The normal vascular pedicle width is 4.8 cm ± 5 mm, acknowledging that in general larger people have a wider pedicle than thin people (66). The vascular pedicle should be measured from two points. On the right side, it should be measured from where the upper border of the right main bronchus crosses the superior vena cava. On the left side, it should be measured from the aortic arch at the left subcla-

Vascular pedicle width is used to evaluate circulating blood volume.

Changes in vascular pedicle width are more important than a single measurement at one point in time.

Table 10.8: Measures of Cardiovascular Status that Can Be Evaluated on Radiography

Parameter	Indicators
Circulating blood volume	Vascular pedicle width
	Transverse cardiac diameter
	Azygos vein diameter
	Pulmonary blood volume
Central venous pressure	Azygos vein diameter
	Vascular pedicle width
Pulmonary blood volume	Pulmonary artery-to-bronchus ratio
	Pulmonary vascular recruitment
Pulmonary arterial pressure	Central vs. peripheral pulmonary artery diameter
	Vessel tortuosity
	Increased pulmonary artery: vein diameter
Capillary wedge pressure (LV function)	Pulmonary vascular cephalization
	Interstitial edema
	Alveolar edema
Systemic extravascular water	Chest wall thickness

LV, left ventricular.

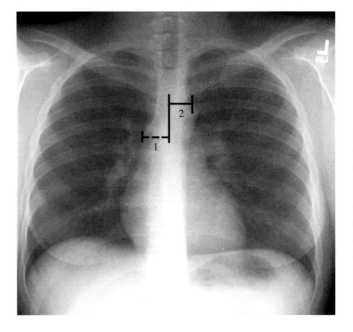

Figure 10.10 Measuring the vascular pedicle. Step 1: right side *(dotted horizontal line)*: measure from where the upper border of the right main bronchus crosses the superior vena cava to midline (1). Step 2: left side *(solid horizontal line)*: measure from the aortic arch at the left subclavian artery origin to midline (2). Step 3: add measurements from steps 1 and 2 above.

vian artery origin (Figs. 10.10 and 10.11). A line is drawn vertically down from the left point to meet a line drawn horizontally from the right point. The meeting point of the two lines to the right point is the vascular pedicle width. The supine position increases the width of the vascular pedicle by increasing venous return. Expiration increases the width of the mediastinum relative to the width of the thorax but has little effect of the vascular pedicle, because expiration is accompanied by increased intrathoracic pressure and pumping of blood out of the thoracic vessels (70).

The transverse diameter of the heart, the azygos vein diameter, and PBV also change with CBV but are less predictable than the vascular pedicle width. Unequivocal radiographic change in left ventricular chamber size occurs reproducibly only with a 66% increase in volume (67). Changes in the distance from the right heart border to midline correlate better with changes in CBV than the total transverse cardiac diameter.

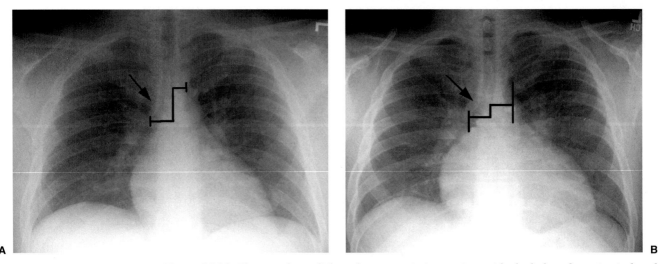

Figure 10.11 The vascular pedicle and azygos vein in a patient with alcohol- and cocaine-induced cardiomyopathy. *A.* Normal vascular pedicle *(lines)* and azygos vein *(arrow)*. *B.* Enlarged vascular pedicle *(lines)*, enlarged azygos vein *(arrow)*, and increased heart size.

CENTRAL VENOUS PRESSURE

CVP is the pressure of blood returning to the right side of the heart, in either the superior or inferior vena cava, immediately adjacent to the heart. CVP reflects right ventricular function, fluid balance, and peripheral vascular resistance. CVP can be invasively and directly measured using a CVP catheter placed into the superior vena cava, usually through either a subclavian vein or internal jugular vein or through the proximal port of a pulmonary arterial catheter (a.k.a. Swan-Ganz catheter). Because there is no valve between the superior vena cava and the right atrium, the pressure is the same. In the absence of tricuspid valve disease, CVP reflects right ventricular end-diastolic pressure, as measured when the tricuspid valve is open. The catheter is attached to either a transducer/monitor system or a manometer set to 0 when held at bedside at the level of the right atrium. Normal CVP measures 4 to 12 mm Hg. CVP is commonly monitored in evaluating the need and effectiveness of fluid replacement or resuscitation. Trends in CVP are more important than an absolute single measurement.

Noninvasively, the azygos vein diameter can be used as an indicator of CVP. On a frontal radiograph, the azygos vein is seen end-on just above the right main bronchus in the right tracheobronchial angle in approximately 85% of chest radiographs (Fig. 10.11) (72). The azygos vein is a distensible structure that responds directly to changes in right atrial pressure (64). It also responds to changes in CBV, paralleling changes in the vascular pedicle width, but less consistently. The azygos vein increases in diameter 7% for every 1% increase in the vascular pedicle width. If the azygos vein is disproportionately large, it should prompt evaluation for causes of inferior vena cava obstruction, acquired or congenital, such as azygos continuation of the inferior vena cava. Normal azygous vein diameter is usually 1 cm or less. Changes in the relative width of the azygos vein on serial chest images can be used as an indicator of CVP. When switching from a posteroanterior to an anteroposterior chest view, there will be a slight increase in the azygos vein diameter. Clinical evidence of elevated CVP includes neck vein distension, peripheral edema, and hepatomegaly.

Causes of elevated and reduced CVP are listed in Table 10.9. Left ventricular failure and mitral valvular disease can both cause increased pressure in the left atrium, subsequently extending into the pulmonary veins, pulmonary arteries, and right heart, resulting in an elevated CVP. Constrictive pericarditis and cardiac tamponade both impair systemic venous return and thereby increase CVP. Peripheral vasoconstriction and the Trendelenburg position both increase CVP by increasing systemic venous return. Chronic

Azygos vein diameter is used to evaluate CVP.

Table 10.9: **Causes of Abnormal Central Venous Pressure**

Increased	Reduced
Right ventricular failure	Low cardiac output
Left ventricular failure	Low circulating blood volume
Pulmonary arterial hypertension	
Increased circulating blood volume	
Mitral valve disease	
Constrictive pericarditis	
Cardiac tamponade	
Peripheral vasoconstriction	
Chronic lung disease	
Trendelenburg position	
Tricuspid valve disease	
Pneumothorax	
Atrial fibrillation/complete heart block	
Abdominal distension	
Pregnancy	

lung disease resulting in decreased lung compliance results in increased pulmonary resistance and elevated CVP. Low cardiac output associated with decreased venous return decreases CVP. Similarly, low CBV, as may be seen in trauma or surgery patients with blood loss or with a large gastrointestinal bleed, also reduces CVP (73). Positive pressure ventilation, pneumothorax, abdominal distension, atrial fibrillation, complete heart block, and tricuspid valve disease all lead to inaccurate falsely elevated CVP readings.

PULMONARY BLOOD VOLUME AND FLOW DISTRIBUTION

Pulmonary vascular capacity is almost twice as large as PBV.

The pulmonary circulation is a high capacity low resistance system positioned between the right and left sides of the heart. Normal PBV is the total amount of blood within the pulmonary vascular circulation. PBV is much smaller than the total pulmonary vascular bed capacity by approximately 30% to 50%, allowing the accommodation of changes in cardiac output that occur physiologically between rest and exercise (resting cardiac output, 6 L/min; exercise cardiac output, up to 16 L/min). PBV varies with patient size, position, respiration, and fluid status. For example, intrathoracic pressure decreases with inspiration, increasing PBV; the reverse occurs with expiration, resulting in the pumping of blood in and out of the pulmonary circulation. Larger patients have larger PBV than smaller patients (74). Overhydration increases PBV, whereas dehydration decreases it. Causes of altered generalized PBV are listed in Table 10.10. The excess pulmonary vascular capacity allows for acute or chronic increases in PBV without an increase in right ventricular or PAP (75). Pathologic changes in the pulmonary vascular bed, as seen with primary pulmonary arterial hypertension and chronic mitral stenosis, and primary lung diseases, such as emphysema and fibrosis, decrease the total capacity of the pulmonary vascular bed, with resultant increase in pulmonary arterial and right ventricular pressures.

The artery-to-bronchus ratio, the A:B ratio, is used to evaluate pulmonary blood flow.

PBV can be estimated by examining the relative diameter of pulmonary vessels to each other and to the adjacent bronchi. The ratio of the diameter of adjacent pulmonary arteries and bronchi seen on end, the A:B ratio, aids in determining whether vessels are abnormally enlarged (64,68). The ratio can be easily estimated on a frontal radiograph by looking at the end on anterior segmental artery and bronchus of the upper lobes (Fig. 10.12). The normal A:B ratio is 1:1 or less. It is closer to 1:1 in the supine position and 0.6 to 0.8:1 when upright. Normally, the A:B ratio is smaller in the upper lobes, 0.6 to 0.8:1, and equal in the lower lobes, because the upper lobes are relatively oligemic. Changes in PBV change both the A:B ratio and the balance of that ratio throughout the lungs. An increase or decrease in the A:B ratio throughout the lungs indicates a generalized increase or decrease in PBV, respectively (64). As PBV increases, the ratio in the upper and lower lungs may become balanced at 1:1 throughout the lungs as all the pulmonary vessels dilate. This is referred to as pulmonary vascular recruitment of addi-

Table 10.10: Causes of Altered Generalized Pulmonary Blood Volume

Increased	Decreased
Inspiration	Expiration
Fluid overload	Fluid deficiency
Overhydration	Dehydration
Renal failure	Third spacing
Increased right ventricular output	Cardiac tamponade
Left-to-right cardiac shunt	
Arteriovenous malformations	
Anemia	Addison disease
Thyrotoxicosis	Hypothyroidism
Fever	Positive pressure ventilation
Pregnancy	
Exercise	

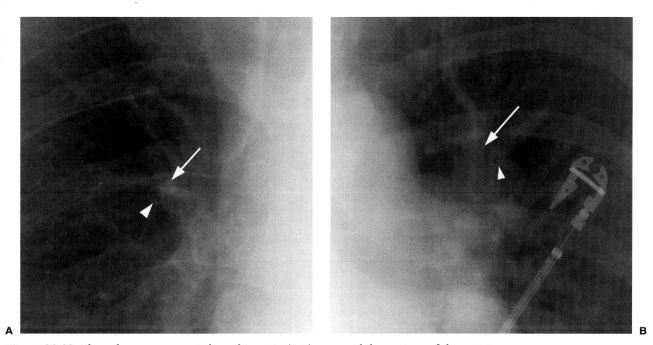

A   B

Figure 10.12 The pulmonary artery-to-bronchus ratio (A:B) on coned down views of the anterior segmental pulmonary artery and bronchus in the upper lobes. *A.* Normal ratio in the right upper lobe, with artery *(arrow)* slightly smaller than the bronchus *(arrowhead)*. *B.* Abnormal ratio in the left upper lobe, with artery *(arrow)* larger than the bronchus *(arrowhead)*.

tional pulmonary vascular bed capacity (Fig. 10.13). Regional changes in PBV and flow may also be seen. For example, there may be a focal increase in the A:B ratio associated with partial anomalous venous return or pulmonary sequestration or a focal decrease with pulmonary embolism, focal emphysema or bulla, or bronchial occlusion/mucous plugging; the latter are associated with a mosaic perfusion pattern on CT (Chapters 14 and 21).

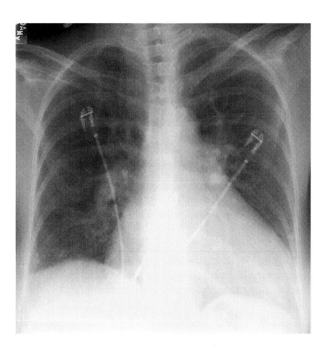

Figure 10.13 Pulmonary vascular redistribution, also known as cephalization, on a portable chest radiograph.

Putting Circulating Blood Volume, Central Venous Pressure, Pulmonary Blood Volume, and Heart Size Together

By evaluating all the indicators of cardiovascular status described above, conclusions can be drawn from chest images regarding fluid status and underlying disease processes. For example, an increase in vascular pedicle width, transverse cardiac diameter, and PBV indicates fluid overload. A wide vascular pedicle accompanied by decreased PBV should suggest cardiac tamponade; the decreased PBV is due to reduced right ventricular output and the wide vascular pedicle due to obstructed central venous return. Finally, increased PBV with normal or decreased systemic blood volume suggests a left-to-right shunt such as a septal defect or acquired rupture of the ventricular septum after myocardial infarction.

Pulmonary Arterial Pressure

Central and peripheral pulmonary artery size can be used to evaluate pulmonary arterial pressure.

The normal PAP is 15 to 30 mm Hg systolic, 6 to 12 mm Hg diastolic, and 14 to 18 mm Hg mean. Causes of elevated PAP include primary pulmonary vascular disease, pulmonary thromboembolic disease, cardiac disease, and chronic lung disease (Chapter 21).

The pressure in the pulmonary arterial circulation can be estimated by comparing the diameter of central and peripheral pulmonary arteries (64,68). Unfortunately, these observations do not distinguish acute variations in PAP that occur in unstable ICU patients but predict a range of pressures in the steady state usually due to chronic increased vascular resistance. With a mild increase of PAP up to 40 mm Hg, there may be mild enlargement of the central pulmonary arteries and suggestion of increased tortuosity of the peripheral pulmonary arteries. These findings are consistently seen with elevations of PAP over 40 mm Hg. Pruning of arteries immediately beyond the hilum may be seen with elevations over 60 mm Hg and is more consistently seen with PAP over 80 mm Hg (76,77). As PAP increases, there is also a gradual increase in the pulmonary artery-to-vein ratio, which can reach 3 or more with elevations in PAP of more than 80 mm Hg. Initially, right ventricular hypertrophy develops in response to elevated PAP, with right ventricular chamber enlargement occurring later and often rapidly once the right ventricle begins to fail.

Left Ventricular Function

PCWP estimates left ventricular end-diastolic pressure.

An assessment of left ventricular function can be made by analyzing the pulmonary vessels and the lung interstitium. In upright normal individuals, the diameter of the lower lobe vessels is larger than in the upper lobes (and therefore the A:B ratio is larger in the lower lungs) with preferential blood flow to the lung bases due to gravity; vessel margins are sharply delineated. In this normal state, total extravascular lung water is approximately 50 mL/L at total lung capacity (64,65). PCWP is used to reflect left-sided heart function. It is a surrogate measurement of left ventricular end-diastolic pressure, as when the mitral valve is open during diastole the pressure between the left ventricle, left atrium, and valveless pulmonary veins equilibrates. PCWP as a reflection of left ventricular function will be invalid in the setting of mitral valve disease; for example, with mitral stenosis PCWP will be artificially elevated. More details about how PCWP is measured can be found in Chapter 11. With elevations in PCWP, changes in both blood vessel size and distinctness occur (78,79). These abnormalities can be divided into three stages: cephalization or pulmonary vascular redistribution (Fig. 10.13), interstitial edema (Fig. 10.14), and alveolar edema (Fig. 10.15).

Normal PCWP is 6 to 12 mm Hg.

Normal PCWP is 6 to 12 mm Hg. As PCWP rises above normal, vessel diameter in upper and lower lung zones first equalizes, with an A:B ratio of 1 throughout the lungs. With further increases in PCWP, redistribution of pulmonary blood flow to the upper lungs occurs, with both an increase in upper lung vessel diameter and a decrease in lower lung vessel diameter (Fig. 10.13). This is recognized radiographically as larger vessels in

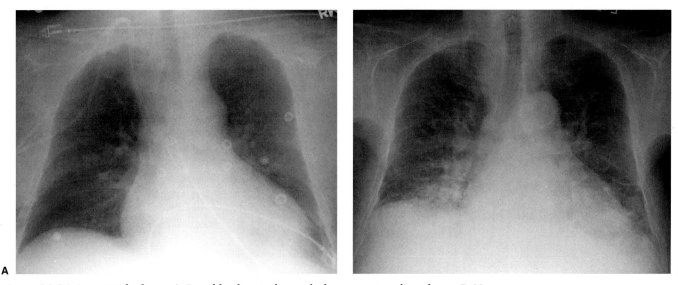

A   B

Figure 10.14 Interstitial edema. *A.* Portable chest radiograph demonstrates a large heart. *B.* New interstitial edema with Kerley B lines, indistinct pulmonary vessels, peribronchial cuffing, and subpleural edema manifesting as a thick minor fissure, in addition to pulmonary vascular redistribution.

the upper lungs compared with lung bases and is often referred to as "cephalization" of pulmonary blood flow. A word of caution is in order when using this sign of elevated PCWP: It can only be applied when the patient is fully upright, has taken sufficient inspiration for the lungs to be near total lung capacity, and when the lung bases are normal. When there is basilar lung disease, such as atelectasis or pneumonia, cephalization will occur secondary to these disease processes to maintain ventilation-perfusion matching and gas exchanged. During this stage there is microscopic interstitial edema that is not yet visible radiographically but is enough to reduce gas exchange. The microscopic edema occurs in a gravity-dependent distribution, resulting in basilar vasoconstriction and shunting of blood flow to the upper lobes to preserve gas exchange and matching of ventilation and perfusion.

Elevated PCWP leads to cephalization, interstitial edema, and alveolar edema.

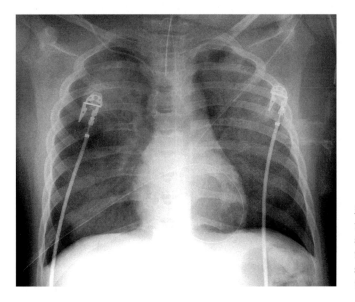

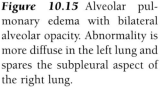

Figure 10.15 Alveolar pulmonary edema with bilateral alveolar opacity. Abnormality is more diffuse in the left lung and spares the subpleural aspect of the right lung.

As PCWP rises further to 18 to 25 mm Hg, it exceeds the normal colloid osmotic pressure of blood, and a fluid transudate develops in the lung interstitium edema. The interstitium of the lungs has both a central compartment that surrounds the bronchovascular bundles and a peripheral compartment that includes the interlobular and intralobular septa. Interstitial fluid in the central compartment results in indistinct vessel margins and peribronchial cuffing. Fluid in the interlobular septa creates linear opacities that extend to the pleural surface, known as Kerley B lines, and fluid in the intralobular septa creates finer basilar reticular opacities, known as Kerley C lines (Fig. 10.14). Kerley A lines are longer and more central. At this stage, total lung water is approximately 60 to 100 mL/L measured at total lung capacity (78,79).

When PCWP reaches 25 mm Hg or greater, fluid transudates collect in larger amounts within both the interstitium and alveoli, producing alveolar pulmonary edema. Radiographically, this manifests as diffuse, symmetric, bilateral, ill-defined, or fluffy lung opacity, often in a perihilar and basilar predominant distribution edema (Fig. 10.15). When alveolar edema begins to appear, lung water is estimated to be 110 to 130 mL/L, increasing to 160 mL/L or more with widespread edema (78,79).

Hemodynamic measurements reflect a moment in time. In contrast, the movement of water in and out of the extravascular compartment may take hours to days. For example, the resorption of fluid from the lung and clearance of lung opacity on radiographs may lag behind normalization of PCWP by hours to a day. There may be a discrepancy in the estimate of left ventricular failure evident on chest radiographs and the measured PCWP. For example, in one series 38% of patients with left ventricular end-diastolic pressures greater than 20 mm Hg had no radiographic evidence of left heart failure (80). Others have noted discrepancies in the estimation of PCWP in patients with acute myocardial infarction or acute left ventricular power failure (80, 81). Possible explanations for these discrepancies include preexisting lung disease (emphysema or interstitial lung disease) or poor inspiration on the radiograph. Furthermore, many of the radiographic estimations described above were made on nonportable radiographs, which are technically superior to ICU portable radiographs performed an sick patients. On such portable radiographs, estimation of blood flow in the upper versus the lower lungs cannot be made because critically ill patients are often imaged in a semiupright position, and the vessel diameter measurements described above were done in fully upright patients. Woodring (82) attempted to circumvent this by studying the relationship of pulmonary artery diameter to the adjacent bronchus in supine and upright patients. When supine, hydrostatic differences occur from the dorsal to ventral aspect of the lungs rather than from the lung bases to apices. Under normal conditions, the A:B ratio is equalized throughout the lungs. When PCWP is elevated, the ratio increases throughout the lungs, allowing distinction between left ventricular failure and normal physiology. This ratio cannot distinguish increased PBF (cardiac shunt) from left ventricular failure, because both produce an increase in the A:B ratio. However, in practice this comparison is often limited by the inability to identify adjacent end on arteries and bronchi.

> Kerley B lines are a classic finding in interstitial edema.

SYSTEMIC EXTRAVASCULAR WATER

> Chest changes in wall soft tissue thickness are used to evaluate systemic extravascular water.

Total fluid balance is a combination of intravascular and extravascular components. Changes in systemic extravascular water, or soft tissue water, can be estimated by changes in chest wall thickness on chest images obtained with consistent patient position. On a frontal radiograph, a useful location for measurement is between the lateralmost rib and the overlying skin. On a lateral view, the distance from the anterior border of the sternum to the skin may be used. A retrospective study correlating changes in chest wall thickness with body weight in renal failure patients showed good correlation (64).

CARDIOGENIC EDEMA VERSUS NONCARDIOGENIC EDEMA VERSUS OTHER CAUSES OF LUNG OPACITY

As described already, there are many etiologies of lung parenchymal opacity in the critically ill patients, including pulmonary edema, atelectasis, pneumonia, and ARDS. It may be difficult to distinguish between these on a single chest radiograph, particularly if the abnormality is diffuse bilateral alveolar opacity. A predominantly perihilar "batwing" or "butterfly" appearance to the opacity is characteristic of pulmonary edema (Fig. 10.16) and atypical for ARDS or pneumonia. On serial chest radiographs, cardiogenic edema usually changes over hours to a day or so (Fig. 10.17), as the etiology of left ventricular failure is clinically identified, whereas ARDS gradually progresses over several days to complete opacification of the lungs.

Causes of pulmonary edema are listed in Table 10.11 and include both cardiac and noncardiac causes. The etiologies of noncardiogenic pulmonary edema are varied (83). For example, high-altitude pulmonary edema is a potentially fatal condition that occurs with rapid ascent (84). It has been estimated that as many as three of four climbers may have subclinical high-altitude pulmonary edema after a modest climb, whereas 15% in one prospective series had either rales or interstitial edema on radiographs after ascent (85). High-altitude pulmonary edema is believed to be secondary to altered permeability of the alveolar-capillary barrier due to intense pulmonary vasoconstriction, resulting in fluid in the lungs of climbers with a high-protein content, in the absence of inflammatory cells. Life-threatening edema may develop secondary to airway obstruction. For example, negative pressure pulmonary edema may occur as a consequence of postintubation laryngospasm due the generation of high negative intrathoracic pressures against a closed airway (86). This characteristically occurs in young men with well-developed thoracic musculature (Fig. 10.3).

Neurogenic pulmonary edema may develop within hours of a neurologic insult, such as stroke, subarachnoid hemorrhage, or traumatic injury, in association with elevated intracranial pressure, systemic and pulmonary arterial hypertension, and elevated left ventricular pressure (87). Patients with subarachnoid hemorrhage have been shown to have

Cardiogenic edema usually changes quickly on several radiographs, over days if not hours.

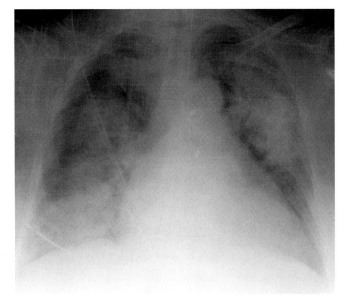

Figure 10.16 Batwing or butterfly acute alveolar pulmonary edema on chest radiograph in a patient who has undergone coronary artery bypass graft surgery in the past.

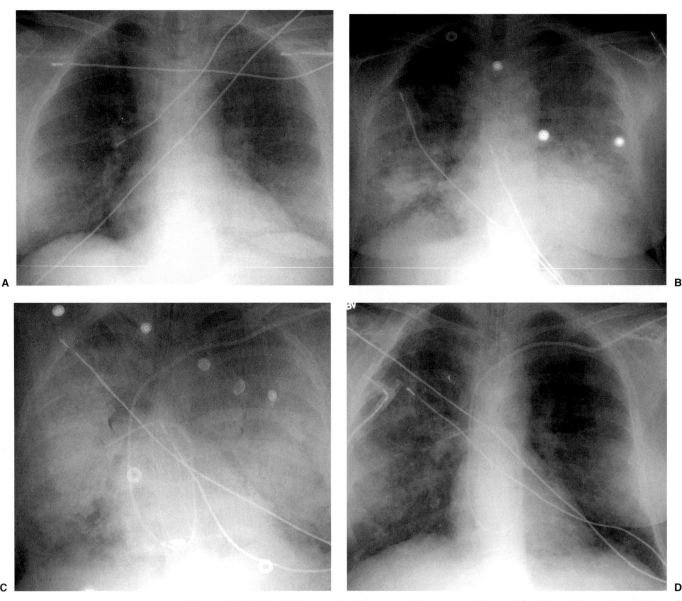

Figure 10.17 Rapid changes in pulmonary edema on serial portable chest radiographs. *A.* Normal chest radiograph. *B.* Alveolar edema with new mid and lower lung alveolar opacities 37 hours later. *C.* Extensive alveolar edema with diffuse lung opacification 4 hours after *B. D.* Only interstitial edema remains 33 hours after *C.*

abnormal left ventricular wall motion and myocardial enzyme release; in severe cases reduction in cardiac output may further exacerbate cerebral ischemia due to ongoing vasospasm (88). In one series, 21% of patients with subarachnoid hemorrhage had moderate or severe cardiac injury and 29% had mild cardiac injury, whereas half had no cardiac injury. The mechanism by cardiac impairment develops is poorly understood and may include endothelial injury with increased pulmonary capillary permeability and hydrostatic changes with increase left atrial pressure and pulmonary venous constriction due to increased sympathetic tone.

There are many toxic substances that when inhaled may cause pulmonary edema. Examples include chlorine-containing bleaching agents; sodium hypochlorite found in disinfectants and spot remover; petroleum distillates or mineral spirits found in furniture polish, wood stain, and varnish; car wax and polish; motor oil and gasoline; selenium

Table 10.11: Causes of Pulmonary Edema

Left ventricular failure
   Myocardial infarction
   Cardiomyopathy
   Aortic or mitral valve disease
Noncardiogenic
   Fluid overload
   Renal failure
   Hepatic failure
   Brain injury
   Near drowning
   Acute respiratory distress syndrome
   High altitude
   Drug reaction
   Drug overdose (cocaine)
   Carbon monoxide toxicity
   Radiation therapy
   Negative pressure pulmonary edema
      Postextubation laryngospasm
      Acute airway obstruction
   Reexpansion pulmonary edema

found in hazardous waste sites; and ash from burning coal or metal industries (89,90). Detail on the effects of specific toxic agents can be found at the website for the Agency for Toxic Substances and Disease Registry (ATSDR), an agency of the U.S. Department of Health and Human Services, at *www.atsdr.cdc.gov.* Some ingested drugs also cause pulmonary edema, such as freebase cocaine (91).

It is important to recognize atypical manifestations of pulmonary edema (Table 10.12). Because pulmonary edema changes with gravity and therefore patient position, a patient in the Trendelenburg position may have more severe edema in the upper lobes (Fig. 10.18) compared with an upright patient, and a patient who preferentially lies on their right side will develop more severe edema in the right lung than in the nondependent left lung. Patients with severe upper lobe predominant emphysema preferentially have most of their pulmonary artery blood flow going to the lower lobes at baseline to maintain gas exchange. When left ventricular failure occurs, pulmonary edema may manifest as bibasilar alveolar consolidation, radiographically mimicking pneumonia or aspiration. The reverse is true in patients with α_1-antiprotease deficiency and lower lobe predominant emphysema. Similarly, patients with either pulmonary embolism or tumor occluding a pulmonary artery will not develop edema in the lung parenchyma supplied by the occluded vessel. Because venous thromboembolism usually involves the lower lobes to

Pulmonary edema is common. Atypical manifestations of common diseases are more common than typical manifestations of rare diseases.

Table 10.12. Causes of Atypical Pulmonary Edema Distribution

Location	Etiology
Unilateral	Persistent decubitus position
	Rapid drainage of large pleural effusion
	Rapid drainage of large pneumothorax
Bibasilar	Upper lobe predominant emphysema
Biapical	Lower lobe predominant emphysema
	Chronic pulmonary embolism
Spares a lobe	Artery occluded by tumor or thromoembolism

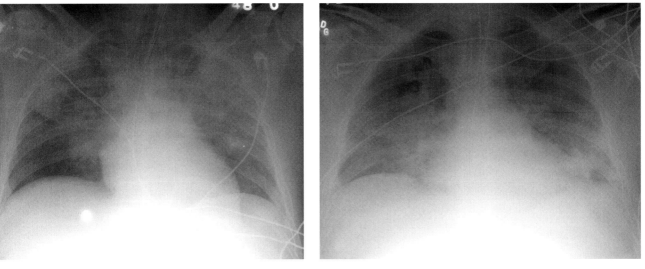

Figure 10.18 Gravitational shift in pulmonary edema distribution with changes in patient position. *A.* Initial chest radiograph demonstrates bilateral upper lung edema when the patient was imaged after being in the Trendelenburg position. *B.* Within 24 hours another radiograph taken after upright positioning demonstrates edema that is now more severe in the lower lungs.

a greater extent that the upper lobes, because of the greater distribution of blood flow to the lower lungs, patients with chronic pulmonary embolism may develop bilateral upper lung edema when left ventricular failure occurs (Fig. 10.19). Unilateral pulmonary edema may develop after the rapid drainage of pleural fluid or air and is referred to as reexpansion pulmonary edema (Fig. 10.20). Lobar sparing of pulmonary edema may be seen if the pulmonary artery to that lobe is occluded by tumor, such as with bronchogenic carcinoma or a lobar artery embolus.

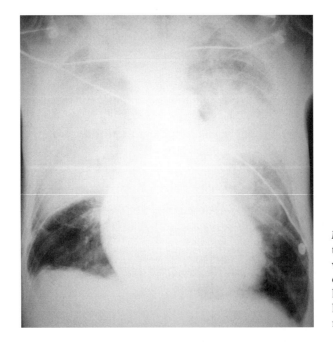

Figure 10.19 Upper lobe distribution of pulmonary edema in a patient with chronic pulmonary emboli occluding blood flow to the lower lobes, manifesting as bilateral upper lung consolidation on posteroanterior chest radiograph.

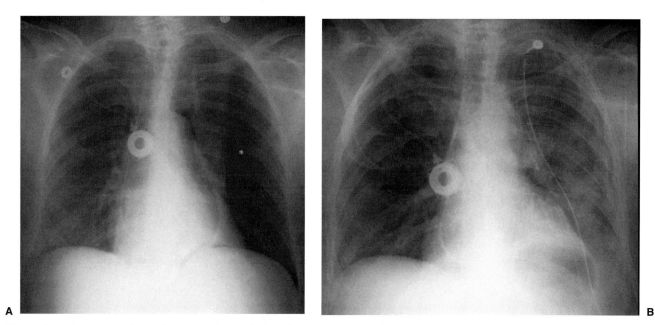

Figure 10.20 Reexpansion pulmonary edema. *A.* Initial posteroanterior chest radiograph demonstrates a large left pneumothorax (*asterisk*) with complete collapse of the left lung. *B.* After chest tube placement with rapid reexpansion of the left lung, there is new diffuse alveolar opacity throughout the left lung.

ABNORMAL AIR COLLECTIONS

There are many locations of abnormal thoracic air collections, as listed in Table 10.13. Some air collections arise as a complication of barotrauma in patients with stiff noncompliant lungs, such as patients with advanced ARDS. Some air collections are iatrogenic, such as after central venous or pulmonary arterial catheter placement (Chapter 11). Other air collections may be a clue to injury or a disease process, such as pneumomediastinum and pneumothorax in the setting of traumatic airway rupture (Chapter 12), or small pockets of air within a pleural fluid collection secondary to infection with gas-forming organisms. In many cases the air collection itself is of little consequence; rather, it is the reason for the development of the air collection that is important. However, in some circumstances the air itself can be a cause of morbidity and even mortality. For example, a tension pneumothorax may result in collapsed lung and even impaired systemic venous return to the heart due to the compression of the superior vena cava. The latter is more common with a right tension pneumothorax than a left one, because the large low-pressure venous structures of the mediastinum are right sided. Many causes of these air col-

A right tension pneumothorax impairs central venous return more than a left tension pneumothorax.

Table 10.13. Abnormal Thoracic Air Collections

Pneumothorax
Pneumomediastinum
Pneumopericardium
Pneumatoceles
Pulmonary interstitial emphysema
Subcutaneous emphysema

lections are discussed in greater detail in chapters related to the specific disease or underlying anatomy. (See Chapter 8 with regard to metastases; also Chapters 11, 12, 14, 17, and 22.) A review of the air collections themselves and etiologies to consider for each are discussed here.

PNEUMOTHORAX

A pneumothorax is defined as "the presence of air or gas in the pleural space" (92). Because of the elastic recoil of the lung, the alveolar pressure is always greater than pleural pressure. When a communication between lung and pleural space develops, air flows from the lung into the pleural space until equilibrium occurs. The larger the pneumothorax, the smaller the lung becomes. As the lung becomes smaller in size, vital capacity of the lung becomes smaller. Symptoms are usually acute ipsilateral chest pain that is exacerbated with breathing and dyspnea. This may be accompanied by tachypnea and hypoxia and even tachycardia, hypotension, and cyanosis when severe. For individuals with normal lungs, symptoms may be minimal even with what may be considered a large pneumothorax (Chapter 12, Fig. 12.14). However, in patients with underlying lung disease with already reduced lung function, this additional reduction can be a cause of significant respiratory distress (Fig. 10.21). Also, a large pneumothorax may cause mediastinal shift and impaired venous return to the heart due to compression of the superior vena cava and inferior vena cava. This is more common on the right side, where these venous structures are located, than on the left side. This is referred to as a tension pneumothorax and should always be suspected when mediastinal shift accompanies a pneumothorax (Fig. 10.22) (Fig. 12.20). Treatment of pneumothorax depends on size and patient stability and ranges from observation to aspiration, chest tube placement, and even surgical treatment in the setting of recurrent bleb rupture or bronchopleural fistula (93)

Causes of pneumothorax are listed in Table 10.14 (94). Air combined with fluid is a hydropneumothorax, with pus is a pyopneumothorax, and with fecal material, as has been reported on the setting of traumatic diaphragmatic rupture, is a fecopneumothorax (95,96).

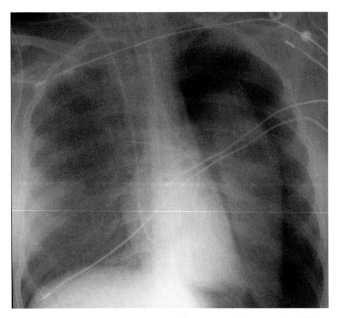

Figure 10.21 Acute respiratory distress syndrome with diffuse lung alveolar opacity and a left pneumothorax on a portable chest radiograph.

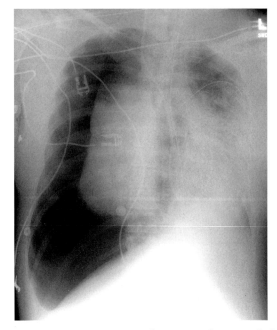

Figure 10.22 Acute respiratory distress syndrome with diffuse lung alveolar opacity and bilateral pneumothoraces on a portable chest radiograph.

Table 10.14: Causes of Pneumothorax

Primary
    Ruptured bleb or bulla
Secondary
    Trauma
        Penetrating (knife, gunshot)
        With rib fracture(s)
        Biopsy/aspiration (lung, pleura, transbronchial, breast, abdominal)
        Iatrogenic (central venous access)
        Ex vacuo (space-occupying process removal and stiff lung)
        Cardiopulmonary resuscitation
        Acupuncture
        Surgery (thoracic, abdominal, neck)
    Interstitial lung disease
        Fibrosis
        Sarcoidosis
    Obstructive lung disease
        Emphysema
        Bronchiectasis
        Langerhans cell histiocytosis
        Lymphangioleiomyomatosis
        Bronchiolitis obliterans/graft-versus-host disease
    Cavity metastases
        Squamous
        Sarcoma
    Increased intrathoracic pressure
        Barotraumas (mechanical ventilation)
        Blunt abdominal trauma
    Other
        Catamenial

A primary spontaneous pneumothorax is usually due to the rupture of an apical bleb (Fig. 10.23); it more commonly occurs in tall individuals and is six times more common in men than women (97). These blebs are actually intrapleural, that is, they are located within the visceral pleural lining of the lung that is made up of a layer of mesothelial cells and submesothelial connective tissue. On imaging studies we recognize blebs as discrete air collections with a well-defined thin wall, usually at the lung apices. Another common location to look for blebs that rupture is the superior segments of the lower lobes, which

Apical blebs that cause spontaneous pneumothorax are actually within the pleural lining.

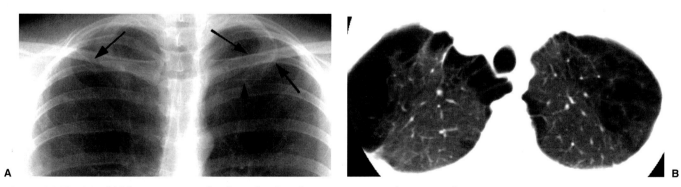

Figure 10.23 Apical blebs in a patient that later developed a spontaneous right pneumothorax. *A.* Chest radiograph demonstrates thin apical lines representing the walls of blebs, seen in more detail on (*B*) computed tomography.

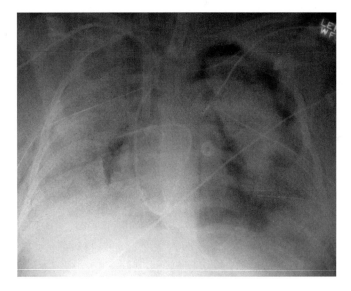

Figure 10.24 Bilateral balanced pneumothoraces on computed tomography with no mediastinal shift.

can be thought of as the apex of the lower lobes. An acute elevation in intrathoracic pressure, as may be seen in trauma or weight lifting, may lead to bleb rupture. Secondary spontaneous pneumothorax is due to underlying lung disease, such as fibrosis, emphysema, or malignancy (98,99), particularly metastatic sarcoma (Fig. 8.24). Trauma is an important cause of pneumothorax, including both blunt and penetrating trauma, as well as iatrogenic pneumothorax secondary to central venous access. Catamenial pneumothorax occurs in synchrony with the menstrual cycle (Fig. 17.19) (100).

Although in most cases a small pneumothorax resolves without treatment, in patients with ARDS a small pneumothorax is evidence of barotraumas and may rapidly enlarge, further reducing oxygenation. Bilateral pneumothoraces usually occur in patients with underlying lung disease and are usually balanced by the pressure across the thorax (Fig. 10.24) (101). Patients with underlying lung disease have a higher mortality with secondary pneumothorax than patients with primary pneumothorax. In patients with chronic obstructive pulmonary disease, the mortality risk is 3.5 times higher. Another important consideration in patients with ARDS and stiff noncompliant lungs is an *ex vacuo* pneumothorax that may occur with the drainage of pleural fluid because of the inability of the small collapsed lung to reexpand into the space previously occupied by the fluid that has been removed (Fig. 10.25). This phenomenon may also be observed when there is rapid lobar collapse due to acute bronchial obstruction (101).

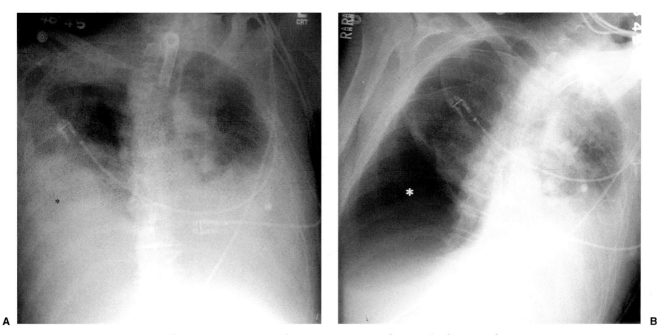

Figure 10.25 *Ex vacuo* pneumothorax in a patient with acute respiratory distress syndrome and stiff noncompliant lungs. A. Initial radiograph demonstrates a large right pleural effusion (*asterisk*). B. After chest tube drainage there is a large pneumothorax (*asterisk*) conforming to the location of the prior pleural effusion.

Radiographically, pneumothorax appears as a thin white line (the visceral pleura) surrounded by lucency (air) in the pleural space on one side and the lung on the other side. Air in the pleural space is found in the most nondependent portion of the thorax. In an upright patient this will be at the apex of the lung. Care should be taken in interpreting semiupright and supine radiographs for pneumothorax, common positions of trauma or ICU chest radiographs, because the location of the pneumothorax will be different. When supine, air collects in the basilar aspect of the pleural space and may be seen between the hemidiaphragm and the lower edge of the lung, at the cardiophrenic angles, and at the lateral costophrenic angle that appear expanded caudally; the latter is known as the deep sulcus sign (Figs. 12.17 and 17.13). It is not uncommon to find a pneumothorax on CT in trauma patients that was not visible on a supine portable chest radiograph. In the decubitus position, air will collect adjacent to the lateral rib margins (Fig. 17.11). Uncommonly, air may be located within a fissure (Figs. 17.14 and 17.15).

Expiratory radiographs are of limited value. On expiration, the lung becomes smaller whereas the pneumothorax is unchanged; hence, the relative size of the pneumothorax is larger. Careful study of this has shown that the odds of missing a small pneumothorax on inspiratory or on expiratory radiographs is equal and likely related to where the thin visceral pleural edge fortuitously overlies the ribs. An expiratory radiograph should be reserved for patients with a normal inspiratory radiograph when there is a high clinical suspicion for pneumothorax and should not be used routinely (102). Ultrasound can identify pleural air and may be particularly useful in ICU patients by bringing the machine to the patient bedside. Pleural air can be recognized as the absence of lung sliding toward the chest wall with separation of the normal lung–chest wall interface, usually viewed anteriorly through the intercostal spaces (103).

> Always "hot light" or magnify the lung apices when looking for a pneumothorax in an upright patient.

> In a supine position, pneumothorax collects anteriorly at the lung base.

PNEUMOMEDIASTINUM

Pneumomediastinum is defined as "escape of air into mediastinal tissues, usually from interstitial emphysema or from a ruptured pulmonary bleb" (104). The sources of air in

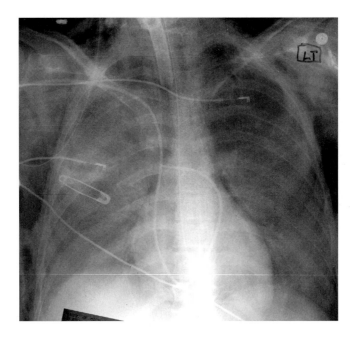

Figure 10.26 Pneumomediastinum manifesting as lucency along both heart borders on a chest radiograph of a patient with acute respiratory distress syndrome. Note the subcutaneous air in the chest wall bilaterally.

pneumomediastinum include the lung, airway, esophagus, neck, and abdomen. Excessive intraalveolar pressure, as may be seen when ventilating stiff noncompliant lungs in ARDS or from blunt trauma with compression of the thorax, results in the rupture of alveoli along the bronchovascular bundles with air dissecting into the adjacent connective tissue (known as the central or axial interstitium of the lung) and then into the mediastinum. Air can subsequently extend from the mediastinum into the neck and then into the body wall soft tissues, manifesting as subcutaneous air and intramammary air (Figs. 10.26, 10.27, and 10.28). Air may also extend caudally from the mediastinum into the retroperitoneum, extraperitoneal compartments, and even the peritoneal cavity. Similarly, air in the

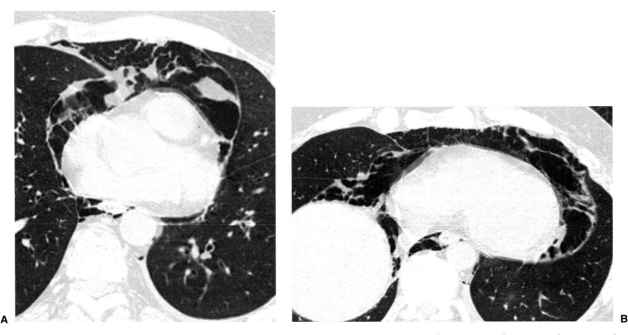

Figure 10.27 Pneumomediastinum on computed tomography. Two axial computed tomography images, *A* and *B*, demonstrate lucency throughout the mediastinum, with intervening strands of opacity caused by mediastinal fat, small neurovascular structures, and lymph nodes.

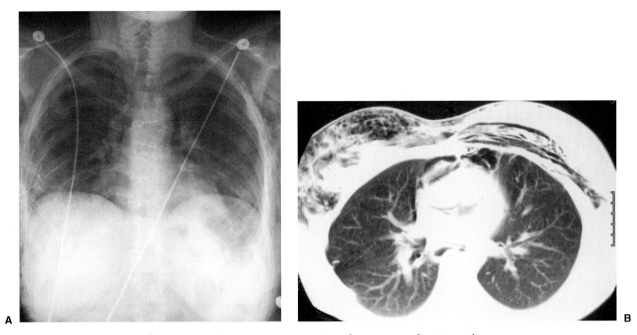

Figure 10.28 Extensive subcutaneous air, intramammary air, and pneumomediastinum due to Munchausen syndrome, as seen on (*A*) posteroanterior chest radiograph and (*B*) computed tomography. Air was self-injected into the chest wall.

neck or retroperitoneal soft tissue can dissect into the mediastinum, as may be seen with neck trauma or surgery or with bowel rupture into the retroperitoneum. Uncommonly, a pneumomediastinum can lead to a pneumothorax, usually when mediastinal pressure rises abruptly or when there is massive pneumomediastinum.

The air in the mediastinum itself is usually of little consequence, and patients often have no symptoms. When present, symptoms include substernal chest pain that is exacerbated by deep breathing, coughing or the supine position, dyspnea, dysphagia, and dysphonia. These may be accompanied by crepitus from subcutaneous emphysema and the Hamman sign (precordial crunching sound with each heart beat). More important than the air is the cause of the air. Causes of pneumomediastinum are listed in Table 10.15 and

Whereas the radiographic appearance of pneumomediastinum may be dramatic, the air causes little problems. The cause of pneumomediastinum is more important.

Table 10.15: Causes of Pneumomediastinum

Asthma
Trauma
    Airway rupture
    Esophageal rupture
    Oropharynx trauma
    Blunt chest trauma
Barotrauma (mechanical ventilation)
Substance abuse
    Smoking marijuana
    Inhalation of cocaine
Athletic competition
Respiratory tract infection
Child birth
Emesis
Severe cough
Seizures
Valsalva maneuver

are generally related to conditions in which there is an acute elevation of thoracic pressure, as may be seen with an acute asthmatic attack or severe coughing or trauma. In the setting of blunt chest trauma, alveolar rupture and dissection of air along the central interstitium into the mediastinum is known as the Macklin effect, first described in 1939. In one series it was responsible for 39% of the cases of pneumomediastinum in patients with severe blunt chest trauma (105). Pneumomediastinum secondary to Boerhaave syndrome, esophageal rupture in the setting of extensive or violent vomiting, carries a high mortality. Pneumomediastinum secondary to traumatic airway or esophageal rupture also carries a high mortality rate, particularly if the diagnosis is not recognized early.

Radiographically, pneumomediastinum appears as thin lucent lines or bubbles of gas along the mediastinal contours, such as the heart, aorta, and superior vena cava, and as streaks of lucency in the superior mediastinum extending toward the neck (Fig. 10.27) (106). On the lateral view, attention should be paid to the retrosternal region when searching for pneumomediastinum and to gas surrounding the aorta and pulmonary artery. Air can also be seen to surround the aortic knob, central pulmonary arteries, airway, and esophagus on radiographs; however, this is usually more appreciated on CT. Air around the right pulmonary artery is known as the ring around the artery sign on the lateral radiograph (Fig. 12.18). Mediastinal gas may insinuate between the parietal pleura and either lung apex or diaphragm, external to the parietal pleura. CT is more sensitive than radiography for the presence of mediastinal gas and for delineating the location of that gas (Fig. 10.27) (Fig. 12.21). The V sign of Naclerio is seen when mediastinal gas is located between parietal pleura and left hemidiaphragm (107). The continuous diaphragm sign with air outlining the central tendon of the diaphragm is seen when mediastinal gas is located between the heart and the diaphragm (108). Changes in position, such as being placed decubitus or supine, does not usually change the distribution of air in the mediastinum, which is in contrast to air in the pleural and pericardial spaces or peritoneal cavity.

> Changes in position usually do not change the appearance of pneumomediastinum radiographically.

PNEUMOPERICARDIUM

Pneumopericardium is defined as the "presence of gas in the pericardial sac" (109). Pneumopericardium is much less common that pneumothorax or pneumomediastinum. Causes of pneumopericardium are listed in Table 10.16. It is usually secondary to trauma,

Table 10.16: Causes of Pneumopericardium

Trauma
    Penetrating trauma
    Surgery
Infection with gas-forming organism
Increased intrathoracic pressure
    Asthma
    Barotrauma
    Valsalva maneuver
Lung disease
    Bronchogenic carcinoma
    Lung infection
Esophageal rupture (severe emesis, Boerhaave syndrome)
Other
    Forceful coughing
    Cocaine abuse
    Gastric perforation (ulcer, tumor)
    Liver abscess
    Pancreatic pseudocyst
    Postpartum

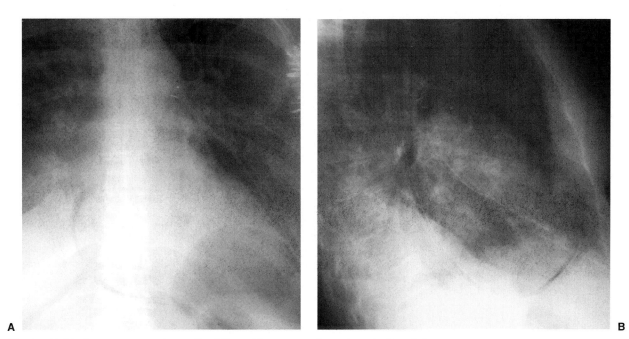

A   **B**

Figure 10.29 Pneumopericardium after bilateral lung transplantation. *A.* Coned down posteroanterior and *(B)* lateral radiograph demonstrate lucency conforming to the pericardial sac that does not extend above the aortic knob. Lucency extending above the aortic knob would indicate a pneumomediastinum.

often penetrating trauma, or may be seen after cardiac surgery (Fig. 10.29) (110–112). Pneumopericardium may also be spontaneous, although this is less common (113), and may also be a cause of cardiac tamponade (114). The latter should be suspected whenever the heart becomes small in the setting of pneumopericardium. Rarely, in Boerhaave syndrome there may be rupture of the esophagus into the pericardial sac, resulting in pneumopericardium. Lung disease may erode into the pericardium, such as bronchogenic carcinoma or invasive aspergillosis. Even cocaine abuse, laparoscopy, ruptured gastric ulcers, and amebic liver abscesses have been reported to cause pneumopericardium (110,115).

Radiographically, pneumopericardium appears as lucency confined to the pericardial sac (Figs. 10.29 and 20.33). It should not extend above the aortic knob, because that is the cephalad aspect of the pericardial space. This can be used to distinguish pneumopericardium from pneumomediastinum. On echocardiography, pneumopericardium has the distinct appearance of swirling echogenic bubbles (116).

Pneumopericardium should not extend above the aortic knob.

PNEUMATOCELES AND INTERSTITIAL EMPHYSEMA

Pneumatoceles and interstitial emphysema are abnormal air collections within the lung. A pneumatocele is defined as "an emphysematous or gaseous swelling" and "a thin-walled cavity within the lung, one of the characteristic sequelae of staphylococcal pneumonia" (117). Most pneumatoceles secondary to staphylococcal pneumonia are found in children. They may be seen with other infections, including *Streptococcus pneumoniae, Haemophilus influenzae, E. coli,* group A streptococci, *Serratia marcescens, Klebsiella pneumoniae,* tuberculosis, and adenovirus and also with trauma, barotrauma, or hydrocarbon inhalation (Figs. 5.15 and 5.16) (118). In the setting of trauma, rapid compression of the lung creates shearing forces due to the negative intrathoracic pressure upon decompression, with rupture of normal lung architecture to create air-filled cyst-like spaces (Figs. 10.5 and 12.16). In infection, peribronchial abscesses may create a ball–valve phenomenon, obstructing a bronchial lumen, with distal hyperexpansion into an air-filled cyst-like space. Pneumatoceles may rupture and are associated with pneumothorax.

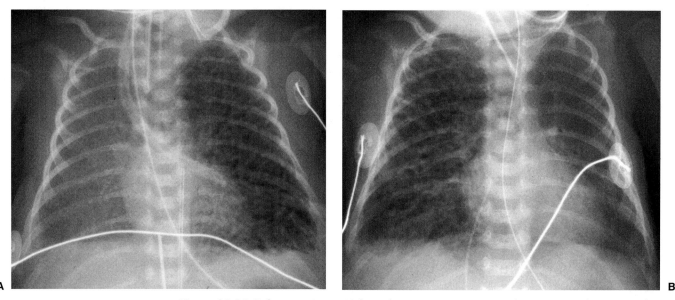

Figure 10.30 Pulmonary interstitial emphysema in a neonate with respiratory distress syndrome (RDS) changing in appearance within a few days. *A.* Portable chest radiograph demonstrates diffuse ground glass opacity of RDS throughout the right lung and diffuse round lucencies representing extensive pulmonary interstitial emphysema throughout the left lung. *B.* Portable chest radiograph 5 days later shows RDS throughout the left lung and diffuse round lucencies representing extensive pulmonary interstitial emphysema throughout the right lung.

Interstitial emphysema is defined as "the presence of air in the pulmonary tissues consequent upon rupture of the air cells; presence of air or gas in the connective tissue" (119). It is commonly referred to as pulmonary interstitial emphysema (PIE). Interstitial emphysema is more commonly seen in neonates with lung disease than in adults. Noncompliant lungs and the use of positive pressure ventilation are both associated with PIE in premature infants requiring mechanical ventilation for respiratory distress syndrome, meconium aspiration, infection, or amniotic fluid embolism (120). Two percent to 3% of all neonatal ICU patients and up to 30% of premature neonatal ICU patients develop PIE. On radiographs, air in alveolar spaces and air in the interstitium are indistinguishable unless there is abnormality of the intervening lung to provide sufficient contrast to detect the interstitial emphysema. Small rounded or linear lucencies are usually seen along the bronchovascular bundles but may also involve the peripheral or septal interstitium and the subpleural connective tissue. PIE ranges from a single focus to diffuse pulmonary involvement and is associated with the subsequent development of pneumomediastinum, pneumothorax, pneumopericardium, and pneumoperitoneum. In neonates, interstitial emphysema may be extensive and change quickly, as in the example given in Fig. 10.30 of a neonate with respiratory distress syndrome.

REFERENCES

1. Bekemeyer WB, Crapo RO, Calhoon S, et al. Efficacy of chest radiography in a respiratory intensive care unit: a prospective study. *Chest* 1985;88:691–696.
2. Henschke CI, Pasternack GS, Schroeder S, et al. Bedside chest radiography: diagnostic efficacy. *Radiology* 1983;149:23–26.
3. Janower ML, Jennas-Nocera Z, Mukai J. Utility and efficacy of portable chest radiographs. *AJR Am J Roentgenol* 1984;142:265–267.
4. Cantwell KG, Press HC JR, Anderson JE. Bedside radiographic examinations: indications and contraindications. *Radiology* 1978;129:383–384.
5. Leong CS, Cascade PN, Kazerooni EA, et al. Bedside chest radiography as part of a postcardiac

surgery critical care pathway: a means of decreasing utilization without adverse clinical impact. *Crit Care Med* 2000;28:383–388.

6. Bitetti J, Zimmerman JE. A clinician's perspective of critical care imaging. In: Goodman LR, Putman CE, eds. *Critical care imaging*, 3rd ed. Philadelphia: WB Saunders, 1992:29.

7. Gross BH, Spizarny DL. Computed tomography of the chest in the intensive care unit. *Crit Care Clin* 1994;10:267–275.

8. Miller WT Jr, Tino G, Friedburg JS. Thoracic CT in the intensive care unit: assessment of clinical usefulness. *Radiology* 1998;209:491–498.

9. White CS, Meyer CA, Wu J, et al. Portable CT: assessing thoracic disease in the intensive care unit. *AJR Am J Roentgenol* 1999;173:1351–1356.

10. Jacobs JE, Birnbaum BA. Abdominal computed tomography of intensive care unit patients. *Semin Roentgenol* 1997;32:128.

11. Guerrero-Lopez F, Vazquez-Mata G, Alcazar-Romero PP, et al. Evaluation of the utility of computed tomography in the initial assessment of the critical care patient with chest trauma. *Crit Care Med* 2000;28:1370–1375.

12. Schurawitzki H, Karnel F, Stiglbauer R, et al. CT-guided percutaneous drainage and fluid aspiration in intensive care patients. *Acta Radiol* 1992;33:131–136.

13. Hurst JM, Davis K Jr, Johnson DJ, et al. Cost and complications during in-hospital transport of critically ill patients: a prospective cohort study. *J Trauma Injury Infect Crit Care* 1992;33: 582–585.

14. Stearley HE. Patients' outcomes: intrahospital transportation and monitoring of critically ill patients by a specially trained ICU nursing staff. *Am J Crit Care* 1998;7:282–287.

15. McCunn M, Mirvis S, Reynolds N, et al. Physician utilization of a portable computed tomography scanner in the intensive care unit. *Crit Care Med* 2000;28:3808.

16. Gunnarsson T, Theodorsson A, Karlsson P, et al. Mobile computerized tomography scanning in the neurosurgery intensive care unit: increase in patient safety and reduction of staff workload. *J Neurosurg* 2000;93:432–436.

17. Lichtenstein D, Axler O. Intensive use of general ultrasound in the intensive care unit. Prospective study of 150 consecutive patients. *Intens Care Med* 1993;19:353–355.

18. Yu CJ, Yang PC, Chang DB, et al. Diagnostic and therapeutic use of chest sonography: value in critically ill patients. *AJR Am J Roentgenol* 1992;159:695–701.

19. Kundel HL, Gefter W, Aronchick J, et al. Accuracy of bedside chest hard-copy screen-film versus hard- and soft-copy computed radiographs in a medical intensive care unit: receiver operating characteristic analysis. *Radiology* 1997;205:859–863.

20. Kundel HL, Seshadri SB, Langlotz CP, et al. Prospective study of a PACS: information flow and clinical action in a medical intensive care unit. *Radiology* 1996;199:143–149.

21. Ashbaugh DG, Bigelow DB, Petty TL, et al. Acute respiratory distress in adults. *Lancet* 1967;2: 319–323.

22. Bernard GR, Artigas A, Brigham KL, et al. The American-European Consensus Conference on ARDS: definitions, mechanisms, relevant outcomes, and clinical trial coordination. *Am J Respir Crit Care Med* 1994;149:818–824.

23. Petty TL. Adult respiratory distress syndrome: definition and historical perspective. *Clin Chest Med* 1982;3:3–7.

24. Bone RC, Balk RA, Cerra FB, et al. ACCP/SCCM Consensus Conference: definitions for sepsis and organ failure and guidelines for the use of innovative therapies in sepsis. *Chest* 1992;101: 1644–1655.

25. Hudson LD, Milberg JA, Anardi D, et al. Clinical risks for development of the acute respiratory distress syndrome. *Am J Respir Crit Care Med* 1995;151:293–301.

26. Milberg JA, Davis DR, Steinberg KP, et al. Improved survival of patients with acute respiratory distress syndrome (ARDS): 1983–1993. *JAMA* 1995;273:306–309.

27. Bachofen M, Weibel ER. Alterations of the gas exchange apparatus in adult respiratory insufficiency associated with septicemia. *Am Rev Respir Dis* 1977;116:589–561.

28. Greene R. Adult respiratory distress syndrome: acute alveolar damage. *Radiology* 1987;163: 57–66.

29. Holter JF, Weiland JE, Pach ER, et al. Protein permeability in adult respiratory distress syndromes. *J Clin Invest* 1986;78:1513–1522.

30. Albelda SM, Gefter WB, Kelley MA, et al. Ventilator-induced sub-pleural air cysts: clinical, radiographic and pathologic significance. *Am Rev Respir Dis* 1983;127:360–365.

31. McLoud TC, Barash PG, Ravin CE. PEEP: radiographic features and associated complications. *AJR Am J Roentgenol* 129:209–213, 1977.

32. Gattinoni L, Caironi P, Pelosi P, et al. What has computed tomography taught us about the acute respiratory distress syndrome? *Am J Respir Crit Care Med* 2001;164:1701–1711.

33. Gattinoni L, Pelosi P, Pesenti A, et al. CT scan in ARDS: clinical and physiopathological insights. *Acta Anaesth Scand* 1991;95:87–96.

34. Goodman LR, Fumagalli R, Tagliabue P, et al. Adult respiratory distress syndrome due to pulmonary and extrapulmonary causes: CT, clinical, and functional correlations. *Radiology* 1999; 213:545–552.

35. Gattinoni L, Presenti A, Torresin A, et al. Adult respiratory distress syndrome profiles by computed tomography. *J Thorac Imag* 1986;1:25–36.

36. Tagliabue M, Casella TC, Zincone GE, et al. CT and chest radiography in the evaluation of adult respiratory distress syndrome. *Acta Radiol* 1994;35:230–234.

37. Desai SR, Hansell DM. Lung imaging in the adult respiratory distress syndrome: current practice and new insights. *Intens Care Med* 1997;23:7–15.

38. Gattinoni L, Pelosi O, Vitale G, et al. Body position changes redistribute lung computed-tomographic density in patients with acute respiratory failure. *Anesthesiology* 1991;74:15–23.

39. Nobauer-Huhmann IM, Eibenberger K, Schaefer-Prokop C, et al. Changes in lung parenchyma after acute respiratory distress syndrome (ARDS): assessment with high-resolution computed tomography. *Eur Radiol* 2001;11:2436–2443.

40. Desai SR, Wells AU, Rubens MB, et al. Acute respiratory distress syndrome: CT abnormalities at long term follow up. *Radiology* 1999;210:29–35.

41. Meaney JF, Kazerooni EA, Garver KA, et al. Acute respiratory distress syndrome: CT findings during partial liquid ventilation. *Radiology* 1997;202:570–573.

42. Hamman L, Rich AR. Fulminating diffuse interstitial fibrosis of the lungs. *Trans Am Clin Climat Assoc* 1935;51:154–163.

43. Katzenstein AL, Myers JL, Mazur MT. Acute interstitial pneumonia. A clinicopathologic, ultrastructural, and cell kinetic study. *Am J Surg Pathol* 1986;10:256–267.

44. Olson J, Colby TV, Elliott CG. Hamman-Rich syndrome revisited. *Mayo Clin Proc* 1990;65: 1538–1548.

45. Vourlekis JS, Brown KK, Cool CD, et al. Acute interstitial pneumonitis. Case series and review of the literature. *Medicine* 2000;79:369–378.

46. Roberts J, Barnes W, Pennoch MHS, et al. Diagnostic accuracy of fever as a measure of postoperative pulmonary complications. *Heart Lung* 1988;17:166–170.

47. Rubin SA, Winer-Muram HT, Ellis JV. Diagnostic imaging of pneumonia and its complications in the critically ill patient. *Clin Chest Med* 1995;16:45–59.

48. Mock CN, Burchard KW, Hasan F, et al. Surgical intensive care unit pneumonia. *Surgery* 1988;104:494–499.

49. Keita-Perse O, Edwards JR, Culver DH, et al. Comparing nosocomial infection rates among surgical intensive-care units: the importance of separating cardiothoracic and general surgery intensive-care units. *Infect Control Hosp Epidemiol* 1998;19:260–261.

50. Baker AM, Meredith JW, Haponik EF. Pneumonia in intubated trauma patients. Microbiology and outcomes. *Am J Respir Crit Care Med* 1996;153:343–349.

51. Andrews CP, Coalson JJ, Smith JD, et al. Diagnosis of nosocomial bacterial pneumonia in acute diffuse lung disease. *Chest* 1981;80:254–258.

52. Norwood SH, Civetta JM. Evaluating sepsis in critically ill patients. *Chest* 1987;91:137–144.

53. Fagon JY, Chastre J, Domart Y, et al. Nosocomial pneumonia in patients receiving continuous mechanical ventilation. Prospective analysis of 52 episodes with use of a protected specimen brush and quantitative culture techniques. *Am Rev Respir Dis* 1989;139:877–884.

54. Tejada Artigas A, Bello Dronda S, Chacon Valles E, et al. Risk factors for nosocomial pneumonia in critically ill trauma patients. *Crit Care Med* 2001;29:304–309.

55. Barkhausen J, Stoblen F, Dominguez-Fernandez E, et al. Impact of CT in patients with sepsis of unknown origin. *Acta Radiologica* 1999;40:552–555.

56. Iwasaki Y, Nagata K, Nakanishi M, et al. Spiral CT findings in septic pulmonary emboli. *Eur J Radiol* 2001;37:190–194.

57. Huang RM, Naidich DP, Lubat E, et al. Septic pulmonary emboli: CT-radiographic correlation. *AJR Am J Roentgenol* 1989;153:41–45.

58. Kuhlman JE, Fishman EK, Teigen C. Pulmonary septic emboli: diagnosis with CT. *Radiology* 1990;174:211–221.

59. Bartlett JG, Gorbach SL. The triple threat of aspiration pneumonia. *Chest* 1975;68:560–566.

60. Landay MJ, Christensen EE, Bynum LJ. Pulmonary manifestations of acute aspiration of gastric contents. *AJR Am J Roentgenol* 1978;131:587–592.

61. Benjamin JJ, Cascade PN, Rubenfire M, et al. Left lower lobe atelectasis and consolidation fol-

lowing cardiac surgery. The effect of topical cooling on the phrenic nerve. *Radiology* 1982;142: 11–14.

62. Zylak CJ, Littleton JT, Durizch ML. Illusory consolidation of the left lower lobe: a pitfall of portable radiography. *Radiology* 1988;167:653–655.

63. Harris RS. The importance of proximal and distal air bronchograms in the management of atelectasis. *Can Assoc Radiol J* 1985;36:103–109.

64. Milne ENC. A physiological approach to reading critical care unit films. *J Thorac Imag* 1986;1: 60–90.

65. Pistolesi M, Miniati M, Milne ENC, et al. The chest roentgenogram in pulmonary edema. *Clin Chest Med* 1985;6:315–344.

66. Milne ENC, Pistolesi M, Miniati M, et al. The vascular pedicle of the heart and the vena azygos. Part I. The normal subject. *Radiology* 1985;152:1–158.

67. Rose CP, Stolberg HO. The limited utility of the plain chest film in the assessment of left ventricular structure and function. *Invest Radiol* 1983;17:139–144.

68. Milne ENC. Correlation of physiologic findings with chest roentgenology. *Radiol Clin North Am* 1973;11:17–47.

69. Ely EW, Haponik EF. Using the chest radiograph to determine intravascular volume status: the role of vascular pedicle width. *Chest* 2002;121:942–950.

70. Milne ENC, Pistolesi M. Assessing systemic intra- and extravascular water. In: *Reading the chest radiograph*. St. Louis: Mosby-Year Book, 1993:80–119.

71. Pistolesi M, Milne EN, Miniati M, et al. The vascular pedicle of the heart and the vena azygos. Part II. Acquired heart disease. *Radiology* 1984;152:9–17.

72. Heitzman ER. Radiologic appearance of the azygos vein in cardiovascular disease. *Circulation* 1973;47:628–634.

73. Woodrow P. Central venous catheters and central venous pressure. *Nurs Stand* 2002;16:45–51.

74. Giuntini C. Pulmonary blood volume and its relationship to total blood volume and central hemodynamics in man. In: *International Symposium on Pulmonary Circulation. Progress in respiratory research*. Vol. 5. New York: Karger, 1970.

75. Milne ENC. Some new concepts of pulmonary blood flow and volume. *Radiol Clin North Am* 1978;16:515–536.

76. Milne ENC, Pistolesi M. Quantification of pulmonary blood volume, flow and pressure: practice. In: *Reading the chest radiograph*. St. Louis: Mosby-Year Book, 1993:202–241.

77. Ravin CE. Pulmonary vascularity: radiographic considerations. *J Thorac Radiol* 1988;3:1–13.

78. McHugh TJ, Forrester JS, Adler L, et al. Pulmonary vascular congestion in acute myocardial infarction: Hemodynamic and radiologic correlations. *Ann Intern Med* 1972;76:29–33.

79. Simon M. The pulmonary vessels: their hemodynamic evaluation using routine radiographs. *Radiol Clin North Am* 1963;2:363–375.

80. Herman PG, Khan A, Kallman CE, et al. Limited correlation of left ventricular end-diastolic pressure with radiographic assessment of pulmonary hemodynamics. *Radiology* 1990;174: 721–724.

81. Cascade PN, Kantrowitz A, Wajszczuk WJ, et al. The chest x-ray in acute left ventricular power failure: an aid to determining prognosis of patients supported by intraaortic balloon pumping. *AJR Am J Roentgenol* 1976;126:1147–1154.

82. Woodring JH. Pulmonary artery-bronchus ratios in patients with normal lungs, pulmonary vascular plethora, and congestive heart failure. *Radiology* 1991;179:115–122.

83. Gluecker T, Capasso P, Schnyder P, et al. Clinical and radiologic features of pulmonary edema. *Radiographics* 1999;19:1507–1531; discussion 1532–1533.

84. Swenson ER, Maggiorini M, Mongovin S, et al. Pathogenesis of high-altitude pulmonary edema: inflammation is not an etiologic factor. *JAMA* 2002;287:2228–2235.

85. Cremona G, Asnaghi R, Baderna P, et al. Pulmonary extravascular fluid accumulation in recreational climbers: a prospective study. *Lancet* 2002;359:276–277.

86. Cascade PN, Alexander G, Mackie DS. Negative pressure pulmonary edema following endotracheal intubation. *Radiology* 1993;186:671–675.

87. Di Pasquale G, Andreoli A, Lusa AM, et al. Cardiologic complications of subarachnoid hemorrhage. *J Neurosurg Sci* 1998;4:33–36.

88. Mayer SA, Lin J, Homma S, et al. Myocardial injury and left ventricular performance after subarachnoid hemorrhage. *Stroke* 1999;30:780–786.

89. Household Hazardous Products and Ingredients. *www.healthgoods.com/Shopping/Household_Products/Household_Hazardous_Products.htm*. © 2002 Healthgoods.com. Accessed August 12, 2002.

90. Agency for Toxic Substances and Disease Registry (ATSDR). *www.atsdr.cdc.gov*.

91. Forrester JM, Steele AW, Waldron JA, et al. Crack lung: an acute pulmonary syndrome with a spectrum of clinical and histopathologic findings. *Am Rev Respir Dis* 1990;142:462–467.

92. Pneumothorax. *Stedman's medical dictionary*, 26th ed. Philadelphia: Lippincott, Williams & Wilkins, 1995:1394–1395.

93. Baumann MH, Strange C, Heffner JE, et al. AACP Pneumothorax Consensus Group. Management of spontaneous pneumothorax: an American College of Chest Physicians Delphi consensus statement. *Chest* 2001;119:590–602.

94. Sahn SA, Heffner JE. Spontaneous pneumothorax. *N Engl J Med* 200;342:868–874.

95. Vermillion JM, Wilson EB, Smith RW. Traumatic diaphragmatic hernia presenting as a tension fecopneumothorax. *Hernia* 200;5:158–160.

96. Di Giorgio A, Al Mansour M, Cardini CL, et al. Congenital cystic adenomatoid malformation of the lung presenting as pyopneumothorax in an eighteen-year-old woman. *J Thorac Cardiovasc Surg* 2001;122:1034–1036.

97. Melton LJ 3rd, Hepper NG, Offord KP. Incidence of spontaneous pneumothorax in Olmsted County, Minnesota: 1950 to 1974. *Am Rev Respir Dis* 1979;120:1379–1382.

98. Srinivas S, Varadhachary G. Spontaneous pneumothorax in malignancy: a case report and review of the literature. *Ann Oncol* 200;11:887–889.

99. Wait MA, Estrera A. Changing clinical spectrum of spontaneous pneumothorax. *Am J Surg* 1992;164:528–531.

100. Joseph J, Sahn SA. Thoracic endometriosis syndrome: new observations from an analysis of 110 cases. *Am J Med* 1996;100:164–170.

101. Berdon WJ, Dee GJ, Abramson ST, et al. Localized pneumothorax adjacent to a collapsed lobe. *Radiology* 1984;150:691–694.

102. Seow A, Kazerooni EA, Pernicano PG, et al. Comparison of upright inspiratory and expiratory chest radiographs for detecting pneumothoraces. *AJR Am J Roentgenol* 1996; 313–316.

103. Lichtenstein DA, Menu Y. A bedside ultrasound sign ruling out pneumothorax in the critically ill. Lung sliding. *Chest* 1995;108:1345–1348.

104. Pneumomediastinum. *Stedman's medical dictionary*, 26th ed. Philadelphia: Lippincott, Williams & Wilkins, 1995:1392.

105. Wintermark M, Schnyder P. The Macklin effect: a frequent etiology for pneumomediastinum in severe blunt chest trauma. *Chest* 2001;120:543–547.

106. Bejvan SM, Godwin JD. Pneumomediastinum: old signs and new signs. *AJR Am J Roentgenol* 1996;166:1041–1048.

107. Naclerio E. The "V" sign in the diagnosis of spontaneous rupture of the esophagus (an early roentgen clue). *Am J Surg* 1957;93:291–293.

108. Levin B. The continuous diaphragm sign. A newly-recognized sign of pneumomediastinum. *Clin Radiol* 1973;24:337–338.

109. Pneumopericardium. *Stedman's medical dictionary*, 26th ed. Philadelphia: Lippincott, Williams & Wilkins, 1995:1390.

110. Hipona FA, Paredes S. The radiology of pericardial disease. *Cardiovasc Clin* 1976;7:91–12.

111. Cochrane LJ, Mitchell ME, Raju S, et al. Tension pneumopericardium as a complication of single-lung transplantation. *Ann Thorac Surg* 1990;50:808–810.

112. Demetriades D, Charalambides D, Pantanowitz D, et al. Pneumopericardium following penetrating chest injuries. *Arch Surg* 1990;125:1187–1189.

113. Katzir D, Klinovsky E, Kent V, et al. Spontaneous pneumopericardium: case report and review of the literature. *Cardiology* 1989;76:305–308.

114. Mirvis SE, Indeck M, Schorr RM, et al. Posttraumatic tension pneumopericardium: the "small heart" sign. *Radiology* 1986;158:663–669.

115. Leitman BS, Greengart A, Wasser HJ. Pneumomediastinum and pneumopericardium after cocaine abuse. *AJR Am J Roentgenol* 1988;151:614.

116. Bedotto JB, McBride W, Abraham M, et al. Echocardiographic diagnosis of pneumopericardium and hydropneumopericardium. *J Am Soc Echocardiogr* 1988;1:359–361.

117. Pneumatocele. *Stedman's medical dictionary*, 26 ed. Philadelphia: Lippincott, Williams & Wilkins, 1995:1390.

118. Atlas AB, Boyer D. Pneumatocele. E-Medicine, Instant Access to the Minds of Medicine. *www.emedicine.compedtopic1829.htm.* Last Updated July 2, 2002; access date September 9, 2002.

119. Emphysema, interstitial. *Stedman's medical dictionary*, 26th ed. Philadelphia: Lippincott, Williams & Wilkins, 1995:562.

120. Bhatt AJ, Ryan RM. Pulmonary interstitial emphysema. E-Medicine, Instant Access to the Minds of Medicine. *www.emedicine.compedtopic2596.htm.* Last Updated May 29, 2002; access date September 9, 2002.

LINES, TUBES, AND DEVICES

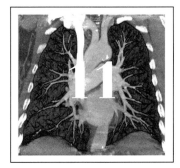

- Venous
- Aorta
- Cardiac
- Airway
- Esophagus
- Chest Tubes

Intrathoracic lines, tubes, and devices are commonly placed, either temporarily or permanently, for the diagnosis, monitoring, or treatment of thoracic disease processes (Table 11.1). Although some are more mundane than others, such as central venous catheters and endotracheal tubes, others are more exotic, such as extracorporeal life support (ECLS) cannulas or left ventricular assist devices. New devices continue to be developed. As radiologists, it is important to recognize the normal position of these lines, tubes, and devices and abnormal positioning with knowledge of the complications that may subsequently arise. In some cases, the very lines, tubes, or devices placed into the thorax for patient care reasons may be the source of patient morbidity and even mortality.

More often than not, the many catheters, tubes, and indwelling monitoring devices used in patient care are initially placed in the correct position. However, this should not lull either the radiologist or clinician into complacency. Catheters may be incorrectly positioned when first placed or may move from their original position into an improper position. Most catheter misplacements are readily correctable and without consequence, whereas others are serious and require immediate intervention. Bekemeyer et al. (1) reported that 27% of lines and tubes were malpositioned on portable radiographs taken after initial placement and that the radiograph was instrumental in deciding whether or not to reposition the catheter in 20%.

Always review the location of all lines, tubes, and devices.

VENOUS

PERCUTANEOUS INDWELLING CENTRAL CATHETER

In the past few years the percutaneous intravascular central catheter (PICC) has been used with increasing frequency (2). A PICC is placed percutaneously into an antecubital, basilic, or brachial vein in much the same way a peripheral intravenous line is placed but using a longer catheter that extends into the large central veins of the thorax. It is used in lieu of a central venous line, often when longer term venous access is required, for up to 3 months. PICCs are made of silicone rubber and vary in size from 2.0 to 5.0 French in diameter. Because of their small diameter, they are of relatively low radiographic opacity and are often difficult to visualize with standard chest radiographic technique (Fig.11.1A).

Table 11.1: Diagnostic, Monitoring, and Therapeutic Thoracic Lines, Tubes, and Devices

Venous
    Percutaneous indwelling central catheter
    Central venous catheter
    Pulmonary artery catheter
    Venovenous or venoarterial extracorporeal life support
    Stents
Arterial
    Intraaortic balloon pump
    Venoarterial extracorporeal life support
    Stents
Cardiac
    Pacemaker
    Implantable cardiac defibrillator
    Left venticular assist device
    Atrial septal defect closure device
Airway
    Endotracheal tube
    Tracheostomy tube
    Intratracheal oxygen catheter
    Stents
Esophagus
    Feeding tube
    Nasogastric or oral-gastric tubes
    Intraesophageal manometer
    Temperature probe
    pH probe
    Stent
    Antireflux devices
    Gastric banding
Pleural
    Chest tubes

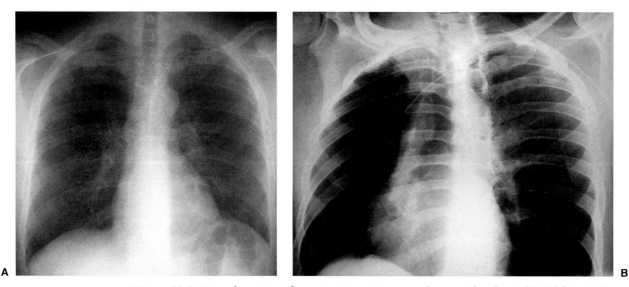

Figure 11.1 Normal position of a percutaneous intravascular central catheter (PICC) line. *A.* Standard posteroanterior chest radiograph demonstrates the left upper extremity PICC with tip in the distal left brachiocephalic vein. *B.* Note the greater conspicuity of the same percutaneous intravascular central catheter on the right anterior oblique radiograph at low kVp technique.

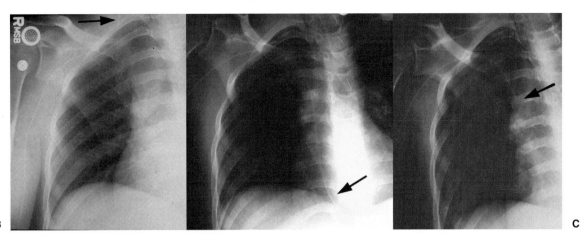

Figure 11.2 Abnormal and normal right upper extremity percutaneous intravascular central catheter position in the same patient after repositioning several times. *A.* Extending up the right internal jugular vein (*arrow*). *B.* Extending through the superior vena cava into the right atrium (*arrow*). *C.* Correct position in the superior vena cava (*arrow*).

Because the PICC is usually placed blindly at the bedside, a postplacement chest radiograph is used to confirm proper position. To make the PICC line more recognizable radiographically, a right anterior oblique radiograph (or if portable left posterior oblique) to rotate the superior vena cava off the thoracic spine, performed using low kVp technique (65 to 70 kVp versus 120 kVp for standard chest radiography) as used for rib detail radiographs, is useful (Fig. 11.1B). Ideally, the catheter tip should be in the superior vena cava or the brachiocephalic veins (Fig. 11.1). Fluoroscopic guidance may also be used to ensure proper positioning. Compared with central venous lines, there is a lower complication rate. The risk of pneumothorax is avoided as the entry site is remote from the pleura. There is also a lower incidence of both thrombosis (Fig. 21.10) and infection. PICCs more frequently become displaced than conventional central venous lines because of their flexibility, requiring repositioning and additional imaging to confirm position (Fig. 11.2).

> Low kVp radiographs taken in an oblique position make it easier to see the position of PICC lines.

CENTRAL VENOUS CATHETER

Central venous access is used for both diagnosis, such as the measurement of central venous pressure and blood draws, and therapy, for the delivery of medications. Central venous catheters are placed percutaneously, usually through an internal jugular or subclavian vein. Less commonly, they are placed using a femoral approach, avoiding the risk of pneumothorax. The subclavian approach is less accepted because of concerns for increased infection and thrombosis and patient mobility. More permanent versions include the Hickman catheter (named after Dr. Hickman; silicone catheter with one, two, or three lumens), and various ports such as the Port-A-Cath (titanium port with a polyurethane catheter) (Sims-Deltec, Inc., St. Paul, MN). The Hickman catheter was developed in the late 1970s as a modification of the Broviac catheter developed by Dr. Broviac in 1973 for infusing total parenteral nutrition. The Hickman catheter is more widely used today, having a wider tube and thicker wall than the Broviac catheter. These are usually placed through a neck vein, tunneled under the skin, with an access point just below the clavicle. The end of the Hickman catheter is outside the patient, with a small Dacron cuff 1 inch before the exit site that acts as a barrier to infection and as an anchor. For the Port-A-Cath, access is gained after cleaning and anesthetizing the skin and then using a needle to puncture through both the skin and the rubber wall of the port's reservoir (Fig. 11.3). Large double-lumen catheters, such as the Sorenson catheter, may be placed for temporary renal dialysis (Fig. 11.4).

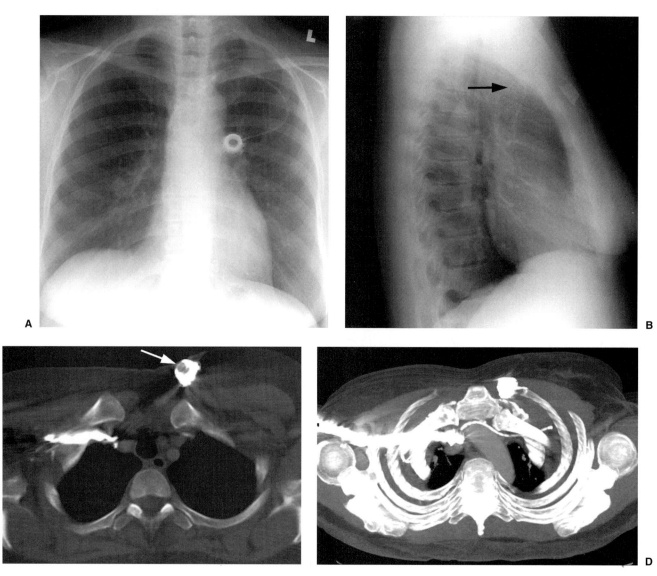

Figure 11.3 Port-A-Cath. *A.* Posteroanterior and *(B)* lateral chest radiographs demonstrate the port reservoir in the left anterior chest wall and catheter entering the left subclavian vein with tip in the superior vena cava. Note the anterior curvature of this left-sided venous catheter on the lateral view *(arrow)*. A right-sided venous catheter does not make this curve. *C.* Computed tomography demonstrates the port reservoir with rubber wall *(white arrow)*. *D.* Computed tomography thick maximum intensity project demonstrates the course of the catheter in the chest wall, heading underneath the clavicle. Note that the catheter curves anteriorly in the left brachiocephalic vein as it crosses anterior to the aortic arch, corresponding to the curvature seen on the lateral chest radiograph, whereas the right-sided vein has a straight course.

A central venous catheter tip should be in the superior vena cava or a brachiocephalic vein.

When used for blood draws and medication delivery, the catheter tip should be located in a brachiocephalic vein or the superior vena cava. When used to measure central venous pressure, the ideal position is in the superior vena cava to avoid inaccurate measurements that may be obtained if the catheter tip abuts or is near valves within the brachiocephalic veins. When located too distally in the right atrium, there is an increased risk of atrial arrhythmias and rarely cardiac perforation. Portable radiographs are obtained after central venous catheter placement, both to confirm that the catheter is in good position (Fig. 11.4) and to look for the possible complication of pneumothorax. Table 11.2 lists the complications that may occur secondary to central venous

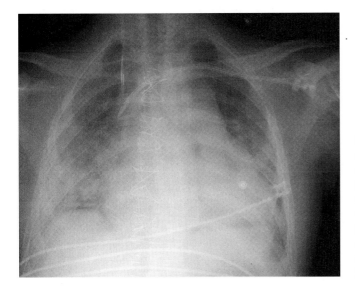

Figure 11.4 Normal position of central venous catheters. Catheter entering from right internal jugular vein with tip in the distal right brachiocephalic vein, and catheter (double lumen) entering from left subclavian vein with tip in the superior vena cava illustrates location of venous anatomy.

catheters (3). Pneumothorax occurs in up to 5% of central venous catheter placements and is more common with the subclavian approach than the jugular approach. Because these catheters are usually placed blindly at the bedside, they can end up in almost any vein within the thorax, neck, or upper extremity. It is important to know the normal venous anatomy and common variants to correctly identify catheter position. Atypical placements include extension cephalad into a jugular vein, across the mediastinum into contralateral veins, down the axillary vein, into the azygous or internal mammary veins, a left-sided superior vena cava, or even the inferior vena cava and hepatic veins (Fig. 11.5). Inadvertent arterial puncture can be confirmed radiographically by location of the catheter over the aorta (Fig. 11.6). However, it is usually recognized clinically by the withdrawal of bright red blood or recognizing pulsatile blood flow from the catheter.

A catheter tip pointing at the wall of the superior vena cava may lead to rupture if not repositioned.

Other complications visible radiographically include venous perforation with mediastinal and/or neck hematoma and infusion of fluid into the mediastinum that may be confused radiographically for hematoma or hemothorax (Figs. 11.7A and 11.7B). Catheter fracture that may result in fragments embolizing into the pulmonary arterial circulation occurs in less than 1% of cases and may be first recognized by the radiologist (Fig. 11.7C and 11.17D). The fragments may be removed percutaneously by the interventional radiologists. The complications of thrombosis (Fig. 11.8) and infection are uncommon and usually without findings on chest radiographs; uncommonly, dilatation of the azygos vein may be found as a collateral pathway if there is thrombosis of the superior vena cava (4). The reasons behind injury or death secondary to central venous catheter placement reported to the Federal Food and Drug Administration (FDA) medical device reporting system revealed that 55% of cases were related to health care professionals (technique); 12% were due to device failure, 3% patient-related factors, 3% pathologic/physiologic

Table 11.2: Complications Secondary to Central Venous Catheters

Malposition
Pneumothorax
Vascular laceration (hemothorax, chest wall/neck/mediastinal hematoma)
Infection (possible source of septic emboli)
Catheter fragmentation and embolization
Venous thrombosis
Venous stenosis

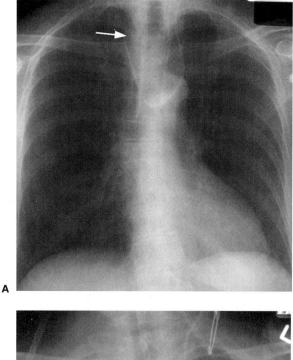

A

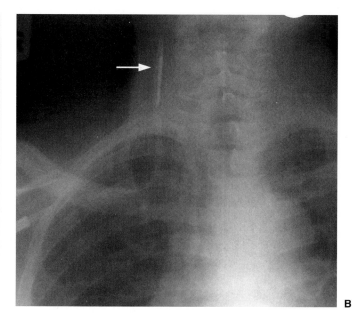

B

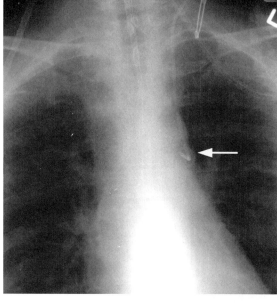

C

Figure 11.5 Malpositioned central venous catheters. *A.* Catheter placed in left internal jugular vein extends across the left and right brachiocephalic veins of the mediastinum and then cephalad into the right internal jugular vein (*arrow*). *B.* Catheter placed in right subclavian vein extends up the right internal jugular vein (*arrow*). *C.* Catheter placed in left internal jugular vein is positioned with tip in the left superior intercostal vein, seen radiographically as the "aortic nipple" (*arrow*). Posteroanterior (*D*) and lateral (*E*) radiographs demonstrate a central venous catheter in the azygos vein (*arrowheads*).

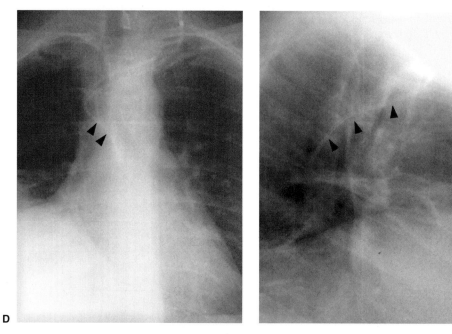

D

E

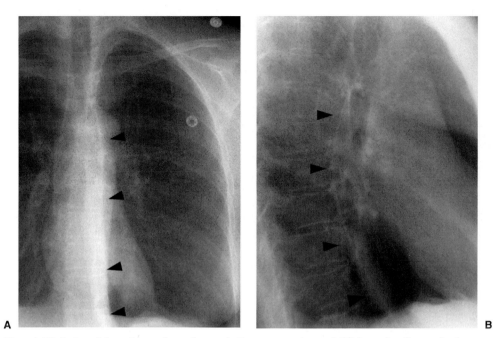

Figure 11.6 Arterial position of a catheter. *A.* Posteroanterior and *(B)* lateral radiographs demonstrate a catheter placed through a brachial artery extending into the left subclavian artery (above the clavicular head) and down the descending thoracic aorta *(arrowheads)*.

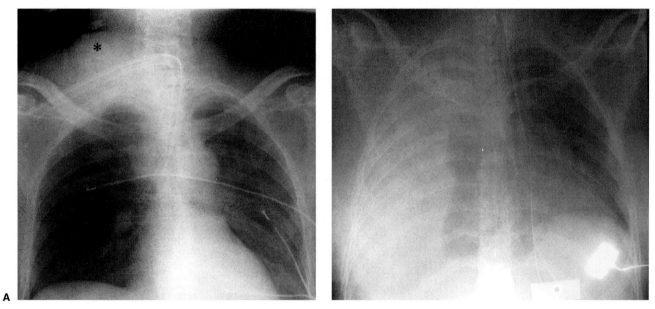

Figure 11.7 Complications of central venous catheter placement. *A.* Neck hematoma *(asterisk)* after right internal jugular line placement attempt. Note the endotracheal tube tip is in the right main bronchus. *B.* Fatal right hemothorax after right internal jugular line placement attempt in a patient with undiagnosed idiopathic thrombocytopenic purpura.

(continued on next page)

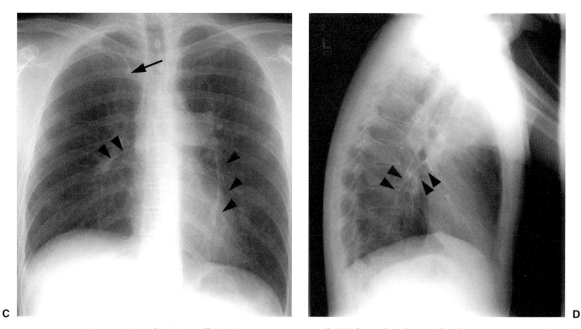

Figure 11.7 (continued) *C.* Posteroanterior and *(D)* lateral radiographs demonstrate a right sub-clavian catheter with tip overlaying the right clavicular head *(arrow)*, as well as catheter fragments in both the right and left pulmonary arteries *(arrowheads)*.

(thrombosis or thromboembolism), and 28% unknown (3). Vascular perforation was responsible for 94% of the fatalities and 54% of injuries. Common reasons implicated for catheter fracture were excessive force during catheter placement or removal, excess syringe pressure when attempting to open an occlusion, shearing the catheter with an insertion needle, catheter puncture with a surgical needle, and failure to follow insert directions.

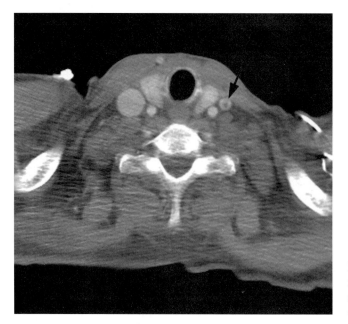

Figure 11.8 Thrombus in left internal jugular vein *(arrow)* in a patient with several recent central venous catheters.

PULMONARY ARTERY CATHETER

Pulmonary artery pressure and resistance, cardiac output, and pulmonary capillary wedge pressure can be measured with a balloon-tipped flow-directed catheter, providing information on cardiac function and hemodynamic status. The pulmonary capillary wedge pressure reflects left atrial and ventricular filling pressures, and left ventricular volume. When positive end-expiratory pressure is being delivered or when left ventricular compliance is reduced, the pulmonary capillary wedge pressure may not accurately reflect left ventricular preload and yield a false impression of fluid status. Although the concept of using a balloon-assisted catheter for this purpose was published 15 years earlier, cardiologist H. J. C. Swan observed a sailboat moving quickly despite the calm weather at the beach in California, leading to the initial idea of devising a catheter attached with a parachute or sail-like device. Initial testing was made with a balloon-tipped catheter, which was easier to make than a sail-like device; due to its success, the parachute idea was abandoned. Cardiologist William Ganz was working on the thermodilution method of measuring cardiac output at the same time, which was incorporated into the catheter. Pulmonary artery catheters are therefore commonly referred to as Swan-Ganz catheters (5).

The basic design has remained unchanged for over 30 years (5). Ideally, the tip of a pulmonary arterial catheter should reside within a large pulmonary artery and should not be located peripheral to the interlobar pulmonary artery that forms each hilum (Fig. 11.9). The balloon should only be inflated during placement and pressure measurement and not left wedged in a small artery. Given the length of these catheters, it is not uncommon for catheters to become coiled in the heart (Fig. 11.10). Redundancy of the catheter in the right atrium and ventricle increases the risk of thrombus formation and thromboembolism (Fig. 11.10C). In addition to the complications listed in Table 11.2 for central venous catheters, there are several complications unique to flow-directed pulmonary arterial catheters, as listed in Table 11.3. They include pulmonary artery perforation with pulmonary hemorrhage, pulmonary infarcts, and pulmonary artery pseudoaneurysms (Fig. 11.11) (6). Chronic positioning of a catheter in a small pulmonary artery branch may also result in pulmonary infarction.

Pulmonary artery pseudoaneurysms occur due to either direct rupture of the artery by the inflated balloon or the catheter tip. Correct pressure in the inflated balloon is about

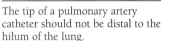

The tip of a pulmonary artery catheter should not be distal to the hilum of the lung.

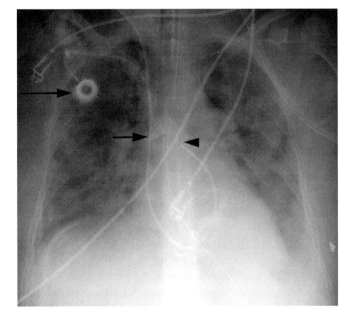

Figure 11.9 Normal position of a pulmonary artery catheter placed through the right internal jugular vein, with tip in the proximal right pulmonary artery *(arrowhead)*. Note the right chest wall port *(large arrow)* with tip in the superior vena cava *(small arrow)*.

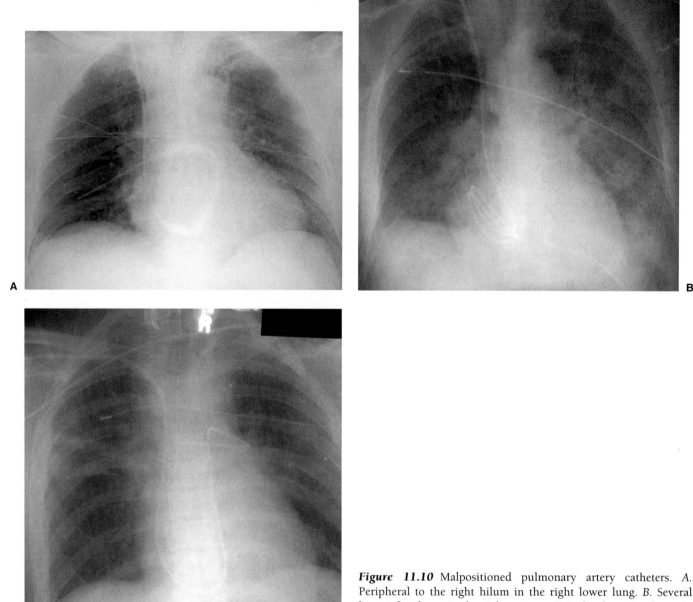

Figure 11.10 Malpositioned pulmonary artery catheters. *A.* Peripheral to the right hilum in the right lower lung. *B.* Several loops of catheter in the right atrium. *C.* Redundancy in the main pulmonary artery.

Pulmonary artery pseudoaneurysms secondary to catheter injury have a high risk of rupture.

300 mm Hg; excess pressure while inflating the balloon may lead to rupture. After the artery is lacerated and blood extends into the alveolar spaces and airway, pulmonary hemorrhage manifests radiographically as alveolar consolidation and hemoptysis clinically. Rupture through the visceral pleura may lead to hemothorax. If the vessel is injured, leaving an incomplete vessel wall, a delayed pseudoaneurysm may be found, often seen later as a pulmonary nodule adjacent to the lung hila. Because of the high risk of pseudoaneurysms rupturing, they require treatment, usually using a percutaneous approach (Fig. 11.11, B and C). Contrast-enhanced computed tomography is usually performed for diagnosis, before catheter-guided treatment.

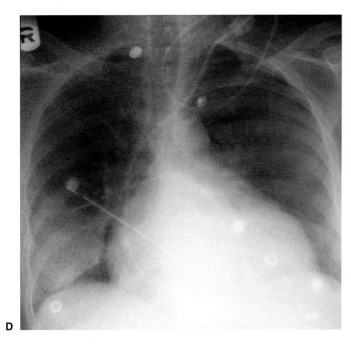

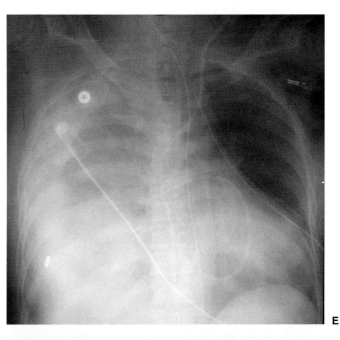

Figure 11.10 (continued) *D* and *E.* Peripheral to the right hilum in the right lower lung with focal pulmonary hemorrhage on (D) the initial postcatheter placement radiograph, followed by (E) extensive pulmonary hemorrhage and hemothorax six hours later. *F.* Placed through right internal jugular vein, perforated a central intrathoracic vein and the parietal pleura with resultant hemothorax. Catheter coiled in the inferior aspect of the right pleural space.

Table 11.3: Complications Secondary to Pulmonary Artery Catheters

Malposition
Redundancy or coiling in heart, pulmonary artery or across cardiac valves
Pneumothorax
Pulmonary infarction
Vascular laceration (hemothorax, chest wall/neck/mediastinal hematoma)
Infection (possible source of septic emboli)
Catheter fragmentation and embolization
Venous thrombosis and thromboembolism
Venous stenosis
Pulmonary artery laceration (hemorrhage, pseudoaneurysm)

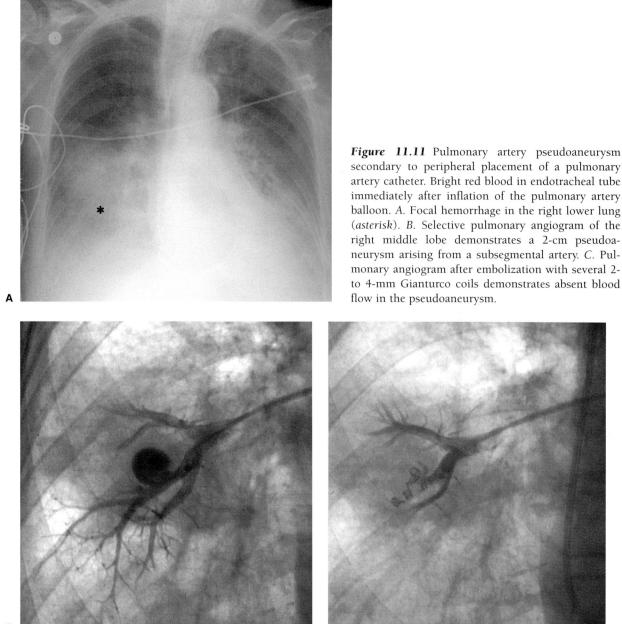

Figure 11.11 Pulmonary artery pseudoaneurysm secondary to peripheral placement of a pulmonary artery catheter. Bright red blood in endotracheal tube immediately after inflation of the pulmonary artery balloon. *A.* Focal hemorrhage in the right lower lung (*asterisk*). *B.* Selective pulmonary angiogram of the right middle lobe demonstrates a 2-cm pseudoaneurysm arising from a subsegmental artery. *C.* Pulmonary angiogram after embolization with several 2- to 4-mm Gianturco coils demonstrates absent blood flow in the pseudoaneurysm.

EXTRACORPOREAL LIFE SUPPORT

ECLS is a form of bedside cardiopulmonary bypass used primarily for the treatment of neonatal respiratory distress. It is used less commonly in adults with acute, severe, and potentially reversible respiratory failure, with or without cardiac failure (7,8). Deoxygenated blood is removed from the venous system through a venous cannula, usually placed in the right internal jugular vein. The blood then undergoes extracorporeal oxygenation and can be returned either through a large vein or artery. In venovenous ECLS, blood is usually returned via the right internal jugular vein and less commonly a femoral vein. In venoarterial ECLS, blood is returned into a large artery, usually the common carotid artery, which is ligated in the process. Although venovenous ECLS is used for oxygenation, venoarterial ECLS is used when left ventricular cardiac support is also necessary.

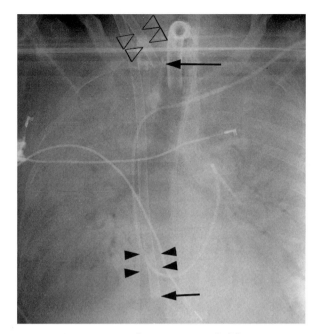

Figure 11.12 Venoarterial extracorporeal life support in a patient with acute respiratory distress syndrome secondary to streptococcal pneumonia. The tip of the venous cannula (*arrowheads*) is in the right atrium (*arrow*) and the tip of the arterial cannula (*open arrowheads*) is in the distal common carotid artery (*large arrow*).

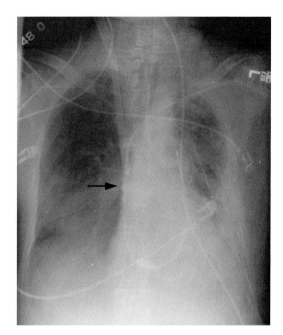

Figure 11.13 Venovenous extracorporeal life support. A single venous cannula is visible on the chest radiograph with tip at the junction of the superior vena cava and the right atrium (*arrow*). Note the normal position of the pulmonary artery catheter in the main pulmonary artery. There are two left chest tubes for the treatment of barotrauma in the form of pneumothorax.

On a chest radiograph the normal location of the venous cannula tip should be in the distal superior vena cava or right atrium (Figs. 11.12 and 11.13). The arterial cannula should be at the top of the aortic arch or in the innominate artery immediately adjacent to the aortic arch (Fig. 11.12). It should be noted that some cannulas have a 1 to 2 cm non-radiopaque tip, so the actual position of the cannula tip is not where it appears to be radiographically. Because ECLS patients are anticoagulated and commonly have chest tubes secondary to barotrauma, it is not surprising that the thoracic complications associated with ECLS are usually related to bleeding, such as hemothorax.

Some ECLS cannulas have a nonradiopaque portion at the tip.

AORTA

INTRAAORTIC BALLOON PUMP

The intraaortic balloon pump (IABP) provides mechanical circulatory support and is able to supplement cardiac output by approximately 20% to 30%. Originally introduced in the late 1960s by Dr. Adrian Kantrowitz, it initially required minor surgery to insert (9), with later design improvements allowing percutaneous placement through the common femoral artery with fluoroscopic guidance, as performed today. It is commonly used for patients with acute cardiogenic shock, unstable angina, and myocardial infarction. The balloon inflates during diastole, increasing pressure in the ascending aorta and thereby increasing coronary perfusion. The balloon deflates in systole to reduce left ventricular afterload and myocardial oxygen requirements. Balloon inflation and deflation is linked to the electrocardiogram. Contraindications to placement include aortic valve regurgitation, aortic aneurysm, severe peripheral vascular disease, and coagulopathy.

The only radiopaque portion is the IABP tip, which should be located in the proximal descending thoracic aorta, at the inferior aspect of the aortic knob (Fig. 11.14). Occa-

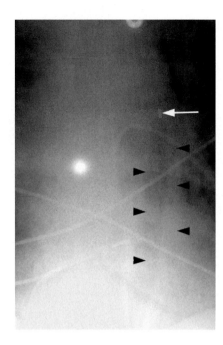

Figure 11.14 Normal position of an intraaortic balloon pump with metallic tip at the inferior aspect of the aortic knob (*arrow*). Note the radiolucency of the inflated balloon (*arrowheads*).

The tip of an IABP should be at the inferior aspect of the aortic knob.

sionally, the lucency of the inflated balloon may be seen as well (Fig. 11.15). If the tip is positioned too proximal, it may extend into the aortic arch branch vessels, potentially injuring or occluding the left subclavian or left vertebral artery, with embolization and stroke (Fig. 11.15) (10). When the tip is positioned too distally in the descending thoracic aorta, the IABP loses its effectiveness (Fig. 11.16). It may also occlude the ostia of the renal and mesenteric arteries, which may be complicated by renal embolism or bowel ischemia (11). Complications secondary to IABPs are listed in Table 11.4. In a retrospective review of complications secondary to IABP in 580 patients, vascular complications occurred in 72 patients (12.4%). The most common complication was ipsilateral leg ischemia in 69 patients; ischemia resolved in 82% of patients, usually by IABP removal or thrombectomy,

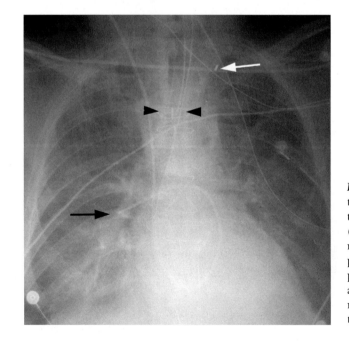

Figure 11.15 Abnormal intraaortic balloon pump position, with tip in the left subclavian artery (*white arrow*). Note the pulmonary artery catheter in correct position in the right descending pulmonary artery (*black arrow*) and the endotracheal tube in correct position with tip 4 cm above the carina (*arrowheads*).

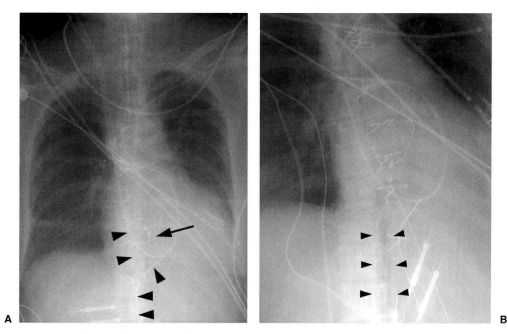

Figure 11.16 Abnormal position of an intraaortic balloon pump in a patient who underwent mitral valve replacement complicated by cardiogenic shock and was placed on extracorporeal life support (cannula tip in distal superior vena cava). She subsequently received a left ventricular assist device as a bridge to heart transplantation. *A.* Tip is in the distal descending thoracic aorta *(arrow).* The pulmonary artery catheter tip is in the right upper lobe artery (truncus anterior). There are two pericardial drains *(arrowheads). B.* Note the inflated balloon *(arrowheads).*

Table 11.4: Complications Secondary to Intraaortic Balloon Pumps
Positioned too high—stroke
Positioned too low–renal or mesenteric ischemia
Aortic perforation
Leg ischemia

with vascular repair and fasciotomy required in 15 patients. Six patients with ischemia died with IABP in place, and 4 patients required amputation for ischemia, but survived. There were three fatal aortic perforations.

CARDIAC

PACEMAKERS

Pacemakers are battery-operated devices used for the treatment of abnormal heart rhythms (12). They may be permanent, with the generator usually implanted in the anterior chest wall under local anesthesia with fluoroscopic guidance and the leads tunneled to the subclavian vein, through which they reach the heart. Temporary pacemakers may also be placed, in which case the generator is external to the patient (Fig. 11.17). Electrical impulses are sent through the wire or wires to the heart. Pacemakers function in demand mode, with a sensing device that turns on the pacemaker when the heartbeat is too slow and turns off the pacemaker when the heart rate is above a predetermined level.

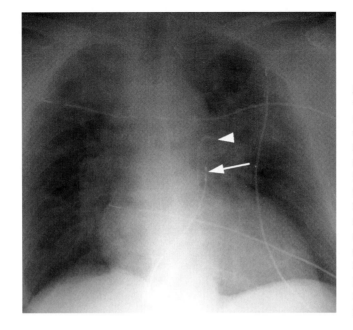

Figure 11.17 Temporary transvenous pacemaker placed through the common femoral vein at the groin, through the inferior vena cava, right atrium across the tricuspid valve and into the right ventricle with tip in the right ventricular outflow tract (*arrow*). There is an adjacent pulmonary artery catheter, also placed from a femoral approach, with tip in the left pulmonary artery (*arrowhead*). The patient had complete heart block that later required a permanent pacemaker.

Pacemakers have considerably decreased in size with advances in technology, as small as 2 to 3 cm. The most common clinical indication for a pacemaker is symptomatic bradycardia. In the setting of atrial fibrillation, a single lead pacemaker is often placed, with tip in the right ventricle (Fig. 11.17). For sick sinus syndrome or advanced atrioventricular heart block, dual-lead systems are used, with leads placed into both the right atrium and the right ventricle (Fig. 11.18). More recently, biventricular pacing is being used for the treatment of heart failure (13). In this setting, there is a third lead for pacing the left ventricle, which is usually positioned in the coronary sinus (Fig. 11.19).

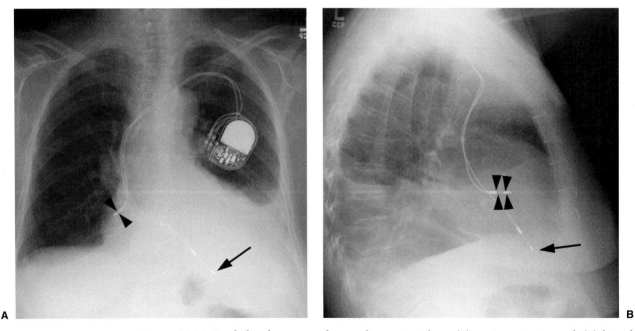

Figure 11.18 Dual-chamber pacemaker as demonstrated on (*A*) posteroanterior and (*B*) lateral radiographs. Device was placed for syncope and bradycardia 14 years earlier. Generator is in the left anterior chest wall with lead tips in the right atrium (*arrowheads*) and right ventricle (*arrows*).

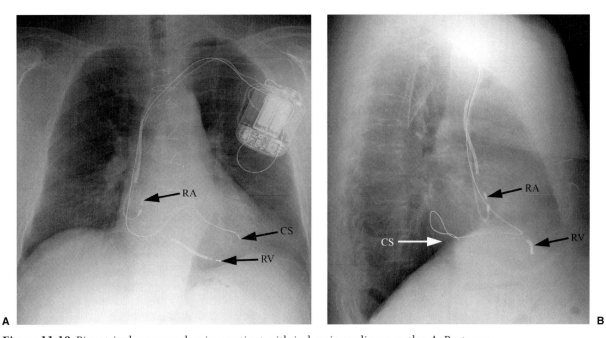

A   **B**

Figure 11.19 Biventricular pacemaker in a patient with ischemic cardiomyopathy. *A*. Posteroanterior and (*B*) lateral radiographs demonstrate a left anterior chest wall generator with three leads, one in the right atrium (*arrow RA*), one in the right ventricle (*arrow RV*), and a third in a venous tributary to the coronary sinus (*arrow CS*). The patient initially presented with syncope, inducible ventricular and supraventricular tachycardia, requiring slow-pathway ablations and a single-chamber defibrillator. Due to progression of heart failure with ejection fraction of 29% and New York Heart Association class III heart failure symptoms, he received a biventricular pacemaker.

The coronary sinus is the major venous drainage for the left ventricular myocardium. It is important to recognize the normal location of the coronary sinus on chest radiographs. Unlike a lead traversing the tricuspid valve from the right atrium into the right ventricle in a horizontal or oblique cranial-to-caudal direction on a front chest radiograph, the coronary sinus lead takes a sharp upward turn over the spine and is more vertically oriented than the oblique course of a catheter in the right ventricular outflow tract that extends into the pulmonary artery. On a lateral chest radiograph, the coronary sinus lead leaves the right atrium and is directed posteriorly, before heading cephalad along the posterior heart border. Figure 11.20 illustrates the normal cardiac venous drainage. Contrast is injected into the coronary sinus under fluoroscopy during lead placement to confirm position.

Most device complications, listed in Table 11.5, are not visible radiographically. However, the chest radiograph sometimes demonstrates the reason for device failure. The most common location of a broken lead is adjacent to the head of the clavicle, likely related to the continuous motion of the shoulder girdle with downward force on the lead (Fig. 11.21). An unwinding of the lead or a crack is evidence of lead failure. Twiddler syndrome refers to a chest wall device that is "twiddled" by the patient, perhaps finding it a source of constant irritation. As the patient rotates the device, the lead may become redundant in the chest wall or wound around the device, with possible retraction of the lead from the location in which it is functional (Fig. 11.22). When leads fail, they are generally severed and left in place, because they become endothelialized within weeks to a few months after placement and are therefore not easily withdrawn. Percutaneous removal of entrenched leads is difficult and not widely practiced. The most common complication seen radiographically related to placement is a pneumothorax (Fig. 11.23).

The most common location of a broken lead is beneath the head of the clavicle.

Nonfunctional leads are usually detached in the chest wall and left in place, because they become covered with endothelium.

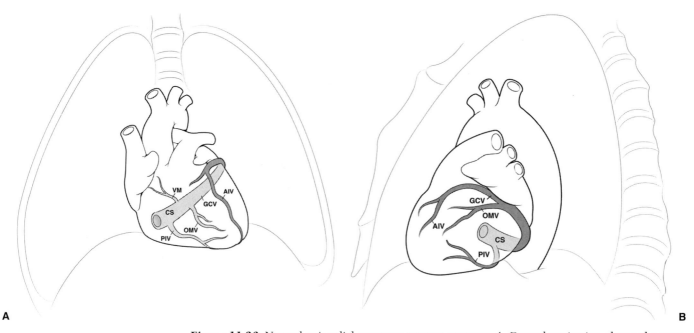

Figure 11.20 Normal epicardial coronary venous anatomy. *A.* Frontal projection shows the anterior interventricular (AIV) and obtuse marginal (OMV) veins draining into the great cardiac vein (GCV). The oblique vein of Marshall (VM) drains into the coronary sinus (CS) at the venous valve of Viessens, marking the point of transition from the coronary sinus into the great cardiac vein at the mid atrioventricular groove. The posterior interventricular vein (PIV) joins the coronary sinus near the ostium to the right atrium. *B.* Lateral projection shows the anterior interventricular vein (AIV) and obtuse marginal vein (OMV) draining into the great cardiac vein (GCV). The posterior interventricular vein (PIV) joins the coronary sinus (CS) near the ostium to the right atrium. (From Cascade PN, Sneider MB, Koelling TM, et al. Radiographic appearance of biventricular pacing for the treatment of heart failure. *AJR Am J Roentgenol* 2001;177:1443-1450, with permission.)

Table 11.5: Complications Secondary to Pacemakers and Implantable Defibrillators
Pneumothorax
Malpositioned leads
Broken leads
Infection
Venous thrombosis
Venous stenosis
Generator migration (Twiddler syndrome)
Generator failure

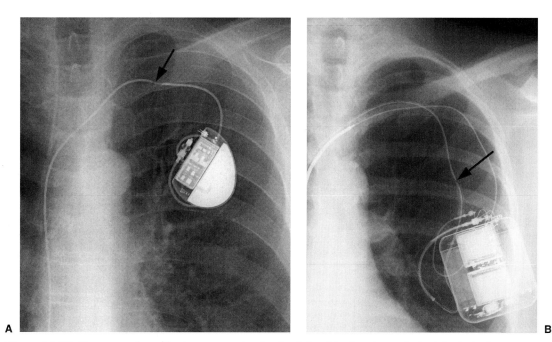

Figure 11.21 Two examples of broken pacemaker leads. *A.* Lead broken beneath the left clavicular head *(arrow)*. *B.* Lead broken *(arrow)* in the chest wall near the generator.

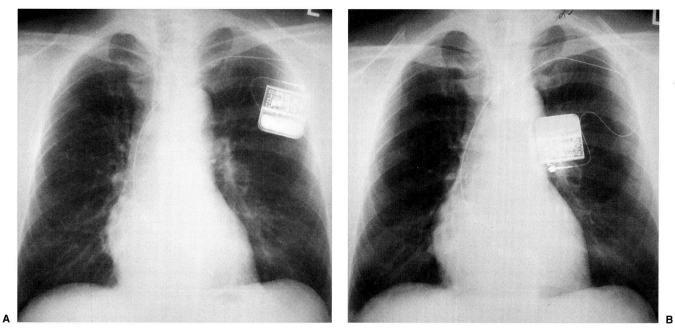

Figure 11.22 Twiddler syndrome. Single lead pacemaker with lead tip in right ventricle. *A.* Note the generator position and the adjacent redundant lead after initial insertion. *B.* Three years later the generator has migrated inferiorly and medially, and the redundant lead in the chest wall has unwound.

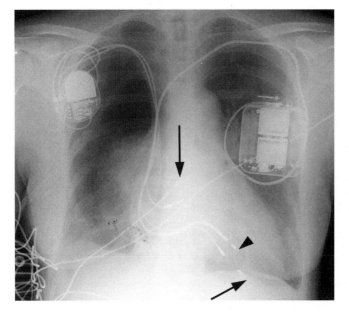

Figure 11.23 Pacemaker and implantable cardiac defibrillators. Pacemaker in the right chest wall with lead tip in the right ventricle *(large arrow, top)* and the larger implantable cardiac defibrillator in the left chest wall with lead tips in the right atrium *(arrow)* and right ventricle *(arrowhead)*. Note the right pneumothorax, a complication of pacemaker placement.

IMPLANTABLE CARDIAC DEFIBRILLATORS

Like pacemakers, defibrillators have also considerably decreased in size with advances in technology, now as small as 4 cm. They were first used in humans in the 1980s (14). An implantable cardioverter defibrillator is used in patients at risk for recurrent sustained ventricular tachycardia or fibrillation and sudden cardiac death (15). Several trials have demonstrated that implantable cardiac defibrillators (ICDs) are better than drug therapy for improving overall survival in patients with severe ventricular arrhythmias (16). One of

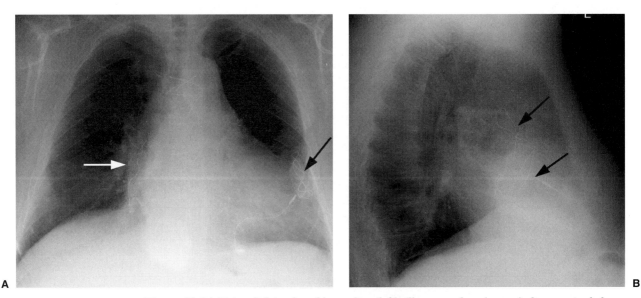

Figure 11.24 Epicardial implantable cardiac defibrillator patches *(arrows)* that required thoracotomy to implant, with epicardial leads that extend to a device in the anterior abdominal wall, as demonstrated on *(A)* posteroanterior and *(B)* lateral radiographs.

the more famous individuals to receive such a device is Dick Cheney, Vice President of the United States in 2002. In one series of 231 consecutive patients receiving ICDs, implantation was successful in all patients with a mean procedure time of 80 ± 32 minutes; after surgery, one pocket hematoma, one seroma, and one pneumothorax required treatment. Only six leads required repositioning at long-term follow-up averaging 453 ± 296 days; no pocket erosions or infections were reported.

When ventricular fibrillation is detected, the ICD delivers an electrical shock that defibrillates the heart and may restore the normal heartbeat. When ventricular tachycardia is detected, the ICD delivers either a smaller electrical shock, referred to as cardioversion, or a series of small rapid pacing impulses, referred to as antitachycardia pacing, to restore the normal heart beat. The ICD will also function as pacemaker and deliver small impulses to the heart during bradycardia until the heart rate returns to normal. Other features of these sophisticated devices include the storage of detected arrhythmic events and performing noninvasive electrophysiologic testing.

Similar to a pacemaker, the generator is placed subcutaneously in the anterior chest wall or, in the case of larger older devices that weighed approximately 290 g, the anterior abdominal wall. By comparison, the current third generation devices weigh in at only 97 g. The leads are either placed transvenously (Fig. 11.23), similar to a pacemaker, or they are positioned on the surface of the heart with the larger devices; the latter requires a thoracotomy for lead placement (Fig. 11.24). The most common complication seen radiographically related to placement is a pneumothorax (Fig. 11.23). Other complications, many not visible radiographically, are listed in Table 11.5 (17).

> Implantable pacemakers and defibrillators are becoming smaller and smaller.

LEFT VENTRICULAR ASSIST DEVICES

Left ventricular assist devices are used to bridge patients with end-stage heart failure until heart transplantation and less commonly for recovery after open heart surgery. Patients have been supported on the device for 1 to 2 years while awaiting transplantation. Based on the results of a recent trial, FDA approval is being sought for destination therapy, which is the implantation of a left ventricular assist device for end-stage heart failure in patients who are not eligible for heart transplantation (18,19). Left ventricular assist devices pull blood from the left ventricle into a pump that then sends the blood back into the aorta, bypassing the weakened left ventricle. The pumping of blood is accomplished by the cyclical inflation of a polyurethane sac adjacent to a blood reservoir. The pump is placed in the upper part of the abdomen, with a tube attached to the pump brought through the abdominal wall to the outside of the body and attached to the external control system.

The first implantable cardiac-assist device to gain FDA approval for commercial sale in the United States was the pneumatically driven HeartMate left ventricular assist system (LVAS) (Thoratec Corporation, Pleasanton, CA), powered by an external drive console. Subsequently, the vented electric LVAS was developed, powered by wearable batteries and carried using a shoulder strap, allowing for greater patient mobility. Both devices have implantable titanium pumps that connect to their drive source by a tube, which exits the body through the skin. The pumping chamber of the LVAS has afferent and efferent cannulas, giving it a unique radiographic appearance (Fig. 11.25). Textured surfaces of the HeartMate devices promote the formation of an adherent tissue lining derived from the patients' own blood, thereby substantially reducing the risk of thromboembolism and stroke. This allows the LVAS to provide hemodynamic support without requiring systemic anticoagulation, as is used for ECLS. As of June 2002, over 6,000 LVASs have been implanted worldwide (19). A new smaller device, the implantable ventricular assist device, has been developed. It is much smaller than the LVAS, weighing approximately 1 pound, designed for use in small adults and children (19).

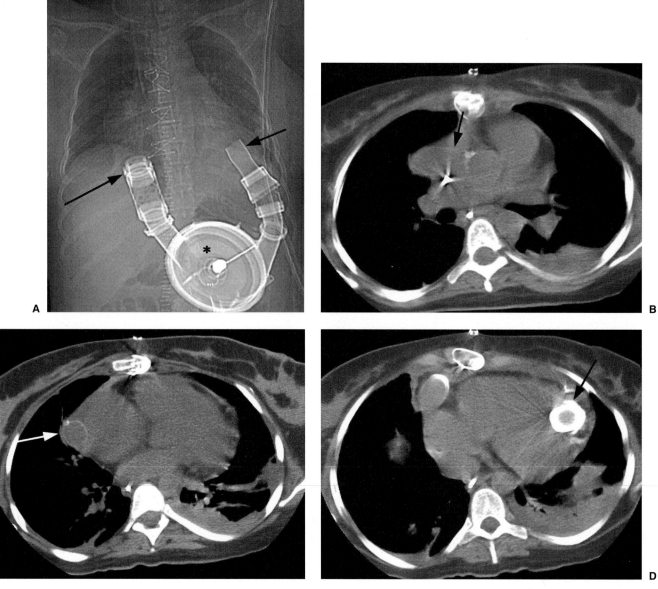

Figure 11.25 HeartMate left ventricular assist system. *A.* Computed tomography scout demonstrates the afferent cannula positioned in the apex of the left ventricle *(small arrow)*. The efferent cannula is positioned in the ascending aorta *(large arrow)* and has a nonvisible radiolucent portion that creates a widened contour to the right side of the mediastinum. The asterisk marks the pump. *B.* Computed tomography image demonstrates the ascending aortic anastomosis *(arrow)* to the nonradiopaque portion of the efferent cannula. *C.* The efferent cannula *(arrow)* corresponds to the widened mediastinum on the frontal projection. *D.* Afferent cannula anastomosis to the left ventricular apex *(arrow)* surrounded by high attenuation suture and reinforcing material.

CORONARY ARTERY BYPASS GRAFT MARKERS

Coronary artery bypass grafting is an effective well-established surgical therapy for relieving angina in patients with symptomatic coronary artery disease and improving mortality in patients with depressed left ventricular function or disease involving the left main trunk (20–22). Autologous vein segments were first used to bypass proximal coronary lesions by Favaloro in 1967 at the Cleveland Clinic (20). Markers on the proximal aorta were introduced in the early 1970s to mark the location of the vein graft anastomosis on the aorta.

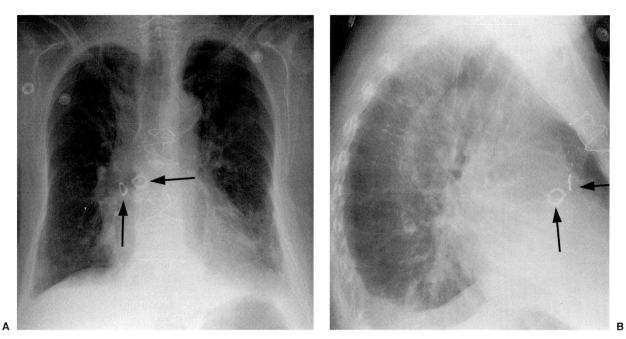

Figure 11.26 Large wire coronary artery bypass graft markers *(arrows)* as seen on *(A)* posteroanterior and *(B)* lateral radiographs.

In a recent prospective study of 182 patients undergoing cardiac catheterization after coronary artery bypass graft surgery with saphenous vein grafts, patients who had markers required significantly less total procedure time, fluoroscopy time, and contrast use than patients without markers (23). This is significant, with 30% to 50% of patients undergoing saphenous vein grafting requiring catheterization within 5 years of surgery.

The markers may either be large wire circles around the ostia of the graft (Fig. 11.26) or small washer-like markers (Fig. 11.27). The latter are preferred, because it is possible

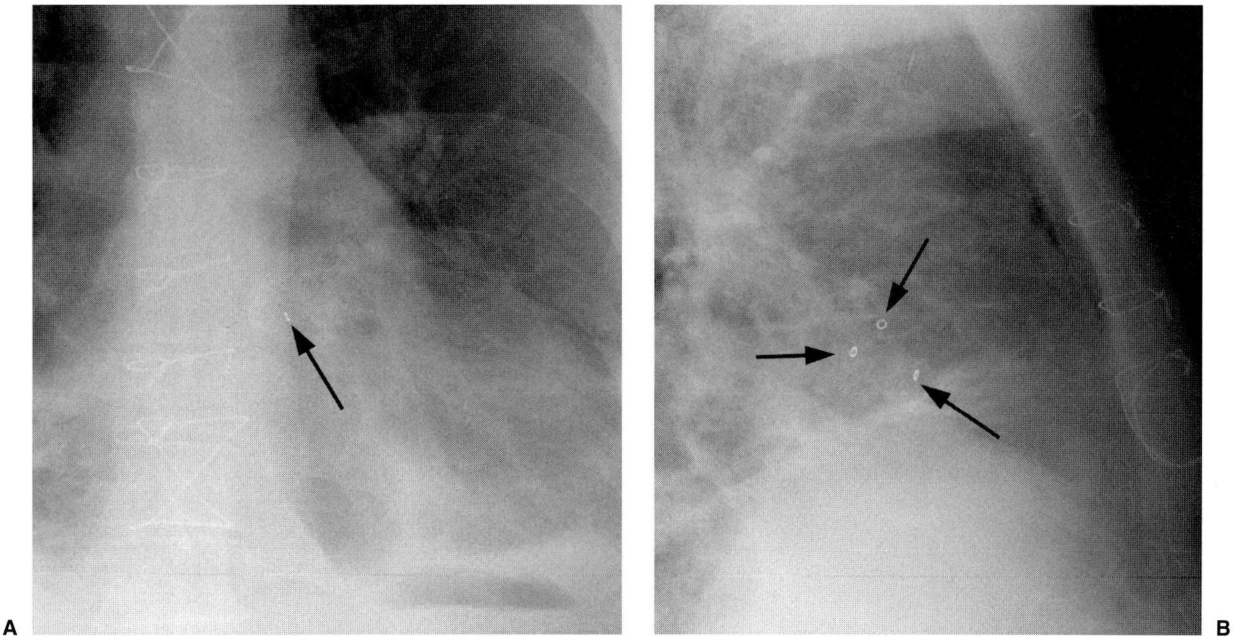

Figure 11.27 Small washer-like coronary artery bypass graft markers *(arrows)* as seen on *(A)* posteroanterior and *(B)* lateral radiographs.

that the larger superior vena cava markers that encircle graft ostia could migrate from the aorta onto the graft itself and cause graft failure. They could impede repeat coronary artery bypass grafting because of the significant amount of surface area they take up on the aorta. There are rare patients in whom placing markers may not be desirable, such as patients with connective tissue disease in whom additional suturing to a fragile aortic wall may not be desirable (24). The use of markers during surgery remains a controversial technique that is not widely practiced.

ATRIAL SEPTAL DEFECT CLOSURE DEVICE

An atrial septal defect is a congential defect in the atrial wall (Chapter 19). Percutaneous atrial septal defect closure was first reported as early as 1976 (25). Design improvements since that time have resulted in smaller retrievable devices that can be implanted with much smaller catheters. Using a catheter inserted into the common femoral vein, the

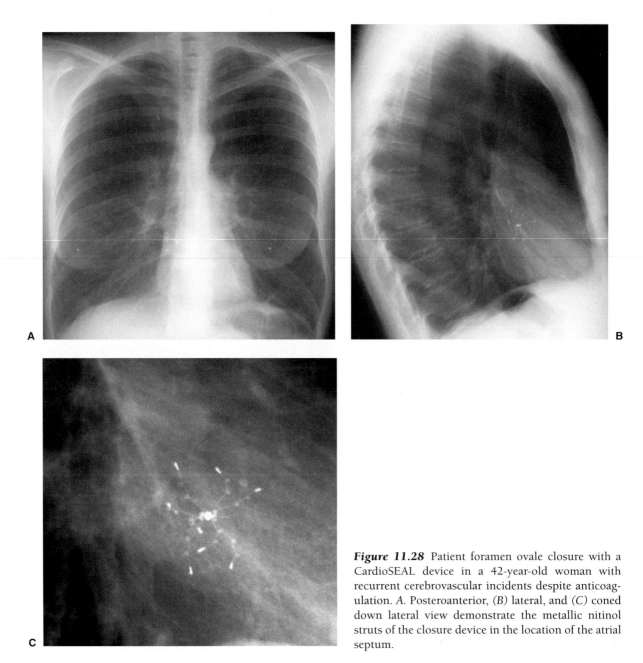

Figure 11.28 Patient foramen ovale closure with a CardioSEAL device in a 42-year-old woman with recurrent cerebrovascular incidents despite anticoagulation. *A.* Posteroanterior, *(B)* lateral, and *(C)* coned down lateral view demonstrate the metallic nitinol struts of the closure device in the location of the atrial septum.

catheter is passed through the cardiac defect into the left atrium, using fluoroscopic and transesophageal echocardiographic guidance. The first portion of the device is pushed out of the catheter and opens in the left atrium. The catheter is backed up across the defect into the right atrium and the second pushed out of the catheter.

Currently used nitinol devices include the CardioSEAL Septal Occlusion System (NMT Medical, Boston, MA) (Fig. 11.28) and the Amplatzer Septal Occluder (AGA Medical Corporation, Golden Valley, MN) (26). Each comes in various sizes depending on the size of the hole. The CardioSEAL is a double-sided umbrella-shaped nitinol device draped with Dacron cloth that resembles a double-sided miniature umbrella or clamshell; the latter is the name by which these are commonly referred. CardioSEAL has been approved by the FDA for selected patients with patent foramen ovale, ventricular septal defects, and fenestrated Fontan defects. The Amplatzer Septal Occluder is a double-disk device made of nitinol mesh connected by a cylindrical waist that can measure 2 to 26 mm, commonly referred to as a button device. The diameter of the waist corresponds to the size of the atrial septal defect; the left atrial disk is 14 mm larger than the waist and the right atrial disk 10 mm larger than the waist. The Amplatzer Septal Occluder is FDA approved for atrial septal defect and fenestrated Fontan defects as well as selected patients with patent foramen ovale. Other percutaneous AGA devices in clinical trials include the Amplatzer Duct Occluder for patent ductus arteriosus closure, the Amplatzer PFO Occluder, and the Amplatzer Muscular Ventricular Septal Occluder.

> Percutaneous devices are rapidly becoming the method of choice for closure of atrial septal defects.

AIRWAY

ENDOTRACHEAL TUBE

Endotracheal tubes are placed through the mouth, less commonly the nose, to maintain an open airway and facilitate ventilation in patients undergoing anesthesia, patients with no gag reflex requiring airway protection, or patients with impaired lung function requiring assisted ventilation. They range in diameter from 2 to 10 mm. In adults, 6 to 9 mm diameter tubes are generally used. The tube is usually secured with tape or a device specifically designed to secure endotracheal tubes to reduce the possibility of upward or downward movement. Adult endotracheal tubes have a balloon cuff, which when inflated serves to both maintain proper placement and prevent aspiration. Cuff pressure should be less than 30 mm Hg to prevent airway damage.

The normal position of an endotracheal tube is with the tip 2 to 6 cm above the carina (Fig. 11.15). A radiopaque stripe on endotracheal tubes is used to make them more visible and confirm position. In 10% to 15% of placements, the tube is malpositioned. This number reaches up to 25% for endotracheal tubes placed in the field by paramedics (27). Complications of endotracheal tube placement are listed in Table 11.6. Abnormal position within the esophageal occurs in 8% of attempted intubations in critically ill patients (Fig. 11.29) (28). When gastric distension is visible on the chest radiography, esophageal intubation should be suspected. Without radiography for confirmation, evaluating tube position at the bedside or prehospital can be very difficult in acutely ill or injured patients. Too distal a position, such as in a main bronchus, may result in ventilation of only one lung,

> The tip of the endotracheal tube should be 2 to 6 cm above the carina.

Table 11.6: Complications Secondary to Endotracheal Tubes

Positioned too high (vocal cord injury, falls out)
Positioned too low (right main bronchus intubation)
Main bronchus intubation (contralateral lung collapse, ipsilateral pneumothorax)
Esophageal intubation
Airway rupture
Airway stenosis

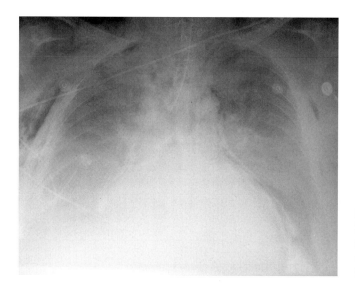

Figure 11.29 Esophageal intubation with esophageal rupture and pneumomediastinum. Gastric contents were refluxing up into the tube.

With neck flexion the tip of the endotracheal tube moves toward the carina. With extension it moves toward the vocal cords.

with collapse of the contralateral lung (Fig. 11.30), and rarely spontaneous pneumothorax of the ventilated lung that is receiving the entire tidal volume of air. Main bronchus intubation is more common on the right than the left. When positioned too proximally, the tube may damage the vocal cords or even fall out of the airway (Fig. 11.31). It should be remembered that the endotracheal tube moves as much as 2 to 4 cm with flexion and extension of the neck with a fulcrum mechanism. With neck flexion, the tube may extend more distally and into a main bronchus, whereas with extension the tube moves more cephalad, potentially across the vocal cords.

Other important positioning problems visible radiographically include chronic positioning of the endotracheal tube tip against the airway wall that may result in airway injury and rupture. If the balloon appears wider that the expected width of the trachea,

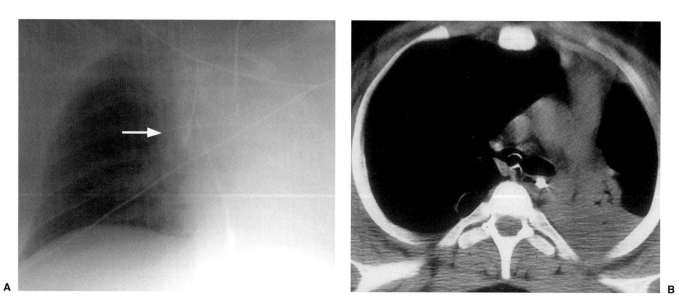

Figure 11.30 Abnormal endotracheal tube position within the right main bronchus. *A.* Chest radiograph with tube tip in right main bronchus *(arrow)*, complete collapse of the left lung with deviation of mediastinum to the left, including the esophagus delineated by a nasogastric tube. *B.* Computed tomography in another patient with tube tip in the right main bronchus, partial collapse of the left lung and shift of mediastinum towards the left.

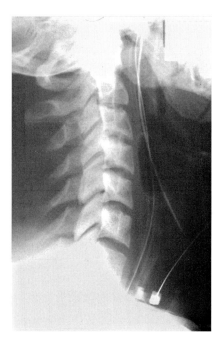

Figure 11.31 Abnormal endotracheal tube with balloon inflated positioned within the pharynx. High position of an endotracheal tube may cause vocal cord injury.

tracheal rupture should be suspected. Pneumomediastinum and subcutaneous emphysema usually accompany it; however, if the balloon itself is occluding the site of rupture, these findings may be absent. Aspiration during intubation is a complication that may be visible on radiographs, with new alveolar opacities typically in the superior or basilar segments of the lower lobes (Fig. 11.32). Postintubation airway stenosis, a late complication after endotracheal tube placement, is discussed in Chapter 16 (Figs. 16.4 and 16.7).

An endotracheal tube balloon that appears wider than the trachea should raise concern for tracheal rupture.

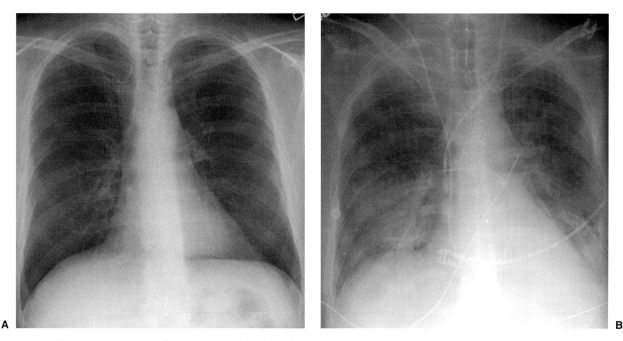

Figure 11.32 Aspiration secondary to endotracheal intubation. *A.* Normal radiograph preintubation. *B.* Postintubation with new bibasilar alveolar opacities. Correct positioning of endotracheal tube, pulmonary artery catheter, and central venous line.

TRACHEOSTOMY TUBE

A tracheostomy is placed during a surgical procedure to create a direct opening into the trachea. Although such procedures may have been documented on Egyptian tablets dating to 3600 BC, the first successful recorded tracheostomy was performed by Prasovala in the fifteenth century. Lorenz Heister coined the term "tracheostomy" in 1718. Clinical indications for a tracheostomy tube include airway obstruction at or above the level of the larynx, mechanical ventilatory support for chronic respiratory failure, and less commonly for sleep apnea. The tubes may be made of metal, plastic, or silicone; the latter two are

Table 11.7: Complications Secondary to Tracheostomy Tubes

Positioned in soft tissues adjacent to airway
Airway stenosis
Trachea-innominate artery fistula

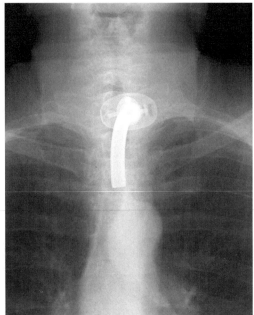

A

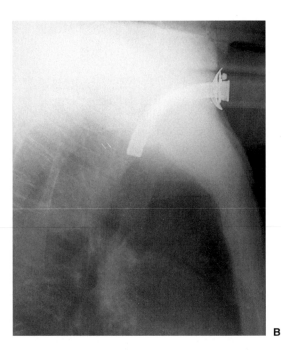

B

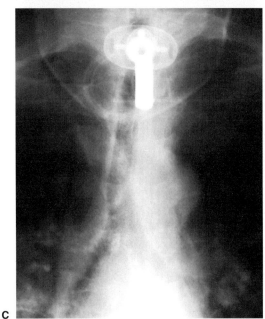

C

Figure 11.33 Tracheostomy tube positioning. *A* and *B.* Correct position. *C.* Incorrect position beside the airway lumen.

popular because they are lightweight and there is less crusting of secretions than with a metal tube. The tubes may be cuffed, like endotracheal tubes, or uncuffed. They may also be fenestrated with an opening to permit speech through the upper airway when the external opening is blocked. There are single and double cannula tubes. Double-cannula tubes have an inner cannula that acts as a removable liner for the more permanent outer tube and can be withdrawn for brief periods to be cleaned. A tracheal button can be placed in a mature tracheostomy tract to maintain the opening; the button itself does not extend into the airway lumen. This is used mostly for sleep apnea treatment and is kept closed during the day and opened when sleeping (29,30).

Table 11.7 lists the complications that may occur with a tracheostomy. Complications visible radiographically are usually related to tube position. When evaluating airway tubes it is important to confirm that they are within, and not in, the soft tissues beside the airway (Fig. 11.33). Postintubation airway stenosis is discussed in Chapter 16 (Figs. 16.4 and 16.7). Rarely, trachea-innominate artery fistula may occur, with an incidence rate of 0.6% to 0.7%, clinically manifesting as bright red arterial blood in the airway (31). It is more commonly associated with the balloon cuff and not the tip of the tube. This complication requires emergency airway control, immediate arterial compression to control the bleeding, and immediate surgical exploration to control and repair the damaged innominate artery. Radiographically, aspirated blood in the airway appears as new alveolar opacities.

TRANSTRACHEAL OXYGEN CATHETER

Direct transtracheal oxygen therapy is used as a more efficient alternative to nasal oxygen delivery in patients requiring long-term oxygen therapy, associated with less discomfort, improved compliance and quality of life, and less morbidity. Patients describe less inconvenience and reduced social stigma usually associated with long-term oxygen therapy and less nasal crusting or obstruction, dry throat, hoarseness, cutaneous allergic reaction, and epistaxis compared with nasal cannula oxygen delivery. Direct transtracheal oxygen therapy can be administered out of the hospital using a much smaller tube than the usual endotracheal tube or tracheostomy (32,33). A polyurethane intratracheal catheter is placed transcutaneously through the anterior aspect of the neck, such as the Heimlich Micro-Trach (Ballard Medical Products Co., Midvale, UT) or the SCOOP model (Transtracheal Systems, Denver, CO), with the device connected to oxygen at the neck (Fig. 11.34). The tip should be 1 to 2 cm above the carina

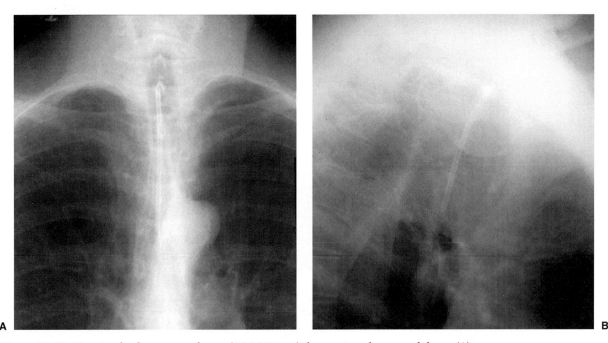

Figure 11.34 Transtracheal oxygen catheter, (SCOOP type) demonstrated on coned down (*A*) posteroanterior and (*B*) lateral radiographs.

(34). One device, the intratracheal oxygen catheter, is tunneled from the anterior abdominal wall under the skin of the chest wall, with the connector to the tubing leading to the oxygen tank located outside the abdominal wall. These catheters measure 7 to 11 French.

ESOPHAGUS

FEEDING TUBES, NASOGASTRIC AND OROGASTRIC TUBES

The position of feeding tubes should be confirmed radiographically before use.

Esophageal tubes are commonly placed to maintain patient nutrition or to decompress the stomach. Feeding tubes are usually positioned in the stomach or duodenum (Fig. 11.35). The duodenum is preferred to minimize gastroesophageal reflux. The most common error in placement is being incorrectly positioned within the gastrointestinal system and may occur anywhere from the pharynx to the jejunum (Figs 11.36A and 11.36B). In the case of suction catheters, it is important that the side port, and not just the tube tip, is located in the stomach.

Complications that may occur with esophageal tubes are listed in Table 11.8 (35). The most serious complication is inadvertent placement into the lung, which may be complicated by pneumothorax, hemorrhage, or the infusion of feeding solution into the tracheobronchial tree and/or pleural space (Fig. 11.36C and 11.36D). Inadvertent passage of the feeding tube into the tracheobronchial tree may be unrecognized if the cough reflex is depressed due to neurologic impairment or sedation. After feeding tube placements, a portable radiograph centered at the diaphragm to include both the lower thorax and upper abdomen should be obtained to confirm correct location before the tube is used. Feeding tubes are much more flexible than nasogastric and orogastric tubes and are therefore more commonly malpositioned. Rarely, tubes may perforate the esophageal wall and even be found in the pleural space (Fig. 17.11).

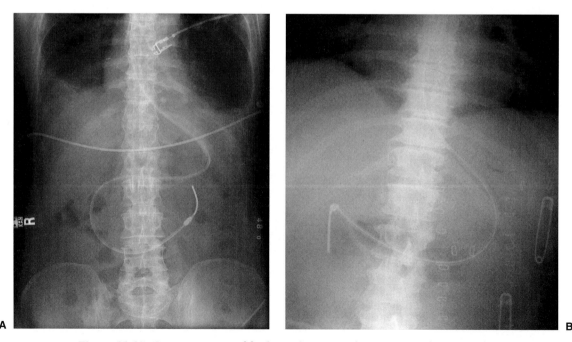

Figure 11.35 Correct position of feeding tubes. *A.* At the Ligament of Treitz. *B.* In the descending duodenum.

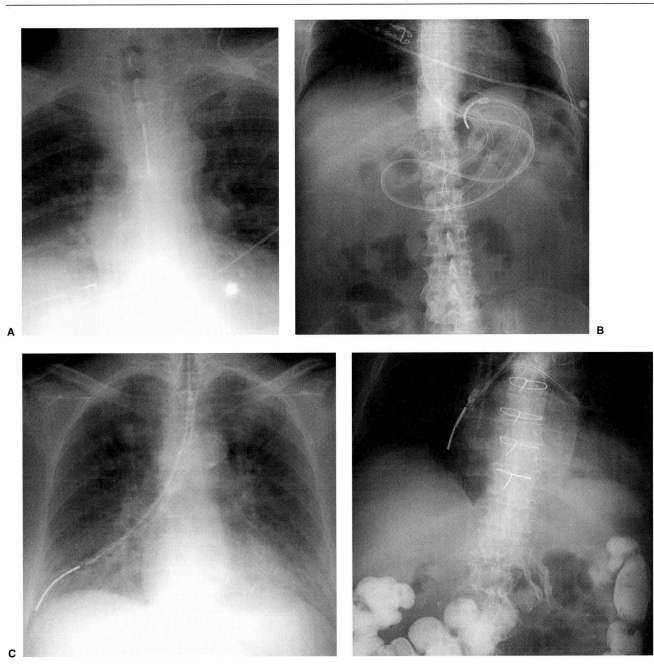

Figure 11.36 Incorrect position of esophageal tubes. *A.* Mid-esophagus. *B.* Excess coils of both feeding tube and nasogastric tube in the stomach. *C.* In the lower right lung. *D.* Looped across the carina and into the bronchus intermedius.

Table 11.8: Complications Secondary to Esophageal Tubes

Malpositioned within gastrointestinal tract
Positioned within airway (pneumothorax, lung laceration/hemorrhage, pleural space)
Esophageal rupture

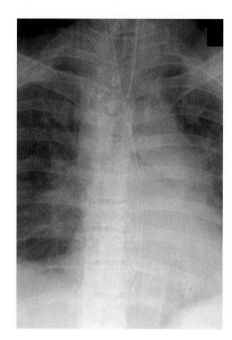

Figure 11.37 Intraesophageal manometer placed for monitoring during a long cervical spine fixation surgery in a trauma patient with a flail chest.

INTRAESOPHAGEAL MANOMETER, TEMPERATURE PROBE, AND pH PROBE

Several different types of esophageal measurement probes may be placed in the esophagus to measure intrathoracic pressure, temperature, and pH. An intraesophageal manometer is a tube with pressure gauges along the surface that measures intrathoracic pressure during the respiratory cycle. It is used to evaluate esophageal contractions in patients with dysphagia and propulsion disturbances, as well as during sleep studies for the diagnosis of upper airway resistance syndrome (36). As the esophagus squeezes on the tube, the pressures are recorded and printed on graph paper similar to an electrocardiogram. The manometer is visible as a thin metallic line along the course of the esophagus, with a slightly larger metallic tip (Fig. 11.37). Temperature probes are used to give a more accurate measurement of body core temperature than the more common oral, axillary, and rectal thermometers. They are used commonly during prolonged surgery and during surgery requiring hypothermic circulatory arrest. The catheter consists of a thermistor sensor attached to a flexible vinyl-covered lead contained within a 9- to 14-French catheter. The tip is usually positioned in the distal esophagus (37). An esophageal temperature probe may be combined with an esophageal stethoscope.

pH probes were first introduced in 1974 and are used routinely to measure pH for the diagnosis of gastroesophageal reflux disease. The 2 mm catheter with an antimony probe is usually positioned with the tip 5 cm above the lower esophageal sphincter for these measurements, with recordings taken continuously for 24 hours (38). Patients are asked to perform activities that evoke symptoms and record the onset of symptoms by pressing a button on a microcomputer data logger (worn around the waist) for correlation with the pH recordings. Simultaneous placement of probes in the distal and proximal esophagus or even intragastric probes may also be used (39).

STENT

Metallic expandable stents are used in the thorax, including the central tracheobronchial tree (Fig. 16.15), aorta (Fig. 18.27), veins (Fig. 11.38), and esophagus (Fig. 11.39) for the treatment of benign and malignant narrowing. Stents may be mesh-type (Fig. 11.38) or coil-type (Fig. 11.39). Stents are either balloon expandable or self-expandable. Tracheo-

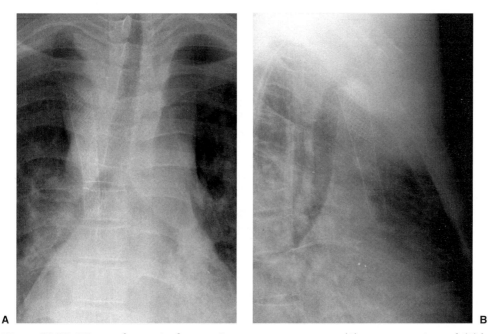

A   B

Figure 11.38 Wire-mesh stent in the superior vena cava as seen on (*A*) posteroanterior and (*B*) lateral radiographs.

bronchial and aortic stents are discussed in Chapters 16 and 18, respectively. Venous and esophageal stents are discussed here.

Venous stents are placed to prevent or treat superior vena cava syndrome (Fig. 11.38), with a greater than 90% success rate in the treatment of superior vena cava syndrome (40). Over 90% of superior vena cava syndrome occurs secondary to malignancy, most commonly bronchogenic carcinoma, followed by lymphoma and metastatic disease. Nonmalignant causes include thrombosis or stenosis secondary to central venous catheters or pacemaker leads, radiation-related strictures, and fibrosing mediastinitis (41).

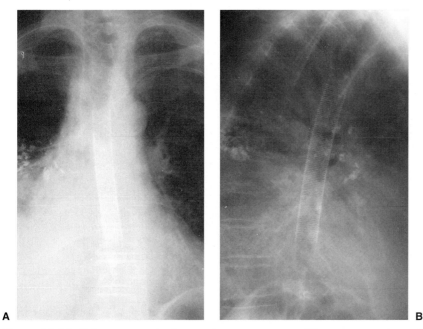

A   B

Figure 11.39 Coil-type stent in the esophagus as seen on (*A*) posteroanterior and (*B*) lateral radiographs.

Esophageal stents may be placed under endoscopy using either local or general anesthesia for the treatment of benign and malignant esophageal strictures, including caustic ingestion or reflux-induced strictures, and esophageal carcinoma (Fig. 11.39) (42). For esophageal cancer patients, stents provide palliative relief from dysphagia and aspiration, for a disease that has a very poor prognosis. Over 90% of esophageal stents are self-expanding metallic stents; plastic stents are less commonly used. Esophageal stents come in a variety of lengths (4 to 9 cm) and are usually 2 cm in diameter. Stents placed across the gastroesophageal junction may be accompanied by severe reflux and subsequent aspiration, leading to the development of the stents with an antireflux valve that are now widely available. Stent complications include perforation, malposition, migration, and food impaction. Dilation or the insertion of a longer stent may be necessary if the reflux induces a stricture. Once in place, stent migration is difficult to correct. Stent occlusion by tumor ingrowth, as well as fistula development, can be prevented by using covered stents. Chronically, pressure necrosis of the esophageal wall with erosion may result in an esophagobronchial fistula. Erosion may also occur into the aorta, heart, or a bronchial artery.

ANTIREFLUX DEVICES AND GASTRIC BANDING

Approved by the FDA in 1979, the silicone gel–filled Angelchik reflux prosthesis may be placed around the gastroesophageal junction for the prevention of gastroesophageal reflux, usually after reduction of a hiatal hernia (Fig. 11.40). It has an internal diameter of 3.1 cm and is secured around the gastroesophageal junction by two reinforced Teflon straps. The Angelchik prostheses are associated with frequent complications, including dysphagia in up to 75% of patients, migration, erosion, or disruption of the ring. In up to 25% of patients they are later removed, and they are not commonly used today (43–45). Medical therapy and surgical therapy, including the various fundoplication procedures, are more commonly used than such prostheses.

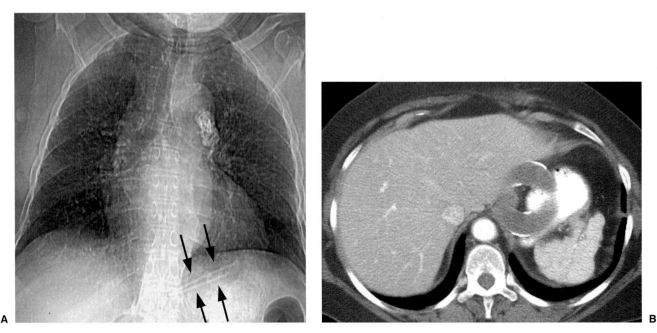

A

B

Figure 11.40 Angelchik prostheses placed 18 years earlier during hiatal hernia repair for gastroesophageal reflux and esophagitis. *A.* Computed tomography scout demonstrates the two Teflon reinforced straps (*arrows*) and (*B*) axial computed tomography image shows the fluid attenuation donut around the gastroesophageal junction.

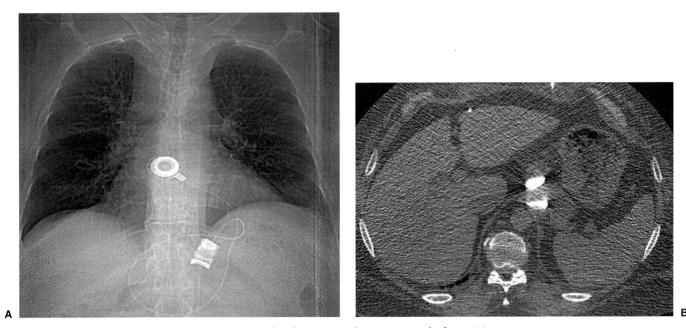

Figure 11.41 Gastric banding for morbid obesity with subsequent reduction in weight from 498 to 344 pounds over the following 18 months, as demonstrated on (A) computed tomography scout and (B) axial computed tomography image.

Gastric banding is performed for the treatment of morbid obesity. The LAP-BAND Adjustable Gastric Banding (LAGB) System (INAMed Health, Santa Barbara, CA) is an example of a gastric banding device available in the United States, approved by the FDA in 2001. Placed laparoscopically, it consists of a band placed around the gastric fundus to create a small upper gastric pouch. The ring diameter can be adjusted and controls the amount of food that enters the remainder of the stomach (46). A reservoir located in the subxiphoid region is used for percutaneous inflation or deflation of the ring. Figure 11.41 is an example of a gastric band.

CHEST TUBES

A chest tube or tube thoracostomy may be placed to remove fluid or air from the pleural space. Tube drainage of fluid is referred to as closed thoracostomy drainage, as opposed to a surgical or open drainage procedure. For example, after lobectomy a pleural tube is usually left in place, and after open heart surgery one or two pericardial drains are usually left in place (Fig. 11.16A). Surgically placed tubes are usually straight semistiff tubes. A variety of other tubes may be placed, including soft and pigtail varieties. For nonloculated pleural effusions, the tube is usually positioned in the caudal aspect of the pleural space, whereas for loculated collections the tube is positioned within the loculation.

Complications secondary to thoracostomy tubes are listed in Table 11.9. Radiography is used to confirm correct tube position. If a thoracostomy tube appears to be in an

Chest tubes are usually positioned in the lower portion of the thorax to drain fluid and in the upper thorax to drain air.

Table 11.9: Complications of Thoracostomy Tubes

Malposition (chest wall, mediastinum, lung, fissure)
Infection (empyema)
Vascular laceration (intercostal artery/vein)
Cardiac laceration
Abdominal viscera laceration (liver, spleen, stomach)

Chest tubes located in a fissure may or may not function correctly.

unusual position and overlies the lower mediastinum, it may be pericardial (Fig. 11.42). Pleural tubes may be incorrectly positioned in the chest wall, lung, mediastinum, or pleural fissures. Such malpositions may result not only in tube malfunction but also damage of adjacent structures, such as lung hematoma secondary to tube puncture, requiring lobectomy (Fig. 11.43). Tubes positioned within fissures may or may not function correctly. In a trauma setting, one series reported that 58% of tubes were positioned in a fissure (47). Computed tomography is useful in the evaluation of malfunctioning or malpositioned tubes (48). Rarely, tubes may lacerate an intercostal artery or vein during placement or from chronic erosion, with subsequent hemothorax or extrapleural hematoma, or may perforate the right ventricle or the upper abdominal viscera if the tube inadvertently is placed through the diaphragm. Infection of a previously noninfected fluid collection is a complication that is usually not visible radiographically, except for failure of drainage or the development of loculation.

Non–image guided thoracostomy drainage may fail due to tube malposition, fluid debris and viscosity, loculation, or a thick pleural peel. In these cases, percutaneous image-guided catheter placement for fluid drainage, using either ultrasound or computed tomography guidance, is particularly helpful for accurate localization of the loculated fluid collection to be treated. Percutaneous drainage is an alternative to more invasive surgical drainage and uses smaller drains, ranging from 8 to 16 French, than closed tube thoracostomy, which are better tolerated by patients. Imaging also can determine whether there are multiple loculations, requiring multiple drains. Intracavitary fibrinolytic therapy is a useful adjunct to tube placement when fluid collections fail tube drainage alone by breaking up adhesions and debris. Percutaneous tube drainage works well for effusions up to 4 to 6 weeks; however, for older fluid collections success is considerably less, usually due to the development of a pleural peel (49). Image-guided placement has success rates of 67% to 83% (50).

Chest tubes for the treatment of pneumothorax are usually placed in the lateral chest wall between the fifth and seventh ribs, with tip extending cephalad toward the apex of the lung (Fig. 11.13). Smaller tubes are commonly used to treat pneumothorax after percutaneous lung biopsy and may be attached to a Heimlich valve. A Tru-Close vent is a self-contained system with a small diameter soft silicone catheter placed through the upper thorax below the clavicle, attached to a small box that contains a one-way valve (Fig. 22.11).

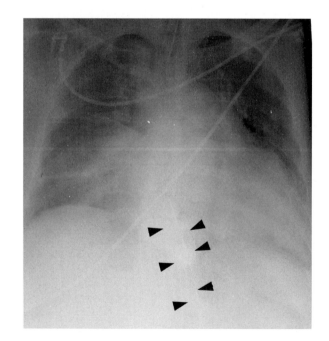

Figure 11.42 Pericardial drain (*arrowheads*) placed for pericardial infection secondary to adjacent large right middle lobe lung abscess.

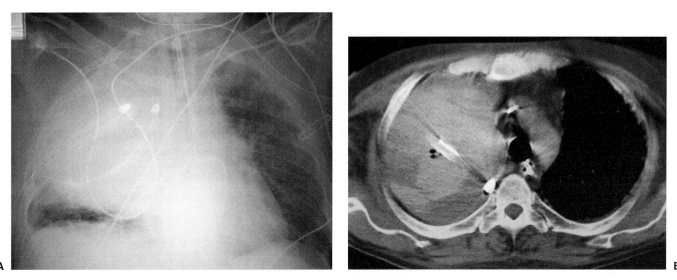

Figure 11.43 Two chest tubes. One punctured the lung, with resulting large pulmonary hematoma. *A.* Chest radiograph shows a large hematoma in the right lung. *B.* Computed tomography demonstrates the high attenuation hematoma surrounding the intraparenchymal chest tube, and a second chest tube in the pleural space posteromedially.

REFERENCES

1. Bekemeyer WB, Crapo RO, Calhoon S, et al. Efficacy of chest radiography in a respiratory intensive care unit: a prospective study. *Chest* 1985;88:691–696.
2. Andrews JC, Marx VM, Williams DM, et al. The upper arm approach for placement of peripherally inserted central catheters for protracted venous access. *AJR Am J Roentgenol* 1992;158: 427–429.
3. Scott WL. Complications associated with central venous catheters. *Chest* 1988;94:1221–1224.
4. Wechsler RJ, Sprin PW, Conant EF, et al. Thrombosis and infection caused by thoracic venous catheters: pathogenesis and imaging findings. *AJR Am J Roentgenol* 1993;160:461–467.
5. Paunovic B, Sharma S, Miller A. Swan-Ganz catheterization. www.emedicine.com; March 19, 2003.
6. De Lima LG, Wynands JE, Bourke ME, et al. Catheter-induced pulmonary artery false aneurysm and rupture: case report and review. *J Cardiothorac Vasc Anesth* 1994;8:70–75.
7. Frazier OH, Rose EA, Macmanus Q, et al. Multicenter clinical evaluation of the HeartMate 1000 IP left ventricular assist device. *Ann Thorac Surg* 1992;53:1080–1090.
8. Anderson HL III, Delius RE, Sinard JM, et al. Early experience with adult extracorporeal membrane oxygenation in the modern era. *Ann Thorac Surg* 1992;53:553–563.
9. Kantrowitz A, Tjonneland S, Freed PS, et al. Initial clinical experience with intraaortic balloon pumping in cardiogenic shock. *JAMA* 1968;203:113–118.
10. Karlson KB, Martin EC, Bregman D, et al. Superior mesenteric artery obstruction by intraaortic counterpulsation balloon simulating embolism: a case report. *Cardiovasc Intervent Radiol* 1981; 4:236–238.
11. Barnett MG, Swartz MT, Peterson GJ, et al. Vascular complications from intraaortic balloons: risk analysis. *J Vasc Surg* 1994;19:81–87.
12. ACC/AHA practice guidelines for implantation of cardiac pacemakers and antiarrhythmia devices. *Circulation* 1998;31:1175–1209.
13. Cascade PN, Sneider MB, Koelling TM, et al. Radiographic appearance of biventricular pacing for the treatment of heart failure. *AJR Am J Roentgenol* 2001;177:1447–1450.
14. Mirowski M, Reid PR, Mower MM, et al. Termination of malignant ventricular arrhythmias with an implanted automatic defibrillator in human beings. *N Engl J Med* 1980;303:322–324.
15. Wolfe DA, Kosinski D, Grubb BP. Update on implantable cardioverter-defibrillators: new, safer devices have led to changes in indications. *Postgrad Med* 1998;103.
16. Multicenter Automatic Defibrillator Implantation Trial Investigators. Improved survival with an

implanted defibrillator in patients with coronary disease at high risk for ventricular arrhythmia. *N Engl J Med* 1996;335:1933–1940.

17. Pacifico A, Wheelan K, Nasir N, et al. Long-term follow-up of cardioverter-defibrillator implanted under conscious sedation in prepectoral subfascial position. *Circulation* 1997;95: 946–950.

18. Rose EA, Gelijns AC, Moskowitz AJ, et al. for the Randomized Evaluation of Mechanical Assistance for the Treatment of Congestive Heart Failure (REMATCH) Study Group. Long-term use of a left ventricular assist device for end-stage heart failure. *N Engl J Med* 2001;345:1435–1443.

19. Thoratec says nearly 6,000 of its heart assist devices have now been implanted in patients worldwide. Press Release, Thoratec Corporation, Pleasanton, CA. June 20, 2002.

20. European Coronary Surgery Study Group. Long-term results prospective randomized study of coronary artery bypass surgery in stable angina pectoris. *Lancet* 1982;2:172–1180.

21. Principal Investigators of CASS and Their Associates. National Heart, Lung, and Blood Institute Coronary Artery Surgery Study. *Circulation* 1981;63:1.

22. CASS Principal Investigators and Their Associates. Coronary Artery Surgery Study (CASS): a randomized trial of coronary artery bypass surgery: survival data. *Circulation* 1983;68:939–950.

23. Peterson LR, McKenzie CR, Ludbrook PA, et al. Value of saphenous vein graft markers during subsequent diagnostic cardiac catheterization. *Ann Thorac Surg* 1999;68:2263–2266.

24. Saffitz JE, Ganote CE, Peterson CE, et al. False aneurysm of ascending aorta after aortocoronary bypass grafting. *Am J Cardiol* 1983;52:907–912.

25. King T, Mills M. Secundum atrial septal defects: non-operative closure during cardiac catheterization. *JAMA* 1976;235:2305–2309.

26. Fischer G, Kramer HH, Stieh J, et al. Transcatheter closure of secundum atrial septal defects with the new self-centering Amplatzer Septal Occluder. *Eur Heart J* 1999;20:541–549.

27. Katz SH, Falk JL. Misplaced endotracheal tubes by paramedics in an urban emergency medical services system. *Ann Emerg Med* 2001;37:32–37.

28. Knapp S, Kofler J, Stoiser B, et al. The assessment of four different methods to verify tracheal tube placement in the critical care setting. *Anesth Analg* 1999;766–770.

29. *www.tracheostomy.com.* July 7, 2002.

30. Kacker A. Tracheostomy. MEDLINE plus Health Information. Updated 10/31/01 *www.nlm.nih. gov/medlineplus/ency/article/002955.htm* Access date July 7, 2002.

31. Siobal M, Kallet RH, Kraemer R, et al. Tracheal-innominate artery fistula caused by the endotracheal tube tip: case report and investigation of a fatal complication of prolonged intubation. *Respir Care* 2001;46:1012–1018.

32. Orvidas LJ, Kasperbauer JL, Staats BA, et al. Long-term clinical experience with transtracheal oxygen catheters. *Mayo Clin Proc* 1998;73:739–744.

32. Hyson EA, Ravin CE, Kelley MJ, et al. Intraaortic counterpulsation balloon: radiographic considerations. *AJR Am J Roentgenol* 1977;128:915–918.

33. Kampelmacher MJ, Deenstra M, van Kesteren RG, et al. Transtracheal oxygen therapy: an effective and safe alternative to nasal oxygen administration. *Eur Respir J* 1997;10:828–833.

34. *SCOOP®* Transtracheal Oxygen Therapy Systems. *www.transtracheal.com/product/scoop.htm.* July 10, 2002.

35. Amato EJ. A nursing reference: gastrointestinal tubes and drains. Part II. Esophageal tubes. *Crit Care Nurse* 1983; 46–48.

36. Shah JN. Esophageal manometry. MEDLINE plus Health Information. Updated 05/25/01. *www.nlm.nih.gov/medlineplus/ency/imagepage/8776.htm.* Access date July 10, 2002.

37. Pearson RC, McCloy RF, Cutler WC, et al. Multichannel digital recording of intraluminal temperature in the upper gastrointestinal tract of man: techniques and analyses. *Clin Phys Physiol Measure* 1988;9:243–248.

38. Richard B, Colletti RB, Christie DL, et al. Indications for pediatric esophageal pH monitoring: a medical position statement of the North American Society for Pediatric Gastroenterology and Nutrition. *J Pediatr Gastroenterol Nutr* 1995;21:253–262.

39. Bailey MA, Katz PO. Gastroesophageal reflux disease in the elderly. *Clin Geriatr* 2000;8. (See also *www.mmhc.comcgarticlesCG0008bailey.html.*)

40. Irving JD, Dondelinger RF, Reidy JF, et al. Gianturco self-expanding stents: clinical experience in the vena cava and large veins. *Cardiovasc Intervent Radiol* 1992;15:328–333.

41. Yellin A, Rosen A, Reichert N, et al. Superior vena cava syndrome: the myth—the facts. *Am Rev Respir Dis* 1990;141:1114–1118.

42. Moores DWO, Ilves R. Treatment of esophageal obstruction with covered, self-expanding esophageal wallstents. *Ann Thorac Surg* 1996;62:963–967.

43. Underwood RA, Weinstock LB, Soper NJ, et al. Laparoscopic removal of an Angelchik prosthesis. *Surg Endosc Ultrasound Intervent Techn* 1999;13:615–617.

44. Stuart RC, Dawson K, Keeling P, et al. A prospective randomized trial of Angelchik prosthesis versus Nissen fundoplication. *Br J Surg* 1989;76:86–89.

45. Maxwell-Armstrong CA, Steele RJ, Amar SS, et al. Long-term results of the Angelchik prosthesis for gastro-oesophageal reflux. *Br J Surg* 1997;84:862–864.

46. O'Brien PE, Brown WA, Smith A, et al. Prospective study of a laparoscopically placed, adjustable gastric band in the treatment of morbid obesity. *Br J Surg* 1999;86:113–118.

47. Curtin JJ, Goodman LR, Quebbeman EJ, et al. Thoracostomy tubes after acute chest injury: relationship between location in a pleural fissure and function. *AJR Am J Roentgenol* 1994;163: 1339–1342.

48. Gayer G, Rozenman J, Hoffmann C, et al. Computed tomography diagnosis of malpositioned chest tubes. *Br J Radiol* 2000;73:786–790.

49. Moulton JS. Image-guided management of complicated pleural fluid collections. *Radiol Clin North Am* 2000;38:345–374.

50. Moulton JS, Benkert RE, Weisiger KH, et al. Treatment of complicated pleural fluid collections with image-guided drainage and intracavitary urokinase. *Chest* 1995;108:1252–1259.

THORACIC TRAUMA

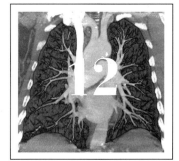

- Biomechanics
- Aortic Injuries
- Osseous Injuries
- Lung and Pleural Injuries
- Tracheobronchial Injuries
- Esophageal Injuries
- Cardiac Injuries
- Diaphragm Injuries
- Upper Abdominal Injuries
- Iatrogenic Injuries
- Summary

Trauma is one of the leading causes of death and disability, often affecting young otherwise healthy individuals (1,2). Chest injuries are a significant contributor to trauma-related deaths and disability. After head and neck injuries, which affect the brain and cervical spinal cord, thoracic injuries affect the next most vital structures, including the heart, aorta, lungs, and thoracic spinal cord. This chapter reviews some of the mechanisms of injury to the various organs and structures within the thorax, along with their imaging features and evaluation.

BIOMECHANICS

Thoracic trauma is the result of either penetrating or blunt injuries or a combination of the two. Knife and gunshot wounds are typical examples of penetrating injuries. Motor vehicle accidents, falls from a great height, and direct blows to the chest are common examples of blunt injuries. Explosions can cause combined injuries, with flying debris causing penetrating injuries and the shock wave of the blast causing blunt injuries. Velocity is an important factor contributing to both penetrating and blunt injuries. Relatively slow moving objects, such as knives and clubs, cause limited local injuries along the path of the blade or at the site of impact. Faster moving objects, such as bullets, not only cause damage along their flight paths but can also create compression shock waves, which travel through adjacent tissues and cause additional injuries. High-speed blunt impacts, such as those resulting from motor vehicle accidents or falls, not only cause direct blow injuries, but also result in the variable deceleration of internal structures, leading to shearing stresses and torsional forces at sites of fixation that can lacerate tissues and tear vessels. In addition, sudden or rapid compression of the chest or abdomen can cause an abrupt pressure increase, resulting in rupture of viscera (1,2).

AORTIC INJURIES

Acute traumatic aortic injury (ATAI) is a devastating and often lethal consequence of thoracic trauma. Proposed mechanisms of injury include the following:

1. Variable deceleration of the thoracic aorta producing shearing stresses, particularly at points of fixation such as the aortic root, the aortic isthmus (just distal to the left subclavian artery origin near the attachment of the ligamentum arteriosus), and the diaphragmatic hiatus;

2. Chest or abdominal wall compression, resulting in a sudden increase in the intraaortic pressure;
3. Chest compression, crushing the aorta between the sternum and spine.

Eighty-five percent of patients with an ATAI will suffer a complete full-thickness tear or rupture of the aortic wall, exsanguinate, and die before reaching the hospital. The remaining 15% of patients with an ATAI will have incomplete partial tears of the aortic wall, forming a pseudoaneurysm. Approximately 50% of these survivors will develop pseudoaneurysm rupture within the first 24 hours after the traumatic event if untreated.

The most common location of traumatic aortic rupture is the aortic root; however, these patients usually do not survive to reach the hospital.

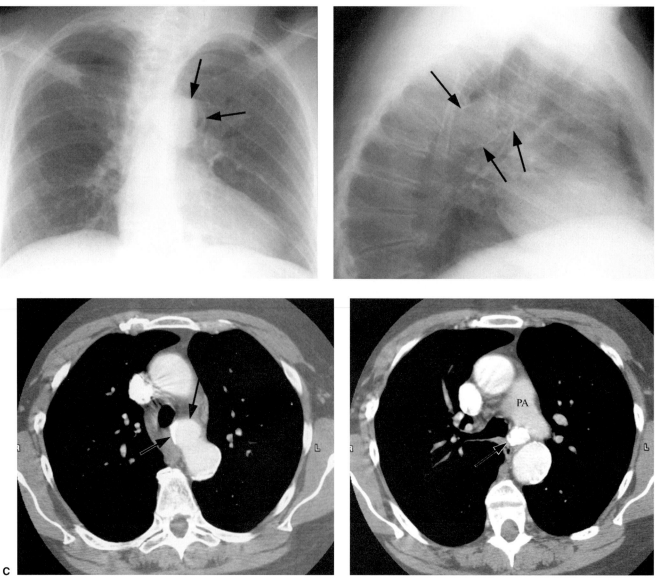

Figure 12.1 Chronic aortic pseudoaneurysm. *A and B.* Frontal and lateral chest radiographs of a patient with a remote history of motor vehicle accident. Note the lobulated contour in the region of the aortic isthmus with mural calcification and a double density in the region of the aortic knob on the frontal view (*arrows*). *C and D.* Contrast enhanced computed tomography demonstrates a chronic pseudoaneurysm in the region of the aortic isthmus with mural calcification (*arrows*). Note the location of the pseudoaneurysm (*arrow*) adjacent to the pulmonary artery (PA) near the attachment of the ligamentum arteriosus in *D*.

Table 12.1: Chest Radiograph Signs of Mediastinal Hematoma

Widening of the superior mediastinum
Obscuration of the aortic arch
Abnormal aortic contour
Fullness, opacification, or loss of definition of the aorticopulmonary window
Caudal displacement of the left main bronchus
Rightward deviation of the trachea
Rightward deviation of a nasogastric tube in the esophagus
Widening of the paraspinal stripe in the absence of a vertebral fracture
Widening of the right paratracheal stripe
Left apical cap and left pleural fluid

Less than 5% of patients will survive long term with a pseudoaneurysm (3). The chest radiograph and computed tomography (CT) of one such patient with a chronic pseudoaneurysm are shown in Fig. 12.1.

ATAI is strongly associated with mediastinal hemorrhage; however, this blood does not arise from the aortic tear itself because the intact adventitia of the pseudoaneurysm maintains aortic integrity and blood flow. The mediastinal hematoma results from concomitant injury to other mediastinal, paraspinal, and intercostal vessels, usually veins and small arteries. Plain chest radiographs do not directly image an aortic tear; only CT and aortography can do this. However, plain films can detect mediastinal hematoma, an indirect sign of ATAI. Therefore, plain films are a useful screening tool and may help guide further imaging evaluation. Although no single plain film finding is totally sensitive or specific for a mediastinal hematoma, the following abnormalities have the greatest diagnostic value: (a) widening of the superior mediastinum; (b) obscuration of the aortic arch; (c) abnormal aortic contour; (d) fullness, opacification, or loss of definition of the aorticopulmonary window; (e) caudal displacement of the left main bronchus; (f) rightward deviation of the trachea; (g) rightward deviation of a nasogastric tube in the esophagus; (h) widening of the paraspinal stripe in the absence of a vertebral fracture; (i) widening of the right paratracheal stripe; and (j) left apical cap and left pleural fluid (Table 12.1) (4). Detection of one or more of these findings should prompt further evaluation with CT aortography. This requires helical CT at a collimation no greater than 3 mm with overlapping reconstructions, coupled with rapid intravenous contrast administration at 4 mL/s.

Direct CT signs of ATAI should be specifically sought and include (a) intraluminal irregularities or areas of low attenuation (polypoid clot, linear-intimal flap), (b) change in caliber of the aorta (pseudoaneurysm, pseudocoarctation), (c) abnormal or irregular aortic wall or contour, (d) abnormal contour of great vessels, and (e) intramural hematoma or dissection (Table 12.2) (5,6). Approximately 90% of these ATAIs should be in the

Table 12.2: CT Signs of Acute Traumatic Aortic Injury

Direct Signs	Indirect Signs
Intraluminal irregularities or areas of low attenuation (polypoid clot, linear-intimal flap)	Mediastinal fat stranding
Change in caliber of the aorta (pseudoaneurysm, pseudocoarctation)	Mediastinal hemorrhage
Abnormal or irregular aortic wall or contour	Perivascular hematoma
Abnormal contour of great vessels	Periaortic hematoma
Intramural hematoma or dissection	

CT, Computed tomography.

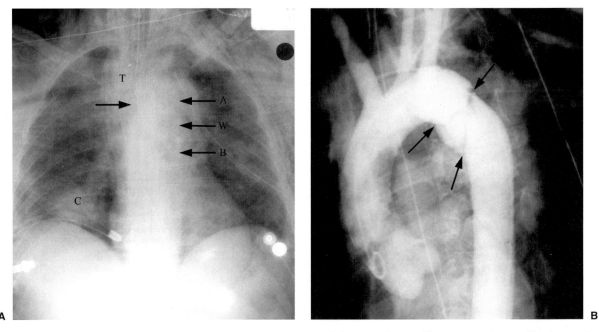

Figure 12.2 Acute traumatic aortic injury with large mediastinal hematoma. *A.* Portable chest radiograph with extensive subcutaneous emphysema, multiple lines and tubes, and a pulmonary contusion (C). The initial "busy" appearance of this study must not distract from the more salient findings of mediastinal hematoma. These findings include widening of the mediastinum, obscuration of the aortic arch (A), fullness of the aortopulmonary window (W), caudal displacement of the left main bronchus (B), rightward deviation of the trachea (T), and rightward deviation of the nasogastric tube (*arrows*). *B.* Aortogram demonstrates partial tear (*arrows*) of the aortic wall, forming a pseudoaneurysm at the aortic isthmus.

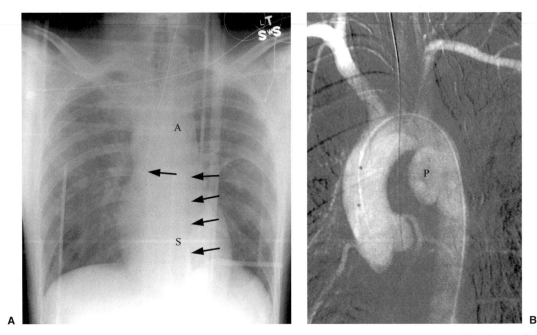

Figure 12.3 Acute traumatic aortic injury with a mediastinal hematoma. *A.* Portable chest radiograph with findings of mediastinal hematoma including obscuration of the aortic arch (A), rightward deviation of the nasogastric tube (*arrow*), and widening of the paraspinal stripe (S, *arrows*). *B.* Aortogram demonstrates pseudoaneurysm (P) at the aortic isthmus.

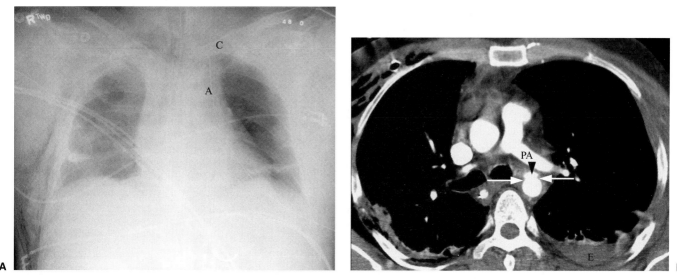

Figure 12.4 Acute traumatic aortic injury. *A*. Portable chest radiograph with finding of mediastinal hematoma including widening of the mediastinum, obscuration of the aortic arch (A), and apical cap (C). *B*. Contrast enhanced computed tomography demonstrates direct signs of aortic injury including abnormal aortic wall contour (*arrows*) and small pseudoaneurysm adjacent to the pulmonary artery (PA) near the attachment of the ligamentum arteriosus. Also, note a left pleural effusion (E).

region of the aortic isthmus (3). CT findings of mediastinal fat stranding, mediastinal hemorrhage, perivascular hematoma, and periaortic hematoma are indirect signs of ATAI and are also seen with nonaortic mediastinal injuries. Nonetheless, these findings require clinical follow-up or, in the case of periaortic hematoma, further evaluation with catheter aortography (5). Figures 12.2 through 12.5 are the chest radiographs and accompanying CTs and/or aortograms from four cases of ATAI. The cases in Figs. 12.2 to 12.4 demonstrate the typical location of ATAI at the aortic isthmus, whereas the case in Fig. 12.5 is from the 10% of ATAIs that occur in other locations.

The most common location of aortic rupture seen clinically is the proximal descending thoracic aorta at the ligamentum arteriosum.

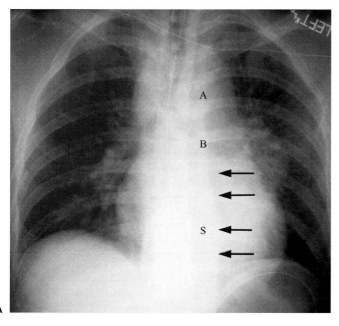

Figure 12.5 Acute traumatic aortic injury. After this young man's motor vehicle accident, he walked to a nearby house to phone for help and then rode in the tow truck to the garage with his car before presenting to the hospital complaining of back pain. *A*. Chest radiograph demonstrates widening of the mediastinum, obscuration of the aortic arch (A), caudal displacement of the left main bronchus (B), and widening of the paraspinal stripe (S, *arrows*).

(continued on next page)

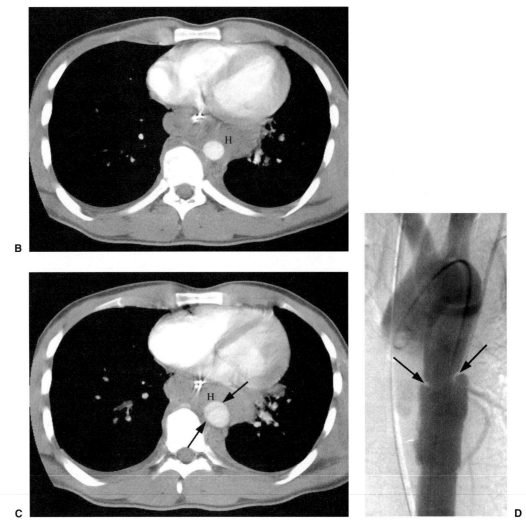

Figure 12.5 (continued) *B and C.* Contrast enhanced computed tomography demonstrates both direct and indirect signs of aortic injury. The direct signs are best seen in *C* and include intraluminal curvilinear low attenuation *(arrows)*, abnormal aortic wall contour, and caliber change when comparing the dilated descending aorta in *C* with the normal size descending aorta in *B*. Both *B* and *C* demonstrate the indirect sign of periaortic hematoma (H). *D.* Aortogram demonstrates partial tear *(arrows)* of the aortic wall, forming a pseudoaneurysm involving the descending thoracic aorta.

OSSEOUS INJURIES

Fractures of thoracic bones are an indication of the force of trauma and are commonly associated with organ injury.

Rib fractures are the most common sequela of chest trauma, occurring in over half of blunt trauma cases (7–9). However, many of these injuries are not initially detected because they are uncomplicated nondisplaced fractures or involve radiographically undetectable costochondral separation (2,7,8,10). This is acceptable because the goal of imaging is not so much to detect the rib fracture itself, but rather the potential associated complications of rib fractures (10). These complications include injury to the intercostal vessels, which can lead to hemothorax or an extrapleural hematoma; lung contusion or laceration; pneumothorax; and subcutaneous emphysema (Figs. 12.6 and 12.7) (2,9,10). The most serious consequence of rib fractures is flail chest (2,7). Flail chest is the result of five or more adjacent rib fractures or more than three segmental rib fractures (a single rib fractured in two or more locations) (Figs. 12.8 and 12.9) (2,7,8). This

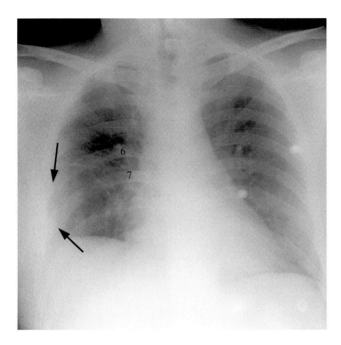

Figure 12.6 Rib fractures with associated hemothorax. Chest radiograph demonstrates minimally displaced fractures (*arrows*) of the right sixth and seventh ribs. There is a also hazy opacity obscuring the right costophrenic angle with blunting consistent with a small associated hemothorax.

creates an abnormally mobile segment of the chest wall that will move paradoxically with respiration (2,7,8). Flail chest can lead to respiratory failure in part secondary to associated lung and pleural injuries and in part secondary to pendelluft (2). Pendelluft is the pendulum-like movement of gas from the normal hemithorax to the flail hemithorax during expiration and then back again during inspiration due to the paradoxical motion of the flail segment. In other words, when the normal hemithorax exhales, the flail hemithorax will paradoxically inhale and vice versa. This results in impaired ventilation due to rebreathing of the same air back and forth between the hemithoraces. This can be treated with mechanical ventilation (2,7,8).

A fail chest is the fracture of three or more ribs in two or more locations each, or the fracture of five or more adjacent ribs.

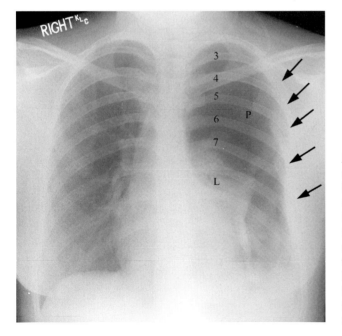

Figure 12.7 Rib fractures with associated pneumothorax and hemothorax. Chest radiograph demonstrates displaced fractures (*arrows*) of the left third through the seventh ribs. There is a large associated left pneumothorax (P) with significant collapse of the left lung (L). There is also blunting of the left costophrenic angle consistent with a small associated hemothorax.

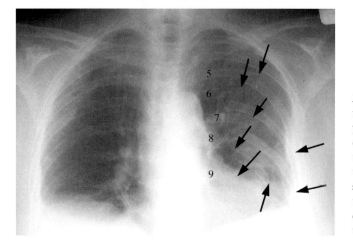

Figure 12.8 Flail chest. Chest radiograph demonstrates displaced fractures (*arrows*) of five consecutive left ribs (fifth through ninth), with three of the ribs (5, 7, and 8) exhibiting segmental fractures. Blunting of the left costophrenic angle indicates a small associated hemothorax.

Lower rib fractures are associated with injury to the liver, spleen, and kidneys.

Fractures of the first three ribs, particularly the first rib (Fig. 12.10), are a marker of severe trauma (2,7,10). Considerable force is required to break these ribs because they are protected by the clavicle, shoulder, scapula, and heavy surrounding musculature (2,7). These fractures are often associated with airway, spinal, vascular, and brachial plexus injuries. Fractures of the lower three ribs are associated with injuries to the spleen, liver, or kidneys (2,10).

Sternal fractures are associated with mediastinal vascular injury.

Sternal fractures can result from steering wheel injuries, seat-belt injuries, crush injuries, and aggressive resuscitation (2,8). Sternal fractures can be important because they are associated with other mediastinal injuries; however, they are virtually impossible to detect on frontal radiographs (10). Lateral views or CT are required to detect sternal fractures, which are usually transverse and near the manubrium (2,8,10). Sagittal and/or coronal reconstructions can be useful (8). An associated retrosternal hematoma

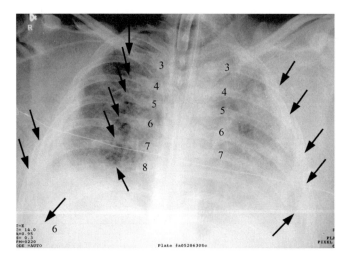

Figure 12.9 Bilateral flail chest. This patient sustained a severe crush injury. Chest radiograph demonstrates displaced fractures (*arrows*) of six consecutive right ribs (third through eighth), all of which are segmental fractures. In fact, the right sixth rib is actually fractured in three locations. There are also displaced fractures (*arrows*) of five consecutive left ribs (third to seventh). Blunting of both costophrenic angles, pleural thickening, and diffuse hazy increased opacity of both hemithoraces (left greater than right) indicate bilateral associated hemothoraces.

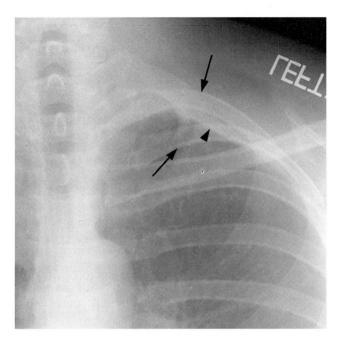

Figure 12.10 First rib fracture. Coned down view of the left apex demonstrates a left first rib fracture *(arrows)*. Also, note the adjacent left apical pleural thickening *(arrowhead)* indicating an associated extrapleural hematoma.

is often noted, which if separated from the aorta by a fat plane suggests that the hematoma is not aortic in origin (2,11). Sternoclavicular dislocations can also be detected with CT (8,9).

Thoracic vertebral fractures can result from motor vehicle accidents or falls from a great height. They are produced by hyperflexion and/or axial loading and account for 25% to 30% of all spine fractures (1). Most injuries occur at the functional thoracolumbar junction, which extends from T-9 to T-11 (1,7,8,12). The thoracic spinal cord is unusually susceptible to injury. This vulnerability is the result of two main factors. First, the thoracic spinal cord is tightly packed in the spinal canal, predisposing it to injury by displaced fragments of bone or disc material and compression by hematoma and cord edema. Second, the vascular supply to the mid-thoracic cord is quite tenuous and can be disrupted easily, resulting in cord ischemia or infarction with associated neurologic impairment (1). The radiographic findings of thoracic spine fractures can be subtle and difficult to identify (8). Initial evaluation should include the frontal chest radiograph and a cross-table lateral view of the spine. There are both direct and indirect plain film signs of thoracic fractures (Table 12.3). Direct signs include cortical disruption and abnormal vertebral body size, shape, opacity, and location (Fig. 12.11) (1). Indirect signs are secondary to paravertebral hematoma (Fig. 12.5) and can overlap with signs of aortic injury. Indirect signs include widening of the paraspinal stripe, mediastinal widening, left apical cap, and deviation of a nasogastric tube (1,7,8,13). If a thoracic spine fracture is suspected, then further evaluation with CT and/or magnetic resonance imaging (MRI) is indicated. Reformatted sagittal and coronal CT images are helpful (1,8). A mediastinal hematoma that is confined to the posterior compartment suggests a vertebral fracture (8).

A portable chest trauma radiograph may suggest thoracic spine fracture but is insufficient to exclude it.

Table 12.3: Radiographic Findings of Thoracic Spine Fractures

Direct	Indirect
Cortical disruption	Widening of the paraspinal stripe
Abnormal vertebral body size	Mediastinal widening
Abnormal vertebral body shape	Apical cap
Abnormal vertebral body opacity	Deviation of a nasogastric tube
Abnormal vertebral body location	

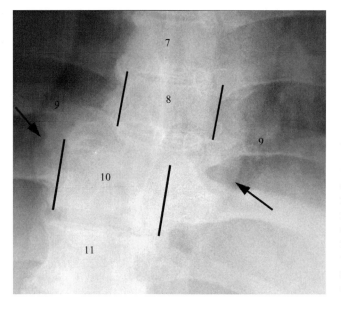

Figure 12.11 Vertebral fracture. Coned down view of the lower thoracic spine demonstrates direct signs of a T-9 compression fracture dislocation, including markedly decreased height of T-9 and malalignment of T-8 with respect to T-10. Paraspinal stripe widening *(arrows)*, an indirect sign of spinal injury, is also present.

LUNG AND PLEURAL INJURIES

Lung contusions usually develop and reach maximum size with 24 hours of trauma.

Contusion in the most common pulmonary parenchymal injury, occurring in approximately half of patients after blunt trauma (2,8,11). The mechanism of injury is local comprehensive and recoil forces within the lung that disrupt small vessels, leading to intraalveolar hemorrhage or a parenchymal bruise (2,9,10,11,14). Interstitial injury with associated capillary leak and edema can also occur but is usually seen with more severe trauma accompanied by blast or shock wave injuries (Fig. 12.12) (14). Contusion appears rapidly and usually reaches its full extent within the first day after trauma (Fig. 12.13). Contusion tends to occur adjacent to solid structure such as the ribs, spine, and solid organs like the heart and liver (2). Contusions may have a varied radiographic appearance, ranging from coarse irregular nodular opacities that may be confluent or discrete to homogenous consolidation with diffuse hazy or focal, poorly defined, fluffy lung opacities, or a combination of these findings (Figs. 12.14 and 12.15) (9,11,14). The presence and extent of

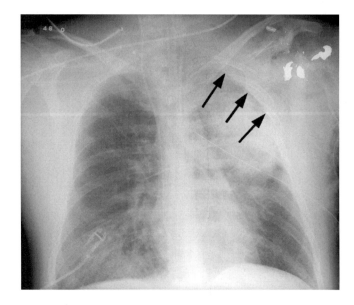

Figure 12.12 Pulmonary contusion. Chest radiograph demonstrates findings of a self-inflicted gunshot wound to the left axilla, including multiple metallic bullet fragments. A large area of focal increased opacity is seen occupying the left upper lung representing alveolar hemorrhage and edema secondary to pulmonary contusion and interstitial injury caused by the shock wave associated with the adjacent gunshot blast. Also note the left apical pleural thickening *(arrows)* secondary to an associated hemothorax.

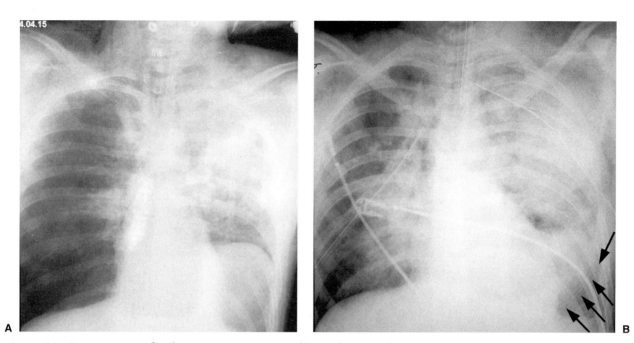

Figure 12.13 Progression of pulmonary contusion. *A.* Chest radiograph demonstrates increased opacity in the left mid and upper lung secondary to pulmonary contusion. There is also hyperlucency on the right secondary to a pneumothorax, subcutaneous emphysema in the supraclavicular regions, and apparent elevation of the left hemidiaphragm secondary to a diaphragmatic rupture. *B.* Chest radiograph 1 day later demonstrates further opacification of the left lung and new opacity in the right medial lung secondary to progression of the contusion. Also, note the up-turned nasogastric tube *(arrows)* in the herniated stomach and resolution of the right pneumothorax after chest tube insertion.

contusion are much better defined with CT than chest radiographs (Figs. 12.14 and 12.15) (2,8,11,14). Contusion may be difficult to distinguish from or may be obscured by other forms of posttraumatic consolidation, including aspiration, edema, and atelectasis (2). Contusion usually begins to resolve within a few days, completely resolving within 1 to 2 weeks (2,8).

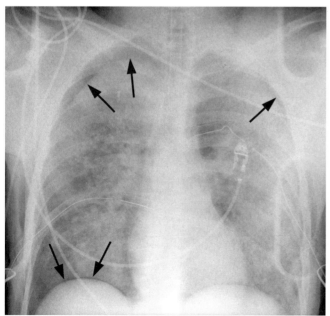

Figure 12.14 Pulmonary contusion and pneumothoraces. *A.* Chest radiograph demonstrates coarse irregular nodular opacities predominantly in the right lung and more diffuse, hazy to focal, poorly defined, fluffy lung opacities predominantly in the left lung consistent with the varied radiographic appearance of contusion. Also, there is a right pneumothorax *(arrows)*, but much less apparent is a small left pneumothorax *(single arrow on right).*

(continued on next page)

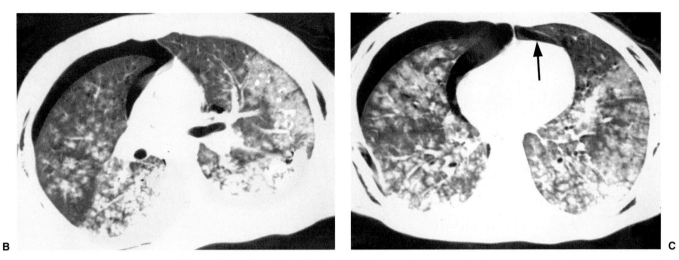

Figure 12.14 (continued) *B and C.* Computed tomography images more clearly demonstrate similar findings of irregular nodular opacities, areas of homogenous consolidation, and areas of fluffy focal opacity. Notice the distribution of some of these opacities adjacent to solid structures, such as the ribs peripherally and the spine medially, in *B.* The right pneumothorax is readily apparent in both *B* and *C*; in addition, notice the ease of detection of the small left pneumothorax (*arrow*) in *C.*

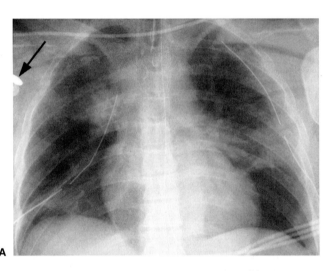

Figure 12.15 Pulmonary contusion. *A.* Chest radiograph demonstrates areas of focal hazy opacity in the left mid lung and right mid-upper lung medially. Also, note the metallic bullet fragment in the right axillary region (*arrow*) and subcutaneous emphysema. *B and C.* Computed tomography images demonstrate focal opacities with bubbly lucency's anteriorly on the right in *B* and on the left in *C.* These contusions/lacerations relate to the flight paths of the patient's gunshot wounds. Areas of confluent homogenous consolidation are seen posteriorly in *C* adjacent to solid structures (i.e., the ribs and spine). These contusions relate to the shock wave injuries secondary to the gunshot wounds. Also, notice the subcutaneous emphysema, which is readily apparent in both *B* and *C.*

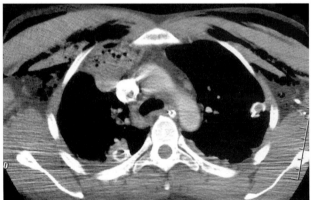

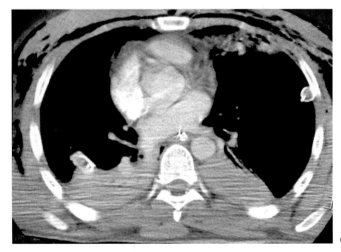

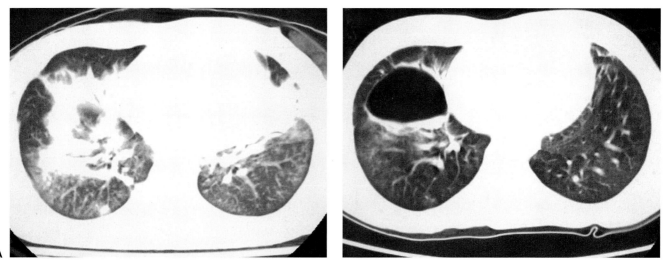

Figure 12.16 Pulmonary laceration/hematoma and contusion evolving into a pneumatocele. *A.* Computed tomography image demonstrates areas of focal and band-like opacities predominantly in the right lung. These represent a combination of pulmonary laceration/hematoma and contusion. *B.* Computed tomography image of the same patient 3 weeks later demonstrates a predominantly air-filled space in the same location. Over time, as the contusion and hemorrhage in the hematoma resolved, they were replaced with air, forming a pneumatocele.

Pulmonary laceration results from shearing forces caused by blunt trauma or direct puncture secondary to penetrating trauma (Fig. 12.15) (2, 9,10,14). The initial linear tear of the laceration rapidly becomes an ovoid space secondary to the elastic recoil properties of the adjacent normal lung (2,14). Lacerations can be obscured by surrounding contusion and may not become apparent until the contusion begins to resolve (2). The postlaceration space can fill with blood, becoming a pulmonary hematoma or air resulting in a pneumatocele (8,10,11,14). A pneumatocele can also form as the hemorrhage in a pulmonary hematoma begins to resolve and is replaced by air (Fig. 12.16) (11,15). Radiographically, hematomas and pneumatoceles will appear as well-circumscribed round areas of focal opacity or lucency (11). Again, CT is much more sensitive for detecting lacerations than plain films (2,8,14).

A pulmonary laceration can extend through the visceral pleura and with associated air leak result in a pneumothorax (14). Compression injuries can cause alveolar rupture and air leak, which can also lead to pneumothorax (2). Figure 12.17 demonstrates a

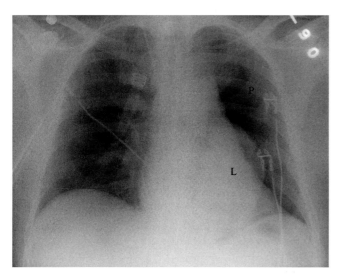

Figure 12.17 Large left pneumothorax. Chest radiograph demonstrates a large left pneumothorax (P) with significant collapse of the left lung (L). There were no rib fractures or history of penetrating trauma; therefore, this pneumothorax must be the result of a parenchymal or airway injury.

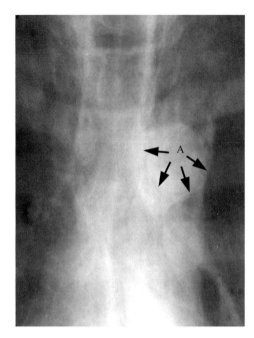

Figure 12.18 Pneumomediastinum. Coned down view of the mediastinum demonstrates streaky linear lucency's throughout the mediastinum and lucencies surrounding the aortic knob (A, *arrows*), the so-called ring around the artery sign. These findings indicate a pneumomediastinum.

On portable supine trauma chest radiographs, pneumothorax collects at the lung bases and is often occult radiographically.

large left pneumothorax that could have resulted from either of these mechanisms. If the air leak from alveolar rupture tracts along the bronchovascular bundles, pneumomediastinum can result (Fig. 12.18) (9,16,17). Similarly, if the air leak tracts along the adventitia of the pulmonary veins, pneumopericardium can occur (16). Obviously, penetrating injuries can violate the pleura and cause pneumothorax. Pneumothorax can be difficult to detect in the posttrauma patient because they are often radiographed in the supine position with the intrapleural air collecting nondependently along the anterior chest wall (1,10). Signs of a pneumothorax on a supine chest radiograph include a deep costophrenic sulcus (the so-called deep sulcus sign; Fig. 17.13), basilar hyperlucency, and unusually sharp delineation of the mediastinal contour (Figs. 12.13A and 12.19) (1,10). Occasionally, decubitus or cross-table lateral views can be helpful to detect pneumothorax (1,10). CT is the most accurate method for detecting a pneumothorax (Fig. 12.14) and should be considered if the patient is to be placed on positive pressure mechanical ventilation, because this can cause even the tiniest pneumothorax to rapidly

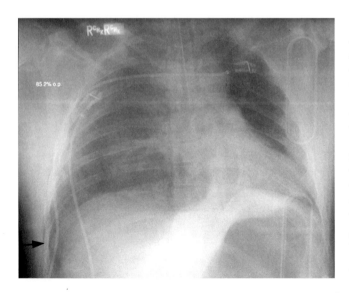

Figure 12.19 "Deep sulcus" sign. Supine chest radiograph demonstrates a deep lucent costophrenic sulcus on the right (*arrow*), the so-called deep sulcus sign. This indicates a right pneumothorax. Also, note contralateral shift of the heart and mediastinum to the left and inferior displacement of the right hemidiaphragm. These findings indicate that this pneumothorax is under tension. The generalized hazy opacity in the right hemithorax is secondary to a dependently layering right hemothorax.

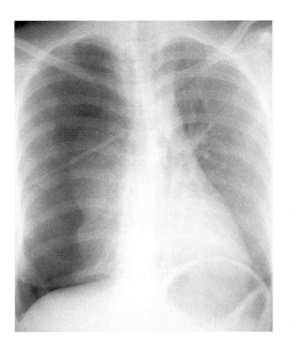

Figure 12.20 Tension pneumothorax. Chest radiograph demonstrates a hyperlucent right hemithorax with significant collapse of the right lung, inferior displacement of the right hemidiaphragm, and contralateral displacement of the mediastinal structures to the left. These findings indicate a right tension pneumothorax, despite the presence of a small bore right chest tube.

increase in size and possibly become a tension pneumothorax (1,2,10). Tension pneumothorax can be a life-threatening situation. Radiographic signs of tension pneumothorax include contralateral displacement of mediastinal structures, inferior displacement of the diaphragm, hyperlucent hemithorax, and ipsilateral collapse of the lung (Figs. 12.19 and 12.20).

Just as air can accumulate in the pleural space after parenchymal injuries, so can blood secondary to hemorrhage at the site of injury, resulting in a hemothorax (1,2,10). Bleeding from low pressure pulmonary vessels is usually self-limited; however, injury to large central pulmonary vessels, systemic thoracic veins or arteries, or lacerated viscera can lead to a large potentially life-threatening hemothorax requiring surgical intervention (1). Again, similar to pneumothorax, hemothorax can be difficult to detect on supine radiographs, in this case due to dependent posterior layering. Signs of hemothorax on a supine chest radiograph include apical cap, hazy increased opacity projected over the hemithorax, and confluent lateral pleural thickening (Figs. 12.4, 12.9, 12.12, and 12.19) (1,10). Again, CT is the most accurate way to detect even small amounts of pleural fluid (Fig. 12.4) (10). Fibrothorax can be the late result of an untreated undrained hemothorax (2). The delayed or late appearance of pleural fluid that continues to slowly accumulate over several days, particularly after a penetrating injury or recent thoracic surgery, raises the possibility of a chylous effusion secondary to thoracic duct disruption (2,10).

Rare complications of thoracic trauma include lung herniation through a defect in the chest wall and torsion of the lung about the hilar structures secondary to disruption of the inferior pulmonary ligament, which normally anchors the lung (2,10).

TRACHEOBRONCHIAL INJURIES

Tracheobronchial injuries (TBIs) occur in about 1% of major chest traumas and have a high mortality, about 30% (2,7,8). Intrathoracic TBIs can occur as a result of compression of the trachea against the spine, shearing forces, or by sudden increased intraluminal pressure. Most injuries (80%) occur within 2.5 cm of the carina and favor the right main bronchus (7). TBIs are often associated with fractures involving one or more of the first three ribs (Fig. 12.10), clavicle, sternum, or scapula (8,18). The clinical and radiographic

Most tracheobronchial injuries occur within 2.5 cm of the carina.

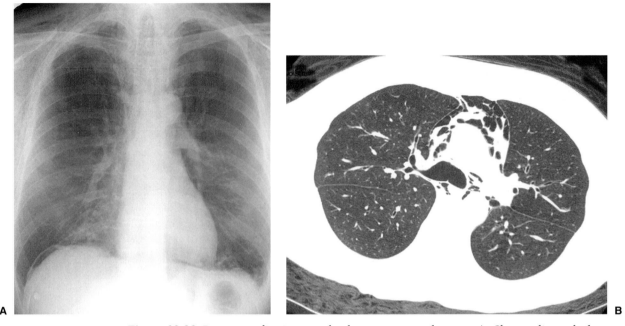

A   B

Figure 12.21 Pneumomediastinum and subcutaneous emphysema. *A.* Chest radiograph demonstrates streaky linear lucencies throughout the mediastinum and subcutaneous tissues in the supraclavicular and axillary regions. These gas collections are the result of an air leak secondary to a tracheal injury. *B.* Computed tomography image of the same patient demonstrates extensive pneumomediastinum.

manifestations of TBIs depend on the location and extent of the airway tear. Airway tears can be partial or incomplete and may remain occult. Diagnosis may be delayed until high-pressure mechanical ventilation is instituted, leading to pneumomediastinum and/or pneumothorax (2). Delayed diagnosis of an airway injury can result in airway stenosis secondary to partial healing. This can lead to air trapping, recurrent atelectasis, or postobstructive pneumonia (2,8). It is unusual to directly visualize the site of airway injury, even with CT. If an airway injury is suspected, then bronchoscopy is indicated.

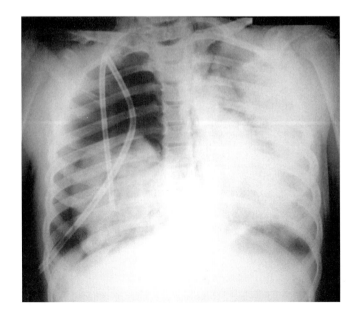

Figure 12.22 "P" and "fallen lung" signs. Chest radiograph demonstrates a right tension pneumothorax despite the presence of a right chest tube. The right lung exhibits significant collapse and has "fallen" inferiorly secondary to complete disruption of the right main bronchus.

Table 12.4: Chest Radiograph Findings of Airway Injury

Pneumomediastinum
Pneumothorax
"P" sign (persistent, progessive, pneumothorax)
"Fallen lung" sign
Interstitial air within the airway wall
Ectopic location of an endotracheal tube
Overdistention of the endotracheal tube cuff balloon

Air leaks associated with tears of the trachea and proximal (extrapleural) left main bronchus tend to be confined to the mediastinum and interstitial planes of the neck and subcutaneous tissues (Fig. 12.21) (2,18). Tears of the right main and distal left main bronchi manifest as pneumothorax (Fig. 12.17). TBIs can cause the so-called P sign (persistent progressive pneumothorax), especially if the pneumothorax persists after chest tube insertion (Figs. 12.20 and 12.22) (7,10). The "fallen lung" sign occurs with complete disruption of a main bronchus. The lung falls inferiorly and laterally to the base of the hemithorax (Fig. 12.22), in contrast to a simple pneumothorax or a pneumothorax from a partial bronchial tear in which the lung collapses medially and centrally (2,8,18). Although the fallen lung sign is specific, it is rare (7). Other signs of airway disruption include interstitial air within the wall of the airway, ectopic location of an endotracheal tube, and overdistention of the endotracheal tube cuff balloon (18) (Table 12.4).

> Persistent or unexplained pneumomediastinum in a trauma patient should raise suspicion of airway rupture or esophageal rupture.

ESOPHAGEAL INJURIES

Esophageal tear after trauma is relatively rare, occurring in less than 1% of patients; however, prompt detection and diagnosis are imperative to avoid the possibility of an ensuing mediastinitis, which carries a high morbidity and mortality (7,8,10). This injury can result from a sudden increase in intraesophageal pressure that may in part be due to the violent ejection of stomach contents into the esophagus, with a pathophysiology similar to Boerhaave syndrome (7,8,10). The resulting tear usually occurs in the left posterolateral wall of the distal esophagus; this is a location where the esophagus is devoid of striated muscle and deficient in extramural support. Other mechanisms of injury can include compression of the esophagus between the sternum and spine, traction from cervical hyperextension, and penetrating injuries, including bone fragments from spinal fractures (8). Chest radiographs cannot directly identify an esophageal tear; therefore, indirect signs must be used. These indirect signs include pneumomediastinum (Figs. 12.18 and 12.21), left pneumothorax, left pleural effusion, and left lower lobe atelectasis (Table 12.5, Fig. 12.23) (8). If an esophageal injury is suspected, an esophagram or endoscopy should be considered. If an esophagram is performed, water-soluble non-ionic contrast should be used initially and, if negative, can be followed by a barium study.

> An esophagram is the test of choice for diagnosing esophageal rupture.

Table 12.5: Chest Radiograph Findings of Esophageal Injury

Pneumomediastinum
Left pneumothorax
Left pleural effusion
Left lower lobe atelectasis

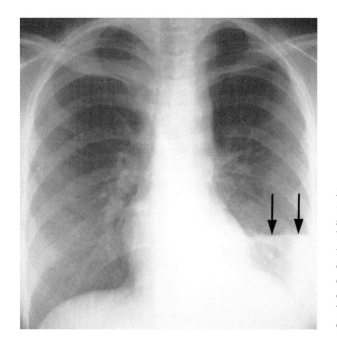

Figure **12.23** Esophageal tear. Chest radiograph demonstrates an air-fluid level *(arrows)* at the left base consistent with a hydropneumothorax. There is also increased opacity at the left base with mild elevation of the left hemidiaphragm compatible with basilar atelectasis. These findings are secondary to an esophageal tear.

CARDIAC INJURIES

Myocardial contusion is the most common cardiac injury in blunt trauma and is occult radiographically.

The heart and pericardium are subject to both penetrating and blunt injuries. Thoracic trauma can induce a variety of cardiac injuries, including myocardial contusion, coronary artery occlusion, myocardial infarction, myocardial rupture or laceration, pericardial tamponade, damage to the valve apparatus, and pericardial rupture or tear, which can lead to cardiac herniation or dislocation (10). Myocardial contusion is common but frequently asymptomatic. Myocardial contusion is difficult to image but is usually evident secondary to elevated creatine phosphokinase enzymes and/or an abnormal electrocardiogram. The right ventricle is most commonly affected because of its immediate retrosternal location. Pericardial tamponade may be secondary to blood or air accumulating in the pericardial sac (8). Pneumopericardium can result from air tracking along the adventitia of pulmonary veins into the pericardial space. Detection of pericardial tamponade secondary to hemopericardium can be challenging radiographically because only a small amount of blood can tamponade cardiac motion acutely without changing the cardiac silhouette size

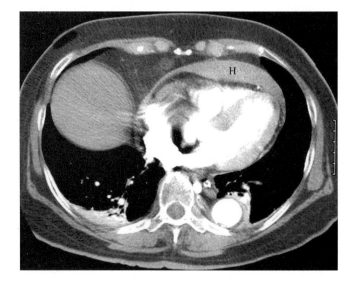

Figure **12.24** Hemopericardium. Computed tomography image demonstrates high attenuation fluid in the pericardial space consistent with a hemopericardium (H).

significantly. However, diagnosis can be made if the cardiac size is noted to be increasing on serial radiographs. Cardiac tamponade can also be secondary to anterior mediastinal hematomas, often resulting from arterial sources, which can compress the myocardium. CT can easily detect both mediastinal hematomas and hemopericardium (Fig. 12.24). Bedside echocardiography can also readily detect the presence of pericardial fluid.

DIAPHRAGM INJURIES

Diaphragmatic rupture occurs in about 5% of patients with blunt trauma (1,19,20–23). Mechanisms of injury in these cases include lateral impact, which distorts the chest wall and creates shearing forces along the diaphragm, and direct frontal impact, which causes increased intraabdominal pressure that "blows out" the diaphragm (19,22). Most diaphragmatic ruptures are associated with significant intraabdominal injuries (22). Although left- and right-sided ruptures likely occur with equal frequency, right-sided ruptures are more often clinically occult, probably because of some protective effect of the liver, and more difficult to diagnose, leading to underreporting of right-sided ruptures (1,20). Therefore, left-sided ruptures are reported in 75% to 90% of cases (8,19). Most of these left-sided tears occur in the posterolateral portion of the diaphragm at the musculotendinous junction, which is the weakest portion of the diaphragm because it is where the pleuroperitoneal membrane finally closes during fetal development (8,19,20,22,23). Most diaphragmatic tears resulting from blunt trauma are greater than 2 cm in length, with many left-sided tears being 10 cm or more in length (8,19,20,22–24).

> An elevated hemidiaphragm in the setting of trauma should raise suspicion for diaphragmatic rupture.

> Left-sided diaphragmatic ruptures are much more common clinically than right-sided ones.

Visceral herniation occurs in approximately half of the cases of diaphragmatic ruptures (8). On the right side the organs most commonly herniated are the liver and occasionally the colon. On the left side the stomach and colon are the most common, but the small bowel, spleen, and kidney can also herniate (23). Herniation is an important complication that can lead to strangulation with associated ischemia, infarction, and/or obstruction (1,19,22,23). Herniation can be delayed after a diaphragmatic injury, but over time negative intrathoracic pressure and positive intraperitoneal pressure lead to progressive enlargement of the diaphragmatic defect, increasing the likelihood of herniation of intraabdominal contents into the thorax (1,19,21–23). This process can be inhibited if the patient requires positive pressure assisted ventilation after the traumatic event, because this will eliminate and actually reverse the pressure gradient between the thorax and abdomen (19,22,24). The period of delay between the diaphragmatic injury and the presentation of herniation is known as the latent phase and can last from months to years. Most cases that result in strangulation occur within 3 years of the traumatic event (1,23).

Plain chest radiography cannot directly image a diaphragmatic tear; therefore, plain film diagnosis of a diaphragmatic rupture depends on secondary signs of herniation of intraabdominal contents into the thorax (10). Chest radiograph findings of diaphragmatic herniation include (a) apparent diaphragmatic elevation; (b) irregular, obscured, or discontinuous diaphragmatic contour; (c) contralateral mediastinal shift; (d) air containing viscera above the hemidiaphragm; (e) basilar opacification; and (f) abnormal U-shaped course of a nasogastric tube with an elevated tip (Table 12.6, Figs. 12.13, 12.25, and 12.26) (1,2,8,10,23,24). However, these findings are nonspecific and can be attributed to or obscured by other abnormalities, such as atelectasis, pulmonary contusion, pleural effusion, posttraumatic lung cysts, pneumothorax, hiatal hernia, and phrenic nerve paral-

---

Table 12.6: Chest Radiograph Findings of Diaphragmatic Herniation

Apparent diaphragmatic elevation
Irregular, obscured, or discontinuous diaphragmatic contour
Contralateral mediastinal shift
Air containing viscera above the hemidiaphragm
Basilar opacification
Abnormal U-shaped course of a nasogastric tube with an elevated tip

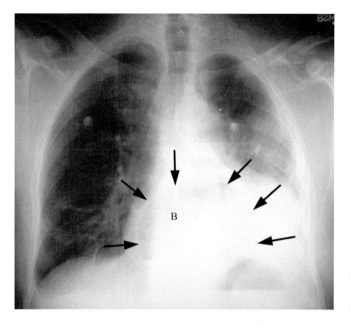

Figure 12.25 Diaphragmatic hernia. Chest radiograph demonstrates apparent elevation and obscuration of the left hemidiaphragm, herniated bowel (B, *arrows*) above the diaphragm, and left basilar opacification. These findings are consistent with a diaphragmatic tear with associated bowel herniation.

Delayed diaphragmatic rupture may present years after trauma, either through radiographic detection or symptoms of bowel strangulation.

ysis (1,8,10). Preexisting diaphragmatic eventration or elevation can also mimic a diaphragmatic injury (8). Thus, the plain film diagnosis of diaphragmatic rupture is difficult. Serial radiographs can be helpful and in particular should be performed after a trauma patient is removed from positive pressure mechanical ventilation (19,22,24).

CT is superior to plain films for the detection and diagnosis of diaphragmatic rupture, and helical CT with multiplanar reformatted images is of further benefit (11,19,21,22). The CT findings of diaphragmatic injury include (a) sharp focal discontinuity of the diaphragm; (b) the "absent diaphragm" sign (nonvisualization of the diaphragm or a large gap between the torn ends of the diaphragm); (c) herniation of peritoneal fat, omentum, bowel, or an organ; (d) the "collar" sign (focal constriction of the bowel or an organ at the site of herniation); (e) the "dependent viscera" sign (herniated organs or bowel no longer supported posteriorly by the ruptured diaphragm fall dependently abutting the posterior ribs); and (f) concomitant pneumothorax and pneumoperitoneum and/or concomitant hemothorax and hemoperitoneum (Table 12.7, Figs. 12.27 and 12.28) (8,11,19,20,21,22).

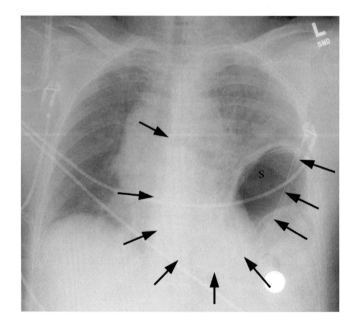

Figure 12.26 Diaphragmatic hernia. Chest radiograph demonstrates apparent elevation of the left hemidiaphragm, herniated gas filled stomach (S) above the diaphragm, and U-shaped course of the nasogastric tube (*arrows*). These findings are consistent with a diaphragmatic tear and gastric herniation.

Table 12.7: CT Findings of Diaphragmatic Injury

Sharp focal discontinuity of the diaphragm
"Absent diaphragm" sign
Herniation of peritoneal fat, omentum, bowel, or an organ
"Collar" sign
"Dependent viscera" sign
Concomitant pneumothorax and pneumoperitoneum
Concomitant hemothorax and hemoperitoneum

CT, computed tomography.

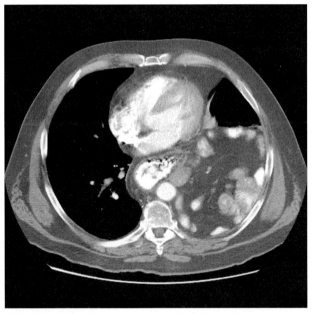

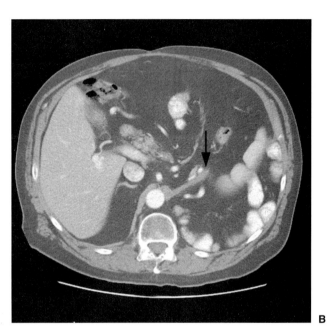

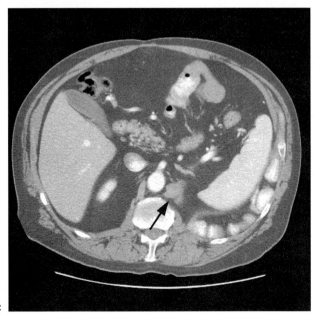

Figure 12.27 Diaphragmatic hernia. *A.* Computed tomography image demonstrates nonvisualization of the diaphragm ("absent diaphragm" sign), herniation of peritoneal fat and bowel, and bowel abutting the posterior ribs ("dependent viscera" sign). *B.* Computed tomography image demonstrates sharp focal discontinuity of the diaphragm (*arrow*) and "dependent viscera" sign. *C.* Computed tomography image demonstrates retraction and bunching of the torn diaphragm at the left crus (*arrow*).

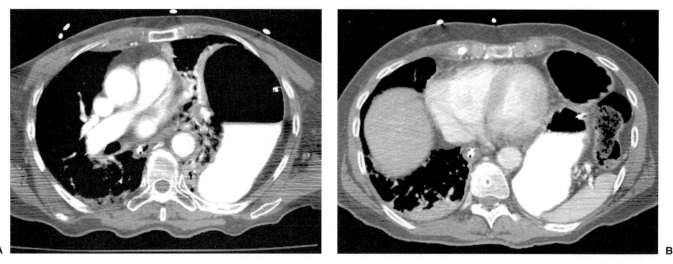

Figure 12.28 Diaphragmatic hernia. *A and B.* Computed tomography images demonstrate the stomach and spleen abutting the posterior ribs consistent with the "dependent viscera" sign secondary to diaphragmatic rupture with associated herniation.

MRI is also helpful for diagnosing diaphragm injuries but is generally not used in the acute trauma setting. MRI is generally used in stable patients with a delayed presentation in whom the CT findings are nondiagnostic or equivocal. (8,19) The MRI findings of diaphragmatic rupture are similar to the CT findings (Fig. 12.29). However, MRI has the advantage of direct coronal and sagittal imaging, allowing evaluation of diaphragm integrity from its insertion site to the dome. Optimal visualization is achieved with T1-weighted images, with the diaphragm appearing as a hypointense band outlined by hyperintense mediastinal and abdominal fat or the liver (8,19,25). Other studies, such as contrast studies of the intestine and radionuclide liver/spleen scans, can occasionally be useful.

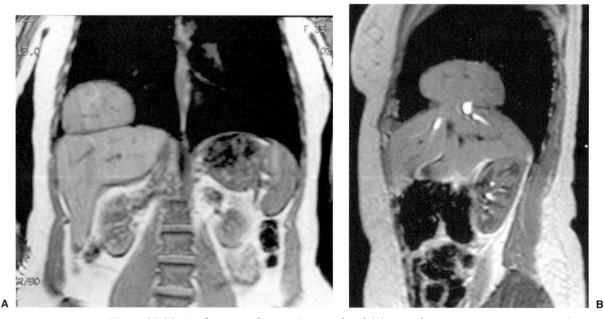

Figure 12.29 Diaphragmatic hernia. *A.* coronal and (*B*) sagittal magnetic resonance images demonstrate focal constriction of the liver as it herniates through a tear in the right hemidiaphragm ("collar" sign).

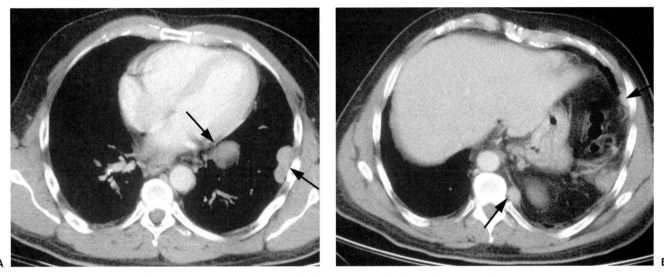

Figure 12.30 Intrathoracic splenosis. This patient was involved in a motor vehicle accident several years before and suffered splenic rupture along with a left diaphragmatic tear. Subsequently, a splenectomy and diaphragmatic repair were performed. *A and B.* Computed tomography images demonstrate an absent spleen consistent with the history of splenectomy and multiple enhancing pleural based nodules *(arrows).* A follow-up radiocolloid liver–spleen scan demonstrated uptake within these pleural based nodules, confirming splenic tissue.

A rare but interesting complication of diaphragmatic rupture is intrathoracic splenosis. This can occur when diaphragmatic rupture is associated with splenic rupture, allowing pieces of spleen to cross the diaphragmatic defect into the thorax and implant on the pleura. This leads to the appearance of pleural-based masses that can be mistaken for a neoplasm (Fig. 12.30). Liver–spleen scans are diagnostic, demonstrating radiocolloid uptake in the masses and confirming splenic tissue (10).

Penetrating injuries of the diaphragm are more common than blunt injuries. The site of injury is more random, depending on the trajectory of the penetrating object. These injuries also tend to be smaller; most are less than 2 cm and many are less than 1 cm, related to the size of the penetrating object. Visceral herniation is uncommon with these smaller injuries. These injuries are usually diagnosed clinically by relying on the entry site and direction of the wound. Patients with penetrating injuries commonly undergo exploratory surgery, at which time the diaphragmatic injury is diagnosed and repaired. Imaging findings include pneumothorax, hemothorax, or radiopaque material associated with the projectile near the diaphragm or indicating a path through the diaphragm (23,24).

UPPER ABDOMINAL INJURIES

It is important to scrutinize the portions of the upper abdomen that are visible at the inferior aspect of the chest radiograph. This is particularly true if fractures of the lower three ribs or signs of diaphragmatic injury are detected, because these findings are associated with significant intraabdominal injuries.

Prominent soft tissue opacity in the left upper quadrant along with medial deviation of the gastric air bubble, medial deviation of a nasogastric tube within the stomach, or inferior displacement of the splenic flexure suggests splenic injury with an associated perisplenic hematoma (26). Rigler sign (visualization of the bowel wall outlined by intraluminal air on the inside and free intraperitoneal air on the outside of a bowel loop) is evi-

An upright chest radiograph is the screening test of choice for detecting free intraperitoneal air.

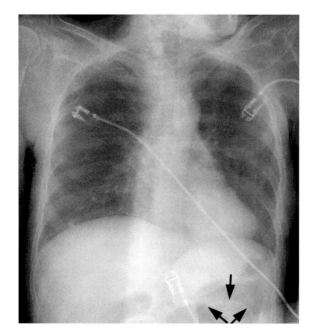

Figure 12.31 Pneumoperitoneum. Supine chest radiograph demonstrates Rigler sign (*arrows*) in the left upper quadrant.

dence of pneumoperitoneum on a supine study (Fig. 12.31). Bowel wall thickening can be a sign of intramural hematoma or ischemia, which in turn can be secondary to hypotension and shock or vascular injury and compromise. Gastric distension can predispose to vomiting and aspiration and can be seen with improper ventilation (Fig. 12.32) or gastric outlet problems related to duodenal injury (26).

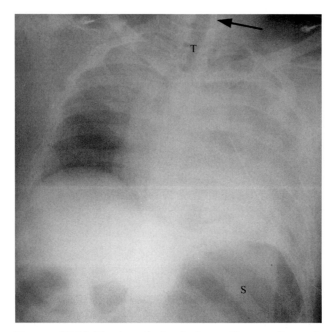

Figure 12.32 Esophageal intubation. Chest radiograph demonstrates significant gaseous distension of the stomach (S). The radiopaque stripe of an endotracheal tube (*arrow*) can be seen projecting outside of the tracheal (T) air column. Also, note the hypoventilatory changes in the lungs.

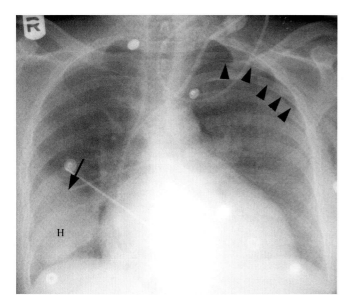

Figure 12.33 Traumatically inserted and malpositioned pulmonary artery catheter. Chest radiograph demonstrates the tip of a pulmonary artery catheter *(arrow)* located peripherally within the right lung. Adjacent parenchymal opacity represents a hematoma (H) caused by rupture of a small pulmonary artery branch secondary to peripheral inflation of the catheter tip balloon. There is also a left apical pneumothorax *(arrowheads)* secondary to previous unsuccessful attempts at placing the catheter into the left subclavian vein. The patient died the next day due to complications of these iatrogenic injuries.

IATROGENIC INJURIES

Iatrogenic injuries are those resulting from or occurring during the course of treatment by a health care professional. Vigorous cardiopulmonary resuscitation can cause sternal and rib fractures (2). Misplaced, malpositioned, or traumatically inserted lines and tubes can cause vascular, airway, esophageal, and lung injuries, resulting in hematomas, hemothorax, pneumothorax, pneumomediastinum, and atelectasis (Figs. 12.32, 12.33, 12.34, and 12.35) (1,7,8).

All lines, tubes, and devices should be checked for correct or incorrect position and complications.

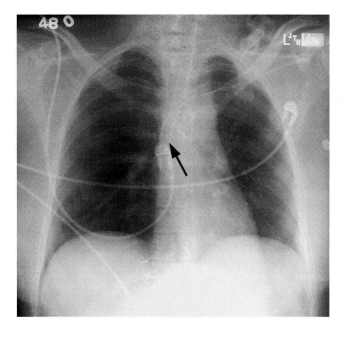

Figure 12.34 Malpositioned endotracheal tube. Chest radiograph demonstrates the endotracheal tube tip *(arrow)* in the right main bronchus. Notice the underinflation of the left lung and the overinflation of the right lung.

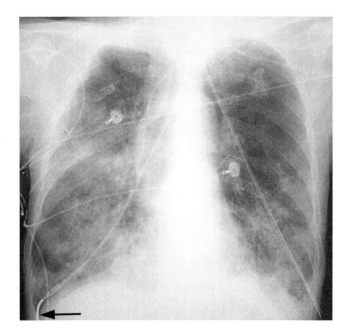

Figure 12.35 Misplaced feeding tube. Chest radiograph demonstrates tip of a feeding tube (*arrow*) in the region of the right costophrenic angle. Fortunately, this was detected before the initiation of tube feeds. However, the patient developed a pneumothorax that required insertion of a chest tube after removal of the feeding tube.

SUMMARY

Many important concepts and radiographic findings of thoracic trauma have been presented and reviewed in this chapter. The challenge is to recall and apply this knowledge quickly and efficiently when interpreting trauma studies in the hectic setting of the emergency room. A simple mnemonic based on the ABCs has been proposed to achieve this goal (7): A, aortic injuries; B, bronchial and tracheal injuries; C, cord and spine injuries; C, contusions and lacerations; D, diaphragm injuries; E, esophageal injuries; F, fractures (ribs, sternum, vertebra, clavicle, scapula); F, flail chest; G, gas (pneumothorax, pneumomediastinum, subcutaneous emphysema, pneumopericardium, pneumoperitoneum); H, heart and pericardial abnormalities (contusion, hemopericardium); H, hemothorax, hematoma, and hemorrhage; I, iatrogenic injuries (Table 12.8). (A multimedia presenta-

Table 12.8: The ABCs of Thoracic Trauma	
A	Aortic injuries
B	Bronchial and tracheal injuries
C	Cord and spinal injuries
C	Contusions and lacerations
D	Diaphragm injuries
E	Esophageal injuries
F	Fractures (ribs, sternum, vertebra, clavicle, scapula)
F	Flail chest
G	Gas (pneumothorax, pneumomediastinum, subcutaneous emphysema, pneumopericardium, pneumoperitoneum)
H	Heart and pericardial abnormalities (contusion, hemopericardium)
H	Hemothorax, hematoma, and hemorrhage
I	Iatrogenic injuries

From Gurney JW. ABCs of blunt chest trauma. In: *Thoracic imaging, 1996*. Reston, VA: Society of Thoracic Radiology, 1996:349–352, with permission.

tion of the "ABCs of Blunt Chest Trauma" can be viewed at Jud Gurney's website, *www.chestx-ray.com.*)

Remember the portable trauma chest radiograph is a screening tool used to guide and determine the need for additional imaging studies, usually CT. Aortic injuries, cardiac tamponade, and tension pneumothorax are the most immediate life-threatening conditions—followed closely by TBIs, esophageal injuries, hemothorax or hematoma caused by systemic arterial injuries, and flail chest. The diagnoses of diaphragmatic injuries, pericardial effusions, and thoracic duct injuries are often initially missed or delayed and may require serial studies. Positive pressure ventilation exacerbates TBIs and pneumothoraces and can also delay the appearance of a diaphragmatic hernia.

REFERENCES

1. Groskin SA. Selected topics in chest trauma. *Radiology* 1992;183:605–617.
2. Greene R. Blunt thoracic trauma. In: *Syllabus: a categorical course in diagnostic radiology, chest radiology*. Oak Brook, IL: Radiological Society of North America, 1992:297–309.
3. Parmley CF, Mattingly TW, Manion WC, et al. Nonpenetrating traumatic injury of the aorta. *Circulation* 1958;17:1086–1101.
4. Mirvis SE, Bidwell JK, Buddemeyer EU, et al. Value of chest radiograph in excluding traumatic aortic rupture. *Radiology* 1987;163:487–493.
5. Patel NH, Stephens KE, Mirvis SE, et al. Imaging of acute thoracic aortic injury due to blunt trauma: a review. *Radiology* 1998;209:335–348.
6. Dyer DS, Moore EE, Mestek MF, et al. Can chest CT be used to exclude aortic injury? *Radiology* 1999;213:195–202.
7. Gurney JW. ABCs of blunt chest trauma. In: *Thoracic imaging, 1996*. Reston, VA: Society of Thoracic Radiology, 1996:349–352.
8. Kuhlman JE, Pozniak MA, Collins J, et al. Radiographic and CT findings of blunt chest trauma: aortic injuries and looking beyond them. *RadioGraphics* 1998;18:1085–1106.
9. Kerns SR, Gay SB. CT of blunt chest trauma. *AJR Am J Roentgenol* 1990;154:55–60.
10. Dee PM. The radiology of chest trauma. *Radiol Clin North Am* 1992;30:291–306.
11. Van Hise ML, Primack SL, Israel RS, et al. CT in blunt chest trauma: indications and limitations. *RadioGraphics* 1998;18:1071–1084.
12. El-Khoury GY, Whitten CG. Trauma to the upper thoracic spine: anatomy, biomechanics, and unique imaging features. *AJR Am J Roentgenol* 1993;160:95–102.
13. Dennis LN, Rogers LF. Superior mediastinal widening from spine fractures mimicking aortic rupture on chest radiographs. *AJR Am J Roentgenol* 1989;152:27–30.
14. Wagner RB, Crawford WO, Schimpf PP. Classification of parenchymal injuries of the lung. *Radiology* 1988;167:77–82.
15. Hollister M, Stern EJ, Steinberg KP. Trauma cases from Harborview Medical Center type 2 pulmonary laceration: a marker of blunt high-energy injury to the lung. *AJR Am J Roentgenol* 1995;165:1126.
16. Bejvan SM, Godwin JD. Pneumomediastinum: old signs and new signs. *AJR Am J Roentgenol* 1996;166:1041–1048.
17. Zylak CM, Standen JR, Barnes GR, et al. Pneumomediastinum revisited. *RadioGraphics* 2000;20:1043–1057.
18. Unger JM, Schuchmann GG, Grossman JE, et al. Tears of the trachea and main bronchi caused by blunt trauma: radiographic findings. *AJR Am J Roentgenol* 1989;153:1175–1180.
19. Killeen K, Mirvis SE, Shanmuganathan K. Helical CT of diaphragmatic rupture caused by blunt trauma. *AJR Am J Roentgenol* 1999;173:1611–1616.
20. Bergin D, Ennis R, Keogh C, et al. The "dependent viscera" sign in CT diagnosis of blunt traumatic diaphragmatic rupture. *AJR Am J Roentgenol* 2001;177:1137–1140.
21. Worthy SA, Kang EY, Hartman TE, et al. Diaphragmatic rupture: CT findings in 11 patients. *Radiology* 1995;194:885–888.
22. Murray JG, Caoili E, Gruden JF, et al. Acute rupture of the diaphragm due to blunt trauma: diagnostic sensitivity and specificity of CT. *AJR Am J Roentgenol* 1996;166:1035–1039.

23. Shackleton KL, Stewart ET, Taylor AJ. Traumatic diaphragmatic injuries: spectrum of radiographic findings. *RadioGraphics* 1998;18:49–59.
24. Gelman R, Mirvis SE, Gens D. Diaphragmatic rupture due to blunt trauma: sensitivity of plain chest radiographs. *AJR Am J Roentgenol* 1991;156:51–57.
25. Shanmuganathan K, Mirvis SE, White CS, et al. MR imaging evaluation of hemidiaphragms in acute blunt trauma: experience with 16 patients. *AJR Am J Roentgenol* 1996;167:397–402.
26. Novelline RA. Abdomen: traumatic emergencies. In: Harris JH, Harris WH, Novelline RA, eds. *The radiology of emergency medicine*, 3rd ed. Baltimore: Williams & Wilkins, 1993:644–649, 659–663.

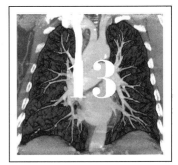

PULMONARY MANIFESTATIONS OF SYSTEMIC DISEASES

- Collagen Vascular Disease
- Polymyositis and Dermatomyositis
- Pulmonary Vasculitides
- Hematologic Disorders
- Metabolic Diseases
- Miscellaneous

Many systemic diseases have thoracic manifestations. In some patients the initial presentation of the disease can be abnormality on chest x-ray (CXR) or chest computed tomography (CT). Only some of the more common diseases are covered in this chapter.

COLLAGEN VASCULAR DISEASE

RHEUMATOID ARTHRITIS

Rheumatoid arthritis is usually insidious in onset, marked by ill health and chronic joint deformity. It has a prevalence of up to 2%, an age at onset of 25 to 55 years, and a male-to-female ratio of 1:3. Rheumatoid factor is positive in 50% to 70% of patients. The term "rheumatoid disease" may be more appropriate. Although the brunt of disease falls on the joints, this is a systemic connective tissue disease with extraarticular manifestations (pulmonary, cardiac, vascular, reticuloendothelial, hematologic, renal, and ocular) in up to 76% of patients (1–7). Rheumatoid lung disease affects 2% to 54% of patients with rheumatoid arthritis, with a male-to-female ratio of 5:1. The manifestations may be subdivided into eight categories (Table 13.1.).

Pleural abnormalities are most frequent (Fig. 13.1A), manifesting as unilateral exudative pleural effusion in 90% of patients and sometimes demonstrating little change over months. Bilateral large effusions can be seen. For pleural disease, the male-to-female ratio is 9:1 (5). There are usually not other pulmonary rheumatoid changes. Pleural disease may antedate the onset of arthritis. The effusion is an exudate with protein content greater than 4 g/dL, a low glucose content (less than 30 mg/dL), and no rise in pleural glucose during intravenous glucose infusion (as opposed to tuberculosis, which also has low pleural fluid glucose). There is generally a low white cell count with many lymphocytes, and pleural fluid is usually positive for rheumatoid factor, lactate dehydrogenase, and rheumatoid arthritis cells (8). Pleural thickening may also occur, usually bilaterally. Pleural fibrosis

Although rheumatoid disease has a 3:1 female predilection, rheumatoid lung disease has a 5:1 male-to-female ratio.

Table 13.1: Radiologic Manifestations of Rheumatoid Arthritis

Pleural abnormalities
Diffuse interstitial fibrosis
Necrobiotic nodules
Caplan syndrome
Bronchial abnormalities
Pulmonary arteritis
Cardiac enlargement
Bone abnormalities on chest radiograph

and adhesions are often found at autopsy. Pneumothorax can occur secondary to rupture of a rheumatoid nodule or end-stage fibrotic lung disease.

Diffuse interstitial fibrosis is seen in 2% to 6% (8), most frequently with seropositive rheumatoid arthritis. It causes a restrictive ventilatory defect with deposition of IgM in alveolar septa and has a lower lobe predominance. The radiographic findings are often indistinguishable from idiopathic pulmonary fibrosis or usual interstitial pneumonitis (Fig. 13.1B). Irregular linear opacities, honeycombing, or a reticulonodular pattern are seen in the lower lobes and occasionally more cephalad. High resolution CT (HRCT) has greatly improved early detection of fibrosis with inter- and intralobular septal thickening and patchy ground glass opacity, mainly in a subpleural distribution. As disease progresses, it eventually results in honeycombing. It is thought that rheumatoid lung disease is more benign than usual interstitial pneumonitis (7–9).

Necrobiotic nodules are identical to subcutaneous nodules. They are well-circumscribed masses in the lungs, pericardium, and visceral organs and are associated with advanced rheumatoid disease. They are a rare manifestation in the lungs. They are usually multiple and noncalcified, measuring 3 mm to 7 cm in size. They are commonly located in the lung periphery. Nodules may cavitate, typically with a thick wall and a smooth outline. They are often found in conjunction with subcutaneous nodules that wax and wane with the activity of the disease (1,3,7–9).

Caplan syndrome consists of multiple nodules due to hypersensitivity reaction to irritating coal dust particles in the lungs of coal miners with rheumatoid. Appearances are similar to necrobiotic nodules without pneumoconiosis. These well-defined nodules of 5 mm to 5 cm may develop rapidly. They tend to appear in clusters, predominantly in the upper lobes and in the lung periphery. Nodules may remain stable but may increase in

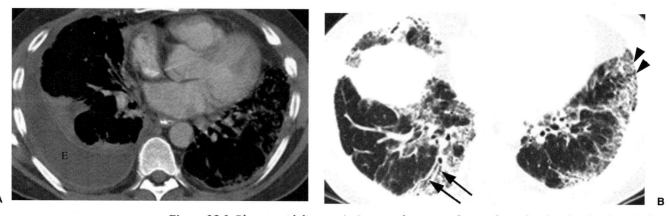

Figure 13.1 Rheumatoid disease. *A.* Computed tomography: moderate loculated right pleural effusion (E). *B.* High resolution computed tomography photographed at lung window settings, more caudal than *A*: peripheral basilar fibrotic change, with traction bronchiectasis (*arrows*) and honeycombing (*arrowheads*).

number, may calcify, or may resolve completely. There is no relationship between severity of arthritis and extent of nodules.

Bronchial abnormalities such as bronchiectasis or bronchiolitis obliterans occasionally occur. Pulmonary arteritis is a rare manifestation of rheumatoid arthritis, with fibroelastoid intimal proliferation of the pulmonary arteries that may result in pulmonary arterial hypertension and/or cor pulmonale (8). Cardiopericardial silhouette enlargement is also unusual and may result from pericarditis with pericardial effusion or myocarditis causing congestive cardiac failure.

Various bone abnormalities may be seen on the CXR. This includes arthritis of visualized joints, ankylosis of vertebral facet joints, and vertebral body collapse secondary to steroid therapy.

SYSTEMIC LUPUS ERYTHEMATOSUS

Systemic lupus erythematosus (SLE) has an incidence of 1 in 2,000, a typical age at onset between 20 and 40 years, and is nine times more common in females than males. It is common in the United States and East Asia, and the incidence is greater in African Americans. Among African-American women the incidence approaches 1 in 250, and disease often has a more severe course. There is an increased incidence of the human leukocyte antigens (HLAs) B8 and DR3. SLE may be exacerbated by sunlight and infection, and a lupus-like syndrome is induced by certain drugs such as hydralazine, oral contraceptives, phenothiazines, and procainamide. The most common early features are fever, arthralgia, general ill health, and weight loss. A characteristic manifestation is the "butterfly" rash on the face, although this does not have to be present. Antinuclear antibodies are present in 95%. The presence of antibodies to double-stranded DNA is diagnostic, although Sm antibodies are more specific for SLE. Hypergammaglobulinemia occurs in 77%, lupus erythematosus (LE) cells in 80%, and a false-positive Wasserman test for syphilis in 24%. SLE affects the joints in 90% of patients, the skin in 80%, the kidneys in 60%, the lungs in 50% to 70%, the cardiovascular system in 40%, the nervous system in 35%, and also the blood and lymphatic system (1,2,5–7). SLE affects the respiratory system more commonly than any other connective tissue disease, with radiologic abnormalities listed in Table 13.2.

Radiographically, the acute form (lupus pneumonitis) is characterized by poorly defined areas of ground glass opacity or consolidation peripherally at the lung bases. In the chronic form there is basal interstitial pulmonary fibrosis, seen in approximately 3% of patients (Fig. 13.2) (5). Bibasal fleeting plate-like atelectasis secondary to infection or infarction can also occur. Alveolar hemorrhage may manifest as ground glass opacity or consolidation. Patients with SLE have an increased incidence of pulmonary emboli secondary to circulating antiphospholipid antibodies. Pulmonary infections due to immunosuppressive therapy are also seen (10,11).

> SLE affects the respiratory system more commonly than any other connective tissue disease.

Table 13.2: Radiologic Manifestations of SLE

Pulmonary abnormalities
    Ground glass opacity (pneumonitis or hemorrhage)
    Consolidation (pneumonitis or hemorrhage)
    Atelectasis
    Pulmonary embolism
Pleural abnormalities
    Effusion (pleuritis)
    Thickening
Cardiovascular abnormalities
    Effusion (pericarditis)
    Cardiomegaly (cardiomyopathy)

SLE, systemic lupus erythematosus

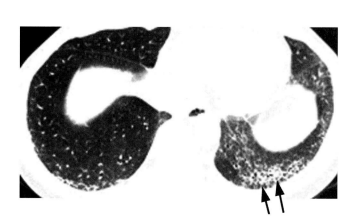

Figure 13.2 Systemic lupus erythematosus. High resolution computed tomography with basilar fibrotic disease, worst in the left lung (*arrows*).

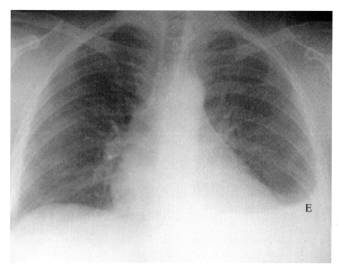

Figure 13.3 Systemic lupus erythematosus, with left pleural effusion (E).

Pleural effusion is the most common radiographic manifestation (Fig. 13.3), with recurrent small bilateral pleural effusions in 70%. Pleural thickening may also occur. Pericardial effusion from pericarditis is also common. Cardiomegaly from primary lupus cardiomyopathy is a rare manifestation (10,11).

PROGRESSIVE SYSTEMIC SCLEROSIS OR SCLERODERMA

Scleroderma has an incidence of 2 to 12 per million, a typical age at onset of less than 45 years, and a male-to-female ratio of 1:3. It is a systemic disease with atrophy and sclerosis of the skin, gastrointestinal tract, musculoskeletal system, lungs, and heart. There is an association with primary biliary cirrhosis. Blood vessels show arteritis and thickening. Generally, the clinical presentation includes fever, lassitude, and weight loss. Antinuclear antibodies are present in 30% to 80%. Anti-topoisomerase or antiScl-70 is present with diffuse cutaneous involvement; anti-centromere antibody is present in one-third of patients with progressive systemic sclerosis and in two-thirds of patients with a more limited form of the disease known as CREST (*c*alcinosis, *R*aynaud, *e*sophageal dysmotility, *s*clerodactyly, and *t*elangiectasias). Progressive systemic sclerosis affects the skin in 90% of patients; the vascular system, esophagus, and intestines in 80%; the lungs in 45%; the heart in 40%; the kidneys in 35%; and the musculoskeletal system in 25% (1,2,7,12).

Basilar interstitial pneumonitis and fibrosis is the usual CXR abnormality, present in up to 80% (3) of patients with lung disease. The basilar distribution is even more pronounced in progressive systemic sclerosis than in other collagen vascular diseases. On CXR there may be fine or coarse reticulations at the bases with low lung volumes. HRCT demonstrates inter- and intralobular septal thickening, subpleural lines and micronodules, ground glass opacity, and honeycombing (Fig. 13.4). Aspiration pneumonia may occur secondary to disturbed esophageal motility. Esophageal dysmotility may result in a dilated air esophagram on CXR or CT. Pleural involvement is rare. Pulmonary arterial hypertension occurs in 6% to 60% (13), and sclerosis of cardiac muscle may result in cor pulmonale. There is an increased risk of lung cancer, especially bronchoalveolar carcinoma.

Basilar distribution of lung disease, typical of most collagen vascular diseases, is especially pronounced in scleroderma.

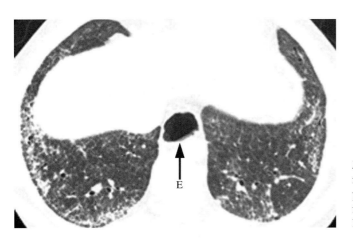

Figure 13.4 Scleroderma. High resolution computed tomography with interstitial abnormality limited to the lung bases. Note esophageal dilation (E).

POLYMYOSITIS AND DERMATOMYOSITIS

These diseases have an incidence of 1 to 8 per million, a bimodal age distribution with an early peak at 5 to 15 years and a later peak at 45 to 65 years, and male-to-female ratio of 1:4. There is an increased incidence of HLAs A1, B8, DR3, and DR5. Clinical presentation may be acute or chronic, with proximal muscle weakness, a heliotrope or violaceous skin rash in dermatomyositis, and telangiectasias over the joints of the hand. Dysphagia occurs in up to 50%. Skin and muscle changes may occur together or 2 to 3 months apart. General ill health and fever are common. Disease is associated with the anti-Jo1 antibody. In 10% there is an underlying malignancy, with carcinomas of lung, breast, stomach, and ovary being the most common. In men presenting over the age of 50, 60% have carcinoma, usually bronchogenic carcinoma (1,2,5). Polymyositis/dermatomyositis presents in one of four ways:

In 10% of polymyositis patients there is an underlying malignancy, often in lung, breast, stomach, or ovary.

1. Primary idiopathic polymyositis/dermatomyositis;
2. Childhood polymyositis/dermatomyositis;
3. Polymyositis/dermatomyositis with neoplasia;
4. Polymyositis/dermatomyositis with collagen vascular disease.

Chest radiographs are often normal. Basal interstitial pulmonary fibrosis indistinguishable from usual interstitial pneumonitis or nonspecific interstitial pneumonitis occurs in up to 10% (Figs. 13.5 and 13.6). Bronchiolitis obliterans and bronchiolitis oblit-

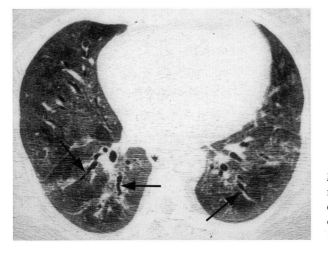

Figure 13.5 Dermatomyositis. High resolution computed tomography demonstrates extensive ground glass opacity with traction bronchiectasis (*arrows*).

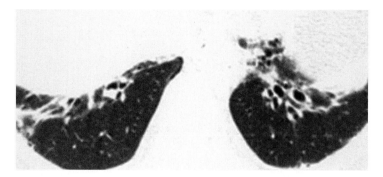

Figure 13.6 Dermatomyositis. High resolution computed tomography predominantly with traction bronchiectasis at the extreme lung bases.

erans organizing pneumonia also occur. When pharyngeal muscle paralysis occurs in polymyositis, aspiration pneumonia may develop. Diaphragmatic elevation with small lung volumes can also be seen (3,7,14).

ANKYLOSING SPONDYLITIS

Unlike other collagen vascular diseases, lung disease in ankylosing spondylitis has an upper lobe predilection.

Of all the seronegative arthritides, ankylosing spondylitis is the main one with chest manifestations. It has an incidence of 1 in 1,000, an age at onset of 15 to 35 years, and male-to-female ratio of 4:1. It is most common in people from the Indian subcontinent. It is more common in whites than blacks and is rare in East Asians. There is a 90% association with HLA B27 (1,2,5). Characteristic findings include synovitis, juxtaarticular osteitis and chondritis with erosion of subchondral bone, and skeletal ankylosis, especially of the sacroiliac joints. Calcification of paraspinal ligaments is noted if there is involvement of the lumbar, thoracic, or cervical spine. Aortic regurgitation is seen in up to 5% of patients. In 1% to 2% of patients, upper lobe pulmonary fibrosis and bullae develop. These fibrobullous lesions may contain mycetomas and are occasionally secondarily infected by *Mycobacterium tuberculosis* (3,7,15).

PULMONARY VASCULITIDES

The pulmonary vasculitides can be categorized according to the size of the vessels primarily involved (Table 13.3) and to whether they are associated with an elevated antinuclear cytoplasmic antibody (ANCA). These disorders have manifestations in many other organ systems, commonly the skin and kidneys, and frequently present with pulmonary hemorrhage (3).

NON–ANTINUCLEAR CYTOPLASMIC ANTIBODY ASSOCIATED VASCULITIDES

Large Vessel (Giant Cell) Vasculitis
Giant cells are a prominent histologic feature of both giant cell (temporal) and Takayasu arteritis. The aorta and great vessels are usually affected, and CT may demonstrate vascular narrowing. Other chest manifestations are extremely rare (1,2,16,17).

Medium-sized Vessel Vasculitis
In polyarteritis nodosa, pulmonary artery involvement is rare, whereas bronchial artery involvement is common. However, thoracic radiologic findings are usually secondary to

Table 13.3: Principle Systemic Vasculitides

Large vessel vasculitides
    Giant cell (temporal) arteritis
    Takayasu arteritis
Medium-sized vessel arteritis
    Polyarteritis nodosa
    Kawasaki disease
Small vessel vasculitis
    ANCA associated (pauci-immune, lacking immune complex)
        Microscopic polyangiitis
        Wegener granulomatosis
        Churg-Strauss syndrome
    Immune complex vasculitis
        Henoch-Schonlein purpura
        Mixed cryoglobulinemia
        Connective tissue disorders
        Hypocomplementemic urticarial vasculitis
        Behçet disease
        Goodpasture syndrome
        Serum sickness/drug/infection

ANCA, Antinuclear cytoplasmic antibody.

cardiac and/or renal failure. A few cases of idiopathic pulmonary fibrosis and cryptogenic organizing pneumonia have been described (1,2,17).

ANTINUCLEAR CYTOPLASMIC ANTIBODY ASSOCIATED VASCULITIDES

Microscopic Polyangiitis

Microscopic polyangiitis is pauci-immune necrotizing small vessel angiitis without granulomatous inflammation. It is a rare disease, has a mean age at onset of 50 years, and a male-to-female ratio of 2:1. It presents with constitutional symptoms, including fever, arthralgias, myalgias, and purpura. pANCA is present in more than 80% of patients. It is the most common cause of a pulmonary–renal syndrome. Common radiologic findings in the chest are pulmonary edema in 6% of patients and pleural effusion in 15% (1,2,3,16).

Wegener Granulomatosis

Classic Wegener granulomatosis is a triad of (a) upper and lower respiratory tract necrotizing granulomatous inflammation, (b) systemic small vessel vasculitis, and (c) necrotizing glomerulonephritis. It has an incidence of 3 per million, a mean age at onset of 40 years, and a male-to-female ratio of 1.3:1. There is an increased incidence of HLAs B8 and DR2. Onset is usually acute or subacute but may be indolent. In patients with Wegener granulomatosis, 85% have a positive cANCA (1–3).

The upper respiratory tract is involved in 100% of cases, affecting the nasal cavity with cartilage destruction and the sinuses with mucosal thickening. Pulmonary involvement is present in 85% to 90% (5). The classic CXR shows widely distributed multiple irregular nodules or masses, varying up to 9 cm, mainly in the lower lungs. Nodules cavitate in 25% to 50% of patients (Fig. 13.7) and are sometimes single. Patchy airspace disease due to pneumonia or pulmonary hemorrhage also occurs (Fig. 13.8). Pleural effusions occur in

Common thoracic manifestations of Wegener granulomatosis are lung nodules or cavities, pulmonary hemorrhage, pleural effusions, and tracheobronchial stenosis.

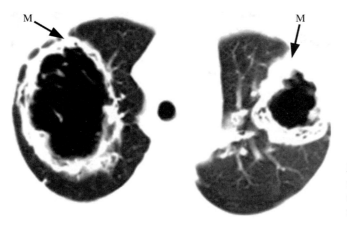

Figure 13.7 Wegener granulomatosis. Computed tomography reveals large bilateral cavitary masses (M).

25% and tracheobronchial stenosis is not uncommon (Fig. 13.9), but lymph node enlargement is rare. Limited Wegener granulomatosis is Wegener granulomatosis without the renal involvement (3,16–18).

Churg-Strauss Syndrome

This consists of a triad of (a) allergic rhinitis and asthma, (b) eosinophilic pneumonia and gastroenteritis, and (c) systemic small vessel vasculitis with granulomatous inflammation. The disease often evolves in this order. It is rare, has a typical age at onset of 38 to 57 years, and affects men and women equally. pANCA is elevated in 70%, cANCA is rarely elevated, tissue eosinophilia occurs in 100% with serum eosinophilia in greater than 30%, and serum IgE is commonly elevated. The cardiac, gastrointestinal, skin, and central nervous systems are commonly involved (1–3,5). CXR manifestations include patchy airspace disease, noncavitary pulmonary nodules, and pleural effusions. Cardiopericardial silhouette enlargement results from pericarditis and/or myocarditis (16,17,19).

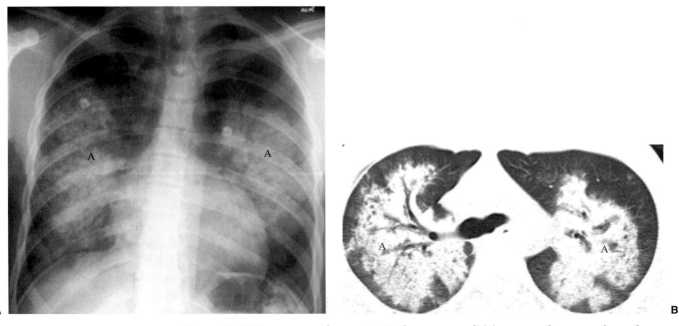

Figure 13.8 Wegener granulomatosis. *A.* Chest x-ray and (*B*) computed tomography: pulmonary hemorrhage manifesting as bilateral central airspace disease (A).

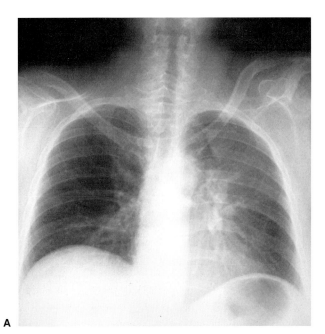

A

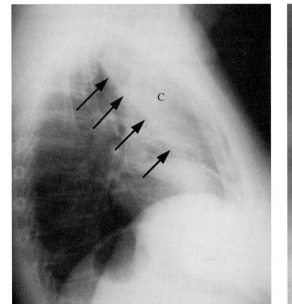

B

C

Figure 13.9 Wegener granulomatosis. A. Posteroanterior and (B) lateral chest x-ray: left upper lobe collapse (C), best seen on the lateral radiograph, where the major fissure is displaced anteriorly (arrows). C. Conventional tomogram through the left upper lobe bronchus: marked bronchial narrowing (arrows).

IMMUNE-COMPLEX VASCULITIS

Necrotizing Sarcoidal Angiitis

Necrotizing sarcoidal angiitis is distinguished from sarcoidosis by the presence of arteritis. It is a rare disorder, has a mean age at onset of 45 years, and a male-to-female ratio of 1:2.5. In general, this is a benign condition that does not require treatment (1–3). Radiologically, the most common pattern is bilateral nodules, occurring in 75% of patients and ranging up to 4 cm in diameter. There is a slight predilection for the lower lobes. Nodules may cavitate and may be miliary. Less common patterns include bilateral airspace disease, basal interstitial abnormality, and pleural effusions (16).

Diffuse Pulmonary (Alveolar) Hemorrhage

Table 13.4 lists the causes of diffuse pulmonary hemorrhage (3).

Table 13.4: Causes of Diffuse Pulmonary Hemorrhage

Antiglomerular basement membrane (Goodpasture disease)
ANCA-associated small vessel vasculitides
Microscopic polyangiitis
Wegener granulomatosis
Churg-Struss syndrome
Immune complex disease/collagen vascular disease
Systemic lupus erythematosus
Other CVD (RA, PSS, Polymyositis, Mixed connective tissue disease)
Henoch-Schonlein purpura
Antiphospholipid syndrome
Behçet's disease
Mixed cryoglobulinemia
Idiopathic pulmonary hemosiderosis
Coagulopathy
Drugs/chemicals

ANCA, Antinuclear cytoplasmic antibody.

Goodpasture disease affects the lungs and kidneys, but hemoptysis typically precedes renal disease.

Antiglomerular Basement Membrane Disease (Goodpasture Disease). Goodpasture disease is a rare disease with an incidence of 1 in two million, a typical age at onset of 20 to 30 years, and a male-to-female ratio of 2 to 9:1. It is rare in African Americans and is essentially a disease of young white males. There is an increased incidence of HLA DR2. When there is pulmonary involvement, it is termed Goodpasture syndrome. Classically, antiglomerular basement membrane disease is a triad of (a) glomerulonephritis, (b) circulating antibodies against the glomerular and alveolar basement membranes, and (c) pulmonary hemorrhage (1,2,20). Usually, IgG causes linear immunofluorescent staining of the basement membranes. Hemoptysis is the most common and earliest feature of Goodpasture disease, typically preceding renal disease by several months. This disease has a poor prognosis, with one series showing 96% mortality and a mean survival of 15 weeks (3). Therapy includes supportive care, plasmapheresis to remove circulating antibodies, and immunosuppression to stop the production of antibodies.

Acute pulmonary hemorrhage causes diffuse or sometimes patchy airspace disease, predominantly in a perihilar distribution (Fig. 13.10) and at the lung bases, with sparing of the costophrenic angles and apices. It is asymmetric and often unilateral. On CT, acute pulmonary hemorrhage is often seen as ground glass opacity or airspace disease, patchy or diffuse. With time this is replaced by a reticular pattern that resolves in less than 2 weeks. If there are repeated hemorrhages, interstitial fibrosis can develop, causing a permanent reticular pattern. Hilar lymph nodes may be enlarged during acute episodes (16,20).

Idiopathic Pulmonary Hemosiderosis. This is a rare disease of childhood with the usual age at onset between 1 and 7 years. Only 20% of cases present over the age of 10. In children males and females are equally affected, but for those older than 20 years of age the male-to-female ratio is 2:1. There is an association with celiac disease and dermatitis herpetiformis. Idiopathic pulmonary hemosiderosis is characterized by a triad of (a) pulmonary hemorrhage, (b) iron-deficiency anemia, and (c) immunoallergic reaction with eosinophilia and mastocytosis (1–4).

Radiologically, abnormalities are identical to those seen in Goodpasture disease, with patchy or diffuse perihilar or basilar airspace disease, in time replaced by a diffuse reticular pattern (Fig. 13.11). With recurrent hemorrhage, generalized fibrosis can occur. HRCT demonstrates patchy or diffuse ground glass opacity or airspace disease in the acute stage, later progressing to fibrosis. Magnetic resonance imaging is particularly useful because of the paramagnetic qualities of intraalveolar hemosiderin, demonstrating high signal on T1

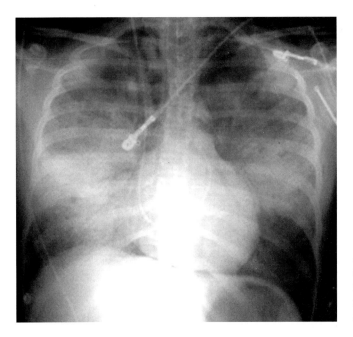

Figure 13.10 Goodpasture disease. Bilateral airspace disease results from pulmonary hemorrhage. Surprisingly, the patient is a woman.

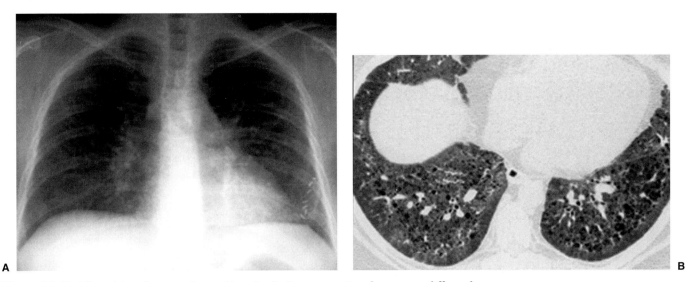

A B

Figure 13.11 Idiopathic pulmonary hemosiderosis. *A.* Posteroanterior chest x-ray: diffuse abnormality of the lungs, not well characterized. *B.* High resolution computed tomography: extensive traction bronchiectasis, honeycombing, and interlobular septal thickening from chronic idiopathic pulmonary hemosiderosis.

and markedly low signal on T2. This allows a diagnosis of hemorrhage that can aid patient management, especially in the very young (3).

HEMATOLOGIC DISORDERS

SICKLE CELL DISEASE

Sickle cell disease is the term given to the group of disorders characterized by the presence of hemoglobin S (HbS). The homozygous form (HbSS) is known as sickle cell anemia and the heterozygous form (HbSA) is known as sickle trait; there are other heterozygous variants. Up to 13% of African Americans have sickle trait (5). The disease only presents after the sixth month of life when fetal hemoglobin (HbF) is replaced by HbS. Red blood cells containing HbS have reduced oxygen transfer capabilities, and at lower oxygen tensions are less plastic, adopting the characteristic sickle shape. This leads to increased blood viscosity and stasis in areas of slow flow or high metabolism. Sickle cell anemia mainly affects the bones and bone marrow, brain, kidney, and spleen but also has manifestations within the chest (1,2). Findings on the CXR may be cardiac, pulmonary, osseous, and abdominal (Table 13.5).

> Autosplenectomy in sickle cell disease increases the risk of infections caused by *S. pneumoniae, H. influenzae, Mycoplasma, Salmonella,* and *Staphylococcus.*

Chronic anemia may result in cardiomegaly and pulmonary plethora. Sickle cell patients may present with "acute chest syndrome." This is a triad of (a) fever, (b) clinical findings of a pulmonary process, and (c) radiologic pulmonary disease. This is a frequent cause for hospitalization. Acute chest syndrome results in lobar or segmental airspace disease, atelectasis, and/or pleural effusions. It is caused by pneumonia or infarction, and distinguishing the two can be difficult. Sickle cell patients are at increased risk of infection, especially with *Streptococcus pneumoniae, Haemophilus influenza,* and *Mycoplasma* due to autosplenectomy. *Salmonella* and *Staphylococcus* infections also occur. Infarction is rare in children, so that acute chest syndrome is usually due to infection. Infarcts are more frequent in adults, although most cases of sickle cell crisis are still due to infection. Imaging for infarction is difficult. Pulmonary angiography is not generally indicated, ventilation-perfusion scanning is often indeterminate, and CT pulmonary angiography may be required. Pulmonary infarct is often associated with evidence of infarction elsewhere, such as in the abdomen, muscle, and bone (3,21–23).

Coarsening and diffuse sclerosis of the thoracic skeleton results from chronic anemia and infarction. Infarcts within the central portions of the vertebral bodies result in H-

---

Table 13.5: Chest Radiographic Manifestations of Sickle Cell Disease

Lung/pleura
    Consolidation (infection or acute chest syndrome)
    Atelectasis
    Pleural effusion
Cardiac
    Cardiomegaly
    Increased pulmonary blood flow
Osseous
    Osteosclerosis
    Humeral head infarcts (focal sclerosis or periosteal reaction)
    H-shaped vertebral bodies
    Short ribs
Abdominal
    Splenomegaly
    Splenic infarction (small and/or calcified spleen)
    Cholelithiasis

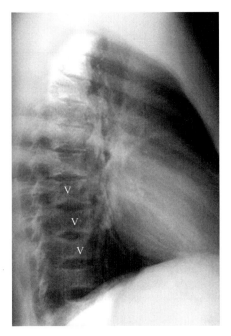

Figure 13.12 Sickle cell disease. Lateral chest x-ray shows typical H-shaped vertebrae (V).

shaped vertebrae (Fig. 13.12). Periosteal reaction may be due to infarction or infection. Infarcts of the humeral head result in focal sclerosis, called "snow-capping." Ribs may be shortened (4). Below the diaphragm cholelithiasis or cholecystectomy clips may be noted, because sickle cell patients have an increased incidence of gallstones secondary to increased hemoglobin turnover. Children may have splenomegaly, whereas adults may have a prominent gastric air bubble as a manifestation of autosplenectomy.

EXTRAMEDULLARY HEMATOPOIESIS

Extramedullary hematopoiesis is the formation of blood outside the bone marrow in the reticuloendothelial organs such as liver, spleen, and lymph nodes. It occurs in severe anemia, usually in congenital anemias such as spherocytosis and sickle cell disease (1,2). The lungs are rarely involved. On CXR or CT, extramedullary hematopoiesis manifests as multifocal smooth paravertebral masses, usually in the lower chest (Fig. 13.13). There may be additional extrapleural masses adjacent to ribs, which may or may not be continuous with the paravertebral masses. Masses can be unilateral or bilateral. They usually do not cause pressure erosion of adjacent bone, a differentiating point from neurogenic tumors (4,24).

Unlike neurogenic tumors, masses of extramedullary hematopoiesis tend not to erode adjacent bone.

LYMPHOPROLIFERATIVE DISORDERS OF THE LUNG

There are many forms of lymphoproliferative disease in the lung (3), with radiologic manifestations including solitary and multiple masses within the lung and/or mediastinum and solitary and multiple lung nodules, areas of ground glass opacity, or consolidation. A list of lymphoproliferative disorders is given in Table 13.6. Lymphoma is discussed in Chapters 8 and 9.

Posttransplant Lymphoproliferative Disorder

Posttransplant lymphoproliferative disorder occurs in 2% of transplant patients, especially heart-lung and renal transplant patients. It is associated with Epstein-Barr infection and immunosuppression. Radiologically, there may be one or multiple nodules and hilar or mediastinal lymph node enlargement (25,26).

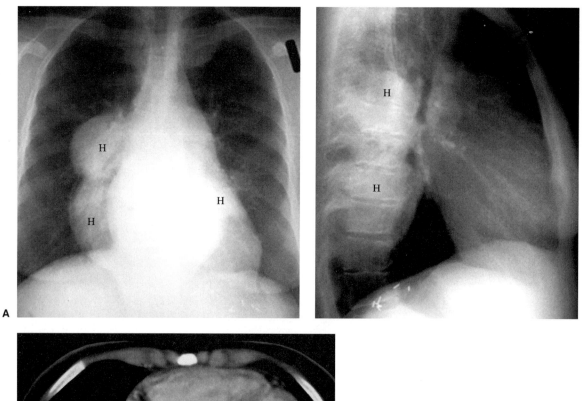

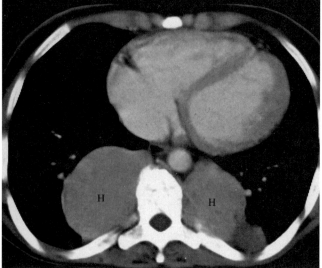

Figure 13.13 Extramedullary hematopoiesis. A. Posteroanterior and (B) lateral chest x-ray: multilobular bilateral posterior mediastinal masses (H). C. Computed tomography: soft tissue attenuation paravertebral masses (H).

Table 13.6: Lymphoproliferative Disorders of the Lung

Plasma cell granuloma
Posttransplant lymphoproliferative disorder
Lymphoid interstitial pneumonitis
Lymphomatoid granulomatosis
Pseudolymphoma
Angioimmunoblastic lymphadenopathy
Castleman disease

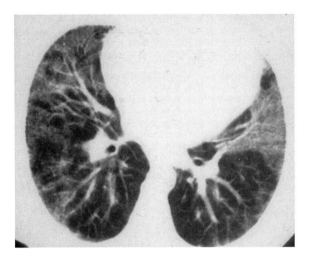

Figure 13.14 Lymphoid interstitial pneumonitis. Ground glass opacity predominantly in the lower anterior lungs.

Lymphoid Interstitial Pneumonitis

Lymphoid interstitial pneumonitis is associated with acquired immunodeficiency syndrome in children and autoimmune and connective tissue disease in adults. Radiologically, it may appear as septal lines, reticulonodular opacities, or nodules. HRCT is particularly useful in its assessment and may demonstrate ground glass opacity (Fig. 13.14). Honeycombing and fibrosis can ultimately occur. Lymphoid interstitial pneumonitis may progress to typical lymphoma (Fig. 13.15). In fact, other than Castleman disease the lymphoproliferative disorders (Fig. 13.16) are now thought to be lymphomas (26).

LEUKEMIA

The leukemias are a heterogeneous group of neoplasms of the hematopoietic cells. They may be of myeloid or lymphoid cell origin and acute or chronic in presentation

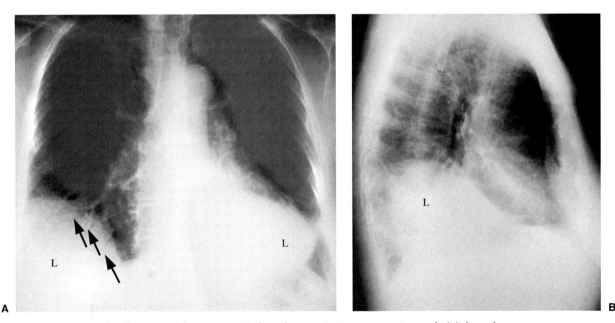

A

B

Figure 13.15 Lymphoid interstitial pneumonitis/lymphoma. *A.* Posteroanterior and *(B)* lateral chest x-ray: mass-like bibasilar airspace disease (L) with air bronchograms *(arrows)*. The biopsy was interpreted as lymphoid interstitial pneumonitis and/or lymphoma, reflecting the overlap of these entities.

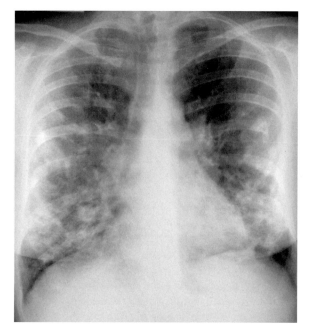

Figure 13.16 Pseudolymphoma. Widespread nodular and patchy opacities, with questionable cavities in the right lung.

(Table 13.7). There is an overall incidence of 13 per 100,000, but this varies depending on the specific type of leukemia and the affected age range. Acute leukemias are more common in children and young adults, whereas chronic leukemias are more common in older adults. Abnormalities seen on chest imaging in leukemia can be divided into three categories, as listed in Table 13.8 (1,2,27,28).

Leukemic infiltration of the lung is common pathologically but is rarely a cause of significant opacities on the chest radiograph. Lung parenchymal abnormalities are better seen on HRCT, but it can be difficult to diagnose the nature of the abnormality. Hemorrhage and infection cannot be distinguished, and both may resemble leukemic infiltrate (Fig. 13.17). Occasionally, leukemic infiltrates can present with a "tree-in-bud" appearance (29).

T-cell leukemias may show massive mediastinal lymph node enlargement that resolves quickly with treatment. Pleural effusions are common. Subpleural and chest wall deposits may occur, causing extraparenchymal masses that may be associated with rib destruction (called chloromas). Chloromas most commonly occur with myeloid leukemias (3).

Pulmonary infection, hemorrhage, and edema are complications of the disease and also of its treatment. Drug reactions may occur, with alveolitis or pulmonary fibrosis. The CXR is very useful for detecting pulmonary abnormality but less useful for distinguishing the specific etiology (29).

Acute graft-versus-host disease occurs 20 to 100 days after bone marrow transplantation. The effects in the lungs are minimal, with the brunt of the disease affecting skin, gastrointestinal tract, and liver. After 100 days it is termed chronic graft-versus-host disease.

Table 13.7: Common Leukemias

Myeloid leukemias
   Acute myeloid leukemia
   Chronic myeloid leukemia
Lymphoid leukemias
   Acute lymphoblastic leukemia
   Chronic lymphocytic leukemia
   Hairy-cell leukemia

Table 13.8: Thoracic Leukemia Categories of Abnormality

Leukemic infiltrates of the lung, intrathoracic lymph nodes, pleura, and/or chest wall
Complications of the disease or its treatment
Graft-versus-host disease

The CXR is frequently normal. When abnormal, there may be diffuse or patchy perihilar airspace disease. More severe disease may result in development of a diffuse interstitial pattern. Bronchiolitis obliterans is the most common finding in chronic graft-versus-host disease and is best appreciated on HRCT with expiratory scanning. This reveals bronchial wall dilation, a mosaic pattern of altered attenuation, and evidence of air trapping on the expiratory scans (30).

Chronic graft-versus-host disease of the lungs is best diagnosed with HRCT that includes expiratory scans.

MULTIPLE MYELOMA

Multiple myeloma is a malignant proliferation of plasma cells from a single clone. It has an incidence of approximately 3 per 100,000, usually presents in the fifth to eighth decade with 98% of patients over the age of 40, and has a male-to-female ratio of 2:1. Blacks have nearly twice the incidence of whites. It is diagnosed by the presence of a monoclonal gammopathy on serum electrophoresis (1,2,5).

Lung involvement is rare. However, thoracic lymph node enlargement and pleural effusions can occur. Myeloma predominantly affects bone; on the CXR this can be seen as generalized osteoporosis of the ribs and vertebral bodies with widespread osteolytic lesions. Expansile lytic rib lesions can occur, as can extrapleural soft tissue masses that erode rib (Fig. 13.18). Plasmacytomas may occur in unexpected locations (Fig. 13.19). In 10% of patients, amyloidosis develops (p. 341).

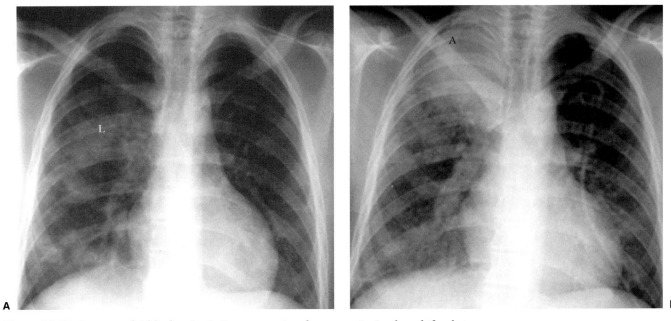

A   B

Figure 13.17 Acute myeloid leukemia. *A.* Posteroanterior chest x-ray in April: multifocal airspace disease, most visible in the right suprahilar lung (L). Biopsy revealed leukemic infiltration, and abnormality resolved after administration of chemotherapy. *B.* Posteroanterior chest x-ray in July: new mass-like opacity at right apex (A) proved to be invasive aspergillosis.

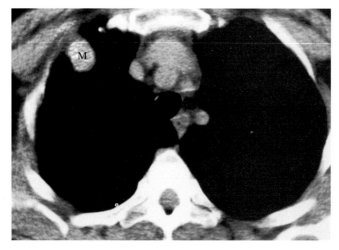

Figure 13.18 Multiple myeloma with extraparenchymal mass (M).

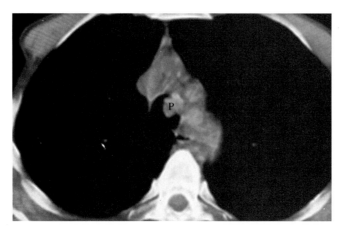

Figure 13.19 Tracheal plasmacytoma (P).

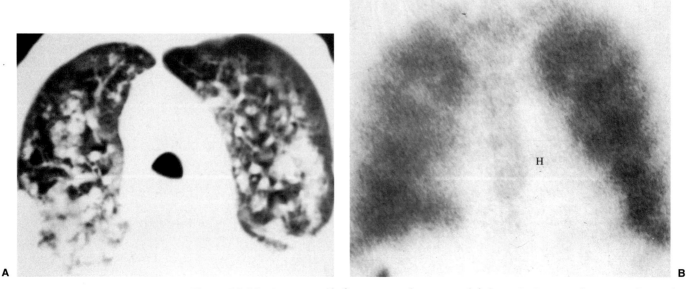

Figure 13.20 Metastatic calcifications in chronic renal failure. *A.* Computed tomography: widespread airspace disease with a somewhat nodular character. *B.* Radionuclide bone scan: image of the chest reveals bilateral uptake throughout the lungs, creating a "negative image" of the heart (H).

METABOLIC DISEASES

RENAL DISEASE

Nephrotic syndrome and renal failure cause a variety of abnormalities on chest imaging. Both can result in pleural effusions, usually bilateral, due to hypoproteinemia or fluid overload. They can also result in airspace disease on CXR due to fluid, red cells, or white cells in the alveoli. Pulmonary edema can occur secondary to fluid imbalance and hypoproteinemia. Hemorrhage can occur as part of diseases such as Goodpasture disease and Wegener granulomatosis (discussed above) or during anticoagulation for dialysis. Renal patients are subtly immunosuppressed and are more prone to infections, including those with atypical organisms. This is especially true of renal transplant patients on immunosuppressive therapy. Patients with renal failure may also develop pericardial effusions due to uremic pericarditis. Metastatic calcification can occur due to renal impairment with secondary hyperparathyroidism (1–4,31).

METASTATIC PULMONARY CALCIFICATION

Metastatic pulmonary or soft tissue calcification can occur in patients with chronic renal impairment, secondary hyperparathyroidism, multiple myeloma, hypervitaminosis D, milk-alkali syndrome, and sarcoidosis. On CXR there is typically persistent airspace disease without clinical evidence of pneumonia or pulmonary edema. In fact, patients are generally minimally symptomatic or asymptomatic. CT may demonstrate that abnormality is high in attenuation. Increased activity on radionuclide bone scan (Fig. 13.20) clinches the diagnosis (1–4,32).

LIVER DISEASE

Liver disease is a rare cause of pulmonary parenchymal abnormalities. Liver disease can result in hypoproteinemia and/or portal hypertension with pleural effusions, unilateral or bilateral. Reduced clotting factors in cirrhosis can cause pulmonary hemorrhage. Hepatomegaly can cause elevation of the right hemidiaphragm and atelectasis at the right lung base (1–4).

AMYLOIDOSIS

Amyloidosis is the extracellular deposition of proteinaceous twisted β-pleated sheet fibrils. It may be localized or systemic. The classification of amyloidosis is listed in Table 13.9 (1,2,5).

Table 13.9: Classification of Amyloidosis

Systemic
    Primary amyloidosis (AL type)
    Amyloidosis associated with multiple myeloma/Waldenstrom macroglobulinemia
      (AL type)
    Amyloidosis secondary or reactive to chronic infection and inflammation (AA type)
    Heredofamilial amyloidosis (AA type)
Localized
    Localized amyloidosis (AL type)
    Amyloidosis associated with aging (AL type)

***Table 13.10: Thoracic Manifestations
of Pulmonary Amyloidosis***

Tracheobronchial
   Diffuse airway narrowing
   Multifocal airway narrowing
   Focal endobronchial mass(es)
Nodular parenchymal
   Nodules(s) (+/− calcification)
   Lymph node enlargement (+/− calcification)
   Pleural effusion
Diffuse parenchymal
   Interstitial lung disease (septal lines, honeycombing)

In systemic amyloidosis there may be pathologic involvement of the lungs, but clinical or radiologic manifestations are rare. Most cases of pulmonary amyloidosis are of the localized type, which affects the lung parenchyma and/or the airways. It usually follows one of three patterns, as given in Table 13.10 (5).

Tracheobronchial amyloidosis is the most common type. It may be diffuse or nodular, but diffuse disease is more common. Radiologically, diffuse disease causes multiple eccentric or concentric areas of stricture, sometimes with calcification and typically affecting the trachea or bronchi to the segmental level. In the nodular form, nodules protrude from the trachea and/or main bronchi. The membranous portion of the trachea is involved, in contradistinction to tracheobronchopathia osteoplastica, where the membranous portion is spared (Figs. 13.21 and 13.22).

The nodular parenchymal form is less common than the tracheobronchial form and usually occurs in patients less than 60 years old. These patients are often asymptomatic. There may be mediastinal or hilar lymph node enlargement or calcification (Figs. 13.23 and 13.24). The nodules may be single or multiple, tend to have a peripheral or subpleural

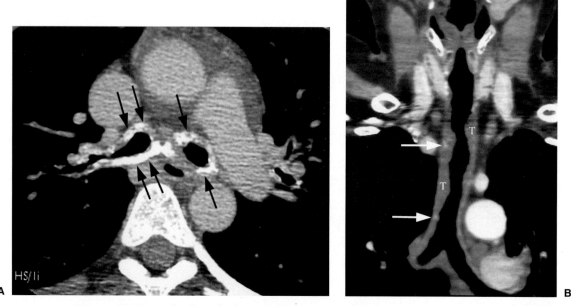

Figure 13.21 Tracheobronchial amyloidosis. *A.* Computed tomography: plaque-like calcification around the entire circumference of the tracheobronchial tree *(arrows)*. *B.* Coronal reconstruction: marked wall thickening (T) with foci of calcification *(arrows)*.

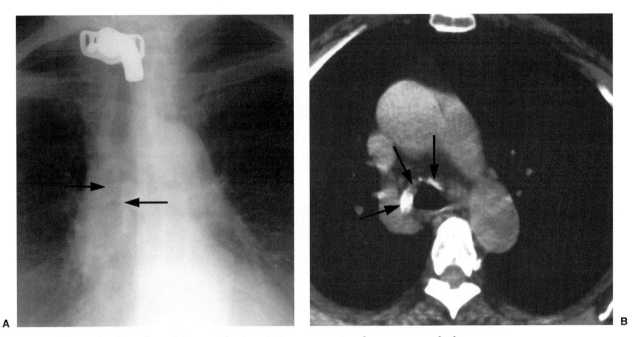

Figure 13.22 Tracheobronchopathia osteoplastica. *A.* Posteroanterior chest x-ray: marked narrowing of bronchus intermedius *(arrows)*. *B.* Computed tomography: calcification *(arrows)* does not extend around the entire tracheal circumference.

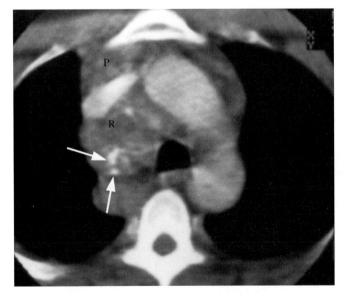

Figure 13.23 Amyloidosis. Enlarged right paratracheal (R) and prevascular (P) lymph nodes with speckled calcification *(arrows)*. (Courtesy of Dr. E. V. Bouffard III, Olney, IL.)

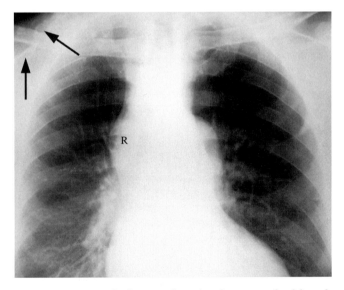

Figure 13.24 Amyloidosis. Enlarged right paratracheal lymph nodes (R) with faintly visible calcification of supraclavicular lymph nodes *(arrows)*.

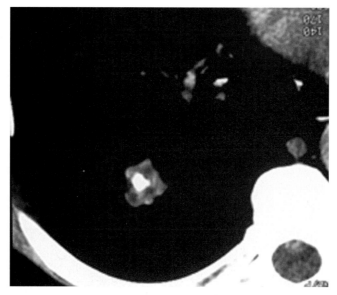

Figure 13.25 Amyloidosis. Calcified right lung nodule.

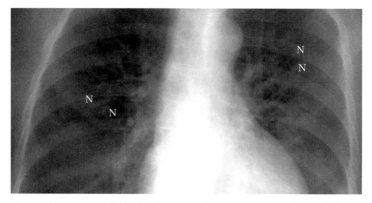

Figure 13.26 Amyloidosis. Multiple bilateral lung nodules (N). At computed tomography, several were faintly calcified.

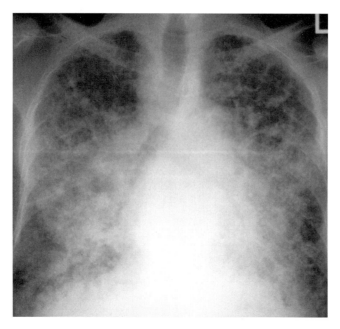

Figure 13.27 Amyloidosis. Extensive bilateral parenchymal involvement. (Courtesy of Dr. Michael Streiter, Huntington, NY.)

distribution, and can calcify or ossify (Figs. 13.25 and 13.26). Nodules range in size from 5 mm to 5 cm and are smooth or lobulated in outline. They can be spiculated and may resemble cancer. Pleural effusion is sometimes associated.

Diffuse parenchymal disease is the least common form and usually occurs in patients over age 60. When systemic amyloidosis affects the lungs it usually does so in this form. With diffuse disease, patients are often asymptomatic with normal imaging. When imaging is abnormal, there are often widespread interstitial opacities that may or may not calcify and can become confluent (Fig. 13.27). Honeycombing has been demonstrated (33,34).

MISCELLANEOUS

LANGERHANS CELL HISTIOCYTOSIS (HISTICYTOSIS X)

This is a poorly understood group of disorders characterized by proliferation of Langerhans cells, possibly due to a defect in immunoregulation. It is subdivided into three separate diseases according to age and severity: Letterer-Siwe disease, an acute disseminated and fulminant form occurring in neonates; Hand-Christian-Schuller disease, a chronic, disseminated, less severe form occurring in children ages 5 to 10 years; and eosinophilic granuloma, the most benign form, occurring in young adults and predominantly affecting the lungs and bones. Lung involvement occurs in 20% of cases and is termed pulmonary Langerhans cell histiocytosis. It has an incidence of 1 to 5 per million and an age at onset of 20 to 40 years. Once thought to be a male-predominant disease, it is now considered equally prevalent in both sexes. This may reflect changing smoking patterns, because there is a strong association with cigarette smoking. It is much rarer among African Americans (1–3,5).

The lungs are initially involved, with multiple upper lobe stellate nodules of 3 to 10 mm, sparing the costophrenic angles. This is the granuloma stage. On HRCT these nodules have a centrilobular peribronchiolar distribution with normal intervening lung. Cavitation is uncommon. Small irregular cysts are also seen. HRCT is extremely useful in the evaluation of the nodules and cysts (Fig. 13.28). Alveolar consolidation is rare but can occur when the alveoli fill with histiocytes and eosinophils. Abnormality progresses to a reticulonodular pattern and finally culminates in fibrosis, large cystic spaces, and honeycombing. Volume loss is uncommon, and one-third actually have increased lung volumes. Spontaneous pneumothorax is very common (35).

Rib involvement results in well-defined osteolytic lesions, which may be expansile (Fig. 13.29). Involvement of vertebral bodies may cause severe collapse with vertebra plana.

Because it is strongly associated with cigarette smoking, eosinophilic granuloma has changed from a male-predominant to a gender-neutral disease.

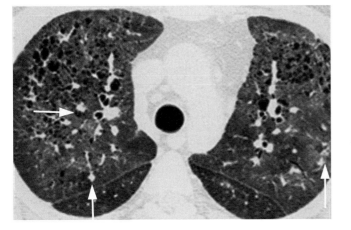

Figure 13.28 Pulmonary Langerhans cell histiocytosis. High resolution computed tomography with multiple upper lobe cysts and scattered irregular lung nodules (*arrows*).

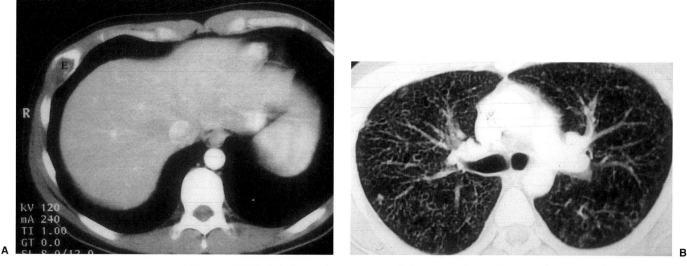

Figure 13.29 Pulmonary Langerhans cell histiocytosis. *A.* Computed tomography at soft tissue window settings: expansile lytic right anterolateral rib lesion (E). *B.* Computed tomography at lung window settings, more cephalad than *A:* numerous lung cysts, with scattered lung nodules.

THE PHAKOMATOSES

Table 13.11 lists these disorders.

Neurofibromatosis (von Recklinghausen Disease)

Neurofibromatosis type 1 (von Recklinghausen disease) is an autosomal dominant disease. It has an incidence of 1 per 3,000, half of cases are sporadic mutations, and there is no gender or racial predominance. The abnormal gene is located on chromosome 17. There is an association with multiple endocrine neoplasia type IIb (pheochromocytoma, medullary thyroid carcinoma, and multiple neuromas). There is also a 10-fold increase in the incidence of congenital heart disease (1,2,5). Neurofibromatosis has a variety of manifestations in the chest and can cause chest wall involvement, mediastinal masses, and lung involvement

Cutaneous tumors can be seen as nodules on the CXR. If they are projected outside the lungs, a diagnosis of cutaneous nodules can easily be made, but otherwise they can be mistaken for pulmonary nodules. Neural tumors can arise from chest wall (Fig. 13.30) or intercostal nerves, and if they are large enough they may erode ribs and cause rib notching (Fig. 13.31). The ribs themselves may be abnormal, being thin and/or twisted (ribbon ribs). Kyphoscoliosis of the thoracolumbar spine occurs in 10% to 60% of patients. There may also be developmental and modeling abnormalities of vertebrae such as posterior vertebral scalloping, enlargement of intervertebral foramina, and absence or remodeling of pedicles (36,37).

Neural tumors, especially neurofibromas, neurilemmomas, schwannomas, and their malignant counterparts, may arise in the middle mediastinum. They can be localized or

Table 13.11: Neurocutaneous Disorders

Neurofibromatosis (von Recklinghausen disease)
Tuberous sclerosis (Bourneville disease)
Cerebelloretinal hemangioblastosis (von Hippel-Lindau syndrome)
Encephalotrigeminal syndrome (Sturge-Weber disease)
Ataxia telangiectasia (Louis-Bar syndrome)
Hereditary hemorrhagic telangiectasia (Osler-Weber-Rendu syndrome)

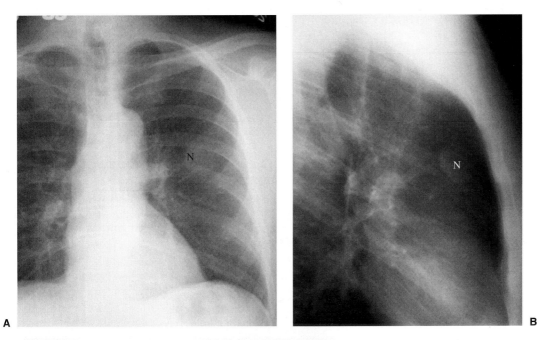

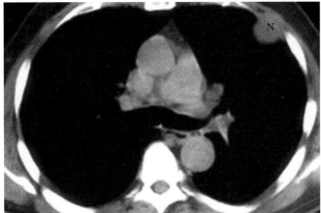

***Figure* 13.30** Chest wall neurofibroma (N) on (A) posteroanterior chest x-ray, (B) lateral chest x-ray, and (C) computed tomography.

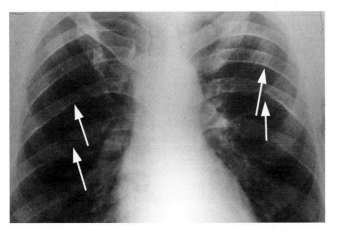

***Figure* 13.31** Neurofibromatosis with rib notching (*arrows*).

diffuse. They are more common on the left. They often arise from the vagus nerve and present as slowly growing, smoothly marginated, middle mediastinal masses that are often low in attenuation on contrast-enhanced CT but may be of muscle attenuation. Nerve sheath tumors are not reliably differentiated on CT. On magnetic resonance imaging neurofibroma and schwannoma are isointense with nerve tissue on T1-weighted imaging and high signal intensity on T2-weighted imaging. Although they may be asymptomatic, large lesions can cause local compression. Malignant transformation is possible (3). Posterior mediastinal masses are even more common and may be neural tumors, lateral meningoceles, or rarely pheochromocytomas. Lateral meningoceles usually occur at the apex of kyphoscoliosis and are more common on the right. They are associated with the vertebral developmental and modeling abnormalities mentioned above.

Lung parenchymal involvement has a prevalence of 20%, affecting men and women equally and taking the form of a basal predominant interstitial fibrosis with upper and mid-lung thin-walled bullae. Neural tumors may simulate lung nodules, and their malignant counterparts may metastasize to the lungs (3,36).

Tuberous Sclerosis (Bourneville Disease)

Tuberous sclerosis is an autosomal dominant disorder with a low penetrance. The abnormal gene is located on chromosome 16, and spontaneous mutations occur in 50% to 80%. Tuberous sclerosis is characterized by a triad of (a) adenoma sebaceum, (b) seizures, and (c) mental retardation. Tuberous sclerosis has an incidence of 7 per million and occurs equally in males and females (1,2).

Pulmonary involvement occurs in 1% to 2% of cases. Pulmonary findings on CXR and HRCT are indistinguishable from those in lymphangiomyomatosis, except for the absence of pleural effusion. Spontaneous pneumothorax often occurs. Tuberous sclerosis causes interstitial disease, with a reticular or reticulonodular CXR appearance (Fig. 13.32). The nodules are small (1 to 2 mm). With time the reticular elements become more marked, with honeycombing and cyst formation. The cysts are usually less than 1 cm and are smooth-walled and uniform. The lung volumes are normal or enlarged due to air trapping and focal emphysema. Bone cysts or sclerotic vertebrae may be seen (36,38,39). Associated renal angiomyolipomas may help to establish the diagnosis in equivocal cases (Fig. 13.32).

> Interstitial lung disease in tuberous sclerosis is indistinguishable from that in lymphangiomyomatosis, except for the absence of pleural effusion in tuberous sclerosis.

Lymphangiomyomatosis

Although not a neurocutaneous disorder, the pulmonary features of lymphangiomyomatosis are virtually identical to tuberous sclerosis. Lymphangiomyomatosis is characterized by a triad of (a) gradually progressive interstitial lung disease with uniform smooth-walled cysts (Fig. 13.33), (b) recurrent chylous pleural effusions, and (c) recurrent pneumothoraces. It is a rare disorder, has an age at onset between 17 and 50 years, and occurs exclusively in women. At HRCT there are numerous small cysts, as in pulmonary Langerhans cell histiocytosis (Fig. 13.34). The cysts in lymphangiomyomatosis are more uniform in size and shape and more diffusely distributed (without the upper lobe predominance of pulmonary Langerhans cell histiocytosis). In addition, pulmonary Langerhans cell histiocytosis often demonstrates associated lung nodules, which are not a feature of lymphangiomyomatosis (1–3).

Ataxia Telangiectasia (Louis-Bar Syndrome)

Ataxia telangiectasia is an autosomal recessive disorder characterized by telangiectasias of the skin and eye, cerebellar ataxia, sinus and pulmonary infections, immunodeficiency, and a propensity to develop malignancies. It has an incidence of 1 in 40,000 and occurs equally in males and females (1,2). On the CXR there may be airspace disease due to infection. With repeated infections, linear fibrotic changes and bronchiectasis tend to occur. Lymph node enlargement is usually absent; its presence may indicate malignancy. Bronchiectasis with respiratory failure is the most common cause of death (36,40).

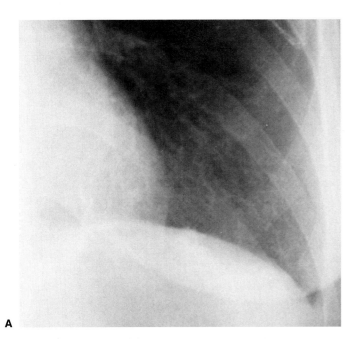

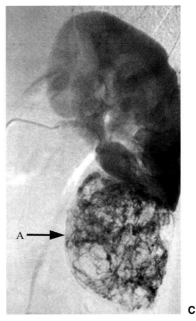

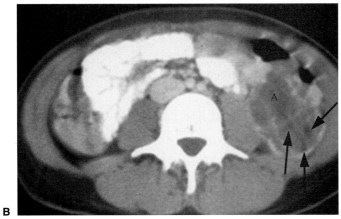

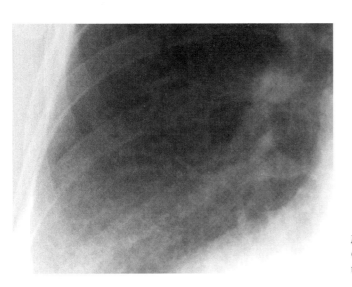

Figure 13.32 Tuberous sclerosis. *A.* Posteroanterior chest x-ray: basilar honeycombing. *B.* Computed tomography: large exophytic left lower pole renal mass (A) with foci of fat (*arrows*) compatible with angiomyolipoma. *C.* Subtraction view of left renal angiogram: vascular mass (A) is angiomyolipoma.

Figure 13.33 Lymphangiomyomatosis. Chest x-ray with multiple cysts, giving the appearance of honeycombing.

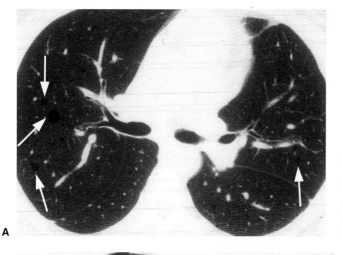

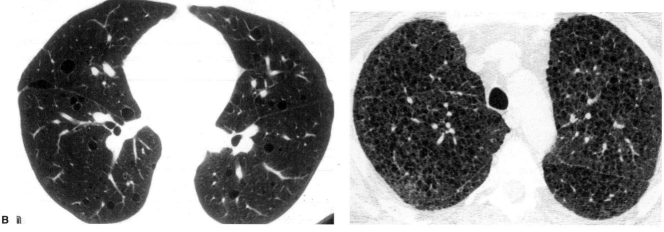

Figure 13.34 Spectrum of severity of lymphangiomyomatosis. *A.* Mild lymphangiomyomatosis: scattered cysts *(arrows)* at high resolution computed tomography, many too small to denote with an arrow. *B.* Moderate lymphangiomyomatosis: more numerous cysts in a different patient. *C.* Severe lymphangiomyomatosis: a third patient with innumerable cysts.

Hereditary Hemorrhagic Telangiectasia (Osler-Weber-Rendu Syndrome)

Nearly 90% of pulmonary arteriovenous malformations occur in the setting of Osler-Weber-Rendu syndrome.

Hereditary hemorrhagic telangiectasia is an autosomal dominant disorder with incomplete penetrance and variable expression. Nearly 90% of pulmonary arteriovenous fistulas (arteriovenous malformations) are associated with this disease, especially if multiple. Arteriovenous malformations and telangiectasias can affect the nasal mucosa, skin, lung, central nervous system, gastrointestinal tract, and liver. Patients may have cyanosis, clubbing, and polycythemia. They frequently present with epistaxis, hemoptysis, or hematemesis. Cerebral abscesses or infarcts commonly occur due to right-to-left shunting. Up to one-third of patients have strokes, either due to a bleeding arteriovenous malformation or infarct (1,2).

On the CXR arteriovenous malformations present as well-demarcated lobulated nodules (Fig. 13.35) (Chapter 21, Fig. 21.29). A draining vein and a feeding artery may be identified, resembling "rabbit ears" or an antenna. Contrast-enhanced CT or pulmonary angiography is helpful in identifying lesions not seen on CXR (Fig. 13.35C). Pulmonary angiography is vital for planning treatment. Although 80% of lesions are simple (one feeding vessel), 20% will have two or more feeding vessels. Feeding vessels less than 3 mm in size are generally not treated. Vessels are occluded with detachable balloons or coils. Larger lesions may require surgery (3,41).

SARCOIDOSIS

Sarcoidosis has an incidence of 2 to 10 per 100,000, with a typical age at onset between 20 and 30 years, with a second peak in the sixth decade, and male-to-female ratio of 1:2 to 3. Although an equal incidence is noted in white men and women, it is up to 10 times

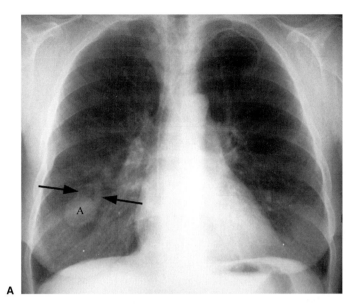

Figure 13.35 Osler-Weber-Rendu syndrome. *A.* Posteroanterior chest x-ray: one right lung nodule (A) with visible feeding artery and draining vein *(arrows).* *B.* Right pulmonary arteriogram: arteriovenous malformation (M) accounts for right lung nodule. *C.* Left pulmonary arteriogram: unexpected small left lung arteriovenous malformation *(arrow).*

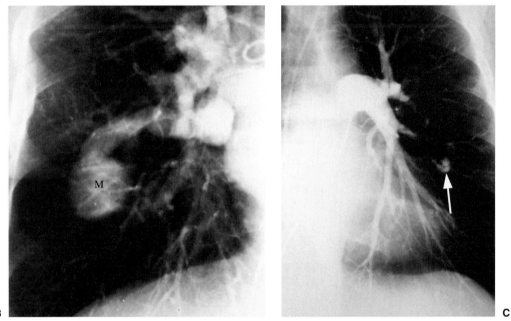

more common in black women than black men and 17 times more common in blacks than whites. There is an increased incidence in people with blood group A. Sarcoidosis may also be familial.

Sarcoidosis is a chronic multisystem disorder of unknown etiology characterized by noncaseating epithelioid cell granulomas, usually presenting with fever, malaise, polyarthralgias (ankles and knees), erythema nodosum, and bilateral hilar and mediastinal lymph node enlargement. Although sarcoidosis predominantly affects the chest, it is a multisystemic disease and affects the skin in up to 70% of cases, with erythema nodosum, lupus pernio, or scar infiltrates. Generalized lymph node enlargement occurs in 30% of patients, with myopathy in 25%. The eyes are involved in 15% (uveitis or keratoconjunctivitis), hepatosplenomegaly is seen in 10%, the bones are involved in 5% to 10%, parotitis occurs in 5%, and the central nervous system is involved in 3% to 5% (1–3,5). On the CXR sarcoidosis may affect lymph nodes, lung parenchyma, airways, vessels, pleura, bones, and liver and spleen. There is a staging system for thoracic sarcoidosis that is based on the chest radiograph (Table 13.12).

Table 13.12: Chest Radiography Staging of Sarcoidosis

	Lymph Node Enlargement	Interstitial Lung Disease
Stage 0	No	No
Stage 1	Yes	No
Stage 2	Yes	Nonfibrotic
Stage 3	No	Nonfibrotic
Stage 4	No	Fibrotic

The triad of bilateral hilar and right paratracheal lymph node enlargement is seen in up to 80% of sarcoidosis patients.

The triad of bilateral hilar lymph node enlargement and (right) paratracheal lymph node enlargement (Garland triad or 1-2-3 sign) is seen in up to 80% of patients, making it the most common intrathoracic manifestation of sarcoidosis. Lymph node enlargement ranges from just detectable to massive and is usually lobulated and well marginated. Symmetry is an important diagnostic feature, because symmetry is not as common a feature of the major diagnostic alternatives (lymphoma, tuberculosis, and metastatic disease) (3,42). In addition to hilar and paratracheal lymph nodes, other lymph nodes may be affected. Anterior mediastinal and subcarinal lymph node enlargement is common but may be difficult to appreciate on the CXR. It is readily apparent on CT. Posterior mediastinal lymph node enlargement is uncommon. Abdominal lymph nodes are occasionally enlarged (Fig. 13.36).

In most patients (60% to 70%), lymph node enlargement completely resolves. This is especially true in patients with erythema nodosum and arthralgias. In the remainder, lung disease develops. Lymph node enlargement is often decreased by the time lung disease is seen. Interstitial lung disease in sarcoidosis is initially not fibrotic, but fibrotic lung disease may develop once lymph node enlargement has resolved. Lymph nodes can show calcification, and this may be in an eggshell pattern (Fig. 13.37) (42). Sarcoidosis is the most common cause of eggshell calcification of lymph nodes after pneumoconiosis (silicosis and coal worker's pneumoconiosis). The radiologic manifestations within the lung parenchyma are discussed in greater detail in Chapter 14.

Sarcoidosis of the larynx occurs infrequently. Thoracic lymph node enlargement may cause compression of the trachea or bronchi. Tracheal involvement is rare, but when it occurs it results in strictures, which may be smooth, irregular, or nodular. Although peribronchial and perivascular granulomatous infiltration is common, symptomatic bronchial obstruction is not. Traction bronchiectasis occurs with pulmonary fibrosis.

Large vessel arteritis is rare; arteritis of small vessels is more common, often with granulomas. This may result in vessel narrowing but usually does not cause vascular

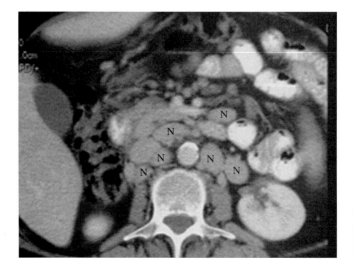

Figure 13.36 Sarcoidosis. Computed tomography with numerous enlarged abdominal lymph nodes (N).

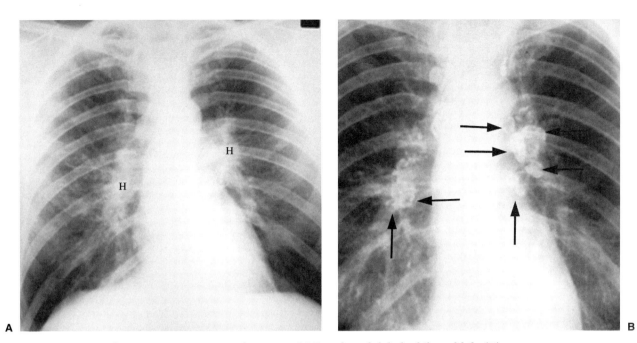

Figure 13.37 Sarcoidosis. *A.* Posteroanterior chest x-ray 1963: enlarged, lobular bilateral hila (H) with ill-defined parenchymal abnormality extending into the perihilar lungs, typical of stage 2 sarcoidosis. *B.* Posteroanterior chest x-ray 1978: lung disease has resolved, and there is now bilateral eggshell calcification of hilar lymph nodes (*arrows*).

necrosis or thrombosis. Coronary artery involvement has been described. Aortic involvement, either aneurysmal dilation or else stenosis and occlusion with a clinical picture similar to Takayasu arteritis, is rare. Pulmonary arteritis or extrinsic compression by enlarged lymph nodes is similarly rare. Although mediastinal lymph node enlargement may be massive, superior vena cava syndrome is very rare. Myocardial involvement may result in ventricular arrhythmias or heart block, cardiomyopathy, and congestive failure (42).

Granulomas may be found on the visceral or parietal pleura, but clinical or radiologic manifestations are uncommon. Pleural effusion occurs in only 2% of patients. Sarcoidosis of bone occurs in 5% to 20% of patients. The phalanges are usually affected, and bone changes on CXR are rare. Although histologic involvement of the liver is common in sarcoidosis (60% to 90%), it is seldom of clinical or radiologic significance (Fig. 13.38). The same applies to the spleen, although splenomegaly occurs in 10% of patients and splenic rupture can occur. Diffuse heterogeneous nodularity of the spleen is also rarely present (3,42).

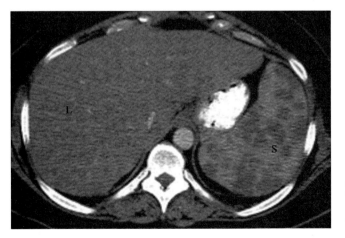

Figure 13.38 Sarcoidosis with numerous tiny lesions throughout the liver (L) and larger lesions in the spleen (S).

REFERENCES

1. Weatherall DJ, Ledingham JGG, Warrell DA. *Oxford textbook of medicine*, 3rd ed. Oxford: Oxford University Press, 1996.
2. Fauci AS, Bracinnald E, Isselbacher KJ, et al. *Harrison's principles of internal medicine*, 14th ed. New York: McGraw-Hill.
3. Armstrong P, Wilson AG, Dee P, et al. *Imaging of diseases of the chest*, 3rd ed. New York: Marby, 2000.
4. Sperber M. *Radiologic diagnosis of chest disease*. New York; Springer-Verlag, 1990.
5. Dahnert W. *Radiology review manual*, 4th ed. Baltimore: Williams & Wilkins, 1999.
6. Hunninghake GW, Fauci AS. Pulmonary involvement in the collagen vascular diseases. *Am Rev Respir Dis* 1979;119:471–503.
7. Wiedemann HP, Matthay RA. Pulmonary manifestations of the collagen vascular diseases. *Clin Chest Med* 1989;10:677–722.
8. Tanoue LT. Pulmonary manifestations of rheumatoid arthritis. *Clin Chest Med* 1998;19:667–685.
9. Remy-Jardin M, Remy J, Cortet B, et al. Lung changes in rheumatoid arthritis: CT findings. *Radiology* 1994;193:375–382.
10. Wiedemann HP, Matthay RA. Pulmonary manifestations of systemic lupus erythematosus. *J Thorac Imaging* 1992;7:1–18.
11. Murin S, Wiedemann HP, Matthay RA. Pulmonary manifestations of systemic lupus erythematosus. *Clin Chest Med* 1998;19:641–665.
12. Owens GR, Follansbee WP. Cardiopulmonary manifestations of systemic sclerosis. *Chest* 1987; 91:118–127.
13. Minai OM, Dweik RA, Arroliga AC. Manifestations of scleroderma pulmonary disease. *Clin Chest Med* 1998;19:713–731.
14. Schwarz MI. The lung in polymyositis. *Clin Chest Med* 1998;19:701–712.
15. Lee-Chiong TL Jr. Pulmonary manifestations of ankylosing spondylitis and relapsing polychondritis. *Clin Chest Med* 1998;19:747–757.
16. Seo JB, Im JG, Chung JW, et al. Pulmonary vasculitis: the spectrum of radiological findings. *Br J Radiol* 2000;73:1224–1231.
17. Sullivan EJ, Hoffman GS. Pulmonary vasculitis. *Clin Chest Med* 1998;19:759–776.
18. Gonzalez L, Van Ordstrand HS. Wegener's granulomatosis. Review of 11 cases. *Radiology* 1973; 107:295–300.
19. Choi YH, Im JG, Han BK, et al. Thoracic manifestation of Churg-Strauss syndrome: radiologic and clinical findings. *Chest* 2000;117:117–124.
20. Ball JA, Young KR Jr. Pulmonary manifestations of Goodpasture's syndrome. Antiglomerular basement membrane disease and related disorders. *Clin Chest Med* 1998;19:777–791.
21. Leong CS, Stark P. Thoracic manifestations of sickle cell disease. *J Thorac Imaging* 1998;13: 128–134.
22. Bhalla M, Abboud MR, McLoud TC, et al. Acute chest syndrome in sickle cell disease: CT evidence of microvascular occlusion. *Radiology* 1993;187: 45–49.
23. Edwards JR, Matthay KK. Hematologic disorders affecting the lungs. *Clin Chest Med* 1989;10: 723–746.
24. Gumbs RV, Higginbotham-Ford EA, Teal JS, et al. Thoracic extramedullary hematopoiesis in sickle-cell disease. *AJR Am J Roentgenol* 1987;149:889–893.
25. Rappaport DC, Chamberlin DW, Shepard FA, et al. Lymphoproliferative disorders after lung transplantation: imaging features. *Radiology* 1998;206: 519–524.
26. Bragg DG, Chor, PJ, Murray KA, et al. Lymphoproliferative disorders of the lung: histopathology, clinical manifestations, and imaging features. *AJR Am J Roentgenol* 1994;163:273–281.
27. Blank N, Castellino RA. The intrathoracic manifestations of the malignant lymphomas and the leukemias. *Semin Roentgenol* 1980;15:227–245.
28. Klatte EC, Yardley J, Smith EB, et al. The pulmonary manifestations and complications of leukemia. *AJR Am J Roentgenol* 1963;89:598–609.
29. Primack SL, Muller NL. High-resolution computed tomography in acute diffuse lung disease in the immunocompromised patient. *Radiol Clin North Am* 1994;32:731–744.
30. Worthy SA, Muller NL. Pulmonary complications after bone marrow transplantation: high-resolution CT and pathologic findings. *Radiographics* 1997;17:1359–1371.
31. Glorioso LW, Lang EK. Pulmonary manifestations of renal disease. *Radiol Clin North Am* 1984;22:647–658.

32. Sanders C, Frank MS, Rostand SG, et al. Metastatic calcification of the heart and lungs in end-stage renal disease: detection and quantification by dual-energy digital chest radiography. *AJR Am J Roentgenol* 1987;149:881–887.

33. Gross BH, Felson B, Birnberg FA. The respiratory tract in amyloidosis and the plasma cell dyscrasias. *Semin Roentgenol* 1986;21:113–127.

34. Urban BA, Fishman EK, Goldman SM, et al. CT evaluation of amyloidosis: spectrum of disease. *Radiographics* 1993;13:1295–1308.

35. Kulwiec EL, Lynch DA, Aguayo SM, et al. Imaging of pulmonary histiocytosis X. *Radiographics* 1992;12:515–526.

36. Aughenbaugh GL. Thoracic manifestations of neurocutaneous diseases. *Radiol Clin North Am* 1984;22:741–756.

37. Klatte EC, Edmund AF, Smith JA. The radiographic spectrum in neurofibrosis. *Semin Roentgenol* 1976;11:17–37.

38. Medley BE, McLeod RA, Houser OW. Tuberous sclerosis. *Semin Roentgenol* 1976;11:35–54.

39. Bell DG, King BF, Hattery RR, et al. Imaging characteristics of tuberous sclerosis. *AJR Am J Roentgenol* 1991;156:1081–1086.

40. Brown LR, Coulam CM, Reese DF. Ataxia-telangiectasia (Louis-Bar syndrome). *Semin Roentgenol* 1976;11:67–70.

41. Swanson KL, Prakash UB, Stanson AW. Pulmonary arteriovenous fistulas: Mayo Clinic experience 1982–1997. *Mayo Clin Proc* 1999;74:671–680.

42. Lynch JP, Kazerooni EA, Gay SE. Pulmonary sarcoidosis. *Clin Chest Med* 1997;18:755–785.

DIFFUSE LUNG DISEASE

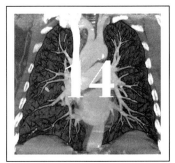

- Chest Radiograph and Pattern Recognition of Diffuse Lung Disease
- Pointers in Pattern Recognition
- High Resolution Computed Tomography Approach to Interstitial Lung Diseases
- Predominantly Reticular Diseases
- Predominantly Nodular Diseases
- Disease Characterized Predominantly by Altered Attenuation
- Disease Characterized Predominantly by Abnormally Increased Attenuation

Imaging has a number of important goals in the patient with diffuse lung disease:

1. Differential diagnosis;
2. Specific diagnosis, if possible;
3. Delineation of extent of disease—may influence choice or locus of therapy, such as in outpatient pneumonia, and may allow subsequent evaluation of response to therapy;
4. Location of disease—may be helpful if biopsy becomes necessary for diagnosis;
5. Demonstration of associated abnormalities (such as in the mediastinum and upper abdomen)

The major diagnostic imaging tools that are generally applied to patients with diffuse lung disease are the chest radiograph (CXR) and chest high resolution computed tomography (HRCT). This chapter focuses on patterns of abnormality using these imaging tools, diagnosis and differential diagnosis (including mnemonics), and the advantages and disadvantages of CXR and HRCT. The radiographic part of this chapter is largely the work of Barry Gross, who as a disciple of Benjamin Felson is more than well qualified for this. The discussion that follows echoes true to the teaching "at the alternator" and comes from teaching conferences for which he has been applauded by his trainees. The second part of this chapter on HRCT focuses on the specific disease processes and patterns of abnormality as they relate to HRCT interpretation.

CHEST RADIOGRAPH AND PATTERN RECOGNITION OF DIFFUSE LUNG DISEASE

There has been a great deal of concern over the past few years about plagiarism in academic circles, especially among historians. I am hoping to dance around that subject by telling everyone in no uncertain terms that everything I know about pattern recognition I learned from Ben Felson. It is, of course, far less than he knew about it. Still, this is the best new material you can get from Ben and me in the twenty-first century.

As I was taught, I do not discuss alveolar (or airspace) and interstitial diseases; I simply discuss CXR patterns of abnormality. There is an interesting overlap of diseases that produce given CXR patterns, some alveolar, some interstitial, and many mixed in anatomic dis-

Table 14.1: Chest Radiographic Findings of Alveolar Disease

Air bronchograms (Fig. 14.1) (and the smaller air alveolograms)
Ill-defined or fuzzy margins
Characteristic distribution
   Focal alveolar disease respects anatomic barriers (lobar or segmental distribution)
   Diffuse alveolar disease ("butterfly" or "batwing" appearance; reverse batwing)
Changes rapidly
Coalescence—when two adjacent areas of alveolar disease approach each other, they tend to blend together
Alveolar nodules—relatively large (1 cm or so), ill-defined nodules with a tendency to coalesce (Fig. 14.3)

tribution. Still, the goal of using a CXR is to generate an appropriate differential diagnosis, and this we can often do. Let us consider various patterns of diffuse lung disease, considering how to recognize the pattern and then how to generate a differential diagnosis.

ALVEOLAR DISEASE

Air bronchograms and ill-defined edges are the hallmark of alveolar disease.

The radiographic hallmarks of alveolar disease are listed in Table 14.1. They include air bronchograms and ill-defined borders. Structures in the lungs are usually well outlined because of air in the alveoli; when the alveoli are filled with abnormality, there is nothing left to provide sharp margination. Alveolar disease may also have a characteristic distribution. For example, focal alveolar disease generally respects the anatomic barriers in the lungs, such as the pleural fissures, therefore demonstrating a lobar or segmental distribution (Fig. 14.1). Other characteristic distributions of more diffuse disease include the "butterfly" or "batwing" appearance (Fig. 14.2), predominantly occupying the central perihilar regions, typical of pulmonary edema, and a reverse batwing appearance of eosinophilic pneumonia. Areas of alveolar disease often coalesce together to form larger areas of alveolar disease (Fig. 14.3). Temporally speaking, alveolar disease processes often change quickly from day to day or even hour to hour.

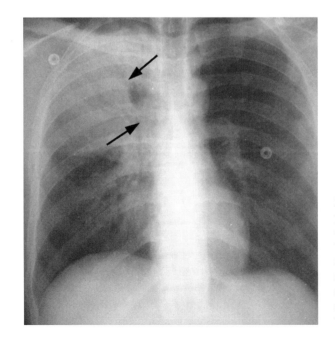

Figure 14.1 Airspace disease in pneumonia, demonstrating air bronchograms and lobar distribution. Posteroanterior chest radiograph reveals branching lucencies (*arrows*) surrounded by right upper lobe airspace disease. Note that disease stops abruptly at its caudal margin, where the minor fissure resides.

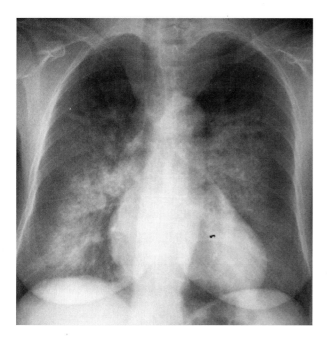

Figure 14.2 Diffuse airspace disease in a "butterfly" distribution, a result of pulmonary hemorrhage in chronic renal failure. Peripheral margins of abnormality are poorly defined.

When alveolar disease is present, the key diagnostic question to ask is whether it is acute or chronic. The answer to that question may be supplied by history; a patient may be able to tell you that he or she was fine until yesterday (acute) or has been symptomatic for 4 months (chronic). Furthermore, a patient who is seriously ill (e.g., an intensive care unit patient) virtually always has acute disease; an asymptomatic patient with significant CXR evidence of alveolar disease usually has chronic abnormality. Old radiographs are another avenue for determining acuteness or chronicity. However, they are sometimes misleading (Fig. 14.4).

Acute alveolar disease has an easy differential diagnosis, as listed in Table 14.2. It is blood or pus or water. Some radiologists like to add cells so they can include adult respiratory distress syndrome in the differential diagnosis; because I think of adult respiratory

Establishing whether alveolar disease is acute or chronic changes the differential diagnosis.

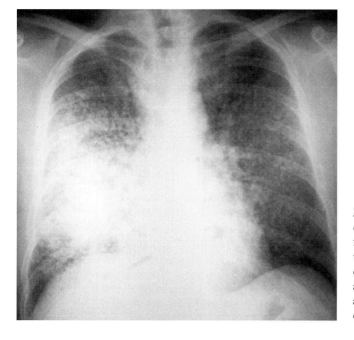

Figure 14.3 Alveolar nodules caused by bronchoalveolar carcinoma, best visualized in the right upper lobe. Nodules become confluent in the right mid-lung, and there are air bronchograms at the cephalad margin of confluent abnormality.

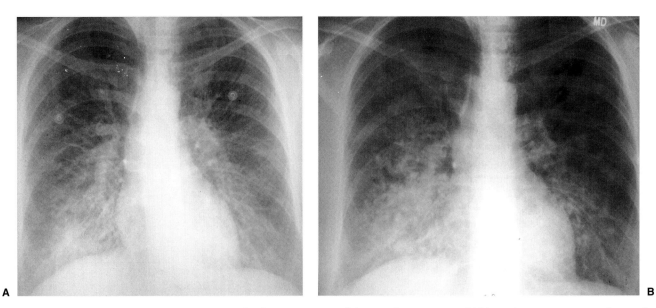

Figure 14.4 Misleading assessment of disease chronicity via old films. *A.* Posteroanterior chest radiograph 12-12: widespread parenchymal abnormality with confluent airspace disease in the right lower lung. *B.* Posteroanterior chest radiograph 1-18, 37 days after *A*: even more airspace disease, seemingly chronic. Clinically, disease had resolved between *A* and *B*, and each episode was thought to represent an acute drug reaction to administered antibiotics. After cessation of antibiotic therapy, the chest radiograph was normal on 1-20.

distress syndrome along the lines of noncardiogenic pulmonary edema, I get to the same end point by a different route. Cells from lymphoma or bronchoalveolar cell carcinoma also fall under that category. Blood or pus or water means that we should consider pulmonary hemorrhage, pneumonia, and edema. Pulmonary hemorrhage is a relatively uncommon cause and is often (although not always) associated with hemoptysis or anemia. Practically speaking, acute alveolar disease is usually pneumonia or pulmonary edema. Finally, some would add a category for protein to cover diseases such as alveolar proteinosis or silicoproteinosis.

It used to be that pneumonia was relatively focal most of the time, and edema was usually diffuse. In the era of acquired immunodeficiency syndrome (Chapter 6), pneumonia can also be diffuse. Edema is often a result of congestive heart failure, which may produce associated cardiomegaly, but there are a number of causes of noncardiogenic edema (Table 10.11) (Fig. 14.5). Furthermore, edema may have unusual distributions (Table 10.12); it may be unilateral (Fig. 14.6) in the upper lobes (with pulmonary hypertension caused by chronic pulmonary emboli) or irregularly irregular (especially in chronic obstructive pulmonary disease). The bottom line is I make my best guess, but I leave it to the clinician caring for the patient to apply my radiographic input to the rest of the available clinical data and thereby to come up with the best diagnosis.

As for chronic alveolar disease, allow me to introduce you to the first of my mnemonics, as listed in Table 14.3. A few words about using mnemonics are in order. I do not want someone to regurgitate such a list at me, demonstrating a complete inability to think and

Table 14.2: Differential Diagnosis of Acute Alveolar Disease ("Blood, Pus, Water, Cells, Protein")

Blood: pulmonary hemorrhage
Plus: pneumonia
Water: edema (cardiogenic and non cardiogenic)
Cells: bronchoalveolar cell carcinoma, lymphoma
Protein: alveolar proteinosis

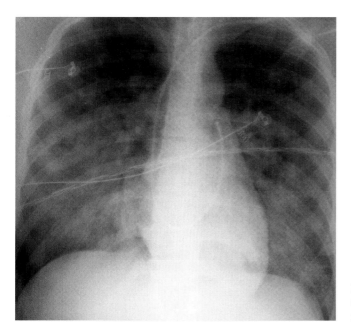

Figure 14.5 Neurogenic pulmonary edema. The patient was found unconscious.

to synthesize information. I want this to be a safety net that allows you to remember the key entities to consider with a given pattern. As you run down the checklist mentally, you should be considering the applicability of each diagnosis to the patient and the pattern at hand. Is the patient a 70-year-old woman? Alveolar proteinosis is generally seen in men from ages 20 to 50, but sarcoidosis is sufficiently widely distributed in the population that almost any age and either gender is perfectly compatible. Is the disease predominantly basilar? That is good for lipoid pneumonia (Fig. 14.7) and desquamative interstitial pneumonitis (DIP), whereas tuberculosis (TB) and fungus are often in the upper lobes, especially with reactivation of previously dormant disease. Are there associated lymph nodes or pleural effusions? If so, lymphoma is a good diagnosis; if not, bronchoalveolar cell carcinoma is a much better bet.

A few more words about mnemonics come to mind. DIP is pretty uncommon; it is really there because "Dallas" is better known than "Allas." When I have visited other pro-

Mnemonics are only helpful if you can remember them.

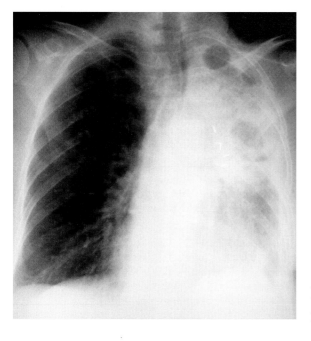

Figure 14.6 Postoperative pulmonary vein thrombosis causing unilateral left pulmonary edema.

Table 14.3: Mnemonic for the Differential Diagnosis of Chronic Alveolar Disease ("TB, Fungus, Dallas")

TB, Fungus Desquamative interstitial pneumonitis Alveolar cell carcinoma Lymphoma Lipoid pneumonia Alveolar proteinosis Sarcoidosis
TB, tuberculosis.

grams I have been told about other mnemonics (as a way to include eosinophilic pneumonia, for instance; I will have more to say about that diagnosis later in this chapter). The best mnemonic is the one you can remember. If you want to include more diagnoses on your checklist, suit yourself. My goal is to include the most common diagnoses, the ones I really do not want to forget. If the answer is not on my list of common entities, I can always consult *Gamuts in Radiology* (1) for more ideas. A variant mnemonic was "STAPLE" for chronic alveolar disease, which some of our residents in the 1980s learned at the Armed Forces Institute of Pathology (sarcoid, TB/fungus, alveolar cell carcinoma, proteinosis, lymphoma, eosinophilic pneumonia, I believe). To the "TB, fungus, Dallas" mnemonic, one of our residents added "*Wins Big*" for Wegener granulomatosis and bronchiolitis obliterans organizing pneumonia (more correctly now known as cryptogenic organizing pneumonia [COP]).

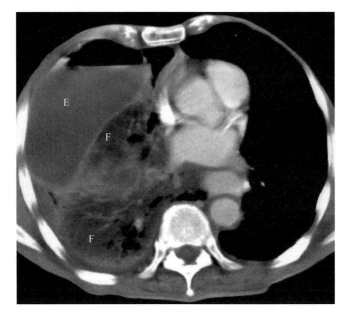

Figure 14.7 Lipoid pneumonia, particularly involving right lower lung. Computed tomography demonstrates fat attenuation filling the alveoli (F). There is an associated *M. fortuitum* empyema (E).

MILIARY NODULES

Turning to the patterns generally thought of as "interstitial," we start with miliary nodules. They are small nodules (under 5 mm in size) that are very uniform in size and sharply defined. Even when they are extremely numerous they do not tend to become confluent. As I often tell residents, the result is the sense that with a pair of tweezers and a lot of patience, you could pick nodules off the radiograph for hours on end. The mnemonic for miliary lung disease is listed in Table 14.4.

Table 14.4: Mnemonic for the Differential Diagnosis of Miliary Lung Disease ("TB, Fungus, SHRIMP")

TB, Fungus *S*arcoid *H*istiocytosis X (eosinophilic granuloma) *R*heumatoid lung *I*diopathic pulmonary fibrosis (usual interstitial pneumonitis) *M*etastases *P*neumoconiosis (especially silicosis)
TB, tuberculosis.

Most tumors that metastasize to the lungs do so a little at a time—one metastasis in January, three in February, two in April, five in May—so that the radiographic picture is nodules varying in size. At the time of detection it would be unusual to have a large number of lesions all under 5 mm in size. The exception would be a very vascular primary neoplasm that could release a shower of metastases all at once. Miliary metastases are mainly seen with thyroid carcinomas; renal cell carcinoma is the next most common source (Fig. 14.8). However, I like to teach that in a given patient, the most likely primary neoplasm to produce a given finding is *that patient's neoplasm*. Miliary nodules in a patient with duodenal leiomyosarcoma could indicate opportunistic infection, but if they prove to be malignant, they will probably be metastatic duodenal leiomyosarcoma (Fig. 14.9).

Usual interstitial pneumonitis (UIP) is on the list not because it tends to cause miliary nodules, but because with diffuse lung disease it is sometimes difficult to decide if the abnormality is the opaque areas (miliary nodules) or the lucent zones in between (honeycombing, see below). On HRCT, which provides better anatomic resolution, UIP is definitely not miliary. Small miliary nodules may also be seen in secondary hemosiderosis due to longstanding mitral valvular disease.

Calcified miliary nodules are a special category. They usually result from histoplasmosis or chickenpox pneumonia. Less commonly, they are seen with silicosis and hemosiderosis. At the far end of the spectrum is alveolar microlithiasis (Fig. 14.10), where tiny calcifications become so numerous they may simulate very opaque alveolar disease; microlithiasis occurs in families, although the inheritance pattern is difficult to discern. Affected patients are often surprisingly asymptomatic.

> Miliary nodules are most commonly due to infection or metastases.

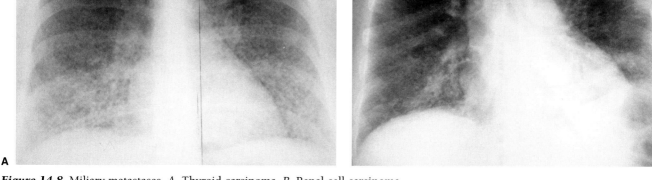

A   B

Figure 14.8 Miliary metastases. *A.* Thyroid carcinoma. *B.* Renal cell carcinoma.

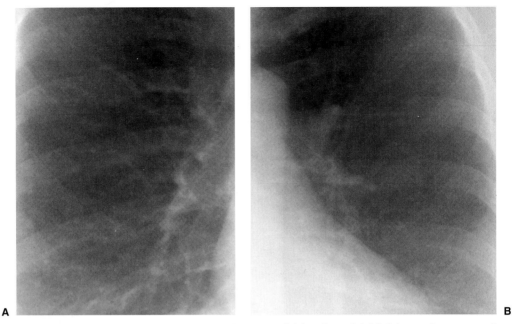

A
B

Figure 14.9 Unusual miliary metastases. Close-ups of (A) right and (B) left lungs demonstrate fine miliary nodules in a patient with duodenal leiomyosarcoma, subsequently proven to be metastases.

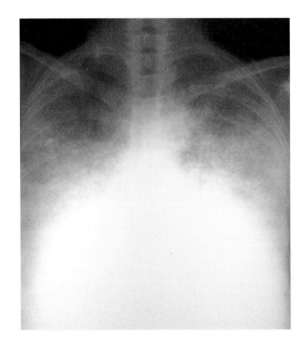

Figure 14.10 Alveolar microlithiasis. Innumerable extremely opaque nodules, resulting in markedly increased opacity of the lungs. (Courtesy of Dr. Michael Streiter, Huntington, NY.)

HONEYCOMBING

This is a pattern of clustered cystic spaces, ranging from 1 to 10 mm in size. Honeycombing tends to occur at the periphery of the lungs, although that may not be easy to appreciate with the CXR. It should also be noted that diseases that do not result in honeycombing at HRCT may nevertheless have a CXR appearance that looks like honeycombing (e.g., lymphangiomyomatosis, with cysts rather than honeycombing at HRCT). The mnemonic for honeycombing is given in Table 14.5. In deference to me, some of our former residents used to make this HIPS ARDS, adding amyloidosis (I was previously obsessed with that disease); because it almost never causes honeycombing, and I am no longer obsessed with amyloidosis, I do not prefer that version.

Table 14.5: Mnemonic for the Differential Diagnosis of Honeycombing ("HIPS RDS")

Histiocytosis X (eosinophilic granuloma)
Idiopathic pulmonary fibrosis or Iatrogenic (drug-induced lung disease)
Pneumoconiosis
Sarcoidosis
Rheumatoid lung
Dermatomyositis
Scleroderma

As previously mentioned, differential diagnosis requires more than a simple recollection of the applicable mnemonic. Disease distribution can be a very helpful piece of ancillary information. A quick glance at a lateral radiograph will convince you that the lungs are somewhat triangular; they are much larger at the bases than at the apices. As a result, disease that is truly uniformly distributed from apices to bases will look somewhat worse at the bases on the CXR. However, some diseases are virtually limited to the lung bases, whereas others will more prominently affect the upper lungs. Examples of upper lung diseases are listed in Table 14.6 and include TB, fungus, sarcoid, ankylosing spondylitis, primary adenocarcinoma of lung, typical emphysema, respiratory bronchiolitis (RB), eosinophilic granuloma (the last four associated with cigarette smoking), and silicosis (and most other inhalational diseases). Lower lung diseases are listed in Table 14.7 and include anything related to blood flow (such as metastases, pulmonary emboli, and most miliary nodules), collagen vascular diseases other than ankylosing spondylitis (RDS in the listed mnemonic), aspiration and lipoid pneumonia, asbestosis, UIP, and emphysema secondary to α_1-antitrypsin deficiency. Please note that this list includes a number of conditions that do not cause honeycombing. Still, honeycombing with upper lung predominance usually boils down to Langerhans cell histiocytosis (a.k.a. eosinophilic granuloma), sarcoidosis, or silicosis (Fig. 14.11); honeycombing with lower lung predominance is often collagen vascular disease, UIP, or asbestosis (Fig. 14.12).

In my experience most drug-induced lung disease is diffuse or at least not lower lung predominant, although amiodarone-induced lung toxicity tends to be basilar. This sometimes allows me to sort out the disease (such as rheumatoid arthritis) from the effect of its treatment (sometimes treated with methotrexate, which can also result in honeycomb lung). Among the collagen vascular diseases, scleroderma in particular is sometimes limited to the extreme lung bases (Fig. 14.13).

Table 14.6: Upper Lung Predominant Diseases

Granulomatous disease
    Tuberculosis
    Fungal infection
    Sarcoidosis
Ankylosing spondylitis
Smoking-related lung diseases
    Primary adenocarcinoma of lung
    Centrilobular emphysema
    Respiratory bronchiolitis
    Langerhans cell histiocytosis (a.k.a. eosinophilic granuloma)
Occupational lung disease
    Silicosis
    Coal workers' pneumoconiosis

Table 14.7: Lower Lung Predominant Diseases

Metastases
Pulmonary emboli and most miliary nodules
Collagen vascular diseases
    Rheumatoid arthritis
    Dermatomyositis
    Scleroderma
Aspiration, including lipoid pneumonia
Asbestosis
Usual interstitial pneumonia
Panlobular emphysema (secondary to α_1-antitrypsin deficiency)

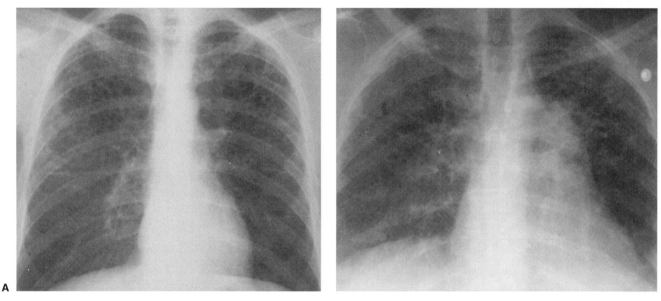

Figure 14.11 Upper lobe honeycombing. *A.* Eosinophilic granuloma. *B.* Sarcoid.

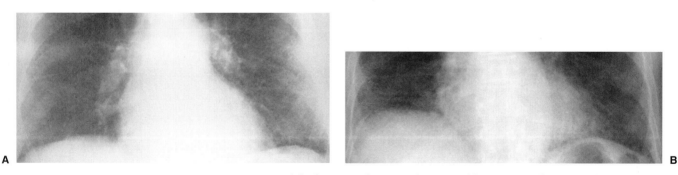

Figure 14.12 Lower lobe honeycombing. *A.* Rheumatoid lung. *B.* Usual interstitial pneumonitis.

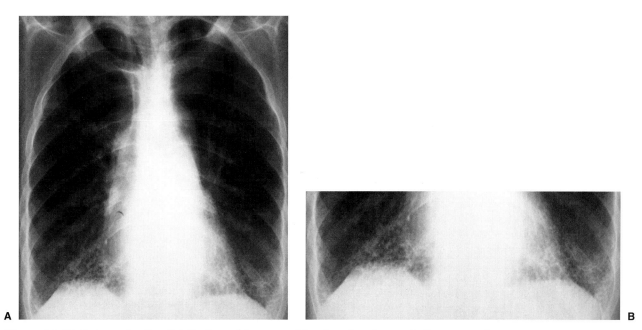

Figure 14.13 Extreme basilar distribution of honeycombing in scleroderma. *A.* Posteroanterior chest radiograph and *(B)* close-up of lung bases.

Gender can also be helpful in sorting among differential diagnostic possibilities. Langerhans cell histiocytosis (a.k.a. eosinophilic granuloma) used to have a significant male predilection (9:1); because it is a cigarette-smoking related disease, it no longer has a pronounced gender preference, likely due to the profound increase in women smoking over the last few decades. Sarcoid has something of a female predominance, but it is so ubiquitous that this turns out not to be helpful in differential diagnosis (many males are also affected). Diseases with continuing significant male predominance include rheumatoid lung (even though rheumatoid arthritis itself has a strong female predominance), ankylosing spondylitis, alveolar proteinosis, silicosis, and asbestosis. Female gender is more typical of lymphangiomyomatosis, dermatomyositis, and scleroderma.

Small Irregular Opacities

This pattern is also referred to as reticulonodular. It describes a complex combination of lines, dots, and spaces and is something of a wastebasket term for thousands of entities that involve the interstitium of the lungs. Although any "interstitial" disease can manifest this way, I particularly try to remember four common entities, as listed in Table 14.8: lymphangitic metastases (Fig. 14.14), sarcoidosis, collagen vascular disease, and pneumoconiosis. It is worth remembering that from a pattern recognition standpoint, this is a less helpful descriptor than miliary or honeycombing.

Table 14.8: Differential Diagnosis of Small Irregular Opacities (a.k.a. Reticulonodular Pattern)

Lymphangitic metastases
Sarcoidosis
Collagen vascular disease
Pneumoconiosis

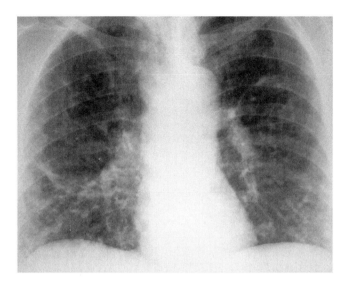

Figure 14.14 Small irregular opacities in lymphangitic spread of uterine sarcoma. Posteroanterior chest radiograph reveals lines, dots, and circles.

BRONCHIAL ABNORMALITY

Bronchiectasis can mimic honeycombing on chest radiographs.

This is a pattern of abnormality of the bronchi, characterized by bronchial enlargement or bronchial wall thickening as manifestations of bronchiectasis, discussed in greater detail in Chapter 15. Bronchial abnormality can be mistaken for honeycombing because enlarged bronchi may result in apparent cystic spaces. However, such bronchi may contain fluid, and they tend not to cluster to quite the same extent as do that honeycomb cysts. Furthermore, careful review of frontal and lateral radiographs will generally demonstrate that abnormal bronchi have a different appearance depending on whether they are viewed in short axis (where they often resemble cystic spaces) or long axis (where their appearance often simulates railroad or tram tracks). As treatment for cystic fibrosis improves and patients survive further and further into adulthood, cystic fibrosis is a more and more common cause of bronchial abnormality (Fig. 14.15).

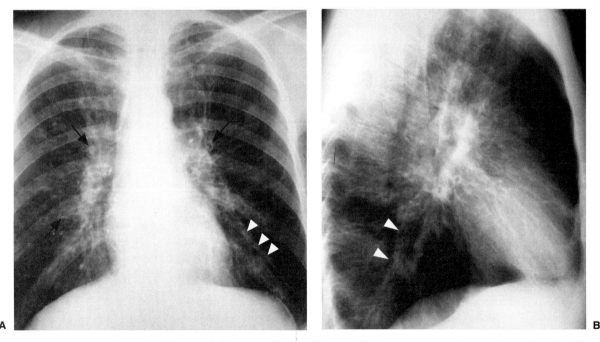

Figure 14.15 Bronchial pattern of cystic fibrosis. (A) Posteroanterior chest radiograph and (B) lateral chest radiograph demonstrate thick-walled bronchi (*arrows*) and tram tracks (*arrowheads*).

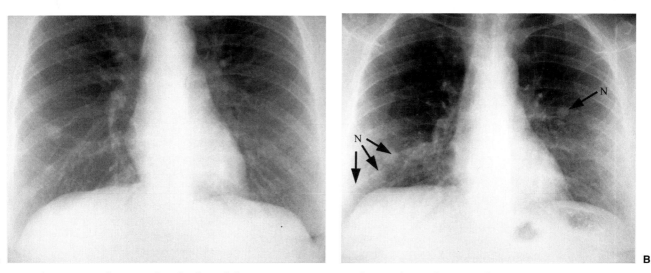

Figure 14.16 Unusual cause of multiple nodules. *A.* Posteroanterior chest radiograph at initial presentation: several lung nodules are best visualized in the right lower lung. *B.* Posteroanterior chest radiograph 31 months after *A*: growing bilateral nodules (N), although growth rate is less than typically seen with lung metastases. Biopsy revealed benign metastasizing leiomyomatosis (pulmonary fibroleiomyomatous hamartomas).

Bronchiectasis may instead be postinflammatory or congenital (Kartagener syndrome). Bronchial wall thickening is also sometimes seen in asthma and chronic bronchitis.

MULTIPLE NODULES AND CAVITARY NODULES

This is a pattern characterized by nodules of varying size. Unlike alveolar nodules, the nodules considered here are sharply outlined. Unlike miliary nodules, they are not uniform in size and they often range well above the 5 mm limit for miliary nodules. The important entities in the differential diagnosis are metastases, metastases, metastases, metastases, and granulomas. This reinforces the fact that metastatic disease is numerically the most common cause and also the most important cause (based on effect on patient outcome) to remember. There are numerous other causes, including Wegener granulomatosis, hamartomas, and arteriovenous malformations; if you have a special interest in the less common causes, this is a good time to go to the Gamut book (Fig. 14.16). Cavitary nodules have a separate mnemonic, as listed in Table 14.9. This mnemonic can be used for a single cavity or for multiple cavities.

In the context of multiple cavities, cancer usually means squamous cell carcinoma metastases. Sarcoma metastases actually have a greater tendency to cavitate, but they are less common (Fig. 14.17). Apart from Wegener granulomatosis, rheumatoid nodules may also cavitate. Vascular reminds us that both bland and septic emboli may cavitate. Infection refers to bacterial lung abscesses and to infections like TB and fungus with a predilection for cavitation. A variety of traumatic lesions presents with cavitations (including lac-

Table 14.9: Mnemonic for the Differential Diagnosis of Cavitary Lung Nodules ("CAVITY")

Cancer
Autoimmune
Vascular
Infection
Trauma
Young (for congenital abnormalities)

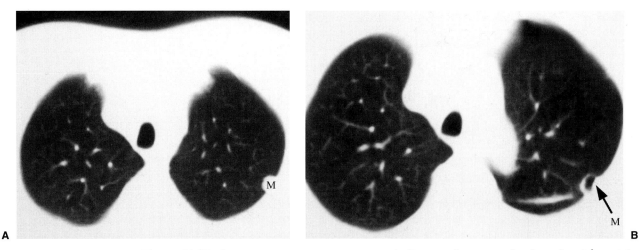

Figure 14.17 Cavitary metastatic osteosarcoma. *A.* Computed tomography december 3rd: peripheral left upper lobe metastasis (M). *B.* Computed tomography 8 weeks after *A*: lesion has cavitated in the interval.

Box 14.1: Summary of Mnemonics

Chronic alveolar disease—TB, fungus, DALLAS
Miliary nodules—TB, fungus, SHRIMP
Honeycombing—HIPS RDS
Cavitary nodule(s)—CAVITY

TB, tuberculosis.

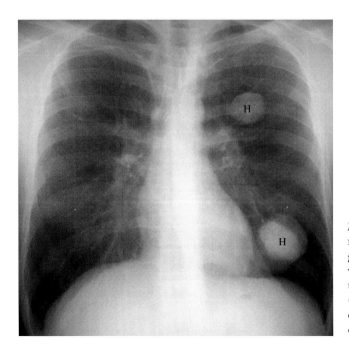

Figure 14.18 Calcified lung nodules (H). This patient also had gastric leiomyosarcoma; together with these calcified hamartomas, this constitutes ⅔ of Carney triad (the other element in the triad is extraadrenal pheochromocytoma, or paraganglioma).

eration, contusion, and pneumatocele). Although congenital abnormalities that cavitate (such as bronchogenic cyst and sequestration) are usually single lesions, they may on occasion be multiple (Box 14.1).

Calcified nodules usually indicate benign disease. Several such nodules are often seen in old TB or histoplasmosis. Hamartomas also calcify and are sometimes multiple, as in Carney triad (Fig. 14.18). However, metastases may also calcify. This is particularly likely after chemotherapy has been administered. *De novo* calcification (or ossification) of metastases is usually a manifestation of sarcomas, especially osteosarcoma (Fig. 14.19). Calcification of lesser magnitude is occasionally seen in adenocarcinoma metastases from the breast or gastrointestinal tract (Fig. 14.20).

POINTERS IN PATTERN RECOGNITION

It takes practice to become proficient at recognizing these patterns and generating differential diagnoses. Personal experience indicates that it is worthwhile to make the effort. Your ability to make diagnoses using pattern recognition will rapidly outstrip that of clinicians, who generally rely on the history and physical examination as guides to the interpretation of the chest radiograph. In practical terms, it is important to know that it is generally easier to recognize a pattern in areas of moderate profusion than in areas of extreme profusion. What I am saying is that although alveolar disease is the pattern that is particularly likely to demonstrate areas of confluent disease, any pattern becomes harder to recognize if you pile on too much of it.

It will assist you enormously to acknowledge one more pattern: "I don't know." Some patients have disease that is not easily sorted into one of the above patterns of abnormality (sometimes the problem is with the pattern, sometimes it is with you as the interpreter of the pattern). In any event, pretending that you know what the pattern is will lead to erroneous differential diagnoses and loss of confidence in the system, both on your part and on the part of your referring clinicians.

> When lung abnormality is extensive, look at the areas least involved to help identify the pattern of abnormality.

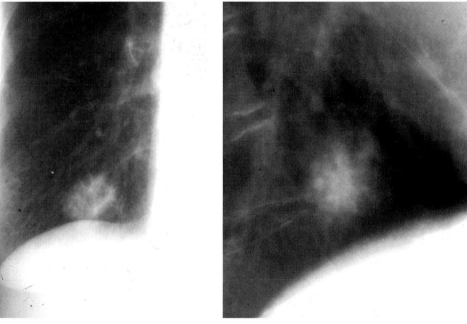

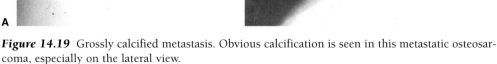

A   B

Figure 14.19 Grossly calcified metastasis. Obvious calcification is seen in this metastatic osteosarcoma, especially on the lateral view.

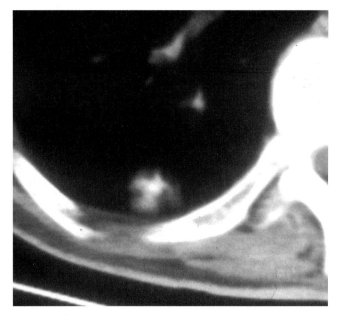

Figure 14.20 Computed tomography demonstration of calcification in metastatic colon carcinoma.

How should you handle a radiograph that demonstrates two (or more) patterns of abnormality (Box 14.2)? There are different answers to that question that apply to different circumstances. If possible, you should try to examine their lists of differential diagnosis for points of overlap (Fig. 14.21). This may result in a very short list of diagnostic possibilities. If one pattern is far more widespread, it is probably better to go with the predominant pattern. If you recognize one pattern and not the other, you should go with the pattern you recognize. If you know a mnemonic (or at least the differential diagnosis) for one and not the other, you should obviously go with the pattern whose differential diagnosis you know. If one pattern has a reasonably focused differential diagnosis and the other is small irregular opacities, go with the pattern with a better differential diagnosis.

I generally approach a radiograph demonstrating two patterns as an example of Osler's Rule (I have also heard this called Occam's Razor): "No matter how you pinch and squeeze, it's got to fit just one disease." It is also worthwhile to remember Hictum's Dictum: "A patient can have as many diseases as he damn well pleases" (Fig. 14.22).

Although this kind of organized analysis will usually work best, there are two other approaches to CXR diagnosis that are sometimes helpful. The first is the "Aunt Minnie" approach. If you happen to have an Aunt Minnie, when she walks in the room you are unlikely to think to yourself, "This is a 65-year-old woman who is 30 pounds overweight, walks with a limp, and wears outrageous color combinations—it is probably my Aunt Minnie." Instead, her overall presentation is sufficiently unique that you get an immediate gestalt impression of her as Aunt Minnie. Similarly, some radiographic presentations are uniquely characteristic of diagnostic entities, and these are labeled as "Aunt Minnies" (Figs. 14.23 and 14.24).

Box 14.2: How to Deal with Two Different Patterns

Cross-check the differential diagnoses
Go with the predominant pattern
Go with the pattern you recognize
Go with the pattern whose differential you know
Go with the more specific pattern
Remember Hictum's dictum

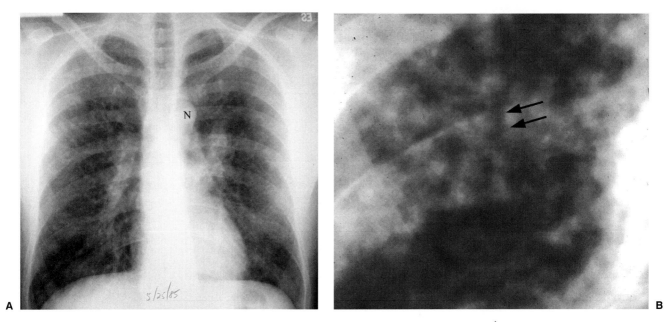

Figure 14.21 Cross-checking multiple patterns. *A.* Posteroanterior chest radiograph May 25th: widespread lung nodules and left hilar lymph node enlargement (N). *B.* Close-up of right perihilar lung two days later: progression of nodules, now with confluence and air bronchograms *(arrows)*. Histoplasmosis is a diagnosis in the differential for nodules, airspace disease, and thoracic lymph node enlargement (and the correct diagnosis).

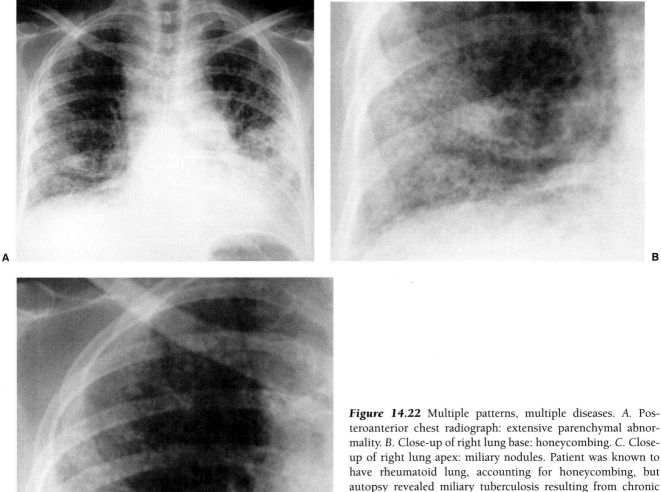

Figure 14.22 Multiple patterns, multiple diseases. *A.* Posteroanterior chest radiograph: extensive parenchymal abnormality. *B.* Close-up of right lung base: honeycombing. *C.* Close-up of right lung apex: miliary nodules. Patient was known to have rheumatoid lung, accounting for honeycombing, but autopsy revealed miliary tuberculosis resulting from chronic steroid therapy for rheumatoid disease, with reactivation of old tuberculosis.

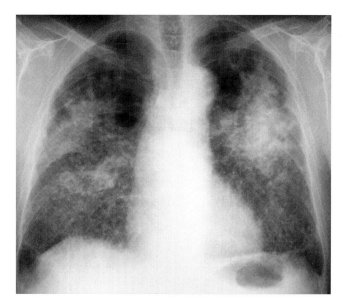

Figure 14.23 Silicosis. Typical appearance of progressive massive fibrosis with upper lobe conglomerate masses. Underlying lungs demonstrate small nodules, and there is emphysematous destruction of upper peripheral lungs adjacent to conglomerate masses.

A second approach is to take into account the patient's clinical presentation and to look for typical radiographic manifestations (Box 14.3). In a patient with severe inherited anemia, this approach makes extramedullary hematopoiesis an important diagnostic consideration for any posterior mediastinal mass. In a patient with prior left upper quadrant abdominal trauma, this makes splenosis a consideration for any left pleural mass(es). Another illustrative example is shown in Fig. 14.25.

The CXR has a number of positive features for assessment of diffuse lung disease. It is widely available and inexpensive. Resultant patient radiation doses are very low. Perhaps most importantly, we (collectively) have an enormous backlog of experience using this tool in this situation. That is how we know that although TB is a common cause of miliary nodules, we do not see calcified miliary nodules after TB.

On the other hand, CXR has disadvantages in the assessment of diffuse lung disease. It is neither sensitive nor specific. Real abnormalities may be missed, and in many patients

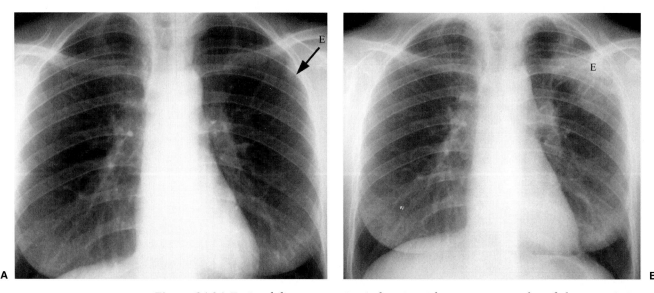

A   B

Figure 14.24 Eosinophilic pneumonia. Asthmatic with recurrent episodes of dyspnea. *A.* Posteroanterior chest radiograph, April 1st: subtle abnormality at periphery of left upper lung (E). *B.* Posteroanterior chest radiograph fifteen days later: left upper lung abnormality has blossomed. Peripheral airspace disease, especially in the upper lungs of atopic patients, is typical.

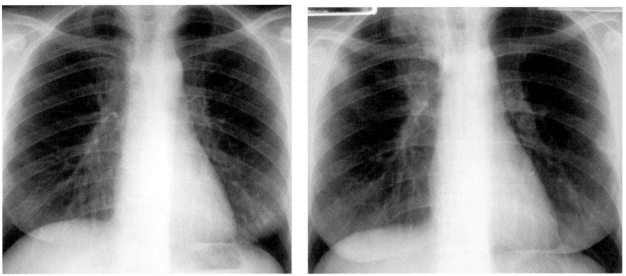

C

D

Figure 14.24 (continued) *C.* Posteroanterior chest radiograph 5-21: complete resolution of abnormality. *D.* Posteroanterior chest radiograph 9-2: recurrence at periphery of both upper lungs (E), also a typical feature if steroid therapy is discontinued.

Box 14.3: Other Tools in the Pattern-Gamut Approach

Gamuts in radiology*
"Aunt Minnies"
Expected abnormalities given the clinical diagnosis

---

*Reader and Felson's *Gamuts in radiology:* Comprehensive lists of roentegen differential diagnosis, 3rd ed. New York, Springer-Verlag, 1993.

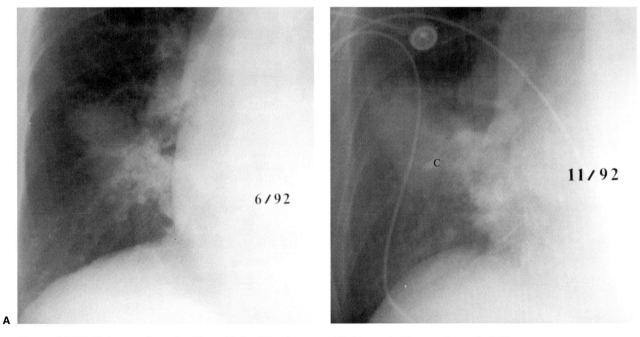

A

B

Figure 14.25 Unknown from the Chest Club of Southeastern Michigan. *A.* Chest radiograph 6-92: patchy right perihilar opacity. *B.* Chest radiograph 11-92: more obvious chronic middle lobe airspace disease (C). *(continued on next page)*

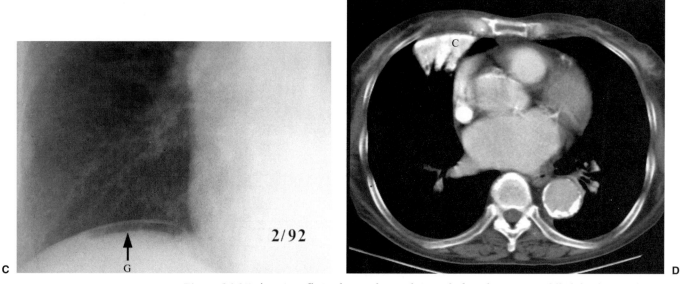

Figure 14.25 (continued) *C.* Chest radiograph 2-92: before there was middle lobe disease there was free intraperitoneal gas (G). Because of the possibility of peritoneal dialysis, metastatic calcification of lung was added to the chronic alveolar differential diagnosis for this patient. *D.* Computed tomography: high-attenuation middle lobe abnormality (C) confirms metastatic calcification of lung. (Courtesy of Dr. David Spizarny, Detroit, MI)

a final diagnosis cannot be established. Disease is not always well localized on the CXR, limiting our ability to guide endoscopists to the best locations for transbronchial lung biopsy in specific patients. Disease activity is also not generally something we can assess. It is thus hard to predict which patients with interstitial lung disease (ILD) will respond to steroids. Although that seems like a trivial distinction, the numerous complications associated with steroid therapy should persuade you otherwise. Finally, associated findings in the mediastinum, axillae, bones, and upper abdomen that might help to explain the etiology of lung disease are generally not well visualized.

HIGH RESOLUTION COMPUTED TOMOGRAPHY APPROACH TO INTERSTITIAL LUNG DISEASES

TECHNIQUE

HRCT differs from conventional CT in that it samples the lung for pattern and distribution of abnormality.

Prone images are useful to distinguish subpleural basilar lung disease from dependent atelectasis.

HRCT is a sampling tool for evaluating the lung parenchyma, during which images are obtained at thin collimation, typically 1 or 1.5 mm (2). HRCT differs from most thoracic CT examinations in two ways. First, during most thoracic CT examinations the entire thoracic volume is captured during the CT acquisition, such as when looking for lung metastases. In contrast, HRCT images are obtained at intervals spaced throughout the lungs. Techniques range from an image every 1 cm to clusters of images at predefined anatomic levels, such as the aortic arch, the carina, and just above the diaphragm. Second, HRCT images are reconstructed using a high spatial frequency reconstruction algorithm that enhances edges, thereby emphasizing the borders of fine lines and nodules, similar (if not identical to) a bone algorithm. In contrast, most thoracic CT examinations use an algorithm for reconstruction that creates a smoother image that is more pleasing to the eye. HRCT images are inherently noisy and suffer from quantum mottle; this usually has little effect on the images reviewed on lung window settings. However, this noise is readily apparent when reviewing on soft tissue window settings. Most HRCT examinations are

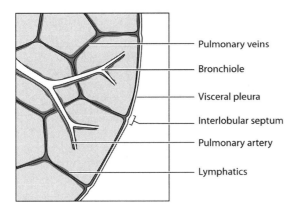

Figure 14.26 Line drawing of a secondary pulmonary lobule. The borders of the lobule are the interlobular septa. At the center of each lobule is a bronchiole and a pulmonary artery branch *(blue)*. The pulmonary vein branches *(red)* run in the interlobular septa. The lymphatics *(green)* are found in the interlobular septa and within the central or axial interstitium that surrounds the bronchovascular bundles. (From Kazerooni EA. High-resolution CT tomography of the lungs. *AJR Am J Roentgenol* 2001;177:501–519, with permission.)

performed at inspiration. Images are often obtained at expiration to evaluate for air trapping that indicates small airway disease. Prone images are useful to exclude lung disease in areas of dependent opacity that is commonly seen in the subpleural posterior portion of the lower lobes, created by atelectasis. This finding is more common with increasing age and in current or former smokers than nonsmokers (3).

ANATOMY

The smallest anatomic unit visible on HRCT is the secondary pulmonary lobule (Fig. 14.26). The walls of these lobules are made up of the interlobular septa, which are typically not seen unless abnormal; they are below the resolution limit of HRCT. The interlobular septa correspond to Kerley B lines on chest radiographs. The occasional visible septum may be normal. The lower limit of resolution on HRCT is approximately 0.1 mm, which is the width of the interlobular septa. Structures 0.2 to 0.3 mm thick can be routinely identified on HRCT. The diameter of the pulmonary artery supplying each lobule is 1 mm, and the diameter of the intralobular acinar arteries is 0.5 mm; both are therefore readily seen on HRCT. Bronchi are visible based on their wall thickness. The 1.0 mm diameter bronchiole supplying the lobule has an approximately 0.15 mm wall, at the limit of HRCT resolution, and is barely if at all visible on HRCT images.

CLINICAL INDICATIONS

The clinical indications for HRCT are summarized in Table 14.10. HRCT is more sensitive and specific for the detection and diagnosis of ILD than both chest radiography and conventional CT (4–9). HRCT is the test of choice for finding and characterizing bronchiectasis. It should be used in cases of suspected diffuse infiltrative lung disease when the chest radiograph is normal or when the pattern of abnormality is unclear on chest radiographs. In cases when the pattern is well characterized at radiography, such as a miliary pattern, HRCT is unlikely to provide additional useful information. Individuals with infiltrative lung diseases, such as usual or nonspecific interstitial pneumonitis (NSIP), benefit

Table 14.10: Clinical Indications for HRCT

Detect and evaluate bronchiectasis
Evaluation of suspected lung disease when chest radiography is normal
Clarify pattern of abnormality from chest radiography to narrow differential diagnosis
Evaluate disease activity
Predict response to therapy and survival
Guide type and location of biopsy
Evaluate effectiveness of medical therapy

further from HRCT, because findings such as ground glass opacity tend to indicate more active and potentially reversible disease against which aggressive, often toxic, pharmaceuticals may be used. In contrast, individuals with predominantly honeycombing have end-stage fibrosis, are unlikely to respond to medical therapy and have a very poor prognosis. HRCT is often repeated over the course of therapy to measure the impact of the therapy. Finally, HRCT can be used to guide the surgeon to the areas of ground glass opacity and away from honeycombing during surgical lung biopsy, thereby improving the ability to characterize the underlying disease process.

DEFINITIONS OF IDIOPATHIC INTERSTITIAL PNEUMONIAS

The definitions of disease used here are taken from new consensus classification of idiopathic interstitial pneumonias developed by the American Thoracic Society and European Respiratory Society, published in 2002 (10). This classification comprises the clinico-pathologic entities in the order of relative frequency, as listed in Table 14.11 (11,12). Each clinical-radiologic diagnosis is paired with a histologic pattern. The clinical terms are most appropriate for clinical description, which includes radiology. The latter terms are used to describe biopsy specimens. COP was formerly known as idiopathic bronchiolitis obliterans organizing pneumonia.

PITFALLS

To interpret HRCT images, it is important to understand the pitfalls (13–15). Unfamiliarity with these pitfalls may cause the interpretation of images as abnormal when the find-

Table 14.11: Classification of Idiopathic Interstitial Pneumonias

Clinical Diagnosis Pattern	Histologic
Idiopathic pulmonary fibrosis/cryptogenic fibrosing alveolitis	Usual interstitial pneumonia
Nonspecific interstitial pneumonia	Nonspecific interstitial pneumonia
Cryptogenic organizing pneumonia	Organizing pneumonia
Acute interstitial pneumonia (Chapter 10)	Diffuse alveolar damage
Respiratory bronchiolitis-interstitial lung disease	Respiratory bronchiolitis
Desquamative interstitial pneumonia	Desquamative interstitial pneumonia
Lymphocytic interstitial pneumonia (Chapter 13)	Lymphocytic interstitial pneumonia

Table 14.12: Pitfalls in the Interpretation of HRCT

Patient related
- Motion artifact (respiratory and/or cardiovascular) creates pseudobronchiectasis, pseudo–ground glass opacity and star artifacts
- Dependent atelectasis mimics or hides early subpleural lung disease
- Image noise in large patients and through the shoulders
- Technical
- Viewing images at incorrect window width and level
- Failure to obtain expiratory images (thereby missing small airway disease)

Interpretive/cognitive
- Failure to detect bronchiectasis due to mucous plugging
- Failure to recognize diffuse air trapping on expiratory images
- Interstitial edema due to left heart failure mimics infiltrative lung diseases
- Edema superimposed on emphysema may mimic honeycombing
- Mosaic perfusion (airway, vascular, or infiltrative lung disease)
- Septal lines and ground glass opacity may be interpreted as an idiopathic interstitial pneumonitis, with infection such as cytomegalovirus or *Pneumocystis carinii* unrecognized

ings can best be attributed to an artifact or interpretation as normal when there is really disease present. These pitfalls can be divided into patient related, technical, and interpretive or cognitive pitfalls, as listed in Table 14.12, with several examples illustrated in Figs. 14.27 through 14.30. A window width that is too narrow or a level that is too low falsely thickens bronchial walls and creates false ground glass opacity by making normal parenchymal structures appear too opaque, whereas a width that is too wide may mask diseases that are characterized by reduced attenuation, including emphysema and cystic lung disease (Fig. 14.29). Serial examinations should always be viewed at the same window width–level combinations to avoid reporting disease as better or worse when it is really an artifact of viewing settings. Although there is no single standard window and level combination, appropriate window width lies between 1,000 and 2,000 Hounsfield units and an appropriate level between −500 and −700 Hounsfield units. Normal lung attenuation is between −600 and −700 Hounsfield units.

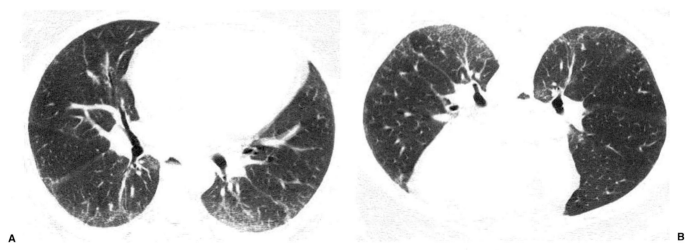

A
B

Figure 14.27 HRCT pitfall: Dependent opacity. *A.* On the supine image there is dependent subpleural ground glass opacity, which can be either be dismissed as dependent opacity or identified as disease, neither of which can be stated confidently without prone images. *B.* On the prone image the abnormality persists, confirming the presence of interstitial lung disease. If the abnormality had resolved, it indicates dependent opacity, a mimic of lung disease.

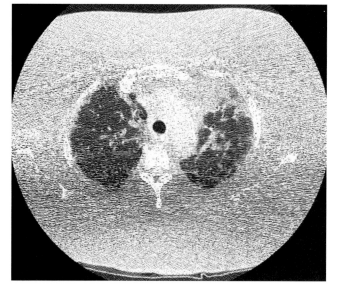

Figure 14.28 HRCT pitfall: Extensive image noise due to large body habitus and relative photon starvation if thin section image, further exaggerated by the use of an edge-enhancing algorithm, rendering this examination nondiagnostic.

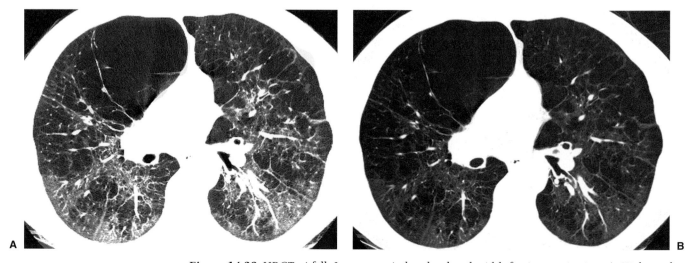

A

B

Figure 14.29 HRCT pitfall: Incorrect window level and width for image viewing. *A.* High resolution computed tomography image at the incorrect window settings appears to demonstrate extensive ground glass opacity, consolidation and septal lines. *B.* In reality, the patient has severe emphysema.

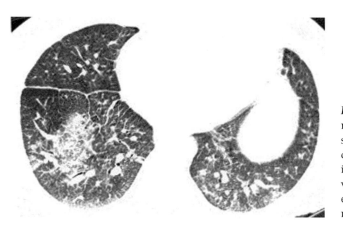

Figure 14.30 Interstitial edema manifesting on HRCT as smooth septal lines and ground glass opacity that is gravity dependent in distribution, with ill-defined vessel margins, and subpleural edema with smoothly thickened right major fissure.

Table 14.13: Patterns of High-Resolution CT Abnormality

Reticular abnormality
- Septal lines
  - Smooth
  - Irregular
  - Nodular
- Honeycombing
- Bronchovascular thickening

Nodular abnormality
- Miliary
- Centrilobular
- Perilymphatic

Altered attenuation
- Increased attenuation
  - Ground glass opacity
  - Consolidation
- Decreased attenuation
  - Cysts
  - Emphysema
- Mosaic attenuation
  - Primary vascular
  - Primary airway
  - Patchy infiltrative lung disease

CT, computed tomography.

MAJOR PATTERNS OF ABNORMALITY

The major patterns of abnormality encountered on HRCT are listed in Table 14.13. As with chest radiographs, these patterns of abnormality may overlap in one examination. It is important to focus on the major or predominant pattern of abnormality when trying to generate a differential diagnosis or a specific diagnosis. For example, a thickened septal line or two can be found on just about any HRCT examination; hence, every disease (as well as normal) could be listed under a gamut for "thickened septal lines." However, to do so would not be practical or useful. Reticular abnormality refers to thickening of inter- and intralobular septa, which when extensive and due to fibrosis form honeycombing. These findings represent abnormal peripheral or "septal" interstitium. There is also a central or axial interstitial compartment, and bronchovascular thickening represents the central equivalent of septal lines. Thickening may be either smooth (as in interstitial pulmonary edema), irregular (as in fibrosis), or nodular (as in lymphangitic tumor spread). Primary nodular abnormality is divided up based on the type and distribution of nodules. Centrilobular nodules that characterize subacute hypersensitivity pneumonitis or RB-associated ILD (RB-ILD) are caused by peribronchiolar inflammation and/or fibrosis. Abnormality that is characterized predominantly by a change in the attenuation of the lung may be either increased, decreased, or mosaic attenuation.

PREDOMINANTLY RETICULAR DISEASES

PULMONARY EDEMA

Interstitial edema appears on chest radiographs as Kerley B lines, which represents edema within the interlobular septa of the "septal" or peripheral interstitial compartment, peribronchial cuffing with perivascular indistinctness due to edema within the central or axial interstitial compartment, and pulmonary vascular redistribution (Fig.

Smooth septal lines in a gravity-dependent distribution should raise the possibility of interstitial pulmonary edema.

> ### Table 14.14: HRCT Findings of Pulmonary Edema
>
> Interlobular septal thickening
> Peribronchovascular interstitial thickening
> Increased vascular caliber
> Pleural effusion
> Thickening of pleural fissures
> Ground glass opacity
>
> From Storto ML, Kee ST, Golden JA, et al. Hydrostatic pulmonary
> edema: high-resolution CT findings. *AJR Am J Roentgenol*
> 1995;165:817–820, with permission.

14.30). The same appearance is seen on HRCT (Table 14.14). Thickened septa in interstitial edema are smooth and usually most severe in a gravity-dependent distribution (16,17). Alveolar opacities are the hallmark of alveolar edema on radiographs; on HRCT this appears as ground glass opacity and even consolidation. Pleural effusions and thickening of fissures may also be a clue that the septal thickening is due to edema and not fibrosis. Edema superimposed on black holes in the lung caused by emphysema may create "pseudo-honeycombing." Note that the distribution will usually be gravity dependent and less subpleural than pulmonary fibrosis. When the major clinical consideration is edema versus ILD, such as UIP or NSIP, repeating the HRCT after diuresis and treatment of heart failure can be useful to demonstrate that the findings have resolved.

LYMPHANGITIC CARCINOMATOSIS

> Polygon formation by thick and nodular septal lines are the hallmarks of lymphangitic carcinomatosis.

Like edema, lymphangitic spread of tumor involves both the peripheral and central interstitial compartments. Involvement of the peripheral compartment is characterized by irregular, nodular, or "beaded" interlobular septa that form polygons and subpleural micronodules (Table 14.15, Fig. 14.31) (18–21). Involvement of the central compartment is characterized by irregular and nodular thickening of the bronchovascular core structures within the secondary lobule and thickening of the central bronchovascular bundles as they extend toward the hila of the lungs. This represents what is known as a perilymphatic distribution of disease. Thick or nodular fissures are common. Early on, these findings may be related to tumor thrombi in lymphatic vessels, accompanied by edema (19). Other findings, such as enlarged lymph nodes and pleural effusions, may accompany the lung findings.

The radiologic findings of lymphangitic carcinomatosis may change slowly or even remain stable for several months, particularly when chemotherapy is being administered. Therefore, stability should not be used to exclude this diagnosis (20). In addition to pulmonary embolism due to a hypercoagulable state, HRCT should be considered in cancer

> ### Table 14.15: HRCT Findings of Lymphangitic Carcinomatosis
>
> Irregular, nodular, or "beaded" interlobular septa
> Polygons
> Subpleural micronodules
> Irregular or nodular thickening of bronchovascular core structures in secondary
>   pulmonary lobules
> Thickening of central bronchovascular bundles
> Pleural effusion
> Thickening and nodularity of pleural fissures
> Enlarged thoracic lymph nodes
>
> From references 18 through 21, with permission.

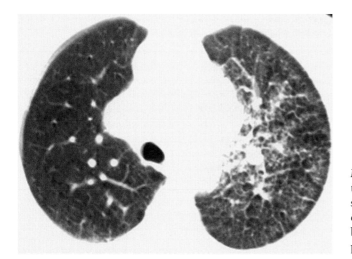

Figure 14.31 Lymphangitic tumor spread in the left lung secondary to bronchogenic carcinoma with nodular and beaded thickened septa forming polygons.

patients with new shortness of breath and a normal chest radiograph to evaluate for radiographically occult lymphangitic carcinomatosis (22). Up to 25% of patients with lymphangitic tumor spread in the lungs may have a normal chest radiograph. In one series, the mean survival of patients with lymphangitic carcinomatosis ranged from 11 to 30 months (median, 13 months).

IDIOPATHIC PULMONARY FIBROSIS

Idiopathic pulmonary fibrosis (10) may appear as a spectrum of abnormalities on HRCT, ranging from ground glass opacity early in the disease course to honeycombing in end-stage disease (Table 14.16). Subpleural lower lobe predominant honeycombing is highly specific for the diagnosis of idiopathic pulmonary fibrosis, a disease process referred to as UIP on histopathologic specimens (Fig. 14.32) (23,24). Traction bronchiectasis and bronchiolectasis accompany areas of honeycombing. Ground glass opacity as the predominant pattern on HRCT has a long differential diagnosis and includes most of the idiopathic interstitial pneumonias, including idiopathic pulmonary fibrosis (25). Reticular and honeycomb abnormalities develop over time in areas that were previously occupied by ground glass opacity. When ground glass opacity is the predominant pattern on HRCT, NSIP and DIP should be suspected.

> Lower lobe predominant subpleural honeycombing is highly specific for idiopathic pulmonary fibrosis.

Table 14.16: HRCT Findings of Idiopathic Pulmonary Fibrosis

Distribution: peripheral, subpleural, basal
Reticular (septal lines)
Honeycombing
Traction bronchiectasis/bronchiolectasis
Architectural distortion
Focal ground glass
Volume loss
Enlarged thoracic lymph nodes
Differential diagnosis
    Asbestosis
    Collagen vascular disease
    Drug toxicity
    Chronic hypersensitivity pneumonitis

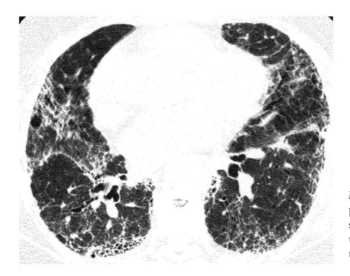

Figure 14.32 HRCT of idiopathic pulmonary fibrosis with subpleural honeycombing, irregular septal thickening, and traction bronchiectasis.

Honeycombing on HRCT represents irreversible fibrosis histologically.

As the name implies, idiopathic pulmonary fibrosis is usually idiopathic in etiology. A similar pattern may also be seen with collagen vascular disease or drug toxicity (26,27). Rarely, idiopathic pulmonary fibrosis is familial. Patients usually present after the age of 50 years with slowly progressive shortness of breath and a nonproductive cough. Most patients with idiopathic pulmonary fibrosis are diagnosed fairly late in the course of the disease and already have honeycombing. The median survival is 2.5 to 3.5 years. Honeycombing represents fibrosis histopathologically and is irreversible (28,29). In contrast, ground glass opacity may represent more active inflammation and is thereby more responsive to therapy (30–32). The pathologic hallmark is heterogeneity and the presence of fibroblastic foci.

ASBESTOSIS

Asbestosis is a basilar predominant reticular lung disease.

This is one of the most common pneumoconioses encountered radiologically, the others being silicosis and coal worker's pneumoconiosis. Although pleural plaques indicate asbestos exposure (Fig. 17.29), the term asbestosis refers to the lung findings in asbestos-exposed individuals. The HRCT findings are listed in Table 14.17. Characteristic findings include inter- and intralobular septal thickening, subpleural and parenchymal bands (the latter akin to a Kerley A line on chest radiographs), and honeycombing in a subpleural posterior and basilar distribution, with or without pleural plaques (Fig. 14.33) (33–35). HRCT is often abnormal in asbestos-exposed individuals patients with normal chest radiographs. Individuals with an abnormal HRCT have lower forced vital capacity and poorer gas exchange than asbestos-exposed individuals with a normal HRCT. Individuals with an abnormal chest radiograph have a longer duration of exposure than those with a normal chest radiograph and abnormal HRCT (36–38).

Table 14.17: HRCT Findings of Asbestosis

Distribution: peripheral, subpleural, basal
Reticular (septal lines)
Subpleural bands
Parenchymal bands
Honeycombing

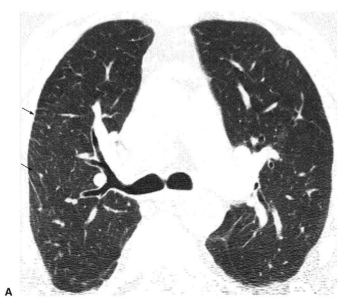

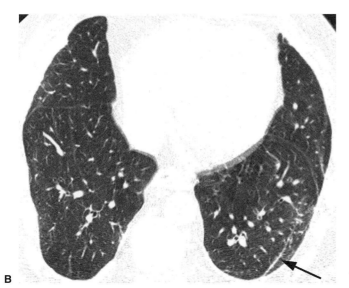

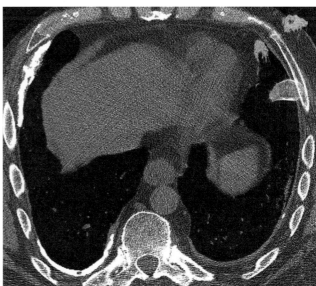

Figure 14.33 HRCT of asbestosis. *A.* Thickened interlobular septa along the periphery of the right lung *(arrows)*. *B.* Subpleural band in the left lower lobe *(arrow)*. *C.* Extensive pleural plaques of asbestos exposure, calcified on the right noncalcified diffuse thickening on the left.

PREDOMINANTLY NODULAR DISEASES

SARCOIDOSIS

This is one of the more commonly encountered chronic infiltrative lung diseases. The clinical presentations, extrapulmonary manifestations, and staging of the disease are discussed in Chapter 13 (Table 13.12, Figs. 13.36, 13.37, and 13.38). The characteristic HRCT findings are peribronchovascular and subpleural nodules in an upper lobe predominant distribution (Table 14.18, Fig. 14.34) (39).

The pathologic lesion of sarcoidosis is the noncaseating granuloma. The granulomas are typically located along lymphatics in the peribronchovascular sheath and to a lesser extent in subpleural and interlobular septal lymphatics (40). This anatomic distribution of abnormality is termed perilymphatic. Nodular upper lobe predominant disease is most commonly sarcoidosis. The major differential diagnosis is silicosis or coal worker's pneumoconiosis if there is an appropriate exposure history. As the disease progresses, irregular

Sarcoidosis is an upper lung predominant nodular lung disease.

Table 14.18: HRCT Findings of Sarcoidosis

Distribution: upper lung predominant
Bronchovascular thickening and peribronchovascular miliary nodules
Subpleural nodules
Irregular mass-like opacities
Architectural distortion and hilar rotation
Honeycombing (late-stage advanced disease)
Multiple pulmonary nodules (uncommon as primary finding)
Alveolar consolidation (uncommon as primary finding)
Enlarged thoracic lymph nodes

opacities, architectural distortion, and honeycombing predominate, as small nodules coalesce into central mass-like opacities (Fig. 14.35) (41). Less common manifestations of pulmonary sarcoidosis include nummular or "coin-like" lesions that resemble metastases and alveolar sarcoidosis that may make the diagnosis challenging. Additional findings include bilateral hilar and mediastinal lymph node enlargement, seen to involve more anatomic locations on CT than at chest radiography.

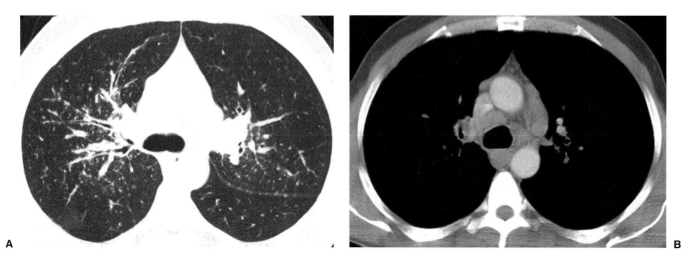

A   **B**

Figure 14.34 HRCT of sarcoidosis. *A.* Small lung nodules surrounding the central bronchovascular structures, which themselves are thickened and beaded. *B.* Enlarged mediastinal lymph nodes.

SILICOSIS AND COAL WORKER'S PNEUMOCONIOSIS

Silicosis is an upper lung predominant nodular lung disease.

Silicosis and coal worker's pneumoconiosis both appear as 2 to 5-mm well-defined discrete nodules that are most extensive in the upper lobes. Over time the nodules may coalesce to form conglomerate masses or progressive massive fibrosis, leaving peripheral emphysema (Fig. 14.36) (42). When this occurs, the profusion of small nodules decreases as they coalesce to form the masses, and emphysema creates increased lucency. Nodules and masses may calcify, and there may be associated eggshell calcified lymph nodes. In early disease when radiographs are still normal, HRCT may reveal the radiographically occult tiny lung nodules. There may be associated lymph node enlargement, calcification of lung nodules, masses and lymph nodes, and a minor component of septal thickening (43–45). Pulmonary function test abnormalities in silicosis correlate more with the amount of underlying emphysema than with the profusion of lung nodules (46). Coalescence of small nodules or conglomerate masses are associated with significant lung volume reduction, reduced gas exchange, and greater airflow obstruction (47).

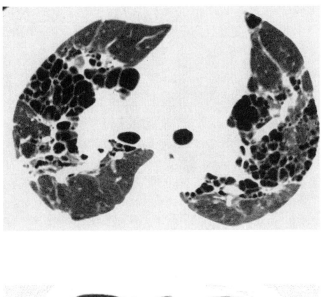

Figure 14.35 HRCT end-stage sarcoidosis with central honeycombing and architectural distortion.

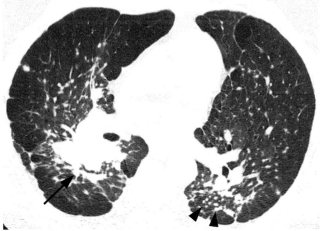

Figure 14.36 HRCT of silicosis with a central right lung conglomerate mass (*arrow*), bilateral small silicotic nodules (*arrowheads*) that coalesce centrally with peripheral emphysema.

HYPERSENSITIVITY PNEUMONITIS

The radiologic appearance depends on the acuity of the exposure. In the subacute stage, diffuse centrilobular nodules, with or without patchy ground glass opacity, and air trapping are seen on HRCT (Fig. 14.37) (48). Clinical history and serologic tests combined with this HRCT appearance are sufficient to make the diagnosis. The HRCT findings are due to a mononuclear cell bronchiolitis and cellular interstitial infiltrate, with poorly defined, scattered, non-necrotizing granulomas (48). Centrilobular nodules have been reported in 40% to 100% of patients with subacute hypersensitivity pneumonitis and patchy ground glass opacity in 52% to 100% (48–50). Ground glass opacity, centrilobular fuzzy nodules, and air trapping are the HRCT hallmarks of subacute hypersensitivity pneumonitis. The abnormality may be more severe in the mid and lower lungs than the lung apices. In a population-based study by Lynch et al. (51) of 31 symptomatic recreation center employees referred because of possible hypersensitivity pneumonitis, 11 were diagnosed with hypersensitivity pneumonitis. Chest radiography was abnormal in only one patient (9%). On contrast, HRCT was abnormal in five patients (45%); in each of these cases poorly defined centrilobular nodules were present.

Ground glass opacity, centrilobular fuzzy nodules, and air trapping are the HRCT hallmarks of subacute hypersensitivity pneumonitis.

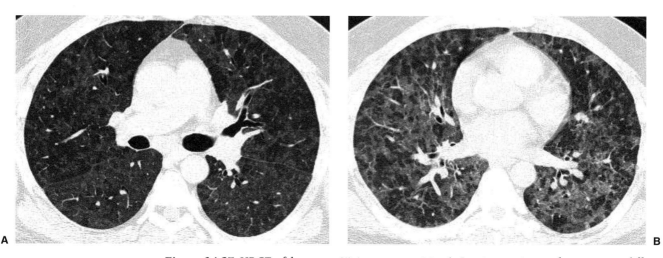

Figure 14.37 HRCT of hypersensitivity pneumonitis. *A.* Inspiratory image demonstrates diffuse ground glass opacity with intervening areas of abnormally low attenuation lung that could loosely be called a mosaic pattern. *B.* Expiratory image demonstrates exaggeration of the mosaic pattern, indicating a component of small airway disease that is commonly seen with hypersensitivity pneumonitis.

Chronic hypersensitivity pneumonitis manifest with patchy reticular abnormality, bronchiectasis, and air trapping that is not in the subpleural lower lung distribution of idiopathic pulmonary fibrosis.

Chronic HP and NSIP may be difficult to separate on HRCT.

The appearance of chronic hypersensitivity pneumonitis is less specific, appearing as fibrosis superimposed on patchy ground glass opacity and centrilobular nodules. It often spares the lung bases or appears patchy with air trapping, findings that can be used to distinguish chronic hypersensitivity pneumonia from UIP (Fig. 14.38) (52,53). Chronic HP and NSIP may be difficult to separate on HRCT. After the antigen that has provoked the lung injury is withdrawn from the patient's environment, ground glass opacity and centrilobular nodules usually improve or resolve, whereas in patients with persistent antigen exposure the HRCT findings persist (49).

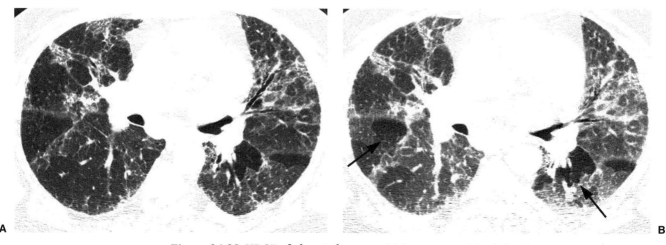

Figure 14.38 HRCT of chronic hypersensitivity pneumonitis. *A.* Inspiratory image demonstrates patchy areas of septal thickening and traction bronchiectasis, which are not in subpleural distribution like usual interstitial pneumonia. Nonspecific interstitial pneumonia can have this appearance as well. *B.* Expiratory image demonstrates a component of air-trapping *(arrows).*

Table 14.19: HRCT Findings of Respiratory Bronchiolitis-associated Interstitial Lung Disease

Distribution: diffuse or upper lung predominant
Centrilobular nodules
Patchy ground glass opacity
Bronchial wall thickening
Air trapping on expiration
Differential diagnosis
    Hypersensitivity pneumonitis
    Desquamative interstitial pneumonia
    Nonspecific interstitial pneumonia

RESPIRATORY BRONCHIOLITIS–ASSOCIATED INTERSTITIAL LUNG DISEASE

RB-ILD is a smoking-related lung disease, with onset usually between ages 30 and 50 years in individuals with an average cigarette smoking history of 30 pack-years. Onset at an earlier age is usually associated with a larger smoking history of shorter duration, such as two to three packs a day for at least 10 years. Men are affected twice as often as women (54,55). Patients with RB-ILD usually have mild slowly progressive dyspnea and a new or increasing chronic cough (10). Some patients are asymptomatic. This abnormality is often an incidental finding in resected lung specimens of patients with bronchogenic carcinoma, another smoking-related disease. Smoking cessation usually results in clinical and radiologic improvement; sometimes corticosteroids are required.

The pathologic features of RB-ILD include the accumulation of pigmented macrophages in a bronchiolocentric distribution with peribronchiolar fibrosis, predominantly involving the first- and second-order respiratory bronchioles. This results in a pattern of centrilobular nodules that is either upper lung predominant or diffuse in distribution. It should be noted that RB-ILD and DIP are a spectrum pathologically, with DIP sharing the association with cigarette smoking as well as macrophage accumulation. The latter is diffuse in DIP and bronchiolocentric in RB-ILD. Other HRCT findings are listed in Table 14.19. There may be superimposed upper lung predominant centrilobular emphysema as well, another smoking-related lung disease (56). Chest radiographs demonstrate bronchial wall thickening and ground glass opacity but may be normal in 14% of patients (10).

> RB-ILD is a smoking-related lung disease characterized by upper lobe predominant centrilobular nodules.

DISEASE CHARACTERIZED PREDOMINANTLY BY ALTERED ATTENUATION

Lung parenchymal attenuation can either be normal, increased (ground glass or consolidation), decreased (emphysema, cysts), or mixed, the so-called mosaic attenuation pattern. Emphysema is discussed in detail in Chapter 15 and so is not discussed here. A mosaic pattern may be seen with small airway disease (Chapter 15), with pulmonary embolism (Chapter 21) or patchy ground glass opacity secondary to an interstitial pneumonia, such as patchy DIP. Expiratory images that either reveal or exaggerate the mosaic pattern indicate small airway disease as the cause.

ABNORMALLY REDUCED ATTENUATION: PREDOMINANTLY CYSTIC LUNG DISEASES

HRCT is very accurate for diagnosing cystic lung disease. Diseases in this category are listed in Table 14.20 and include Langerhans cell histiocytosis (a.k.a. eosinophilic granuloma) and

Table 14.20: HRCT Cystic Lung Diseases
Lymphangioleiomyomatosis
Tuberous sclerosis
Langerhans cell histiocytosis (a.k.a. eosinophilic granuloma)
Chronic *Pneumocytis carinii* infection
Very cavitary metastases

lymphangioleiomyomatosis (LAM), which are both obstructive lung diseases that clinically present with shortness of breath. Other predominantly cystic disease are less common, such as chronic *Pneumocystis carinii* infection or very cavitary thin-walled metastases.

LAM is a very rare cystic lung disease with classic highly specific radiologic findings. This disease is characterized by uniformity and homogeneity. Uniformly sized cysts, uniformly distributed from lung apex to base and center to periphery, uniformly occur in women of childbearing age. Early in the disease the cysts are surrounded by normal lung parenchyma (Fig. 13.34). Over time, no normal parenchyma is visualized (Fig. 14.39) (5,57). The severity of the cysts measured visually or using attenuation-based quantitative CT corresponds to the severity of obstructive pulmonary function abnormalities, the impairment in gas exchange, and the reduction in exercise performance (58,59). The same disease process may also be seen in the lungs of patients with tuberous sclerosis, in which case men can also have the disease. LAM may be a forme fruste of tuberous sclerosis, because patients with LAM have an increased incidence of angiomyolipomas of the kidneys, one of the findings of tuberous sclerosis.

> LAM is a disease of uniformity: uniformly sized cysts, uniformly throughout the lungs, and uniformly in women.

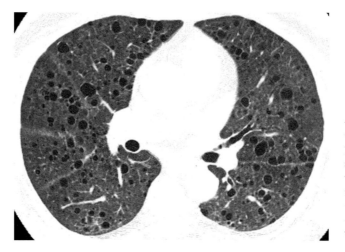

Figure 14.39 High resolution computed tomography of lymphangioleiomyomatosis demonstrates small lung cysts with well-defined walls separated by intervening areas of normal lung that were uniformly distributed through the lungs from apices to bases.

> Langerhans cell histiocytosis is characterized by upper lung predominant irregularly shaped cysts and nodules and is a smoking-related lung disease.

Langerhans cell histiocytosis (otherwise known as histiocytosis X or eosinophilic granuloma) is a cigarette smoking–related lung disease characterized by irregular cysts and nodules that is more severe in the upper lungs than the lower lungs. A history of cigarette smoking is reported in 90% to 100% of cases. Over time, the nodules give way to predominantly cystic lesions. When a combination of cysts and irregular nodules is identified, more severely involving the upper lungs than the lung bases, this diagnosis can be made with confidence (Fig. 14.40) (60–62). The abnormalities may resolve with smoking cessation, but if abnormality and symptoms persist, medical therapy such as corticosteroids may be used. Bone and pituitary gland involvement (diabetes insipidus) are uncommon. In one series of 48 patients, only 2 patients had pituitary involvement

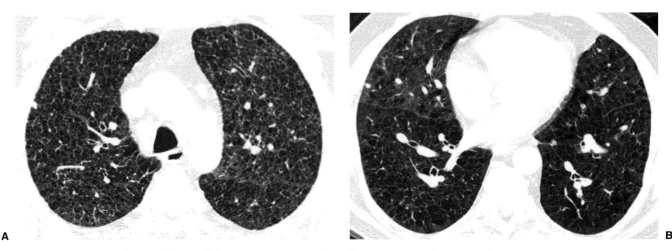

Figure 14.40 HRCT of Langerhans cell histiocytosis. *A.* High resolution computed tomography image through the upper lobes demonstrates the characteristic irregular cysts and small nodules. *B.* Abnormality is less severe in the lower lungs.

and 4 had bone lesions (63). Bronchoalveolar lavage can be used to suggest this diagnosis.

In practice, there should be little difficulty distinguishing between LAM and Langerhans cell histiocytosis. The main differences are outlined in Table 14.21.

Table 14.21: *Langerhans Cell Histiocytosis vs. Lymphangioleiomyomatosis*

	Langerhans Cell Histiocytosis	*Lymphangioleiomyomatosis*
Distribution	Upper lung predominant	Diffuse
Lung findings	Cysts and nodules	Cysts
Other findings	None	Chylous effusions
		Lymph node enlargement
Cyst shape	Irregular	Round and smooth
Associations	Cigarette smoking	Tuberous sclerosis
Gender	Males > females	Females only

DISEASE CHARACTERIZED PREDOMINANTLY BY ABNORMALLY INCREASED ATTENUATION

DESQUAMATIVE INTERSTITIAL PNEUMONIA

DIP was once thought to be due the intraalveolar accumulation of desquamated epithelial cells, hence the name. It is now known to be due to the intraalveolar accumulation of macrophages (64). DIP usually occurs in smokers aged 30 to 50 years and is twice as common in men as in women (10). When DIP occurs in nonsmokers there is usually second-hand smoke exposure. Symptoms include the gradual onset of dyspnea and dry cough over weeks or months and may progress to respiratory failure. DIP is fairly rare compared with UIP and NSIP.

The HRCT findings of DIP are listed in Table 14.22. The characteristic HRCT finding of DIP is ground glass opacity, which is lower lung predominant and subpleural in most cases (Fig. 14.41). In approximately one-fourth of cases the abnormality may be patchy. Reticular lines are a less prominent finding, usually confined to the lung bases (65). Intraalveolar

DIP manifests on HRCT with ground glass opacity that is usually more severe in the lower lungs (it is rarer than most of the interstitial pneumonias).

Table 14.22: HRCT Findings of Desquamative Interstitial Pneumonia

Distribution: basal, peripheral predominance
Ground glass attenuation
Reticular lines
Differential diagnosis
- Respiratory bronchiolitis-interstitial lung disease
- Hypersensitivity pneumonitis
- Infection, such as *Pneumocystis carinii* infection

macrophages create the ground glass opacity, and septal fibrosis creates the reticular lines. In DIP the intraalveolar macrophage accumulation is diffuse, whereas in RB-ILD it is bronchiolocentric. Honeycombing is uncommon. With treatment, ground glass opacity usually resolves (31,66).

NONSPECIFIC INTERSTITIAL PNEUMONIA

NSIP is a recently recognized entity, characterized by a histologic pattern that does not fit into the classification of other interstitial pneumonias, such as UIP, DIP, and lymphoid interstitial pneumonia (LIP) (67). NSIP is often subdivided into cellular and fibrotic forms, the latter being more common (68). NSIP is a heterogeneous group of disorders and may be seen in association with collagen vascular diseases such as scleroderma, hypersensitivity pneumonitis, DIP, drug-induced pneumonitis, infection, and immunodeficiency, including human immunodeficiency virus infection (10). The age at onset is approximately 10 years younger than UIP, it may occur in children, and it has a better prognosis than UIP. There is no gender predominance. Patients present with gradually progressive dyspnea and dry cough, with up to half having weight loss. Most patients either stabilize or improve with therapy; a few die (10). Lymphocytosis may be seen on bronchoalveolar lavage.

The HRCT findings of NSIP are listed in Table 14.23. Ground glass attenuation predominates, with a letter component of irregular lines (Fig. 14.42) (30,32,68–70). Bronchiectasis is commonly seen in areas of ground glass attenuation. Ground glass attenuation corresponds to interstitial thickening pathologically due to inflammation and/or fibrosis. Cellular NSIP is predominantly inflammatory, whereas fibrotic NSIP is predominantly fibrotic. In the setting of bronchiectasis, ground glass opacity represents interstitial fibrosis. Unlike UIP, there are no fibroblastic foci. Honeycombing is very uncommon.

Ground glass opacity with traction bronchiectasis in a lower lung predominant distribution should raise the possibility of NSIP.

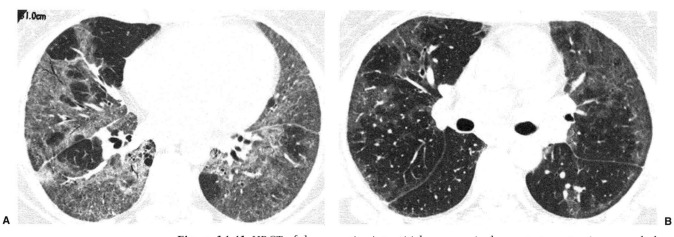

Figure 14.41 HRCT of desquamative interstitial pneumonia demonstrates extensive ground glass opacity that is more severe at the lung bases *(A)* than apices *(B)*.

Table 14.23: HRCT Findings of Nonspecific Interstitial Pneumonia

Distribution: peripheral, subpleural, basal
Ground glass attenuation
Irregular lines
Consolidation
Differential diagnosis
- Usual interstitial pneumonia
- Desquamative interstitial pneumonia
- Chronic organizing pneumonia
- Hypersensitivity pneumonitis

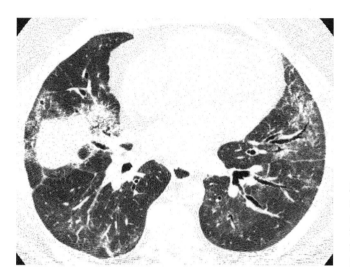

Figure 14.42 HRCT of nonspecific interstitial pneumonia demonstrates basilar predominant ground glass opacity with mild traction bronchiectasis in the absence of honeycombing.

LYMPHOID INTERSTITIAL PNEUMONIA

LIP is characterized by a diffuse lymphoid interstitial infiltrate of lymphocytes, plasma cells, histiocytes, and type 2 cell hyperplasia, dominated by alveolar septal involvement (10). This is in contrast to the peribronchiolar lymphocytic infiltration with germinal centers seen with follicular bronchiolitis (10). Care should be taken to distinguish between LIP and lymphoma histologically, the latter associated with destruction of alveolar architecture, Dutcher bodies, and infiltration of the pleura and along the lymphatics.

LIP is more common in women than men and may present at any age, but most often between 40 and 50 years (71). It has very gradual onset and progression of dyspnea with cough that usually occurs over a few years before clinical presentation, and symptoms are generally milder than other interstitial pneumonias. Idiopathic LIP is rare, with most cases associated with either collagen vascular or autoimmune diseases, as listed in Table 14.24. LIP is also associated with human immunodeficiency virus infection, usually in children. Over 75% of cases are associated with either a polyclonal or monoclonal gammopathy. Once thought to be a premalignant condition, many of the earlier described cases of LIP were reclassified as either low grade lymphoma or NSIP. Using the current histologic definition of LIP, malignant transformation is rare. LIP is less common than UIP and NSIP, and less is known about its natural history or responsiveness to therapy. Corticosteroids are the usual mode of treatment, and some cases may progress to fibrosis. Lymphocytes are seen at bronchoalveolar lavage.

Ground glass opacity and centrilobular nodules are the predominant finding on HRCT, with reticular abnormality in half of patients (72). Findings are usually diffuse in

Table 14.24: Conditions Associated with Lymphocytic Interstitial Pneumonia

Collagen vascular disease
   Sjögren syndrome
   Rheumatoid arthritis
   Systemic lupus erythematosis
Infection
   Hepatitis B
   Pneumocystis carinii
   Ebstein-Barr virus
Immunologic disorders
   Hashimoto thyroiditis
   Chronic active hepatitis
   Primary biliary cirrhosis
   Myasthenia gravis
   Hypogammaglobulinemia
   Severe combined immunodeficiency
   Autoimmune hemolytic anemia
   Pernicious anemia
Drug induced/toxic exposure
HIV infection (in children)

HIV, human immunodeficiency virus.
Adapted from American Thoracic Society/European Respiratory Society International Multidisciplinary Consensus Classification of the Idiopathic Interstitial Pneumonias. *Am J Respir Crit Care Med* 2002;165:277–304.

distribution. Perivascular cysts or honeycombing, nodules and diffuse consolidation have also been reported (73).

CRYPTOGENIC ORGANIZING PNEUMONIA

Multifocal patchy consolidation (sometimes nodular) is the hallmark of COP.

Previously know as bronchiolitis obliterans organizing pneumonia, COP is the preferred term, avoiding confusion with bronchiolitis obliterans (10). COP is characterized by organizing pneumonia within alveolar ducts and alveoli, with or without bronchiolar involvement. COP may be associated with many conditions, as listed in Table 14.25. COP has a

Table 14.25: Conditions Associated with Cryptogenic Organizing Pneumonia

Idiopathic
Infection
Diffuse alveolar damage
Distal to obstruction
Aspiration pneumonia
Drug reaction
Fume and toxic exposures
Collagen vascular diseases
Hypersensitivity pneumonitis
Eosinophilic lung disease
Inflammatory bowel disease
Reparative reaction (to tumor, infection, etc.)

Adapted from American Thoracic Society/European Respiratory Society International Multidisciplinary Consensus Classification of the Idiopathic Interstitial Pneumonias. *Am J Respir Crit Care Med* 2002;165:277–304.

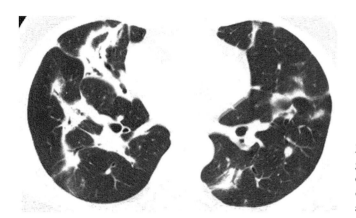

Figure 14.43 HRCT of cryptogenic organizing pneumonia demonstrates multifocal bilateral patchy consolidation with air bronchograms.

mean age at onset of 55 years, occurs equally in men and women, and is twice as common in nonsmokers than smokers (74). Patients present with a short duration of dyspnea and cough, often less than 3 months, which may follow a lower respiratory tract infection. There may be systemic symptoms including sweats and chills, fever, and myalgias. At bronchoalveolar lavage there is a lymphocytosis.

At radiography and HRCT, the hallmark is patchy multifocal and often subpleural alveolar consolidation that does not resolve with antibiotic therapy (Fig. 14.43) (75). Less commonly there are discrete nodular opacities and ground glass opacity. The abnormality is commonly more severe in the lower lungs than the lung apices. The findings rapidly clear with corticosteroid therapy (76).

COP usually responds quickly to corticosteroid therapy with resolution within a few weeks or few months.

PULMONARY ALVEOLAR PROTEINOSIS

Pulmonary alveolar proteinosis (PAP) is a rare disease, characterized by excess surfactant production with the accumulation of phospholipoproteinaceous material within the alveoli that stains pink with periodic acid–Schiff stain. The phospholipids is mostly comprised of lecithin, which is the predominant component of surfactant, and surfactant specific proteins. Over 80% of individuals with PAP are aged 30 to 50 years, and the disease affects men three times more often than women. Patients usually present with dyspnea, cough, and hypoxemia and occasionally with low grade fever. PAP patients are at increased risk of infection with *Aspergillus, Nocardia, Mycobacteria, Cryptococcus neoformans, Histoplasma capsulatum, P. carinii,* and viruses, which may be due to the culture medium created by the phospholipoproteinaceous material and to impaired macrophage function and surfactant abnormalities, which impair host defenses by preventing surfactant from binding to infectious organisms so that they can be phagocytosed by macrophages. The first clinical presentation for patients is often due to the superimposed infection. Most cases are idiopathic; less commonly PAP is associated with chemical inhalation. Whole lung lavage with as many as 20 to 40 L of fluid is the mainstay of therapy, usually performed when dyspnea limits daily activities (77).

The characteristic findings of PAP on HRCT are diffuse or perihilar predominant ground glass opacity with superimposed septal lines that form polygons, giving the "crazy-paving" appearance (Fig. 14.44) (78). The former is due to the phospholipoproteinaceous material within the alveoli, and the latter is usually due to edema (77,79). The abnormality is usually symmetric and is usually out of proportion in extent and severity compared with mild clinical symptoms. The extent of HRCT abnormalities corresponds to the restrictive abnormality seen with pulmonary function testing. Progression to pulmonary fibrosis is rare. Uncommonly, PAP has been reported in children, in whom the appearance on HRCT may also include small miliary nodules (80).

Ground glass opacity with superimposed smooth septal lines forming polygons is the hallmark of alveolar proteinosis and is referred to as "crazy-paving."

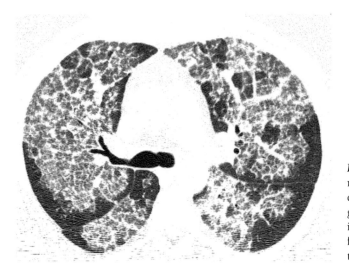

Figure 14.44 HRCT of pulmonary alveolar proteinosis demonstrates diffuse symmetric ground glass opacity with superimposed thickened septal lines, forming polygons and creating the "crazy-paving" appearance.

REFERENCES

1. Reeder MM. *Reeder and Felson's gamuts in radiology: comprehensive lists of roentgen differential diagnosis*, 3rd ed. New York: Springer-Verlag, 1993.
2. Mayo JR, Webb WR, Gould R, et al. High-resolution CT of the lungs: an optimal approach. *Radiology* 1987;163:507–510.
3. Remy-Jardin M, Remy J, Boulenguez C, et al. Morphologic effects of cigarette smoking on airways and pulmonary parenchyma in healthy adult volunteers: CT evaluation and correlation with pulmonary function tests. *Radiology* 1993;186:107–115.
4. Raghu G, Mageto Y, Lockhart D, et al. The accuracy of the clinical diagnosis of new-onset idiopathic pulmonary fibrosis and other interstitial lung disease: a prospective study. *Chest* 1999; 116:1168–1174.
5. Bonelli FS, Hartman TE, Swensen SJ, et al. Accuracy of high-resolution CT in diagnosing lung diseases. *AJR Am J Roentgenol* 1998;170:1507–1512.
6. Potente G, Bellelli A, Nardis P. Specific diagnosis by CT and HRCT in six chronic lung diseases. *Comput Med Imaging Graph* 1992;16:277–282.
7. Nishimura K, Izumi T, Kitaichi M, et al. The diagnostic accuracy of high-resolution computed tomography in diffuse infiltrative lung diseases. *Chest* 1993;104:1149–1155.
8. Leung AN, Staples CA, Muller NL. Chronic diffuse infiltrative lung disease: comparison of diagnostic accuracy of high-resolution and conventional CT. *AJR Am J Roentgenol* 1991;157: 693–696.
9. Mathieson JR, Mayo JR, Staples CA, et al. Chronic diffuse infiltrative lung disease: comparison of diagnostic accuracy of CT and chest radiography. *Radiology* 1989;171:111–116.
10. American Thoracic Society/European Respiratory Society International Multidisciplinary Consensus Classification of the Idiopathic Interstitial Pneumonias. This joint statement of the American Thoracic Society (ATS), and the European Respiratory Society (ERS) was adopted by the ATS board of directors, June 2001 and by the ERS Executive Committee, June 2001. *Am J Respir Crit Care Med* 2002;165:277–304.
11. Kitaichi M. Pathologic features and the classification of interstitial pneumonia of unknown etiology. *Bull Chest Dis Res Inst Kyoto Univ* 1990;23:1–18.
12. Bjoraker J, Ryu J, Edwin M, et al. Prognostic significance of histopathologic subsets in idiopathic pulmonary fibrosis. *Am J Respir Crit Care Med* 1998;157:199–203.
13. Griffin CB, Primack SL. High-resolution CT: normal anatomy, techniques, and pitfalls. *Radiol Clin North Am* 2001;39:1073–1090.
14. Gruden JF, McGuinness G. Subjective pitfalls in HRCT interpretation. *Crit Rev Diagn Imaging* 1996;37:349–434.
15. Primack SL, Remy-Jardin M, Remy J, et al. High-resolution CT of the lung: pitfalls in the diagnosis of infiltrative lung disease. *AJR Am J Roentgenol* 1996;167:413–418.

16. Brasileiro FC, Vargas FS, Kavakama JI, et al. High-resolution CT scan in the evaluation of exercise-induced interstitial pulmonary edema in cardiac patients. *Chest* 1997;111:1577–1582.
17. Storto ML, Kee ST, Golden JA, et al. Hydrostatic pulmonary edema: high-resolution CT findings. *AJR Am J Roentgenol* 1995;165:817–820.
18. Stein MG, Mayo J, Muller N, et al. Pulmonary lymphangitic spread of carcinoma: appearance on CT scans. *Radiology* 1987;162:371–375.
19. Munk PL, Muller NL, Miller RR, et al. Pulmonary lymphangitic carcinomatosis: CT and pathologic findings. *Radiology* 1988;166:705–709.
20. Ikezoe J, Godwin JD, Hunt KJ, et al. Pulmonary lymphangitic carcinomatosis: chronicity of radiographic findings in long-term survivors. *AJR Am J Roentgenol* 1995;165:49–52.
21. Remy-Jardin M, Beuscart R, Sault MC, et al. Subpleural micronodules in diffuse infiltrative lung diseases: evaluation with thin-section CT scans. *Radiology* 1990;177:133–139.
22. Sadoff L, Grossman J, Weiner N. Lymphangitic pulmonary metastases secondary to breast cancer in patients with normal chest radiographs and abnormal perfusion scans. *Oncology* 1975;31:164–171.
23. Tung KT, Wells AU, Rubens MB, et al. Accuracy of the typical computed tomographic appearances of fibrosing alveolitis. *Thorax* 1993;48:334–338.
24. Wells AU, Hansell DM, Rubens MB, et al. The predictive value of appearances on thin-section computed tomography in fibrosing alveolitis. *Am Rev Respir Dis* 1993;148:1076–1082.
25. Collins J, Stern EJ. Ground-glass opacity at CT: the ABCs. *AJR Am J Roentgenol* 1997;169:355–367.
26. Ikezoe J, Johkoh T, Kohno N, et al. High-resolution CT findings of lung disease in patients with polymyositis and dermatomyositis. *J Thorac Imaging* 1996;11:250–259.
27. Devenyi K, Czirjak L. High resolution computed tomography for the evaluation of lung involvement in 101 patients with scleroderma. *Clin Rheumatol* 1995;14:633–640.
28. Muller NL, Colby TV. Idiopathic interstitial pneumonias: high-resolution CT and histologic findings. *RadioGraphics* 1997;17:1016–1022.
29. Muller NL, Miller RR, Webb WR, et al. Fibrosing alveolitis: CT-pathologic correlation. *Radiology* 1986;160:585–588.
30. Katoh T, Andoh T, Mikawa K, et al. Computed tomographic findings in non-specific interstitial pneumonia/fibrosis. *Respirology* 1998;3:69–75.
31. Akira M, Yamamoto S, Hara H, et al. Serial computed tomographic evaluation in desquamative interstitial pneumonia. *Thorax* 1997;52:333–337.
32. Park CS, Jeon JW, Park SW, et al. Nonspecific interstitial pneumonia/fibrosis: clinical manifestations, histologic and radiologic features. *Korean J Intern Med* 1996;11:122–132.
33. Aberle DR, Gamsu G, Ray CS, et al. Asbestos-related pleural and parenchymal fibrosis: detection with high-resolution CT. *Radiology* 1988;166:729–734.
34. Akira M, Yamamoto S, Yokoyama K, et al. Asbestosis: high-resolution CT-pathologic correlation. *Radiology* 1990;176:389–394.
35. Aberle DR. High-resolution computed tomography of asbestos-related diseases. *Semin Roentgenol* 1991;26:118–131.
36. Staples CA, Gamsu G, Ray CS, et al. High resolution computed tomography and lung function in asbestos-exposed workers with normal chest radiographs. *Am Rev Respir Dis* 1989;139:1502–1508.
37. Falaschi F, Boraschi P, Antonelli A, et al. Diagnosis with high-resolution computerized tomography of early asbestos-induced disease. *Radiol Med* 1993;86:220–226.
38. Neri S, Antonelli A, Falaschi F, et al. Findings from high resolution computed tomography of the lung and pleura of symptom free workers exposed to amosite who had normal chest radiographs and pulmonary function tests. *Occup Environ Med* 1994;51:239–243.
39. Brauner MW, Grenier P, Mompoint D, et al. Pulmonary sarcoidosis: evaluation with high-resolution CT. *Radiology* 1989;172:467–471.
40. Muller NL, Kullnig P, Miller RR. The CT findings of pulmonary sarcoidosis: analysis of 25 patients. *AJR Am J Roentgenol* 1989;152:1179–1182.
41. Murdoch J, Muller NL. Pulmonary sarcoidosis: changes on follow-up CT examination. *AJR Am J Roentgenol* 1992;159:473–477.
42. Remy-Jardin M, Degreef JM, Beuscart R, et al. Coal worker's pneumoconiosis: CT assessment in exposed workers and correlation with radiographic findings. *Radiology* 1990;177:363–371.
43. Begin R, Ostiguy G, Fillion R, et al. Computed tomography scan in the early detection of silicosis. *Am Rev Respir Dis* 1991;144:697–705.

44. Remy-Jardin M, Remy J, Farre I, et al. Computed tomographic evaluation of silicosis and coal workers' pneumoconiosis. *Radiol Clin North Am* 1992;30:1155–1176.
45. Talini D, Paggiaro PL, Falaschi F, et al. Chest radiography and high resolution computed tomography in the evaluation of workers exposed to silica dust: relation with functional findings. *Occup Environ Med* 1995;52:262–267.
46. Bergin CJ, Muller NL, Vedal S, et al. CT in silicosis: correlation with plain films and pulmonary function tests. *AJR Am J Roentgenol* 1986;146:477–483.
47. Begin R, Ostiguy G, Cantin A, et al. Lung function in silica-exposed workers. A relationship to disease severity assessed by CT scan. *Chest* 1988;94:539–545.
48. Silver SF, Muller NL, Miller RR, et al. Hypersensitivity pneumonitis: evaluation with CT. *Radiology* 1989;173:441–445.
49. Remy-Jardin M, Remy J, Wallaert B, et al. Subacute and chronic bird breeder hypersensitivity pneumonitis: sequential evaluation with CT and correlation with lung function tests and bronchoalveolar lavage. *Radiology* 1993;189:111–118.
50. Hansell DM, Wells AU, Padley SP, et al. Hypersensitivity pneumonitis: correlation of individual CT patterns with functional abnormalities. *Radiology* 1996;199:123–128.
51. Lynch DA, Rose CS, Way D, et al. Hypersensitivity pneumonitis: sensitivity of high-resolution CT in a population-based study. *AJR Am J Roentgenol* 1992;159:469–472.
52. Grenier P, Chevret S, Beigelman C, et al. Chronic diffuse infiltrative lung disease: determination of the diagnostic value of clinical data, chest radiography, and CT and Bayesian analysis. *Radiology* 1994;191:383–390.
53. Adler BD, Padley SP, Muller NL, et al. Chronic hypersensitivity pneumonitis: high-resolution CT and radiographic features in 16 patients. *Radiology* 1992;185:91–95.
54. Myers J, Veal C, Shin M, et al. Respiratory bronchiolitis causing interstitial lung disease. A clinicopathologic study of six cases. *Am Rev Respir Dis* 1987;135:880–884.
55. Heyneman LE, Ward S, Lynch DA, et al. Respiratory bronchiolitis, respiratory bronchiolitis-associated interstitial lung disease, and desquamative interstitial pneumonia: different entities or part of the spectrum of the same disease process? *AJR Am J Roentgenol* 1999;173:1617–1622.
56. Moon J, DuBois R, Colby T, et al. Clinical significance of respiratory bronchiolitis on open lung biopsy and its relationship to smoking related interstitial lung disease. *Thorax* 1999;54:1009–1014.
57. Templeton PA, McLoud TC, Muller NL, et al. Pulmonary lymphangioleiomyomatosis: CT and pathologic findings. *J Comput Assist Tomogr* 1989;13:54–57.
58. Crausman RS, Lynch DA, Mortenson RL, et al. Quantitative CT predicts the severity of physiologic dysfunction in patients with lymphangioleiomyomatosis. *Chest* 1996;109:131–137.
59. Muller NL, Chiles C, Kullnig P. Pulmonary lymphangiomyomatosis: correlation of CT with radiographic and functional findings. *Radiology* 1990;175:335–339.
60. Taylor DB, Joske D, Anderson J, et al. Cavitating pulmonary nodules in histiocytosis-X high resolution CT demonstration. *Austral Radiol* 1990;34:253–255.
61. Moore AD, Godwin JD, Muller NL, et al. Pulmonary histiocytosis X: comparison of radiographic and CT findings. *Radiology* 1989;172:249–254.
62. Lee WA, Hruban RH, Kuhlman JE, et al. High resolution computed tomography of inflation-fixed lungs: pathologic-radiologic correlation of pulmonary lesions in patients with leukemia, lymphoma, or other hematopoietic proliferative disorders. *Clin Imaging* 1992;16:15–24.
63. Travis WD, Borok Z, Roum JH, et al. Pulmonary Langerhans cell granulomatosis (histiocytosis X). A clinicopathologic study of 48 cases. *Am J Surg Pathol* 1993;17:971–986.
64. Tubbs R, Benjamin S, Reich N, et al. Desquamative interstitial pneumonitis. Cellular phase of fibrosing alveolitis. *Chest* 1977;72:159–165.
65. Hartman TE, Primack SL, Swensen SJ, et al. Desquamative interstitial pneumonia: thin-section CT findings in 22 patients. *Radiology* 1993;187:787–790.
66. Hartman TE, Primack SL, Kang EY, et al. Disease progression in usual interstitial pneumonia compared with desquamative interstitial pneumonia. Assessment with serial CT. *Chest* 1996;110:378–382.
67. Katzenstein A, Fiorelli R. Nonspecific interstitial pneumonia/fibrosis. Histologic features and clinical significance. *Am J Surg Pathol* 1994;18:136–147.
68. Kim T, Lee K, Chung M, et al. Nonspecific interstitial pneumonia with fibrosis: high-resolution CT and pathologic findings. *AJR Am J Roentgenol* 1998;171.
69. Hartman T, Swensen S, Hansell D, et al. Nonspecific interstitial pneumonia: variable appearance at high-resolution chest CT. *Radiology* 2000;217:701–705.
70. Cottin V, Donsbeck A, Revel D, et al. Nonspecific interstitial pneumonia. Individualization of a

clinicopathologic entity in a series of 12 patients. *Am J Respir Crit Care Med* 1998;158: 1286–1293.

71. Koss MN. Pulmonary lymphoproliferative disorders. *Monogr Pathol* 1993:145–194.

72. Johkoh T, Muller NL, Pickford HA, et al. Lymphocytic interstitial pneumonia: thin-section CT findings in 22 patients. *Radiology* 1999;212:567–572.

73. Ichikawa Y, Kinoshita M, Koga T, et al. Lung cyst formation in lymphocytic interstitial pneumonia: CT features. *J Comput Assist Tomogr* 1994;18:745–748.

74. Izumi T, Kitaichi M, Nishimura K, et al. Bronchiolitis obliterans organizing pneumonia. Clinical features and differential diagnosis. *Chest* 1992;102:715–719.

75. Guerry-Force ML, Muller NL, Wright JL, et al. A comparison of bronchiolitis obliterans with organizing pneumonia, usual interstitial pneumonia, and small airways disease. *Am Rev Respir Dis* 1987;135:705–712.

76. Alasaly K, Muller N, Ostrow DN, et al. Cryptogenic organizing pneumonia. A report of 25 cases and a review of the literature. *Medicine* 1995;74:201–211.

77. Shah PL, Hansell D, Lawson PR, et al. Pulmonary alveolar proteinosis: clinical aspects and current concepts on pathogenesis. *Thorax* 2000;55:67–77.

78. Holbert JM, Costello P, Li W, et al. CT features of pulmonary alveolar proteinosis. *AJR Am J Roentgenol* 2001;176:1287–1294.

79. Lee KN, Levin DL, Webb WR, et al. Pulmonary alveolar proteinosis: high-resolution CT, chest radiographic, and functional correlations. *Chest* 1997;111:989–995.

80. McCook TA, Kirks DR, Merten DF, et al. Pulmonary alveolar proteinosis in children. *AJR Am J Roentgenol* 1981;137:1023–1027.

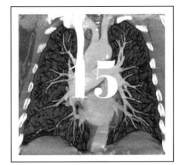

OBSTRUCTIVE LUNG DISEASE

■ Clinical History and Physical Examination
■ Pulmonary Function Testing
■ Radiologic Studies
■ Asthma
■ Chronic Bronchitis
■ Emphysema
■ Giant Bulla
■ Bronchiectasis
■ Impact of Imaging on Therapy

Obstructive lung diseases are characterized by progressive expiratory airway flow limitation and respiratory symptoms, including chronic cough, sputum production, and dyspnea. These diseases are common and associated with significant morbidity and mortality. Clinically, asthma is characterized by reversible airflow obstruction, chronic bronchitis by a productive cough, and emphysema by irreversible airflow obstruction, dyspnea on exertion, pulmonary hyperinflation, and destruction of alveolar walls. Pathologically, asthma is characterized by inflammation and airway remodeling, whereas chronic obstructive pulmonary disease (COPD) is categorized by emphysema, small airway inflammation and fibrosis, and mucous gland hyperplasia (1).

Although there are many similarities among the major pathophysiologic categories of disease causing chronic airflow obstruction, the advent of new therapeutic modalities and differences in patient prognosis highlight the importance of making a specific diagnosis. For example, patients with nonasthmatic airflow obstruction have a greater rate of decline in forced expiratory volume in 1 second (FEV$_1$) and poorer survival than patients with chronic asthmatic bronchitis (2), and patients with a self-reported history of chronic bronchitis have a steeper drop in FEV$_1$ than patients with asthma (3). By using clinical history, physical examination, and pulmonary function testing together with imaging, in particular high resolution computed tomography (HRCT), the subsets of chronic obstructive lung disease can be distinguished and therapy correctly tailored.

Table 15.1 lists the common diseases that are traditionally considered under the heading "COPD." COPD is currently defined as a disease state characterized by airflow obstruction that does not change markedly over months of observation. It is usually pathologically a result of chronic bronchitis or emphysema (1,4). According to a National Heart, Lung and Blood Institute Workshop on the subject, "The term 'COPD' is generally used in

Clinically and radiographically, manifestations of more than one form of COPD may be present in the same patient.

Table 15.1: Chronic Obstructive Pulmonary Diseases

Asthma
Chronic bronchitis
Emphysema
Bronchiectasis

clinical discourse to describe individuals diagnosed with one or more of the following conditions: asthmatic bronchitis, chronic bronchitis, chronic obstructive bronchitis and emphysema" (5). Less common obstructive lung diseases include bronchiolitis obliterans and lymphangioleiomyomatosis. It is estimated that 14 million people in the United States have COPD, of which approximately 12.5 million have chronic bronchitis and 1.65 million have emphysema. COPD is the fourth leading cause of death in the United States (4). Asthma is also common, affecting approximately 11 million people (6). The prevalence of COPD, in particular asthma, is increasing (7,8). Given the strong association of COPD and cigarette smoking, this condition is largely preventable. Within any one patient features of emphysema, chronic bronchitis and asthma may overlap, and distinguishing between them may therefore be confounded. For example, some patients with asthma, particularly longstanding asthma, lack the reversibility of airflow obstruction that characterizes asthma, thereby mimicking COPD (7). Conversely, some patients with chronic bronchitis and emphysema have a significant component of bronchoreversibility, thereby mimicking asthma (9).

CLINICAL HISTORY AND PHYSICAL EXAMINATION

Cough, wheezing, and dyspnea are the common symptoms of obstructive lung disease and overlap between asthma and COPD. History can be useful to identify a specific obstructive lung disease, for example, a history of symptoms first appearing in childhood, a persistent cough after an upper respiratory tract infection, and/or a history of atopic disease or occupational exposure favor asthma (10,11). An episodic cough, perhaps brought on by exercise or allergens, also indicates an asthmatic component to obstructive lung disease. In contrast, patients with COPD generally have more constant and progressive symptoms; many patients with longstanding disease may be asymptomatic even in the face of severe disease (12). Age is an indicator of the type of obstructive lung disease. In one study, the mean age of patients with predominantly asthmatic bronchitis was 29.6 years versus 64.6 years for emphysematous COPD (2). Patients with α_1-antitrypsin deficiency develop premature COPD, with a mean age of dyspnea onset at 40 years for smokers and 53 years for nonsmokers. Therefore, patients less than 50 years of age with moderate or severe chronic airflow obstruction, basilar emphysema, and a strong family history of obstructive disease, should be tested for α_1-antitrypsin deficiency (4).

The most useful signs on physical examination of airflow obstruction are objective wheezing, barrel chest deformity, rhonchi, hyperresonance, subxiphoid apical impulses, and an objective measurement of prolonged expiration (11,13,14). Forced expiratory time may be useful to screen for obstructive lung disease; however, physicians are generally poor at estimating the severity of obstruction from physical examination. In one series, only 38% of physicians' pretreatment estimates were accurate (15). The role of blood studies in the evaluation of obstructive lung disease is limited. An elevated IgE level and increased blood eosinophils may aid in identifying patients with asthmatic airflow obstruction. Patients with any history of asthma have a higher degree of eosinophilia and elevated IgE levels than patients without a history of asthma (3,16). However, patients with newly diagnosed chronic bronchitis may also have elevated IgE and eosinophil levels.

PULMONARY FUNCTION TESTING

The most useful laboratory studies for the evaluation of airflow obstruction are pulmonary function tests. These tests are necessary for diagnosis, evaluating disease severity, and monitoring response to treatment (4,17). Spirometry is a simple screening test for airflow obstruction, with spirometers widely available and simple to use. American Thoracic Society guidelines provide normal standards and the framework for the interpretation of results, with values adjusted for age and gender (Table 15.2) (18). The most valuable measurements include the FEV_1, forced vital capacity (FVC), and peak inspiratory/expiratory flows measured from a maximal expiratory maneuver. A decrease in the FEV_1/FVC ratio from the predicted range is diagnostic of airflow obstruction (18,19). A lower initial FEV_1/FVC ratio in COPD may be associated with greater declines in FEV_1 over time (20). Airflow obstruction severity is judged on FEV_1 expressed as a percent of the predicted value (18). A graphic representation of peak expiratory and inspiratory flow versus lung volume, known as the flow-volume loop, should be examined to exclude potential upper airway obstruction (21).

Measurement of spirometric parameters before and after administration of a short-acting β agonist may aid in establishing bronchoreversibility. A rise in FEV_1 of 12% with an absolute rise of at least 200 mL indicates bronchoreversibility (18). Complete reversibility of airflow obstruction makes the diagnosis of asthma likely and strongly argues against COPD (11). However, a subset of patients with asthma develop irreversible airflow obstruction (7,22–24). Such patients typically have a longer duration of asthma and more symptomatic disease than asthma patients with reversible obstruction (22). Furthermore, asthma patients with irreversible airflow obstruction may have baseline FEV_1, FVC, and postbronchodilator FEV_1 measurements indistinguishable from COPD patients; therefore, the lack of bronchodilator reversibility cannot be used with sufficient specificity to differentiate COPD from asthma (23). Up to 30% of patients with COPD have bronchoreversibility at spirometric testing (25,26). In a series of patients with asthma (n = 287) or COPD (n = 108), the mean increase in FEV_1 from baseline after inhaled albuterol was higher in asthma patients (16.5% versus 10.6%); however, there was significant overlap (9). The best specificity for the diagnosis of asthma (84%) was defined at a threshold of a 20% or greater increase in FEV_1 from baseline; however, sensitivity was poor. The postbronchodilator FEV_1 has been shown to be the single best predictor of survival in patients with COPD, with a value below 30% of predicted associated with marked reduction in long-term survival (25). As a result, the postbronchodilator FEV_1 has become instrumental in establishing an appropriate time for considering surgical therapy in patients with advanced COPD.

Spirometry can also be performed after the administration of an agent to induce bronchial hyperreactivity, such as methacholine (19,27). Patients with asthma have greater airway hyperresponsiveness than patients with COPD (27–29,30), although many patients with COPD also have airway hyperreactivity (27). In the Lung Health Study of almost 6,000 current smokers with borderline to moderate airflow obstruction, nonspecific airway hyperresponsiveness (defined as a drop of at least 20% in FEV_1 after inhalation of no more than 25 mg/mL methacholine) was noted in 85.1% of women and 58.9% of men (31). Baseline airway obstruction, wheeze, cough with or without sputum production, and a past history of asthma or hay fever were associated with hyperresponsiveness.

Table 15.2: Categories of Obstructive Abnormality on Pulmonary Function Testing

	FEV_1 (% Predicted)	FEV_1 / FVC (% Predicted)
Mild obstructive abnormality	70%	<70%
Moderate/moderately severe obstructive abnormality	50–70%	<70%
Severe obstructive abnormality	<50%	<70%

FEV, forced expiratory volume in one second; FVC, forced vital capacity.
From American Thoracic Society. Lung function testing: selection of reference values and interpretative strategies. *Am Rev Respir Dis* 1991;144:1202–1218, with permission.

The measurement of lung diffusing capacity for carbon monoxide (DL_{CO}) is a routine test in the evaluation of chronic airflow obstruction, particularly for more advanced disease. DL_{CO} is a sensitive test for emphysema, a disease process associated with loss of alveolar surface area and pulmonary circulation (32). Decreased DL_{CO} accompanying chronic airflow obstruction suggests at least a component of emphysema (33). The specificity of DL_{CO} for obstructive lung disease is low, and it should be used together with clinical history and physical examination. In large epidemiologic studies, a normal DL_{CO} is associated with asthma rather than COPD (34). DL_{CO} may be also increased in patients with asthma (35, 36). However, when asthma manifests with irreversible airway obstruction, DL_{CO} may be low (23). In patients with emphysema, there is a strong correlation between low DL_{CO} and greater severity of emphysema on CT (37). A decreased DL_{CO} is associated with a more rapid decline in pulmonary function over time (20).

Peak expiratory flow is the maximal flow that can be achieved during maximal expiratory effort. This measurement has been widely accepted and advocated for the monitoring of patients with airflow obstruction, particularly asthma (17). Widespread availability of inexpensive, simple, reliable devices has made the routine measurement of peak expiratory flow rate possible (38). There is a close relationship between the FEV_1 and peak expiratory flow rate; however, in general peak expiratory flow rate is consistently higher (38,39). Limitations of using peak expiratory flow rate include a reduction in peak expiratory flow rate both with obstructive lung disease and upper airway obstruction (21) and a lower sensitivity of peak expiratory flow rate than spirometry for detecting reversibility of airflow obstruction after bronchodilators or detecting bronchial response to challenge with occupational sensitizers (40,41).

RADIOLOGIC STUDIES

Posteroanterior and lateral chest radiographs are part of the initial evaluation of dyspnea. Many of the radiographic signs of obstructive lung disease lack specificity, such that chest radiographs are used predominantly to support a diagnosis of obstructive lung disease and not for primary diagnosis. Radiographic signs of obstructive lung disease also lack sensitivity and should not be used to exclude the diagnosis. The radiographic features of asthma, chronic bronchitis, and emphysema often overlap, similar to the overlap in clinical features. Although CT findings in the different forms of obstructive lung disease are well described and CT is the best tool to evaluate the severity of emphysema *in vivo*, CT has a limited role in the primary diagnosis of obstructive lung disease. In a small subset of dyspnea patients with an isolated reduction in diffusing capacity and otherwise normal pulmonary function tests and a normal chest radiograph, HRCT is useful for establishing the diagnosis of emphysema (42,43). When bronchiectasis is suspected, HRCT is the technique of choice for detecting, localizing, and characterizing bronchiectasis, having replaced bronchography. HRCT examinations can also be performed at end-expiration to add a functional component to the inspiratory HRCT technique. Expiratory CT may demonstrate air trapping in patients with small airway diseases such as asthma and bronchiolitis obliterans, often when inspiratory HRCT images are normal (44).

ASTHMA

CLINICAL FEATURES AND DEFINITION

The diagnosis of asthma is based on clinical history and evidence of reversible airflow obstruction (17). Asthma is typically characterized by airway inflammation, airway hyper-responsiveness, and reversible airflow obstruction (7,45). Accurate diagnosis, monitoring of disease severity, and treatment response are considered the standard of care for asthma (17). Asthma is difficult to diagnose on purely clinical grounds (17,46). In one series of

60 adults with a physician diagnosis of asthma, 40% did not meet objective diagnostic criteria for asthma. Disease severity is often understated by both the patient and physician in the absence of spirometry or peak flow measurement (17).

Asthma is often thought of as a childhood illness, with many outgrowing the disease by adolescence if not adulthood. Asthma may persist into adulthood. Individuals diagnosed with asthma in childhood who ceased wheezing during adolescence have no difference in pulmonary function than normal control subjects, whereas those who continue to wheeze have abnormal pulmonary function. However, 60% of patients who stopped wheezing have evidence of bronchial hyperresponsiveness with histamine challenge (47). The outcome of childhood asthma is predominantly related to the initial level of bronchial obstruction and airway responsiveness. Lack of asthma at follow-up is associated with younger age and less severe airway obstruction when first tested, whereas the absence of bronchial hyperreactivity is associated with younger age, higher FEV_1, and shorter untreated period (48). Milder disease and early intervention are important components to asthma outcome. Tobacco smoke has a deleterious effect on asthma. Asthmatics exposed to greater than 3 hours of smoke per week have greater severity of asthma scores, worse asthma-specific quality of life scores, and decreased SF-36 health status questionnaire scores and increased odds for emergency room visits, urgent doctor visits, and hospitalizations compared with non–smoke-exposed asthma control subjects (49).

The development of asthma is multifactorial and includes family history of asthma and current or former smoking (50). The odds of having a child with asthma are three times greater in a family in which one parent has asthma and six times more likely when both parents have asthma and are greater if the mother has asthma than if the father has asthma (51). In one series of 265 first-degree offspring of asthma patients, 18% of the offspring had definite asthma and 8% had probable asthma (52).

PATHOPHYSIOLOGY

Inflammation is now recognized to have a large role in asthma (7). Even in patients with mild asthma there is collagen deposition beneath the epithelial basement membrane and extensive inflammation in bronchial biopsy specimens (53). There are increased numbers of inflammatory cells and eosinophils in the airway epithelium of asthmatics, and these cells are associated with increased bronchial reactivity. Greater subepithelial thickening correlates with lower FEV_1 and greater peak flow variability, suggesting that the clinical severity of asthma is associated with both the severity of inflammation and also the degree of airway remodeling (54). Patients with COPD who demonstrate corticosteroid reversibility may have features of asthma and inflammation, with COPD responders having a larger number of eosinophils and higher levels of eosinophilic cationic protein in bronchoalveolar lavage fluid and thicker reticular basement membrane than COPD nonresponders (55).

Airway inflammation plays an important role in asthma.

CHEST RADIOGRAPHY AND COMPUTED TOMOGRAPHY

The chest radiographic features of asthma include pulmonary hyperinflation with increased lung lucency and mild bronchial wall thickening (Fig. 15.1). However, the chest radiograph is often normal, particularly in the absence of acute asthma symptoms. Mild pulmonary artery enlargement may occur due to transient pulmonary hypertension (56). During acute exacerbation of asthma, atelectasis, mucous plugging, spontaneous pneumomediastinum, or pneumothorax may develop. The latter occurs due to air trapping with a ball–valve phenomenon, allowing air into the lungs with inspiration but little if any exit of air on expiration. HRCT examinations are frequently abnormal in asthma patients with normal chest radiographs. In one series 71.9% of asthmatics had an abnormal HRCT, whereas only 37.8% of these patients had an abnormal chest radiograph (57). HRCTs may be normal, particularly in mild asthma.

Radiographs are often normal in asthma patients.

HRCT may show bronchial wall thickening or air trapping in asthma not evident on chest radiographs.

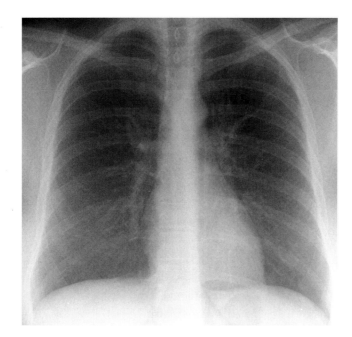

Figure** **15.1 Posteroanterior chest radiograph of a patient with asthma demonstrates pulmonary hyperinflation and peribronchial cuffing.

Bronchial dilatation occurs in 28% to 36% of asthma patients and bronchial wall thickening in 82% to 92% of asthma patients (58,59). Reversible findings on HRCT include mucoid impaction and lobar collapse, present in 10% to 20% of asthmatic patients (57,58). In longstanding asthma, bronchial dilatation and bronchial wall thickening on HRCT are often irreversible (23,57,58,60). Bronchial wall thickening and bronchial dilatation are more common and more severe in asthmatic patients with moderate to severe airflow obstruction and in patients with a prolonged history of asthma than in patients with mild obstruction or normal airflow (61–64).

Air trapping is commonly demonstrated on expiratory HRCT and may precede the development of airway dilatation and thickening (Fig. 15.2) (60). Patients with nonallergic asthma have more extensive airway remodeling on CT than patients with allergic asthma, with a higher frequency of bronchial dilatation, bronchial recruitment, and emphysema (63). In contrast, patients with chronic stable asthma develop a reduction in

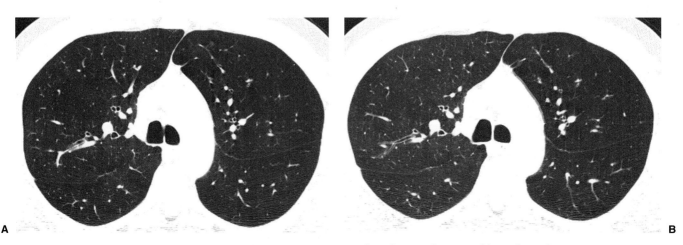

***Figure** 15.2* HRCT in a patient with asthma and irreversible airflow obstruction. *A.* Inspiratory image demonstrate diffuse abnormally low attenuation lung parenchyma. *B.* On the expiratory image the lungs remain inflated, without the usual decrease in size and increase in attenuation that is expected at expiration.

lung attenuation on HRCT that is not due to emphysema. In nonsmoking asthmatic patients, emphysema is not a feature of asthma on HRCT (65,66). This reduction in lung attenuation may represent nondestructive hyperinflation.

Some lung findings on HRCT in mild asthmatics can be provoked and are reversible. After bronchial provocation with methacholine chloride, a reduction in lung attenuation and reduction in the cross-sectional area of small airways (less than 5 mm^2) occurs compared with baseline, accompanied by a 10% to 26% decrease in FEV$_1$. After reversal with albuterol, these findings return to normal (67). After methacholine inhalation, the internal airway lumen diameter has been shown to decrease 17% from baseline, increasing to 18% above baseline after albuterol inhalation (68). Methacholine-induced bronchial constriction occurs in bronchi of all sizes but is most severe in the small bronchi 2 to 4 mm in diameter (69). Although in normal patients a decrease in bronchial wall thickness accompanies bronchoconstriction, bronchial wall thickness does not decrease in asthmatic patients as measured on HRCT (69).

CHRONIC BRONCHITIS

Chronic bronchitis is diagnosed clinically by the presence of chronic productive cough for 3 months in each of 2 successive years in a patient in whom other causes of chronic cough have been excluded (4). Compared with asthma and emphysema, the radiographic features of chronic bronchitis are poorly described. Findings at chest radiography include pulmonary hyperinflation and thickened bronchial walls, resulting in peribronchial thickening or cuffing, and increased "markings" due to superimposition of the thickened small bronchi and bronchiole walls (70). There is little information on the HRCT findings in chronic bronchitis. The most common HRCT finding is bronchial wall thickening, a nonspecific finding (71). In one series of 45 patients with air trapping on expiratory HRCT, 4 patients with chronic bronchitis were reported (44). All four patients had air trapping on expiratory HRCT, and one patient had a normal inspiratory HRCT. In the remaining three patients, the inspiratory HRCT demonstrated bronchial wall thickening, a tree-in-bud appearance secondary to mucoid impaction, and ground glass opacity presumed to be secondary to concomitant infection.

EMPHYSEMA

According to the American Thoracic Society, emphysema is defined as "a condition of the lung characterized by abnormal, permanent enlargement of the air spaces distal to the terminal bronchiole, accompanied by destruction of their walls" and without obvious fibrosis (4). Emphysema occurs due to an imbalance in the proteolytic activity in the lungs, resulting in destruction of alveolar tissue. This may be seen with an overabundance of proteolytic enzymes, a lack of antiproteases, or a combination of both. In smoking-related centrilobular emphysema there is excess protease, whereas in α_1-antitrypsin deficiency there is a deficiency of α_1-antiproteinase.

The pathologic classification of emphysema is based on the secondary pulmonary lobule. The four major categories of emphysema, as listed in Table 15.3, are centrilobular (cen-

Table 15.3: Major Categories of Emphysema

Types of Emphysema	Anatomic Distribution	Associations
Centrilobular (a.k.a. centriacinar)	Upper lung predominant	Cigarette smoking
Panlobular (a.k.a. panacinar)	Lower lung predominant	α_1-Antitypsin deficiency
Paraseptal	Subpleural	Aging
Paracicatricial	Focal	Scar/fibrosis

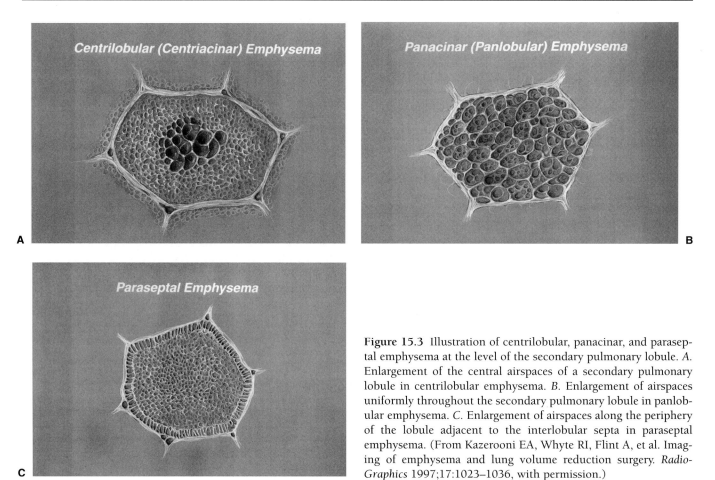

Figure 15.3 Illustration of centrilobular, panacinar, and paraseptal emphysema at the level of the secondary pulmonary lobule. *A.* Enlargement of the central airspaces of a secondary pulmonary lobule in centrilobular emphysema. *B.* Enlargement of airspaces uniformly throughout the secondary pulmonary lobule in panlobular emphysema. *C.* Enlargement of airspaces along the periphery of the lobule adjacent to the interlobular septa in paraseptal emphysema. (From Kazerooni EA, Whyte RI, Flint A, et al. Imaging of emphysema and lung volume reduction surgery. *Radio-Graphics* 1997;17:1023–1036, with permission.)

Centrilobular emphysema is usually most severe in the upper lungs and is secondary to cigarette smoking.

triacinar), panacinar (panlobular), paraseptal, and paracicatricial (Fig. 15.3) (72). Table 15.4 summarizes the differences between centrilobular and panlobular emphysema. *Centrilobular emphysema* is the most common form of emphysema and is usually secondary to cigarette smoking. The destruction of alveolar walls begins in the central portion of the secondary pulmonary lobule (Fig. 15.4) and is heterogeneous, affecting adjacent lobules with varying degrees of severity; it is usually most severe in the upper lobes (Fig. 15.5). The relatively greater ventilation-perfusion ratio in the upper portion of the lungs compared with the lung bases favors greater deposition of the particulate matter from cigarette smoke in the upper lungs. Activated macrophages release the proteolytic enzyme, elastase; free radicals and oxidants in cigarette smoke inactive normally protective antiproteases, leading to greater destruction of the upper lobes than the lower lobes (72).

Panlobular emphysema is usually most severe in the lower lungs and is secondary to α_1-antitrypsin deficiency.

Panlobular emphysema typically occurs in patients with α_1-antitrypsin deficiency and is accelerated by superimposed cigarette smoking. The proteolytic enzyme elastase is found within neutrophils and macrophages in the lung and is kept in check by antiproteases, such as α_1-antitrypsin. More circulating α_1-antiprotease is usually delivered to the lower lungs than the upper lungs due to the greater distribution of blood flow to the lower

Table 15.4: Centrilobular Versus Panlobular Emphysema

	Centrilobular	Panlobular
Within a lobule	Heterogenous	Homogenous
Anatomic distribution	Upper lung predominant	Lower lung predominant
Associations	Cigarette smoking	α_1-Antitrypsin deficiency

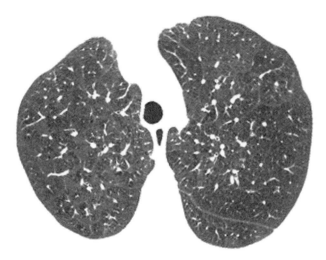

Figure 15.4 Mild centrilobular emphysema on high resolution computed tomography with small rounded areas of low attenuation adjacent to centrilobular arteries.

lungs. When α_1-antiprotease is deficient, the greatest deficiency is therefore seen at the lung bases; the lack of antiproteolytic activity results in greater destruction of lung parenchyma at the lung bases. Therefore, in contrast to centrilobular emphysema, panlobular emphysema is usually more severe in the lower lungs than the upper lungs and homogeneously affects the entire lobule as well as adjacent lobules (Fig. 15.6).

Paraseptal emphysema involves the peripheral or paraseptal portion of the secondary pulmonary lobules (Fig. 15.7), the apices and paramediastinal portion of the upper lobes, and may be related to aging, although it remains poorly understood. Pathologically, the most distal portion of the acinus is involved, explaining why this form of emphysema appears to be most noticeable adjacent to the pleura or interlobular septa. This form of emphysema can lead to spontaneous pneumothorax and even progressively enlarging bulla.

Paracicatricial emphysema, also known as perifocal emphysema, occurs adjacent to areas of scarring, fibrosis, and granulomas (Fig. 15.8). As an example, it may be seen in the periphery of the upper lungs in patients with silicosis and conglomerate masses. In this form of emphysema, airspace enlargement and alveolar septal destruction occur in the vicinity of focal lesions such as fibrotic granulomas. The destruction occurs gradually after the scar has formed. The lesion often has little functional significance, unless multiple foci are present.

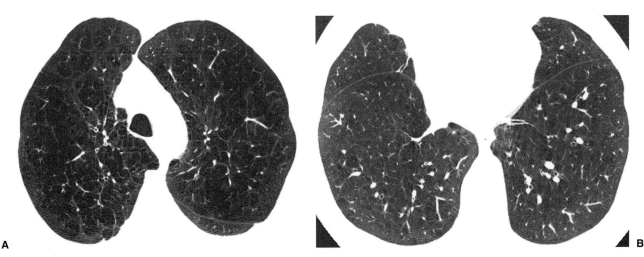

A   B

Figure 15.5 Advanced centrilobular emphysema on high resolution computed tomography with (A) severe emphysema involving the entire upper lobes and (B) less severe emphysema involving the lower lobes, where areas of normal attenuation parenchyma can be found.

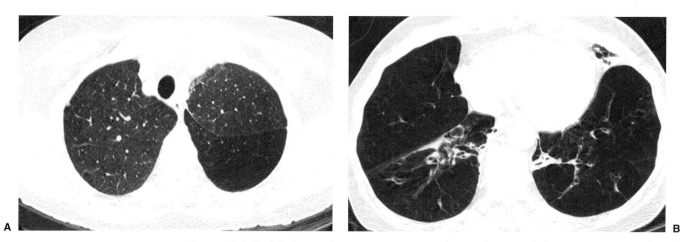

Figure 15.6 Panlobular emphysema in a patient with α₁-antitrypsin deficiency on HRCT. (A) Mild emphysema involving the entire upper lobes and (B) severe emphysema involving the lower lobes.

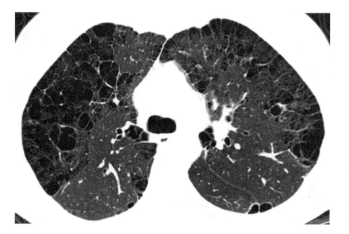

Figure 15.7 Paraseptal emphysema on HRCT with abnormal low attenuation regions along the pleural surface and adjacent to interlobular septa.

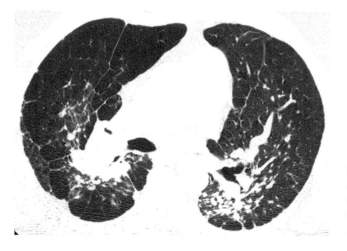

Figure 15.8 Paracicatricial emphysema in a patient with advanced silicosis. Peripheral emphysema surrounds the central conglomerate masses.

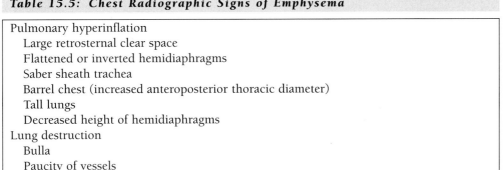

Table 15.5: Chest Radiographic Signs of Emphysema

Pulmonary hyperinflation
  Large retrosternal clear space
  Flattened or inverted hemidiaphragms
  Saber sheath trachea
  Barrel chest (increased anteroposterior thoracic diameter)
  Tall lungs
  Decreased height of hemidiaphragms
Lung destruction
  Bulla
  Paucity of vessels

CHEST RADIOGRAPHY

The chest radiographic features of emphysema include both signs of lung destruction and pulmonary hyperinflation (Table 15.5). Signs of lung destruction include irregular radiolucency of the lungs, arterial depletion, and thin-walled bullae. Signs of hyperinflation include flattening or depression of the diaphragm, enlargement of the retrosternal clear space, increased anteroposterior chest dimension (the so-called barrel chest), increased lung height, and decreased height of the right hemidiaphragm (Fig. 15.9) (56,73,74). These signs alone or in combination have variable sensitivity for emphysema detection ranging from 40% to 80% (56). Additional signs of severe emphysema are due to secondary pulmonary arterial hypertension and right heart overload, with enlargement of central pulmonary arteries and right heart chambers. Although moderate to severe emphysema is generally radiographically detectable, chest radiographs are insensitive for detecting mild emphysema.

Signs of emphysema on radiographs include both lung destruction and hyperinflation.

Radiographs are not sensitive for mild or even moderate emphysema.

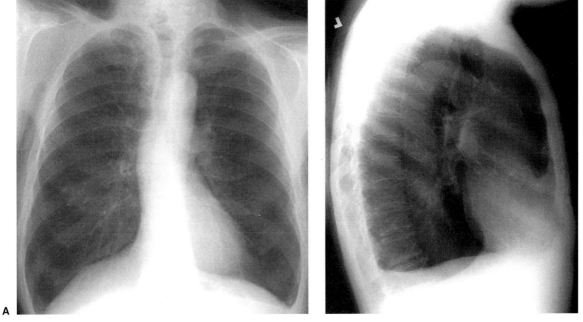

A   B

Figure 15.9 Radiographic manifestations of emphysema on (*A*) posteroanterior and (*B*) lateral chest radiographs include pulmonary hyperinflation manifesting as flattened hemidiaphragms, a large retrosternal clear space, tall lungs, and a saber sheath trachea. Abnormal pulmonary vascular branching pattern is a sign of lung destruction.

Signs of hyperinflation are the most sensitive for emphysema detection but lack specificity when applied to other obstructive lung diseases. For example, Reich et al. (75) demonstrated that when the height of the right hemidiaphragm on the lateral chest radiograph was less than or equal to 2.6 cm, chest radiographs were 67.7% sensitive for detecting patients with obstructive spirometry (75). In the same series, a right lung height of 29.9 cm or more on the posteroanterior chest radiograph was 69.8% sensitive (FP [false positive] rate for both, 5%). By combining signs of both lung destruction and hyperinflation, the specificity of chest radiographs for emphysema improves but at the expense of sensitivity. Only the presence of bullae is specific for emphysema on chest radiographs. Chest radiographs provide supporting evidence of the diagnosis of emphysema and are used to evaluate for complications of emphysema, such as pneumonia or lung cancer; the insensitivity of chest radiographs for detecting mild to moderate emphysema has limited their usefulness as a diagnostic tool (74,76,77).

COMPUTED TOMOGRAPHY

The severity of emphysema on CT correlates very well with the severity of emphysema in pathologic specimens.

CT provides excellent anatomic detail for detecting, characterizing, and estimating the severity of emphysema. Not surprisingly, conventional CT is more accurate than chest radiography, and HRCT is more accurate than conventional CT (78–80). On CT, emphysema appears as abnormal areas of low attenuation lung without definable walls, resulting in a decrease in the mean attenuation value of the lung parenchyma (Figs. 15.4, 15.5, and 15.6) (56). When reporting emphysema on CT, it is important to note the severity, symmetry between lungs, and distribution within the lungs as upper lobe predominant, diffuse, or lower lobe predominant. The presence of giant bullae, bronchiectasis, or nodules (Fig. 15.10) that may represent occult lung cancer in this high risk population should also be reported. Up to 5% of emphysema patients being evaluated for lung transplantation or lung reduction surgery have been found to have incidental lung cancer during their evaluations, many of which are only detected with CT (81). CT plays a major role in selecting candidates for lung volume reduction surgery. Good candidates have target areas of emphysema, usually in both upper lobes. Poor candidates have diffuse emphysema (82).

Focal apical target areas of emphysema are a predictor of good outcome after lung volume reduction surgery.

Several investigators have shown that CT is accurate for quantifying emphysema, using either visual scoring methods or attenuation threshold-based quantitative analysis; both of these methods fail to detect mild emphysema (78,79,83–96). Quantitative analysis of the severity of emphysema has been referred to as the density mask technique and was initially performed on selected axial two-dimensional images (86). The same technique can be applied to three-dimensional helical CT volumetric data sets acquired during a single inspiration for evaluation of the entire lungs (Fig. 15.11) (97,98). Lung volumes, including total lung capacity and residual volume, can also be calculated using

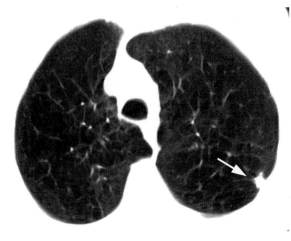

Figure 15.10 One-centimeter nodule (*arrow*) in the left upper lobe represents a clinically and radiographically occult bronchogenic carcinoma in an emphysema patient being evaluated for lung volume reduction surgery.

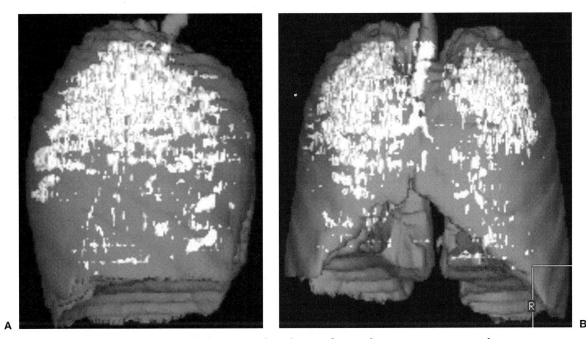

A   B

Figure 15.11 A,B. Three-dimensional density mask technique for emphysema superimposes the emphysema (all voxels less than −900 Hounsfield units as shown in white) on the total lung volume (all voxels less than −700 Hounsfield units as shown in gray) in both the anterior and lateral projections. These represent target areas for resection during lung volume reduction surgery.

inspiratory and expiratory helical CT data, with excellent correlation to static lung volumes (99). The thinner the collimation of the images, the better the correlation of CT attenuation based measurements with the severity of emphysema (79).

Visual and quantitative CT measurements of emphysema severity correlate well with diffusing capacity and pulmonary capillary blood volume in patients with emphysema but only moderately with measures of airflow obstruction, such as FEV_1, FVC, and the FEV_1/FVC ratio. The severity of expiratory airway obstruction may therefore not be related to the severity of alveolar wall destruction alone (33,37,96,100,101). By measuring the lung attenuation on inspiratory and expiratory CT, the ratio of CT attenuation number at expiration to inspiration can be calculated; this has been shown to correlate well with air trapping and less well with the morphologic destruction of emphysema (102).

SCINTIGRAPHY

Planar perfusion scintigraphy and single photon emission CT with technetium 99m ([99m] Tc) macroaggregated albumin display the perfusion to the lungs in multiple projections and planes (103). Lung perfusion can be visually estimated or quantified. Areas of emphysema or bullae are associated with reduced lung perfusion (Fig. 15.12). The perfusion that is demonstrated on perfusion scans is relative perfusion. The lack of perfusion could be related to either a large bulla or to an area of moderate to severe emphysema in lungs that are otherwise normal. Ventilation scintigraphy with [99m] Tc DTPA aerosol is of limited value due to the large amount of central airway distribution that occurs in patients with obstructive lung disease (Fig. 15.13) (104). Ventilation scintigraphy with radiolabeled xenon gas during the wash-in, equilibrium, and wash-out phases may not have the same limitation and may demonstrate areas of air trapping. The extensive perfusion abnormalities seen in patients with emphysema reduce the usefulness of ventilation-perfusion scans in emphysema patients being evaluated for suspected pulmonary embolism.

Perfusion scintigraphy demonstrates relative, not absolute, perfusion within the lungs.

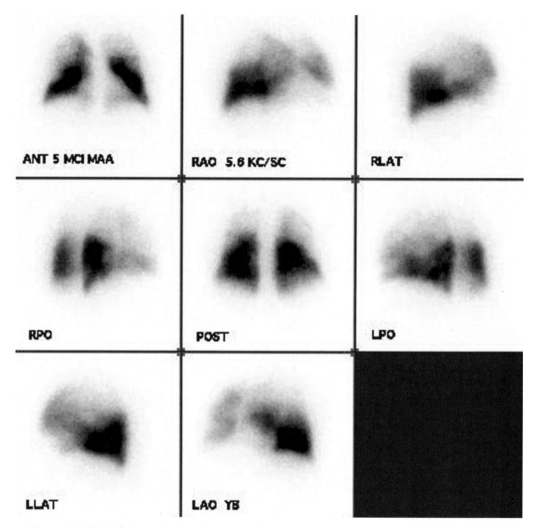

Figure 15.12 Perfusion scintigraphy using technetium 99m macroaggregated albumin in a patient with upper lobe predominant emphysema demonstrates absent perfusion that corresponds to areas of emphysema seen anatomically with computed tomography.

GIANT BULLA

A bulla is defined pathologically as "a sharply demarcated, dilated air space that measures 1 cm or more in diameter and possesses a thin epithelialized wall, which is usually no greater than 1 mm in thickness" and on CT as "a round, focal air space 1-cm or more in diameter, demarcated by a thin wall; usually multiple or associated with signs of pulmonary emphysema" (105). Giant bulla has varying definitions, and they may be as small as 5 cm or as large as the entire hemithorax (106). They are more common in young men than women or older individuals and are more common in smokers than nonsmokers but may been seen in the latter as well. One definition is a bulla involving one-third or more of a lung. Giant bullous disease is often referred to as vanishing lung syndrome. Rarely, a giant bulla may resolve spontaneously, often due to infection (107). More recently, giant bulla has been reported to develop after lung volume reduction surgery (108).

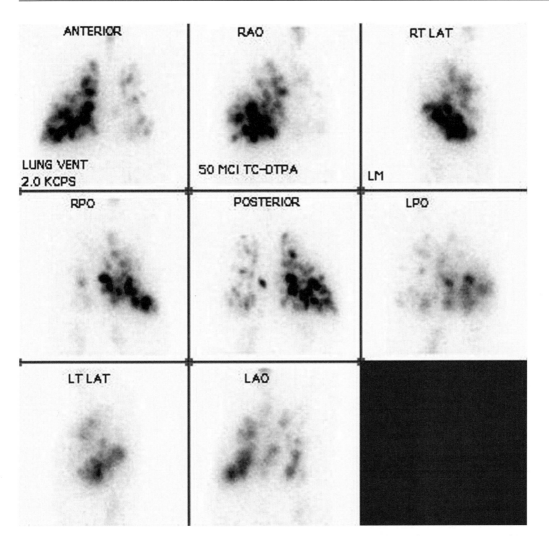

Figure 15.13 Ventilation scintigraphy using technetium 99m DTPA aerosol in a patient with emphysema demonstrates extensive central airway deposition of the radiotracer, hindering evaluation of regional ventilation in the lung parenchyma.

Most giant bullae asymmetrically involve the lungs on both radiographs and CT; bulla predominantly involve the upper lungs (Fig. 15.14) (109). On CT, paraseptal emphysema, centrilobular emphysema, and subpleural bullae are commonly present in addition to the dominant bulla. Bullae in these patients can involve an entire lobe or seemingly an entire lung, with marked compression of adjacent normal lung; the latter is an important criterion for determining if patients will do well with surgical resection. When giant bullae impair pulmonary function and are associated with compressed lung on CT, the usual method of treatment is surgical resection (110,111).

Compressed lung next to giant bulla on CT is used to select patients suitable for bullectomy.

Bronchiectasis

Clinical Features and Definition

Patients with bronchiectasis typically have chronic respiratory symptoms, including cough, recurrent pneumonia, and abundant sputum production. Shortness of breath and hemoptysis may also occur. The causes of bronchiectasis are varied (Table 15.6) (112).

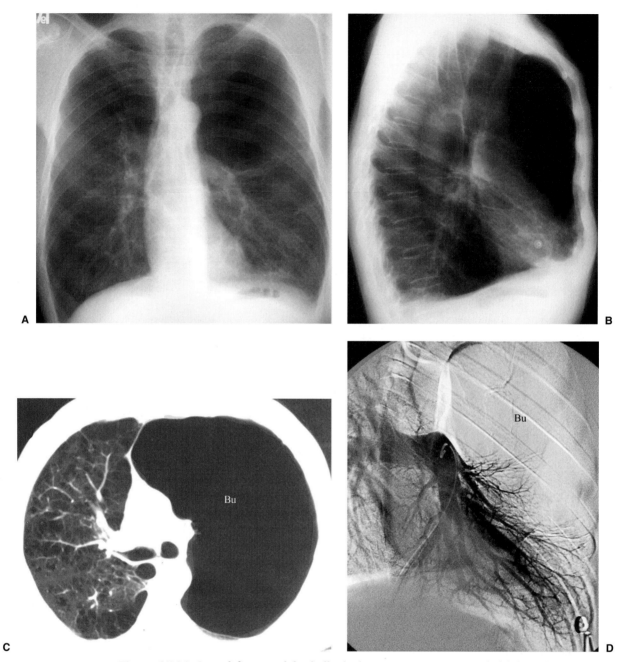

Figure 15.14 Giant left upper lobe bulla (Bu). *A.* Posteroanterior and *(B)* lateral radiographs demonstrate a large, single, air-containing, thin-walled bulla in the left upper lobe with contralateral mediastinal shift. *C.* Computed tomography and *(D)* pulmonary angiography demonstrate compression of adjacent normal lung parenchyma and crowing of pulmonary vessels.

Cystic fibrosis is the classic disease in which bronchiectasis is a major component. It is a genetic disease in which abnormally thick mucus is produced because of an abnormal cystic fibrosis transmembrane conductance regulator protein, resulting in faulty transport of sodium and chloride within cells lining the airway. Approximately 30,000 children and adults in the United States have cystic fibrosis, and 1 in 31 individuals is a carrier of the defective gene. It is diagnosed with a sweat chloride test that measures the amount of salt in the sweat; high levels indicate cystic fibrosis (113). In cystic fibrosis, bronchiectasis is usually more severe in the upper lobes than the lower lobes and is accompanied by pul-

Table 15.6: Causes of Bronchiectasis

Infection
    Tuberculosis
    Mycobacterium avium complex
    Allergic bronchopulmonary aspergillosis
    Recurrent infection
    Human immunodeficiency virus
Bronchial obstruction with mucoid impaction
Asthma
Chronic bronchitis
Pulmonary fibrosis
Hypogammaglobulinemia
Recurrent aspiration
Mounier-Kuhn syndrome
Inherited disorders
    α_1-Antitrypsin deficiency
    Cystic fibrosis
    Williams Campbell syndrome
    Dyskinetic cilia syndromes
Idiopathic

monary hyperinflation (Fig. 15.15). With new therapies for cystic fibrosis that are gene based, it is now not uncommon to see individuals in the fourth decade of life with relatively mild disease. Patients with cystic fibrosis are prone to airway colonization with bacteria, such as *Pseudomonas*, and also to recurrent pulmonary infection. There is a 25-point radiographic scoring system for cystic fibrosis, known as the Brasfield system, that is useful for grading the severity of lung disease and evaluating progression over time; this system has good correlation with pulmonary function (114).

Tuberculosis is a common cause of bronchiectasis worldwide, where it is a common indication for surgical resection of lung, but less so in industrialized nations. Lady Windemere syndrome, due to mycobacterium avium complex infection, is a subacute disease, classically in older women, in which bronchiectasis is usually most severe in the middle

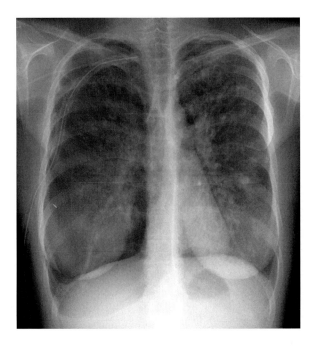

Figure 15.15 Posteroanterior radiograph of a 25-year-old woman with cystic fibrosis and a spontaneous right pneumothorax with a chest tube in place.

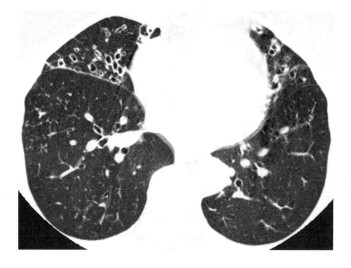

Figure 15.16 Mycobacterium avium complex infection with bronchiectasis that is most severe in the right middle lobe and lingula.

lobe and lingula (Fig. 15.16) (115). Bronchiectasis is also commonly seen with emphysema in α_1-antitrypsin deficiency and in association with human immunodeficiency virus infection (116–118). Traction bronchiectasis often accompanies pulmonary fibrosis and honeycombing and may be seen with nonspecific interstitial pneumonitis and usual interstitial pneumonitis (Chapter 14). In Mounier-Kuhn syndrome, bronchiectasis is associated with tracheomegaly (Chapter 16, Fig. 16.16) (119). In dyskinetic ciliary syndrome, also known as primary ciliary dyskinesia, the cilia within the bronchial epithelium are dysfunctional, leading to an inability to clear mucus from the airways and bronchiectasis. When found in association with situs inversus and recurrent sinusitis, this represents Kartagener syndrome (120). When found in association with infertility and sinusitis, this represents Young syndrome (121). Williams-Campbell syndrome is a rare cause of diffuse bronchiectasis in which there is a deficiency of cartilage in the third- to fifth-order airways (Fig. 15.17) (122).

Focal bronchiectasis with mucoid impaction may be seen due to bronchial atresia (Fig. 16.5) or to an endobronchial lesion, such as a carcinoid tumor (Fig. 15.18) or foreign body (123). Allergic bronchopulmonary aspergillosis classically manifests as dilated bronchi radiating out from the hila of the lungs, filled with mucus, creating a finger-in-glove appearance (Fig. 5.49) (124).

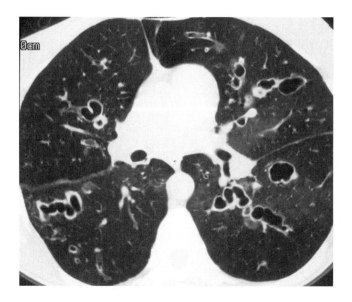

Figure 15.17 Bronchiectasis in Williams-Campbell syndrome. HRCT images demonstrate extensive cystic and varicose bronchiectasis with bronchial wall thickening.

with incomplete reversibility of airflow obstruction compared with those of COPD. *Can Respir J* 1998;5:270–277.

24. Brown P, Greville H, Finucane K. Asthma and irreversible airflow obstruction. *Thorax* 1984;39:131–136.

25. Anthonisen N. Prognosis in chronic obstructive pulmonary disease: results from multicenter clinical trials. *Am Rev Respir Dis* 1989;140:S95–99.

26. Nisar M, Earis J, Pearson M, et al. Acute bronchodilator trials in chronic obstructive pulmonary disease. *Am Rev Respir Dis* 1992;146:555–559.

27. Sterk P. Bronchoprovocation testing. *Semin Respir Crit Care Med* 1998;19:317–324.

28. Woolcock A, Anderson S, Peat J, et al. Characteristics of bronchial hyperresponsiveness in chronic obstructive pulmonary disease and in asthma. *Am Rev Respir Dis* 1991;143:1438–1443.

29. Brand P, Postma D, Kerstjens H, et al. Relationship of airway hyperresponsiveness to respiratory symptoms and diurnal peak flow variation in patients with obstructive lung disease. *Am Rev Respir Dis* 1991;143:916–921.

30. Greenspon L, Gracely E. A discriminant analysis applied to methacholine bronchoprovocation testing improves classification of patients as normal, asthma, or COPD. *Chest* 1992;102:1419–1425.

31. Tashkin D, Altose M, Bleecker E, et al. The Lung Health Study: airway hyperresponsiveness to inhaled methacholine in smokers with mild to moderate airflow limitation. *Am Rev Respir Dis* 1992;145:301–310.

32. Cotton D, Soparkar G, Graham B. Diffusing capacity in the clinical assessment of chronic airflow obstruction. *Med Clin North Am* 1996;80:549–564.

33. Morrison N, Abboud R, Ramadan F, et al. Comparison of single breath carbon monoxide diffusing capacity and pressure-volume curves in detecting emphysema. *Am Rev Respir Dis* 1989;139:1179–1187.

34. Knudson R, Kalternborn W, Burrows B. Single breath carbon monoxide transfer factor in different forms of chronic airflow obstruction in a general population sample. *Thorax* 1990;45:524–529.

35. Collard P, Njinou B, Nejadnik B, et al. Single breath diffusing capacity for carbon monoxide in stable asthma. *Chest* 1994;105:1426–1429.

36. Stewart R. Carbon monoxide diffusing capacity in asthmatic patients with mild airflow limitation. *Chest* 1988;94:332–336.

37. Gelb A, Schein M, Kuei J, et al. Limited contribution of emphysema in advanced chronic obstructive pulmonary disease. *Am Rev Respir Dis* 1993;147:1157–1163.

38. Jain P, Kavuru M, Emerman C, et al. Utility of peak expiratory flow monitoring. *Chest* 1998;114:861–876.

39. Vaughan T, Weber R, Tipton W, et al. Comparison of PEFR and FEV1 in patients with varying degrees of airway obstruction. Effect of modest altitude. *Chest* 1989;95:558–562.

40. Dekker F, Schrier A, Sterk P, et al. Validity of peak expiratory flow measurement in assessing reversibility of airflow obstruction. *Thorax* 1992;47:162–166.

41. Berube D, Cartier A, L'Archeveque J, et al. Comparison of peak expiratory flow rate and FEV1 in assessing bronchomotor tone after challenges with occupational sensitizers. *Chest* 1991;99:831–836.

42. Klein JS, Gamsu G, Webb WR, et al. High-resolution CT diagnosis of emphysema in symptomatic patients with normal chest radiographs and isolated low diffusing capacity. *Radiology* 1992;182:817–821.

43. Chin NK, Lim TK. A 39-year-old smoker with effort dyspnea, normal spirometry results, and low diffusing capacity. *Chest* 1998;113:231–233.

44. Arakawa H, Webb WR. Air trapping on expiratory high-resolution CT scans in the absence of inspiratory scan abnormalities: correlation with pulmonary function tests and differential diagnosis. *AJR Am J Roentgenol* 1998;170:1349–1353.

45. Murray JF, Nadel JA. *Textbook of respiratory medicine*, 2nd ed. Vol. 2. Philadelphia: Saunders, 1994:27–39.

46. Linden-Smith J, Morrison D, Hernandez P, et al. Overdiagnosis of asthma? A community survey. *Am J Respir Crit Care Med* 1999;159[Suppl 3]:A135.

47. Martin A, Landau L, Phelan P. Lung function in young adults who had asthma in childhood. *Am Rev Respir Dis* 1980;122:609–616.

48. Panhuysen C, Vonk J, Koeter G, et al. Adult patients may outgrow their asthma: a 25-year follow-up study. *Am J Respir Crit Care Med* 1997;155:1267–1272.

49. Eisner M, Yelin E, Henke J, et al. Environmental tobacco smoke and adult asthma: the impact of changing exposure on health outcomes. *Am J Respir Crit Care Med* 1998;158:170–175.

50. Ronmark E, Lundback B, Jonsson E, et al. Incidence of asthma in adults—report from the Obstructive Lung Disease in Northern Sweden Study. *Allergy* 1997;52:1071–1078.

51. Litonjua A, Carey V, Burge H, et al. Parental history and the risk for childhood asthma: does the mother confer more risk than father? *Am J Respir Crit Care Med* 1998;158:176–181.

52. Panhuysen C, Bleecker E, Koeter G, et al. Characterization of obstructive airway disease in family members of probands with asthma. *Am J Respir Crit Care Med* 1998;157:1734–1742.

53. Beasley R, Roche W, Roberts J, et al. Cellular events in the bronchi in mild asthma and after bronchial provocation. *Am Rev Respir Dis* 1989;139:806–817.

54. Chetta A, Foresi A, Deldonno M, et al. Bronchial responsiveness to distilled water and methacholine and its relationship to inflammation and remodeling of the airways in asthma. *Am Rev Respir Crit Care Med* 1996;153:910–917.

55. Chanez P, Vignola A, O'Shaugnessy T, et al. Corticosteroid reversibility in COPD is related to features of asthma. *Am Rev Respir Crit Care Med* 1997;155:1529–1534.

56. Webb WR. Radiology of obstructive pulmonary disease. *AJR Am J Roentgenol* 1997;169: 637–647.

57. Paganin F, Trussard V, Seneterre E, et al. Chest radiography and high resolution computed tomography of the lungs in asthma. *Am Rev Respir Dis* 1992;146:1084–1087.

58. Grenier P, Mourey-Gerosa I, Benali K, et al. Abnormalities of the airways and lung parenchyma in asthmatics: CT observations in 50 patients and inter- and intraobserver variability. *Eur Radiol* 1996;6:199–206.

59. Lynch DA, Newell JD, Tschomper BA, et al. Uncomplicated asthma in adults: comparison of CT appearance of the lungs in asthmatic and healthy subjects. *Radiology* 1993;188:829–833.

60. Carr DH, Hibon S, Rubens M, et al. Peripheral airways obstruction on high-resolution computed tomography in chronic severe asthma. *Respir Med* 1998;92:448–453.

61. Park CS, Muller NL, Worthy SA, et al. Airway obstruction in asthmatic and healthy individuals: inspiratory and expiratory thin-section CT findings. *Radiology* 1997;203:361–367.

62. Park JW, Hong YK, Kim CW, et al. High-resolution computed tomography in patients with bronchial asthma: correlation with clinical features, pulmonary functions and bronchial hyperresponsiveness. *J Invest Allerg Clin Immunol* 1997;7:186–192.

63. Paganin F, Seneterre E, Chanez P, et al. Computed tomography of the lungs in asthma: influence of disease severity and etiology. *Am J Respir Crit Care Med* 1996;153:110–114.

64. Awadh N, Muller NL, Park CS, et al. Airway wall thickness in patients with near fatal asthma and control groups: assessment with high resolution computed tomographic scanning. *Thorax* 1998;53:248–253.

65. Biernacki W, Redpath AT, Best JJ, et al. Measurement of CT lung density in patients with chronic asthma (see comments). *Eur Respir J* 1997;10:2455–2459.

66. Kinsella M, Müller NL, Staples C, et al. Hyperinflation in asthma and emphysema. Assessment by pulmonary function testing and computed tomography. *Chest* 1988;94:286–289.

67. Goldin JG, McNitt-Gray MF, Sorenson SM, et al. Airway hyperreactivity: assessment with helical thin-section CT. *Radiology* 1998;208:321–329.

68. Kee ST, Fahy JV, Chen DR, et al. High-resolution computed tomography of airway changes after induced bronchoconstriction and bronchodilation in asthmatic volunteers. *Acad Radiol* 1996;3:389–394.

69. Okazawa M, Muller N, McNamara AE, et al. Human airway narrowing measured using high resolution computed tomography. *Am J Respir Crit Care Med* 1996;154:1557–1562.

70. Takasugi JE, Godwin JD. Radiology of chronic obstructive pulmonary disease. *Radiol Clin North Am* 1998;36:29–55.

71. Hartman TE, Tazelaar HD, Swensen SJ, et al. Cigarette smoking: CT and pathologic findings of associated pulmonary diseases. *Radiographics* 1997;17:377–390.

72. Pratt P. Emphysema and chronic airways disease. In: Dail D, Hammar S, eds. *Pulmonary pathology*. New York: Springer-Verlag, 1988:654–659.

73. Pratt PC. Role of conventional chest radiography in diagnosis and exclusion of emphysema. *Am J Med* 1987;82:998–1006.

74. Thurlbeck WM, Simon G. Radiographic appearance of the chest in emphysema. *AJR Am J Roentgenol* 1978;130:429–440.

75. Reich SB, Weinshelbaum A, Yee J. Correlation of radiographic measurements and pulmonary function tests in chronic obstructive pulmonary disease. *AJR Am J Roentgenol* 1985;144: 695–699.

76. Nicklaus TM, Stowell DW, Christiansen WR, et al. The accuracy of the roentgenologic diagnosis of chronic pulmonary emphysema. *Am Rev Respir Dis* 1966;93:889–899.

77. Thurlbeck WM, Müller NL. Emphysema: definition, imaging, and quantification. *AJR Am J Roentgenol* 1994;163:1017–1025.

78. Bergin C, Müller N, Nichols DM, et al. The diagnosis of emphysema. A computed tomographic-pathologic correlation. *Am Rev Respir Dis* 1986;133:541–546.

79. Miller RR, Müller NL, Vedal S, et al. Limitations of computed tomography in the assessment of emphysema. *Am Rev Respir Dis* 1989;139:980–983.

80. Tanino M, Nishimura M, Betsuyaku T, et al. A comparative study of computed tomographic techniques for the detection of emphysema in middle-aged and older patient populations. *Nihon Kokyuki Gakkai Zasshi* 2000;38:368–372.

81. Kazerooni EA, Chow LC, Whyte RI, et al. Preoperative examination of lung transplant candidates: value of chest CT compared with chest radiography. *AJR Am J Roentgenol* 1995;165: 1343–1348.

82. Flaherty K, Kazerooni E, Curtis J, et al. Short-term and long-term outcomes after bilateral lung volume reduction surgery. Prediction by Quantitative CT. *Chest* 2001;119:1337–1346.

83. Remy-Jardin M, Remy J, Gosselin B, et al. Sliding thin slab, minimum intensity projection technique in the diagnosis of emphysema: histopathologic-CT correlation. *Radiology* 1996;200: 665–671.

84. Hruban RH, Meziane MA, Zerhouni EA, et al. High resolution computed tomography of inflation-fixed lungs. Pathologic-radiologic correlation of centrilobular emphysema. *Am Rev Respir Dis* 1987;136:935–940.

85. Spouge D, Mayo JR, Cardoso W, et al. Panacinar emphysema: CT and pathologic findings. *J Comput Assist Tomogr* 1993;17:710–713.

86. Müller NL, Staples CA, Miller RR, et al. "Density mask." An objective method to quantitate emphysema using computed tomography. *Chest* 1988;94:782–787.

87. Gevenois PA, Yernault JC. Can computed tomography quantify pulmonary emphysema? *Eur Respir J* 1995;8:843–848.

88. Gevenois PA, Zanen J, de Maertelaer V, et al. Macroscopic assessment of pulmonary emphysema by image analysis. *J Clin Pathol* 1995;48:318–322.

89. Gevenois PA, de Maertelaer V, De Vuyst P, et al. Comparison of computed density and macroscopic morphometry in pulmonary emphysema. *Am J Respir Crit Care Med* 1995;152:653–657.

90. Gevenois PA, De Vuyst P, Sy M, et al. Pulmonary emphysema: quantitative CT during expiration. *Radiology* 1996;199:825–829.

91. Sakai F, Gamsu G, Im JG, et al. Pulmonary function abnormalities in patients with CT-determined emphysema. *J Comput Assist Tomogr* 1987;11:963–968.

92. Sakai N, Mishima M, Nishimura K, et al. An automated method to assess the distribution of low attenuation areas on chest CT scans in chronic pulmonary emphysema patients. *Chest* 1994;106:1319–1325.

93. Sanders C, Nath PH, Bailey WC. Detection of emphysema with computed tomography. Correlation with pulmonary function tests and chest radiography. *Invest Radiol* 1988;23:262–266.

94. Foster WL Jr, Pratt PC, Roggli VL, et al. Centrilobular emphysema: CT-pathologic correlation. *Radiology* 1986;159:27–32.

95. Nishimura K, Murata K, Yamagishi M, et al. Comparison of different computed tomography scanning methods for quantifying emphysema. *J Thorac Imaging* 1998;13:193–198.

96. Müller NL, Thurlbeck WM. Thin-section CT, emphysema, air trapping, and airway obstruction (editorial; comment). *Radiology* 1996;199:621–622.

97. Kazerooni E, Martinez F, Quint L, et al. Quantitative helical CT indices of emphysema as predictors of outcome after lung volume reduction surgery. *Radiology* 1996;201:298.

98. Kazerooni EA, Whyte RI, Flint A, et al. Imaging of emphysema and lung volume reduction surgery. *Radiographics* 1997;17:1023–1036.

99. Kauczor HU, Heussel CP, Fischer B, et al. Assessment of lung volumes using helical CT at inspiration and expiration: comparison with pulmonary function tests. *AJR Am J Roentgenol* 1998;171:1091–1095.

100. Gelb A, Zamel N, McKenna R Jr, et al. Mechanism of short-term improvement in lung function after emphysema resection. *Am J Respir Crit Care Med* 1996;154:945–951.

101. Morrison NJ, Abboud RT, Müller NL, et al. Pulmonary capillary blood volume in emphysema. *Am Rev Respir Dis* 1990;141:53–61.

102. Eda S, Kubo K, Fujimoto K, et al. The relations between expiratory chest CT using helical CT and pulmonary function tests in emphysema. *Am J Respir Crit Care Med* 1997;155:1290–1294.

103. Mettler F, Guiberteau M. *Essentials of nuclear medicine*, 3rd ed. Philadelphia: Saunders, 1991.

104. Jamadar DA, Kazerooni EA, Martinez FJ, et al. Qualitative ventilation-perfusion scintigraphy

and SPECT imaging in the evaluation of lung volume reduction surgery candidates: description and prediction of clinical outcome. *Eur J Nuclear Med* 1999;26.

105. Austin JH, Muller NL, Friedman PJ, et al. Glossary of terms for CT of the lungs: recommendations of the Nomenclature Committee of the Fleischner Society. *Radiology* 1996;200: 327–331.

106. Goto H, Yuasa K, Takahashi S, et al. Giant bulla occupying the whole hemithorax. *Chest* 1987; 92:384–385.

107. Shanthaveerappa HN, Mathai MG Jr, Fields CL, et al. Spontaneous resolution of a giant pulmonary bulla. *J KY Med Assoc* 2001;99:533–536.

108. Iqbal M, Rossoff L, McKeon K, et al. Development of a giant bulla after lung volume reduction surgery. *Chest* 1999;116:1809–1811.

109. Stern EJ, Webb WR, Weinacker A, et al. Idiopathic giant bullous emphysema (vanishing lung syndrome): imaging findings in nine patients. *AJR Am J Roentgenol* 1994;162:279–282.

110. Laros CD, Gelissen HJ, Bergstein PG, et al. Bullectomy for giant bullae in emphysema. *J Thorac Cardiovasc Surg* 1986;91:63–70.

111. Martinez F. Surgical therapy for chronic obstructive pulmonary disease: conventional bullectomy and lung volume reduction surgery in the absence of giant bullae. *Semin Respir Crit Care Med* 1999;20:351–364.

112. Aronchick JM, Miller WT, Jr. Bronchiectasis. *J Thorac Imaging* 1995;10:255–267.

113. Orenstein D, Winnie G, Altman H. Cystic fibrosis: a 2002 update. *J Pediatr* 2002;140:156–164.

114. Brasfield D, Hicks G, Soong S, et al. Evaluation of scoring system of the chest radiograph in cystic fibrosis: a collaborative study. *AJR Am J Roentgenol* 1980;134:1195–1198.

115. Hartman TE, Swensen SJ, Williams DE. Mycobacterium avium-intracellulare complex: evaluation with CT. *Radiology* 1993;187:23–26.

116. King MA, Stone JA, Diaz PT, et al. Alpha 1-antitrypsin deficiency: evaluation of bronchiectasis with CT. *Radiology* 1996;199:137–141.

117. King MA, Neal DE, St. John R, et al. Bronchial dilatation in patients with HIV infection: CT assessment and correlation with pulmonary function tests and findings at bronchoalveolar lavage. *AJR Am J Roentgenol* 1997;168:1535–1540.

118. McGuinness G, Naidich DP, Garay S, et al. AIDS associated bronchiectasis: CT features. *J Comput Assist Tomogr* 1993;17:260–266.

119. Roditi GH, Weir J. The association of tracheomegaly and bronchiectasis. *Clin Radiol* 1994;49: 608–611.

120. Kinney TB, DeLuca SA. Kartagener's syndrome. *Am Fam Physician* 1991;44:133–134.

121. Handelsman DJ, Conway AJ, Boylan LM, et al. Young's syndrome. Obstructive azoospermia and chronic sinopulmonary infections. *N Engl J Med* 1984;310:3–9.

122. McAdams HP, Erasmus J. Chest case of the day. Williams-Campbell syndrome. *AJR Am J Roentgenol* 1995;165:190–191.

123. Anonymous. Image interpretation session. Bronchial carcinoid tumor of the left lower lobe with postobstructive bronchiectasis. *Radiographics* 1991;11:134–136.

124. Angus RM, Davies ML, Cowan MD, et al. Computed tomographic scanning of the lung in patients with allergic bronchopulmonary aspergillosis and in asthmatic patients with a positive skin test to *Aspergillus fumigatus*. *Thorax* 1994;49:586–589.

125. Sicard JA, Forestier J. Iodized oil as contrast medium for radioscopy. *Bull Mem Soc Med Hop Paris* 1922;46:463.

126. Christoforidis AJ, Nelson SW, Tomashefski JF. Effects of bronchography on pulmonary function. *Am Rev Respir Dis* 1962;85:127.

127. Goldman JM, Currie DC, Morgan AD, et al. Arterial oxygen saturation during bronchography via the fiberoptic bronchoscope. *Thorax* 1987;42:634–635.

128. Currie DC, Cooke JC, Morgan A, et al. Interpretation of bronchograms and chest radiographs in patients with chronic sputum production. *Thorax* 1987;42:278–284.

129. Morcos SK, Andersen PB, Ward P, et al. The efficacy of bronchography via the flexible bronchoscope using a water soluble non-ionic dimer (iotrolan) in diagnosing airway disease. *J Bronchol* 1996;3:106–111.

130. Cole P, Flower CDR, Lavender JP. Clinical and imaging aspects of bronchiectasis. In: Potchen EJ, Grainger RG, Greene R, eds. *Pulmonary radiology—The Fleischner Society*. Philadelphia: Saunders, 1993:242–258.

131. Cooke JC, Currie DC, Morgan AD, et al. Role of computed tomography in diagnosis of bronchiectasis. *Thorax* 1987;42:272–277.

132. Webb W. Radiology of obstructive pulmonary disease. *AJR Am J Roentgenol* 1997;169:637–647.

133. Carr DH, Oades P, Trotman-Dickenson B, et al. Magnetic resonance scanning in cystic fibrosis: comparison with computed tomography. *Clin Radiol* 1995;50:84–89.
134. Naidich DP, McCauley DI, Khouri NF, et al. Computed tomography of bronchiectasis. *J Comput Assist Tomogr* 1982;6:437–444.
135. Breatnach ES, Nath PH, McElvein RB. Preoperative evaluation of bronchiectasis by computed tomography. *J Comput Assist Tomogr* 1985;9:949–950.
136. Engeler CE, Tashjian JH, Engeler CM, et al. Volumetric high-resolution CT in the diagnosis of interstitial lung disease and bronchiectasis: diagnostic accuracy and radiation dose. *AJR Am J Roentgenol* 1994;163:31–35.
137. Kang EY, Miller RR, Muller NL. Bronchiectasis: comparison of preoperative thin-section CT and pathologic findings in resected specimens. *Radiology* 1995;195:649–654.
138. Kim JS, Muller NL, Park CS, et al. Cylindrical bronchiectasis: diagnostic findings on thin-section CT. *AJR Am J Roentgenol* 1997;168:751–754.
139. Grenier P, Maurice F, Musset D, et al. Bronchiectasis: assessment by thin-section CT. *Radiology* 1986;161:95–99.
140. Phillips MS, Williams MP, Flower CD. How useful is computed tomography in the diagnosis and assessment of bronchiectasis? *Clin Radiol* 1986;37:321–325.
141. Stern EJ, Muller NL, Swensen SJ, et al. CT mosaic pattern of lung attenuation: etiologies and terminology. *J Thorac Imaging* 1995;10:294–297.
142. Bhalla M, Turcios N, Aponte V, et al. Cystic fibrosis: scoring system with thin-section CT. *Radiology* 1991;179:783–788.
143. Lee PH, Carr DH, Rubens MB, et al. Accuracy of CT in predicting the cause of bronchiectasis. *Clin Radiol* 1995;50:839–841.
144. Reiff DB, Wells AU, Carr DH, et al. CT findings in bronchiectasis: limited value in distinguishing between idiopathic and specific types. *AJR Am J Roentgenol* 1995;165:261–267.
145. Collins J, Blankenbaker D, Stern EJ. CT patterns of bronchiolar disease: what is "tree-in-bud?" *AJR Am J Roentgenol* 1998;171:365–370.
146. Hartman TE, Primack SL, Lee KS, et al. CT of bronchial and bronchiolar diseases. *Radiographics* 1994;14:991–1003.
147. Im JG, Itoh H, Shim YS, et al. Pulmonary tuberculosis: CT findings—early active disease and sequential change with antituberculous therapy. *Radiology* 1993;186:653–660.
148. Akira M, Higashihara T, Sakatani M, et al. Diffuse panbronchiolitis: follow-up CT examination. *Radiology* 1993;189:559–562.
149. Poletti V, Zompatori M, Boaron M, et al. Cryptogenic constrictive bronchiolitis imitating imaging features of diffuse panbronchiolitis. *Monaldi Arch Chest Dis* 1995;50:116–117.
150. Skorodin MS. Pharmacotherapy for asthma and chronic obstructive pulmonary disease. Current thinking, practices, and controversies. *Arch Intern Med* 1993;153:814–828.
151. Boyd G, Morice A, Pounsfod J, et al. An evaluation of salmeterol in the treatment of chronic obstructive pulmonary disease (COPD). *Eur Respir J* 1997;10:815–821.
152. Jones P, Bosh T. Quality of life in COPD patients treated with salmeterol. *Am J Respir Crit Care Med* 1997;155:1283–1289.
153. Verberne A, Fuller R. An overview of nine clinical trials of salmeterol in an asthmatic population. *Respir Med* 1998;92:777–782.
154. Vermetten F, Boermans A, Luiten W, et al. Comparison of salmeterol with beclomethasone in adult patients with mild persistent asthma who are already on low-dose inhaled steroids. *J Asthma* 1999;36:97–106.
155. Barnes P. Inhaled glucocorticoids for asthma. *N Engl J Med* 1995;332:868–875.
156. Callahan C, Dittus R, Katz B. Oral corticosteroid therapy for patients with stable chronic obstructive pulmonary disease. A meta-analysis. *Ann Intern Med* 1991;114:216–223.
157. van Grunsven P, van Schayck C, Derenne J, et al. Long term effects of inhaled corticosteroids in chronic obstructive pulmonary disease: a meta-analysis. *Thorax* 1998;54:7–14.
158. Albert R, Martine R, Lewis S. Controlled clinical trial of methylprednisolone in patients with chronic bronchitis and acute respiratory insufficiency. *Ann Intern Med* 1980;92:753–758.
159. Thompson W, Nielson C, Carvalho P, et al. Controlled trial of oral prednisone in outpatients with acute COPD exacerbation. *Am J Respir Crit Care Med* 1996;154:407–412.
160. Burge P. EUROSCOP, ISOLDE and the Copenhagen City Lung Study. *Thorax* 1999;54:287–288.
161. Calverley P, Burge P, Jones P, et al. Effect of 3 years treatment with fluticasone propionate in patients with moderately-severe COPD. *Am J Respir Crit Care Med* 1999;159[Suppl 3]: A524.
162. Spencer S, Anie K, Burge P, et al. Rate of health status decline is reduced in COPD patients

treated with fluticasone compared to placebo. *Am J Respir Crit Care Med* 1999;159[Suppl 3]: A522.

163. American Thoracic Society. Dyspnea mechanisms, assessment, and management: a consensus statement. *Am J Respir Crit Care Med* 1999;159:321–340.

164. Deslauriers J. Surgical management of chronic obstructive pulmonary disease. *Ann Thorac Surg* 1995;60:873–874.

165. Cooper JD, Trulock EP, Triantafillou AN, et al. Bilateral pneumectomy (volume reduction) for chronic obstructive pulmonary disease. *J Thorac Cardiovasc Surg* 1995;109:106–119.

166. Benditt JO, Albert RK. Surgical options for patients with advanced emphysema. *Clin Chest Med* 1997;18:577–593.

167. Utz J, Hubmayr R, Deschamps C. Lung volume reduction surgery for emphysema: out on a limb without a NETT. *Mayo Clin Proc* 1998;73:552–556.

168. Sciurba F. Early and long-term functional outcomes following lung volume reduction surgery. *Clin Chest Med* 1997;18:259–276.

169. Ingenito E, Evans R, Loring S, et al. Relation between preoperative inspiratory lung resistance and the outcome of lung-volume-reduction surgery for emphysema. *N Engl J Med* 1998;338: 1181–1185.

170. Slone R, Pilgram T, Gierada D, et al. Lung volume reduction surgery: comparison of preoperative radiologic features and clinical outcome. *Radiology* 1997;204:685–693.

171. Gierada D, Slone R, Bae K, et al. Pulmonary emphysema: comparison of preoperative quantitative CT and physiologic index values with clinical outcome after lung-volume reduction surgery. *Radiology* 1997;205:235–242.

172. Weder W, Thurnheer R, Stammberger U, et al. Radiologic emphysema morphology is associated with outcome after surgical lung volume reduction. *Ann Thorac Surg* 1997;64:313–319; discussion 319–320.

173. Wisser W, Klepetko W, Kontrus M, et al. Morphologic grading of the emphysematous lung and its relation to improvement after lung volume reduction surgery. *Ann Thorac Surg* 1998;65: 793–799.

THE CENTRAL AIRWAYS

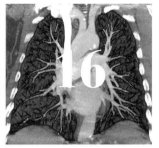

■ Computed Tomography
  Techniques
■ Anatomy
■ Congenital Anomalies
■ Inflammatory Conditions
■ Infectious Conditions
■ Traumatic Rupture
■ Postoperative Stenosis and
  Dehiscence
■ Stents
■ Diffuse Airway Enlargement
■ Saber Sheath Trachea
■ Focal Foreign Body
■ Broncholithiasis
■ Tracheal Diverticula
■ Tracheobronchial Neoplasms
■ Metastases

COMPUTED TOMOGRAPHY TECHNIQUES

Imaging of the upper airways provides information that can lead to safer bronchoscopic evaluation, airway dilatation, or surgical repair for patients with airway compromise. Occasionally, imaging may preclude the need for bronchoscopy as a diagnostic tool. Although multidirectional tomography used to be the mainstay for imaging the upper airways, this equipment is rarely found now in most modern hospitals, and planar tomography is currently used (Fig. 16.1). This type of equipment is best suited for renal and musculoskeletal applications but is not optimal for evaluating the thorax. Moreover, because of its infrequent use in the thorax, there is a general lack of expertise on the part of the radiologic technologists obtaining the studies and the radiologists interpreting the examinations. High kilovoltage (150 kVp or greater) radiography with heavy filtration (using aluminum, brass, or copper) can provide high quality tracheal images, although in practice it is rarely used. Fluoroscopy is sometimes a useful dynamic method to evaluate for tracheomalacia, particularly in pediatric patients (1).

Ultrasound may be helpful in patients who are unable to breath-hold or lie flat for computed tomography (CT) evaluation. However, limitations of this technique include nonvisualization of the intrathoracic trachea, poor visualization of posterior wall lesions, and suboptimal evaluation of calcium. One report suggested that ultrasound may be useful as a follow-up investigation in some patients (2). Magnetic resonance imaging (MRI) produces excellent soft tissue contrast of structures and has the capability of imaging in multiple planes. Typically, T1-weighted images, before and after contrast, are most helpful (3). Unfortunately, limitations of MRI include potentially long imaging times, motion artifact, suboptimal evaluation of calcifications, and suboptimal spatial resolution as compared with CT (Fig. 16.1). Therefore, MRI currently has limited usefulness in this setting. For all intents and purposes, CT has virtually replaced all other modalities for imaging the tracheobronchial tree at the current time. In addition to its ability to image the airways, CT also enables visualization of extraluminal spread of disease.

> CT is the modality of choice for evaluating the tracheobronchial tree.

Most published studies concerning CT evaluation of the central airways have used conventional CT scanners. On such equipment, a limited number of sections (typically three to six) can be obtained during a single breath-hold, necessitating pauses in scanning to allow the patient to breath. There may be significant misregistration between sections obtained on different breath-holds, leading to overlap and/or gaps between adjacent images. Unfortunately, such misregistration leads to highly suboptimal reconstruction of the CT data in other planes, and therefore the data are usually displayed only in the axial plane. In general, due to their orientation along the long axis of the body, the trachea and

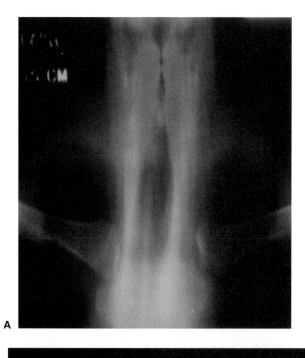

A

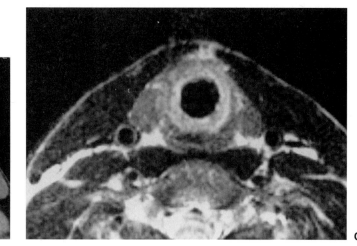

Figure 16.1 Wegener's granulomatosis. *A.* Coronal tomogram of the trachea demonstrates marked subglottic luminal narrowing. *B.* Axial computed tomography through the subglottic trachea demonstrates submucosal thickening and luminal narrowing. *C.* Axial magnetic resonance imaging (TR 2,350, TE 90) shows mucosal thickening of high signal intensity within the tracheal lumen.

B   C

main bronchi are better suited to demonstration in the coronal or oblique planes rather than the axial plane. In addition, the necessity for frequent pauses for breathing leads to the use of relatively thick (5 to 10 mm) sections to cover the area of interest in a timely fashion. Despite these limitations, conventional CT is useful for evaluating focal and diffuse tracheal stenoses and masses and for assessing disease involvement of adjacent structures.

Recent technologic advances have led to the development of helical CT scanners (both single and multislice) that enable rapid aquisition of a large number of thin sections. Thus, an entire study can be performed during a single breath-hold, thereby eliminating misregistration artifacts from varying degrees of respiration. The technique can be particularly useful in patients with multiple stenoses, in whom a proximal stricture is not traversable by a bronchoscope. An entire set of images can be obtained in expiration and in inspiration to look for dynamic changes suggestive of tracheomalacia or bronchomalacia. Helically acquired CT data can be used to produce high quality multiplanar reconstructions (MPRs) (two-dimensional images) oriented along any desired axis and three-dimensional reconstructions and virtual reality bronchoscopic views of the airway lumen. MPRs occasionally provide information that is not evident on the axial images, although generally the addition of MPRs does not lead to significant increase in diagnostic accuracy when assessed by experienced radiologists. However, MPRs may be helpful in detecting mild stenoses, in more accurately depicting the length of tracheal lesions, and in detecting tracheal webs; MPRs are

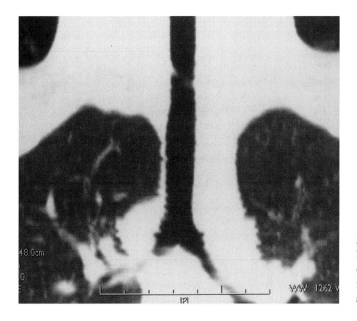

Figure 16.2 Tracheal web. Multiplanar reformat in the coronal plane demonstrates a fine tracheal web that was not apparent on axial images.

extremely useful in demonstrating findings to referring clinicians (Fig. 16.2). Three-dimensional images, including shaded surface displays, minimum intensity projections, volume rendering, and virtual bronchoscopy (endoluminal three-dimensional views) (Fig. 16.3), provide additional ways to display the helically acquired CT data.

All these techniques have potential pitfalls in interpretation, require accurate setting of thresholds to provide a true representation of the data, and may be time consuming to produce at a workstation (4–7). The virtual bronchoscope has the advantage of passing bronchial obstructions and stenoses, and both endobronchial and peribronchial anatomy can be studied. Unlike fiberoptic bronchoscopy, however, virtual bronchoscopy is unable to depict mucosal detail and true color. In general, three-dimensional postprocessing methods are time consuming to perform and are rarely required in routine clinical practice, although they may be complementary in some situations. The true incremental yield of such display techniques has yet to be established. Axial images with the addition of two-

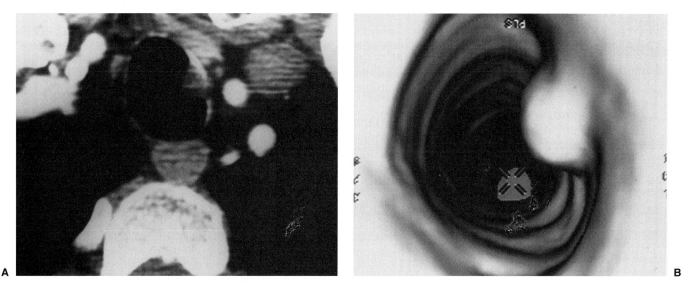

A   **B**

Figure 16.3 Virtual bronchoscopy. *A.* Axial computed tomography and *(B)* virtual bronchoscopic image demonstrate a small adenoid cystic carcinoma.

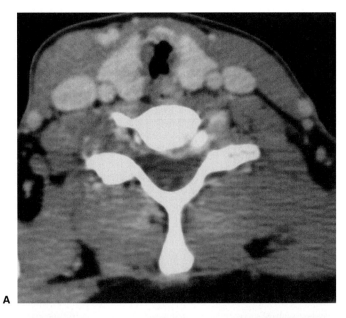

A

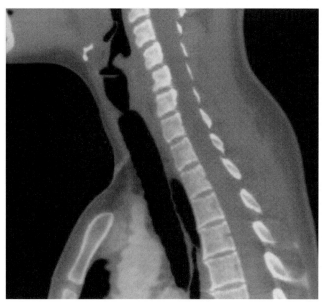

B

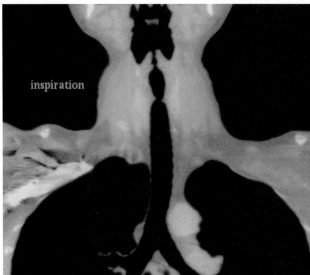

C

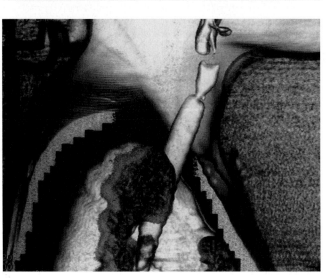

D

Figure 16.4 Postintubation tracheal stenosis. *A.* Axial contrast-enhanced computed tomography demonstrates irregular thickening of the subglottic tracheal wall with luminal narrowing. *(B)* Sagittal and *(C)* coronal multiplanar reformats help show the craniocaudal extent of the stenosis. *D.* Three-dimensional shaded surface display and *(E)* volume rendered reformats demonstrate the abnormality but do not add any further information.

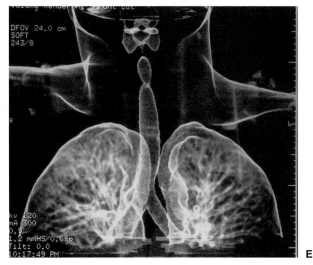

E

dimensional multiplanar reformats are generally sufficient and are quick to produce from the data set (8–12) (Fig. 16.4).

One drawback of helical CT is the necessity for full patient cooperation, including the ability to breath-hold for at least 15 to 20 seconds (using a single slice scanner) and abstain from swallowing or other gross movement. Hyperventilation before scanning often aids the patient in accomplishing a sufficiently long breath-hold. The new, rapid, multi-slice helical scanners are useful in reducing the necessary breath-hold time. Examinations performed during free breathing are generally of limited diagnostic usefulness, and patients unable to suspend respiration during scanning are usually better imaged with conventional tomography. Cardiac motion causes some artifacts, although it usually does not compromise the diagnostic quality of the examination.

A suggested helical imaging protocol would include 1 to 3 mm sections from epiglottis to carina (tracheal study) or from mid-trachea to lower lobe bronchi (central bronchial study), depending on the area of interest. Overlapping images are reconstructed and used to create reformatted planar and three-dimensional images. The patient should be scanned with the neck hyperextended for a tracheal study. If the suspected region of interest is in the neck, the patient's arms should be down; otherwise, the arms should be up. Initially, the patient is scanned in suspended inspiration, using a single breath-hold, if possible, after hyperventilation. The scan is then repeated during expiration. Intravenous contrast material may be given if a mass is suspected and/or if evaluation of the adjacent mediastinal and hilar structures is required (5). Increased pitch leads to increased stair step artifacts, especially in airways that course obliquely, such as the left main bronchus. Thin sections are essential to reduce partial volume averaging, and overlapping reconstructions help to reduce stair-step artifact (13).

ANATOMY

The trachea is a midline structure. On the posteroanterior radiograph there is a slight deviation to the right and a smooth indentation on the left wall of the trachea due to indentation of the aortic arch. Location in the anteroposterior axis is variable but is usually midway between the sternum and spine (14). There is marked variation in cross-sectional shape. The most common shapes are round or oval; less commonly the trachea may be horseshoe shaped with a flat posterior wall, an inverted pear shape, or almost square. The length of the trachea as measured on CT is 6 to 9 cm (15). On chest radiography, the upper limits of normal coronal and sagittal diameter in men is 25 and 27 mm, respectively, and in women is 21 and 23 mm, respectively (16). The lower limit of normal is 13 mm for men and 10 mm for women.

The trachea is made up of horseshoe-shaped bands of hyaline cartilage that support the anterior and lateral walls. Posteriorly is the trachealis muscle, which makes up the posterior tracheal membrane. The layers are the mucosa, submucosa, cartilage or muscle, and adventitia. The tracheal wall consists of 1 to 3 mm of soft tissue on CT. Cartilage may calcify; this is most common in older females. The posterior wall is thicker and may be flat, concave, or convex. The intrathoracic portion of the trachea starts at manubrium (17) and divides into the left and right main bronchi at the carina. The carinal angle, measured as the angle of divergence of the main bronchi along their inferior borders, can vary, with a range between 35 and 91 degrees (average, 55 to 60 degrees). In adults, the right main bronchus has a more vertical course than the left. In children up to age 15 years, the course is similar bilaterally. The right main bronchus is wider (15.3 mm on the right as compared with 13 mm on the left) (18) and shorter (2.2 cm on the right as compared with 5 cm on the left) than the left main bronchus (19,20). Although there are variations in the normal bronchial branching patterns that may be noted incidentally at bronchoscopy, these are mostly of no clinical significance. Generally, the locations of the bronchopulmonary segments are constant. Classification of the bronchial segments is presented in Table 16.1.

The lower limit of normal tracheal diameter is 13 mm in men and 10 mm in women.

Table 16.1: Jackson and Huber Classification of Bronchial Segments

Right upper lobe	Apical
	Anterior
	Posterior
Right middle lobe	Lateral
	Medial
Right lower lobe	Superior
	Medial basal
	Anterior basal
	Lateral basal
	Posterior basal
Left upper lobe	
Upper division	Apical–posterior
	Anterior
Lingular division	Superior
	Inferior
Left lower lobe	Superior
	Anteromedial
	Lateral basal
	Posterior basal

CONGENITAL ANOMALIES

There may be either agenesis or aplasia of bronchi (i.e., with either absent or rudimentary lung tissue) with involvement of an entire lung, a lobe, or a single segment. This may be a primary phenomenon or secondary to factors such as a space-occupying lesion, thoracic cage abnormality, oligohydramnios, or reduced perfusion. In pulmonary agenesis, the carina is absent; in aplasia, there is a blind ending pouch. Congential bronchial anomalies are often associated with VACTERL (Vertebral dysgenesis, Anal atresia, Cardiac anomalies, Tracheo Esophageal fistula, Renal anomalies, Limb anomalies) abnormalities (21).

Focal mucoid impaction with a tubular soft tissue structure surrounded by hyperaerated lung should suggest bronchial atresia.

There are many variants of lobar and segmental agenesis, aplasia, and hypoplasia. Bronchial atresia is uncommon; it is possibly related to a vascular insult after 15 weeks' gestation. There is focal obliteration of a segmental bronchus with normal distal structures. A distal mucoid impaction is generally present, showing an ovoid, round, or branching shape and sometimes containing an air–fluid level (Fig. 16.5). The distal lung, which is aerated via collateral air drift, may be hyperinflated. The most common site is the left upper lobe; 64% involve the left apicoposterior segmental bronchus, 14% the left lower lobe, and 8% the right middle and lower lobes (22). Bronchial atresias are often discovered incidentally, and bronchoscopy is used to exclude an endobronchial lesion (23).

The most congenital variant in tracheobronchial anatomy is the right tracheal (or "pig") bronchus.

Other congenital abnormalities include those of bronchial division. Right-sided isomerism is associated with asplenia, and left-sided isomerism is associated with polysplenia and cardiac abnormalities. The right tracheal bronchus is either a displaced right apical bronchus or a supernumerary bronchus; the incidence of this finding is approximately 0.1% to 2% (24). There may or may not be associated lung tissue; it may be a blind ending pouch. A left tracheal bronchus is rarer (0.3% to 1%) and is always an early origin of the left apicoposterior segmental bronchus. It is often associated with distal lung abnormality such as bronchiectasis, lymphangiectasia, and hyperinflation, possibly due to vascular compression by the left pulmonary artery (25). The bridging bronchus is an ectopic bronchus arising from the left main bronchus, crossing the midline and supplying the right lower lobe; the right main bronchus supplies the right upper and right middle lobes only. The accessory paracardiac bronchus has an incidence of 0.09% to 0.5% (26).

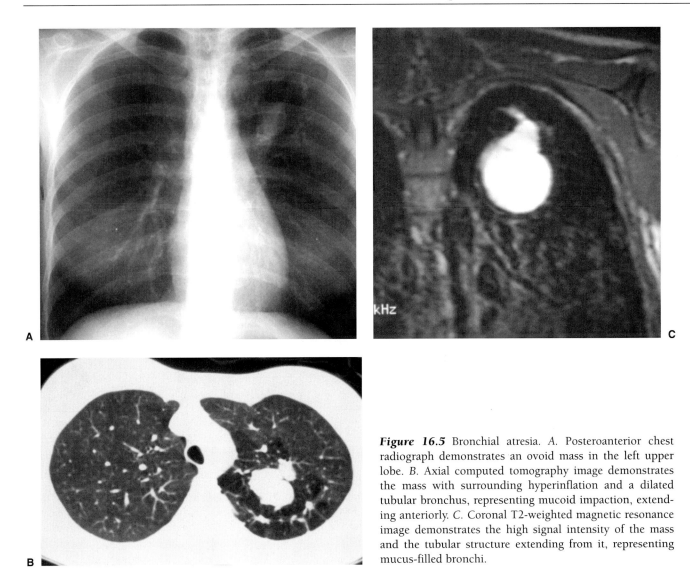

Figure 16.5 Bronchial atresia. *A.* Posteroanterior chest radiograph demonstrates an ovoid mass in the left upper lobe. *B.* Axial computed tomography image demonstrates the mass with surrounding hyperinflation and a dilated tubular bronchus, representing mucoid impaction, extending anteriorly. *C.* Coronal T2-weighted magnetic resonance image demonstrates the high signal intensity of the mass and the tubular structure extending from it, representing mucus-filled bronchi.

Although often asymptomatic, it may cause hemoptysis, infection, cough, or dyspnea. This is a true supernumerary anomalous bronchus and may or may not ventilate a rudimentary or accessory lobe, separated by a fissure. It arises from the medial wall of the bronchus intermedius (Fig. 16.6). Other minor bronchial branching variations are common (23).

INFLAMMATORY CONDITIONS

POSTINTUBATION STENOSIS

Tracheal stricture or stenosis is most commonly a complication of tracheal intubation with a cuffed endotracheal tube; tracheostomy tube placement and trauma are less common etiologies. Postintubation stenosis may occur at the level of the tracheostomy stoma or at the level of the balloon for an endotracheal or tracheostomy tube. A stenosis is more likely with higher balloon cuff pressures, when the capillary pressure may be exceeded, leading to necrosis and fibrosis. Occasionally, stenosis is seen at level of the tube tip. The stricture

The most common cause of focal tracheal stenosis is prior intubation.

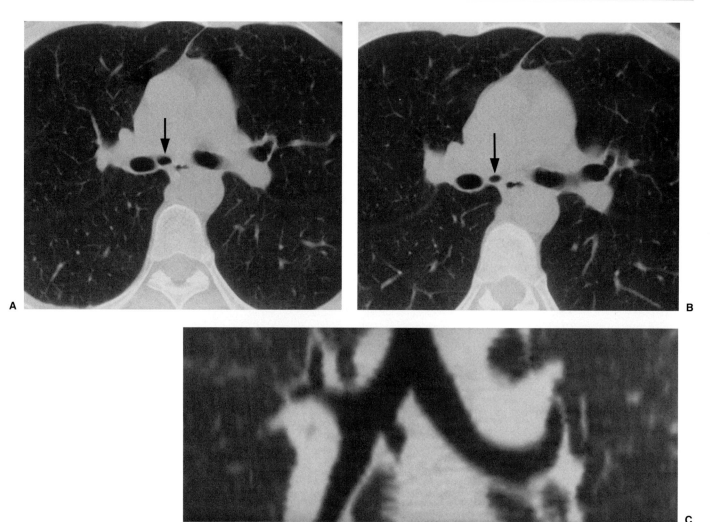

Figure 16.6 Accessory paracardiac bronchus. *(A and B)* Axial computed tomography and *(C)* coronal reformat shows accessory bronchus arising from the medial wall of the bronchus intermedius.

generally results from pressure necrosis, causing ischemia and scarring. Stenosis can also be caused by inflammation with weakening of the tracheal wall (tracheomalacia) or by granulation tissue, especially at the level of the tube tip (27).

Acute stenoses are generally secondary to mucosal edema, granulation tissue, and necrotic pseudomembranes. Mucosal thickening is internal to the cartilage, and there is no change in the size of the tracheal lumen on expiration. Such stenoses may be single or multiple (28) and concentric, eccentric, web-like, or A-shaped, secondary to laterally impacted fractures of cartilage after tracheostomy. Chronic strictures may show cartilage and posterior membrane deformities and associated tracheomalacia (17,29,30).

CT using axial images alone is very accurate (approximately 90%) in detecting benign tracheal stenoses, although thin webs or short segment strictures may be missed. There is little gain to the addition of reformats. Reformats are useful, however, in more accurately depicting the longitudinal extent of the stenosis and may be helpful in detecting thin webs or short segment strictures (31) (Figs. 16.4 and 16.7).

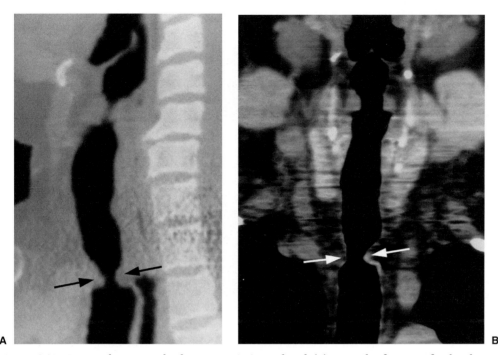

Figure 16.7 Postintubation tracheal stenosis. A. Sagittal and (B) coronal reformats of a distal tracheal stricture after intubation.

TRACHEOBRONCHOMALACIA

Tracheobronchomalacia is a weakness of the tracheal and bronchial walls and cartilage. Wall collapse is present during forced expiration and may be focal or diffuse. The many causes include primary congenital or secondary to tracheal intubation, chronic obstructive pulmonary disease, trauma, infection, relapsing polychondritis, radiation, tumors, surgery, or tracheobronchial fistula. The incidence increases with age, and it is said to be the fifth most common cause of chronic cough (32). Other symptoms are wheeze or unexplained dyspnea. Complications, secondary to the reduced efficiency of the cough mechanism, are retained mucus, infection, and bronchiectasis (33).

Relapsing polychondritis is a rare disease (fewer than 500 cases have been reported) characterized by recurrent inflammation and destruction of cartilage of the ears, nose, larynx, trachea, and peripheral joints; cardiovascular manifestations (aortitis, vasculitis, valvular insufficiency, and aneurysms) occur in 30% of cases. Respiratory involvement, occurring in 50% to 70% of cases, imparts a poor prognosis and causes approximately 50% of deaths from this disease, generally from recurrent pneumonia (31,33–35). The cause of the disease is unknown but appears to be immune mediated. Histologically, the normal collagen is replaced by fibrous tissue. Airway obstruction can occur by three mechanisms. First, inflammatory swelling of the glottic or subglottic area is the most common cause of upper airway obstruction in this disorder. Second, encroachment of the glottic or tracheal lumen due to cicatricial contraction may occur late in the course of the disease. Finally, with dissolution of the cartilaginous supporting structure of the trachea, there is dynamic collapse of the airway, especially with forced inspiration and expiration. Granulation tissue and fibrosis may also lead narrowing of the tracheal lumen (17,34,35). Tracheal stenosis with relapsing polychondritis is usually a late manifestation of the disease and reflects diffuse tracheal involvement; however, localized stenosis occurring in the proximal, middle, or distal trachea may also occur. CT findings include thickening of the tracheal wall with or without calcifications; the posterior membranous wall of the trachea is spared

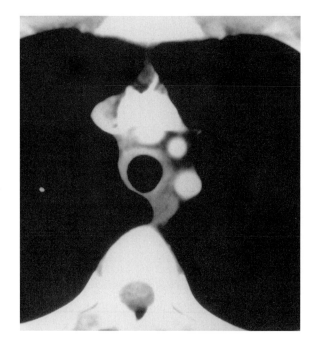

Figure 16.8 Relapsing polychondritis. Axial computed tomography demonstrates thickening of the tracheal wall with sparing of the posterior membrane.

A decrease in airway diameter from inspiration to expiration is a sign of tracheomalacia.

(Fig. 16.8). There may be focal or diffuse tracheal narrowing, with or without expiratory airway collapse (28).

Tracheobronchomalacia can be evaluated using bronchoscopy, fluoroscopy, and CT. Dynamic CT performed during inspiration and expiration may offer a useful alternative to bronchoscopy and fluoroscopy (Fig. 16.9). CT is performed either through the entire trachea with table movement or at a fixed point with the table stationary (note the trachea moves cranially on expiration; therefore, table position needs to compensate for this).

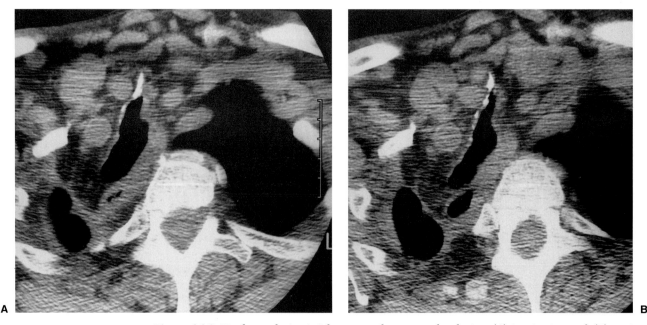

Figure 16.9 Tracheomalacia. Axial computed tomography during (A) inspiration and (B) expiration; multiplanar reformat during (C) inspiration and (D) expiration. Narrowing of the tracheal lumen during expiration, demonstrating tracheomalacia.

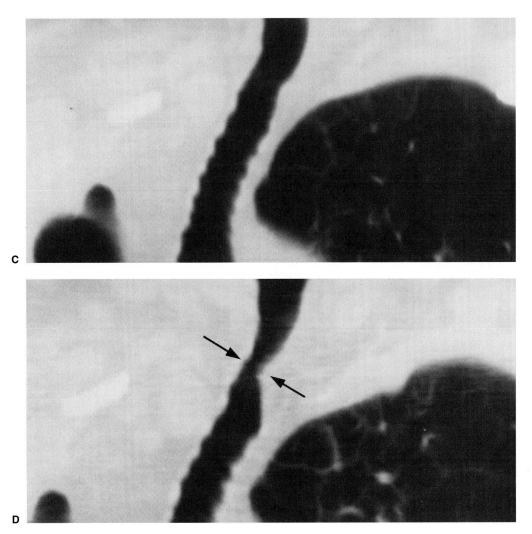

C

D

Figure 16.9 (continued)

Images during full inspiration, followed by dynamic expiration (after patient coaching in the technique) are obtained (36–38). Aquino et al. (39) demonstrated that a reduction in tracheal cross-sectional area of greater than 18% in the upper trachea and 28% in the mid-trachea gave a high probability for malacia (89% to 100%).

WEGENER GRANULOMATOSIS

Wegener granulomatosis (WG) is a vasculitis involving the upper and lower respiratory tract. The kidneys and other organs are usually also involved. It involves the nasal sinuses and less commonly the nasal septum, uvula, subglottic larynx, trachea, and bronchi (Chapter 13) (33). Clinically, patients present with hoarseness, stridor, and upper airway obstruction. The tracheobronchial tree is affected by an ulcerating tracheobronchitis, subglottic stenoses, inflammatory pseudotumors, tracheal and bronchial stenoses without inflammation, bronchiectasis, and hemorrhage. Diffuse involvement is rare and late. Stenoses in the subglottic region may involve the adjacent vocal cords. Tracheal stenoses may extend into the main bronchi and are typically circumferential, either concentric or eccentric; there may be mucosal irregularity or ulceration (Figs. 16.10 and 13.9). Cartilage and paratracheal soft tissues are less commonly involved (40–42).

The classic triad of WG includes lung/airway, sinus, and renal involvement.

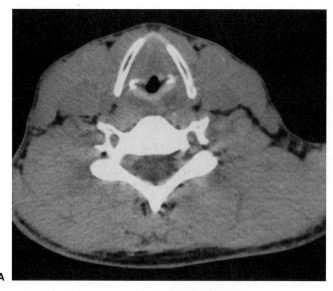

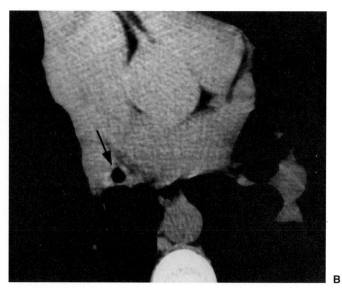

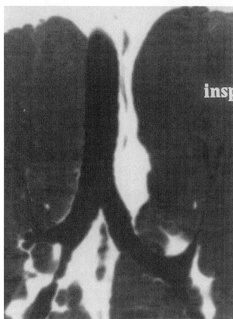

Figure 16.10 Wegener granulomatosis. *A.* Axial computed tomography at the level of the vocal cords demonstrates marked narrowing of the lumen and thickening of the vocal cords. *B.* Axial computed tomography and *(C)* coronal multiplanar reformat at the level of the right lower lobe bronchus demonstrates circumferential thickening of the bronchus wall *(arrow),* with narrowing of the lumen.

Tracheal stenosis in WG is more common in women (more than 90%) than men.

For reasons that are not clear, over 90% of cases of tracheal stenosis complicating WG have occurred in females, even though WG occurs equally in males and females. Tracheal symptoms typically develop months or years after WG has been documented in other sites. However, tracheal obstruction/stenosis may occasionally be the presenting feature of the disease or the first manifestation of relapse. Tracheobronchial WG is usually treated medically. Surgical treatments are sometimes done, although they may fail due to active inflammation, vasculitis, and necrosis, leading to complications such as poor healing at anastomotic sites.

CT findings include focal or diffuse airway narrowing anywhere from the hypopharynx to the lobar bronchi, with circumferential wall thickening (Fig. 16.11). Enlarged, abnormally calcified, tracheal cartilages have been described, and lobar collapse secondary to granulomatous obstruction of an airway may occur (33). Occasionally, there is concomitant mediastinal or hilar lymphadenopathy. These findings are often seen in association with pulmonary parenchymal manifestations of the disease, including multiple nod-

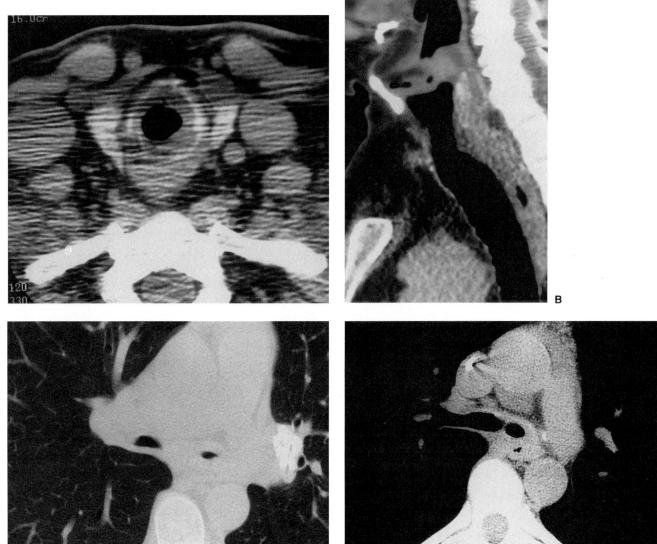

Figure 16.11 Wegener granulomatosis. *A.* Axial computed tomography and *(B)* sagittal multiplanar reformat demonstrates circumferential wall thickening in a subglottic location. *C and D.* Axial computed tomography demonstrates circumferential thickening of the walls of the right and left main bronchi, with luminal narrowing.

ules or consolidation, often with cavitation. MRI findings have been described but are nonspecific, with T1-weighted imaging demonstrating thickening of the submucosal tissues, luminal narrowing, and marked gadolinium enhancement, and T2-weighted imaging demonstrating increased signal intensity (Fig. 16.1) (43).

SARCOIDOSIS

Sarcoidosis is a systemic granulomatous disease of unknown etiology. The nonairway manifestations are described in Chapter 13. Histologically, noncaseating epithelioid granulomas are present. Tracheal or bronchial stenosis may complicate sarcoidosis in 1% to 10% of cases but is rarely severe. Rarely, the proximal airways may be affected without involvement of other body sites. There may be granulomatous lesions within the airways or there may be extrinsic compression due to adjacent enlarged lymph nodes. On occasion, chronic granulomatous infiltration of bronchial submucosa may lead to narrowing of lobar or segmental bronchi, resulting in suppurative complications or postobstructive pneumonitis.

On CT, the most common finding is thickening of the bronchial walls, which may be smooth or nodular. There may be bronchial compression secondary to extrinsic compression from enlarged lymph nodes (33).

AMYLOIDOSIS

Amyloidosis is the extracellular deposition of an insoluble protein that stains with Congo red. Amyloidosis has localized and diffuse forms and may involve many organ systems (Chapter 13). Tracheobronchial amyloidosis is the most common form of localized pulmonary amyloid (44). Males are affected twice as frequently as females (45). Symptoms include cough, dyspnea, hemoptysis, stridor, and wheeze. Laryngeal involvement may present early with hoarseness. Airway involvement is usually diffuse but may be focal. In diffuse disease the larynx, trachea, and main and segmental bronchi can be involved contiguously or with skip lesions. Submucosal amyloid deposits protrude into the airway lumen, and eccentric or concentric stenoses can occur. The chest radiograph can be normal; however, segmental or lobar collapse is seen in 50%. CT will demonstrate areas of collapse or hyperinflation secondary to an endobronchial deposit, creating a check-valve effect. Strictures and submucosal nodular deposits will also be shown. Contrast enhancement and stippled calcifications of the nodular deposits have been identified (33,43). Occasionally, these amyloid deposits develop calcification and even ossification (17), and some investigators believe this is the etiology for tracheobronchopathia osteochondroplastica (see below).

Airway wall thickening with enhancement or calcification should suggest amyloidosis.

TRACHEOBRONCHOPATHIA OSTEOCHONDROPLASTICA

Tracheobronchopathia osteochondroplastica is a rare disorder of unknown etiology. Patients are often asymptomatic, although they may exhibit hemoptysis, cough, hoarseness, stridor, or recurrent lower respiratory tract infections. The disease typically occurs in middle-aged men and is of uncertain etiology (see Amyloidosis, above). Typically, a long segment of trachea, extending to involve the main bronchi, is involved. Multiple submucosal osteocartilaginous nodules involve the anterior and lateral walls; these may occlude the airway lumen, causing distal collapse (33). CT will demonstrate thickened cartilage with 3 to 8 mm irregular nodules and calcifications protruding into the airway lumen, leading to irregular narrowing of the distal trachea and main bronchi. There is characteristic sparing of the posterior membrane (17,31).

ULCERATIVE COLITIS

A tracheobronchitis is occasionally associated with ulcerative colitis. CT demonstrates thickened tracheal or bronchial walls, with luminal narrowing. Bronchiectasis and bronchiolitis obliterans are also seen, affecting the more distal airways. There is concentric fibrosis of the submucosa, with ulceration and inflammation of the mucosa on pathologic analysis (31).

INFECTIOUS CONDITIONS

FIBROSING MEDIASTINITIS

Fibrosing mediastinitis (also termed granulomatous, collagenous, or sclerosing mediastinitis) is a rare disorder in which exuberant proliferation of fibrous and connective tissue compresses and encases vital structures within the mediastinum. Mediastinal lymphadenopathy is invariably present, but clinical manifestations of fibrosing mediastinitis are a result of an exaggerated granulomatous and fibrotic response beyond the confines of lymph nodes. This fibrotic process may continue to accrue over several years, invading, encasing, and obliterating mediastinal vessels (superior vena cava, pulmonary arteries, and veins) (Fig. 21.31); esophagus; trachea; and major bronchi. Most patients present between ages 20 and 40; the process is usually indolent and progresses slowly over months or years. *Histoplasma capsulatum* has been implicated in 50% to 70% of cases, but occasional cases attributable to *Mycobacteria tuberculosis, Coccidioides immitis, Aspergillus flavus,* and other fungi have been described. Narrowing or compression of the trachea occurs in 15% to 30% of cases, usually in association with other regional manifestations; tracheal obstruction may rarely occur as an isolated feature. Tracheoesophageal fistulas have also been described. Bronchial stenosis appears to be among the more common manifestations of fibrosing mediastinitis, although the actual prevalence is not clear. Obstruction of lobar or main bronchi may result in recurrent atelectasis or pneumonitis associated with purulent sputum, cough, wheezing, and fever. Broncholiths may also occur when granulomas erode through the bronchial wall and may result in bronchial obstruction or severe hemoptysis. CT findings include soft tissue masses in the mediastinum that encase and narrow vessels and central airways. Focal calcifications are often, although not always, present (Fig. 16.12).

Fibrosing mediastinitis classically appears as infiltrative mediastinal soft tissue with calcification. If not calcified, infiltrating malignancy must be considered.

Up to half of the cases of fibrosing mediastinitis are considered idiopathic, because no infectious organism is recovered.

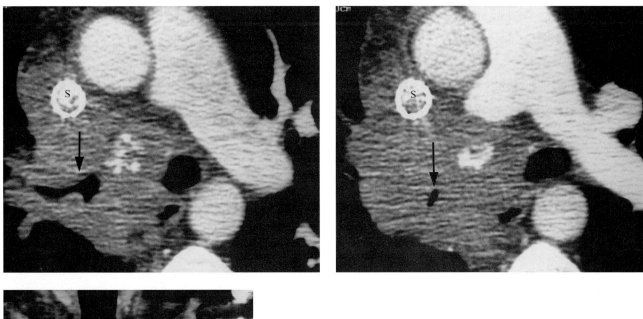

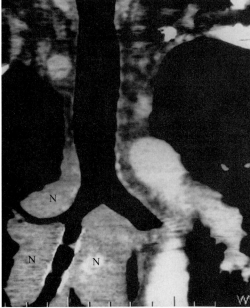

Figure 16.12 Fibrosing mediastinitis *A and B.* Axial computed tomography shows extensive abnormal soft tissue within the mediastinum with calcifications. There is narrowing of the right main bronchus (*arrows*). Note stenting of the superior vena cava (S). *C.* Coronal reformat after stenting of right bronchus intermedius again demonstrates extensive mediastinal lymph node enlargement (N) and subcarinal calcifications.

Unfortunately, the prognosis of fibrosing mediastinitis is poor. Spontaneous resolution does not occur, and no pharmacologic treatment has been shown to be effective. The course is usually chronic, with gradual worsening over 3 to 7 years. Mortality exceeds 30%, with most deaths resulting from cor pulmonale, progressive respiratory failure, or complications of surgery. When a specific infectious agent (such as *H. capsulatum* or *M. tuberculosis*) has been identified, antifungal or antituberculous therapy is recommended, but it is unlikely that these antimicrobial therapies will reverse the fibrotic lesion, once established.

TUBERCULOSIS AND OTHER INFECTIONS

The incidence of tuberculous bronchial stenosis has dropped to 10% after the introduction of antibiotics. Airway disease is caused by granulomatous disease within the tracheal or bronchial wall or by extrinsic pressure or extension from involved peribronchial lymph nodes (33,46,47). There are three stages:

1. Hyperplastic—tubercles present within the submucosal layer;
2. Ulceration and necrosis of the airway wall;
3. Fibrosis and stenosis.

Tuberculosis usually involves the distal trachea and proximal main bronchi. Active tuberculosis leads to irregular (or rarely smooth) circumferential thickening of the airway wall with narrowing or occlusion of the airway (Fig. 16.13). The thickened wall may enhance with contrast material. There may be increased density of adjacent mediastinal fat at CT due to inflammatory infiltration and/or there may be enlarged mediastinal lymph nodes. Lesions in the airway may ulcerate and form fistulas with adjacent structures. In contrast, inactive fibrotic disease leads to smooth narrowing with minimal or no wall thickening or adjacent inflammatory disease. Often, the left main bronchus is involved. Generally, the findings of active disease are reversible with medical therapy.

Bacterial, viral, and fungal infections affecting the airway typically cause subglottic and laryngeal narrowing (31). Rhinosclerosis (scleroma) is a chronic granulomatous disorder of the upper respiratory tract associated with the bacterium *Klebsiella rhinosclero-*

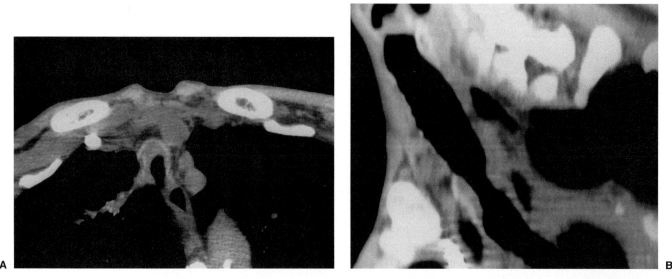

A   **B**

Figure 16.13 Tuberculosis of the trachea. *A.* Axial computed tomography demonstrates irregular narrowing of the mid-trachea with adjacent fibrocalcific lung changes. *B.* Multiplanar reformat showing craniocaudal extension.

matis. It affects the nose, paranasal sinuses, pharynx, and occasionally the trachea (2% to 9%). Diffuse symmetric narrowing or nodular masses may develop. The course is slowly progressive with healing by fibrosis (33,48,49).

TRAUMATIC RUPTURE

Bronchial rupture is rare; the usual mechanism of injury is rapid deceleration with associated shearing forces. Mortality is high (30%). Rupture usually occurs within 2.5 cm of the carina, more commonly on the right (33). The imaging findings depend on the site of rupture. Tracheal or proximal left main bronchus ruptures do not communicate with the pleural space; therefore, pneumomediastinum but not pneumothorax will be present (Fig. 12.21). Right main bronchus or distal left main bronchus ruptures do communicate with the pleural space, and pneumothorax will be present (50). Other signs include air around the bronchus, subcutaneous emphysema, and lung collapse. There may be associated thoracic bone fractures (33).

> Traumatic airway rupture usually occurs within 2.5 cm of the carina.

POSTOPERATIVE STENOSIS AND DEHISCENCE

Postoperative bronchial stenosis may be seen after a partial lung resection with bronchial anastomosis or after lung transplantation. Bronchial stenosis is due to granulation tissue, fibrous stricture, or bronchomalacia. CT accuracy for diagnosis of anastomotic stenosis is very high (approximately 90%) using axial images alone, and there is very slightly higher accuracy when MPR or virtual bronchoscopy images are added (Fig. 16.14).

The most sensitive and specific indicator of a bronchial dehiscence at CT is the demonstration of a bronchial defect, followed by the presence of extraluminal air (this can be seen in the immediate postoperative period without the presence of a defect). An endoluminal flap or spherical air collections can also be a normal feature of a telescoping anastomosis; however, irregular air collections and posterior wall defects suggest dehiscence (51,52). It has been reported that a small dehiscence (less than 4 mm) or a small amount of extraluminal air generally indicates that the anastomosis will heal without adverse sequelae. However, when the CT shows a large dehiscence (greater than 4 mm) or a large amount of extraluminal air, CT is not useful in predicting which patients will require intervention for optimal anastomotic healing. An incomplete dehiscence will heal by fibrosis, typically causing an hourglass stenosis (33).

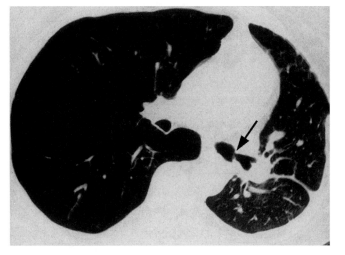

Figure 16.14 Post–lung transplant bronchial stenosis. Axial computed tomography shows focal narrowing (*arrow*) at the anastomosis.

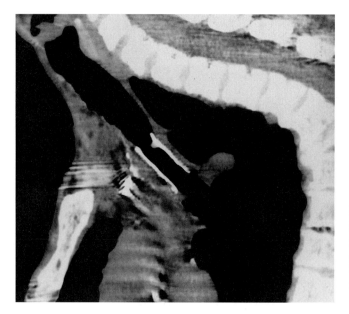

Figure 16.15 Tracheal stent. Sagittal multiplanar reformat through the trachea demonstrates stent position across a benign stricture caused by tuberculosis (same case as Fig. 16.13).

STENTS

Stents are occasionally used in the management of benign tracheal or bronchial stenoses or obstruction. Conditions in which they are used include post–lung transplant anastomotic stricture, tracheomalacia, external compression, and inflammatory conditions such as relapsing polychondritis. They can be located as far as second-order bronchial branches and can be placed via a flexible bronchoscope. The stents eventually become epithelialized, which helps to prevent migration. CT is used to evaluate the present airway, including airway anatomy, diameter, malacia, and distal collapse or air trapping. Poststent CT can assess complications including inflammation, stent migration, airway erosion, stent fracture, and distal lung collapse (Fig. 16.15) (53).

DIFFUSE AIRWAY ENLARGEMENT

Diffuse enlargement of the trachea and main bronchi may be associated with tracheobronchomegaly (see below) or Ehlers-Danlos syndrome. Upper lobe fibrosis secondary to conditions such as sarcoidosis and cystic fibrosis may also enlarge the tracheal lumen due to traction. Allergic bronchopulmonary aspergillosis sometimes causes central bronchiectasis, affecting the main and segmental bronchi (28).

TRACHEOBRONCHOMEGALY

Tracheobronchomegaly is often associated with bronchiectasis.

Tracheobronchomegaly or Mounier-Kuhn syndrome is a rare condition of unknown etiology that presents with marked dilatation of the trachea and main bronchi. The more distal bronchi are of normal caliber; however, repeated infections may lead to bronchiectasis. Histologically, there is atrophy of the tracheobronchial elastic and muscle fibers (54). A congenital defect has been suggested, and associations have been made with the Ehlers-Danlos and cutis laxa syndromes (55). Males are more commonly affected, mostly in the third and fourth decades. Subjects present with a history of repeated chest infection. Chest radiographs characteristically demonstrate a dilated trachea, which has a corrugated appearance secondary to prolapse of atrophied muscle fibers and mucosa through the tracheal rings. This is best appreciated on a lateral chest radiograph. CT also demonstrates

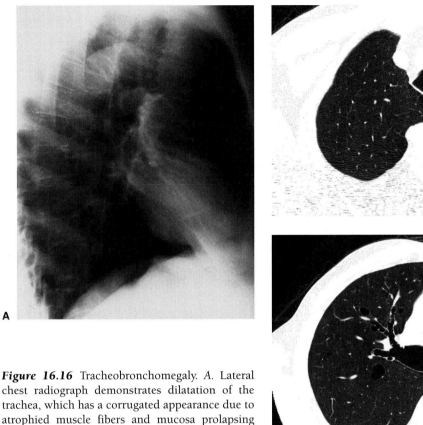

Figure 16.16 Tracheobronchomegaly. *A.* Lateral chest radiograph demonstrates dilatation of the trachea, which has a corrugated appearance due to atrophied muscle fibers and mucosa prolapsing through tracheal rings. *B* and *C.* Axial computed tomography shows marked dilatation of the trachea and central bronchi. The distal bronchi are of normal caliber.

dilatation of the trachea and mucosal prolapse and shows the abrupt transition between dilated central bronchi and normal caliber distal bronchi (Fig. 16.16) (56,57). The diagnosis is confirmed by any tracheal or bronchial diameter exceeding the mean plus 3 standard deviations on standard chest radiograph (trachea greater than 3 cm, right main bronchus greater than 2.4 cm, or left main bronchus greater than 2.3 cm) (54,56).

> A tracheal diameter of more than 3 cm indicates tracheomegaly.

SABER SHEATH TRACHEA

Saber sheath trachea is a condition associated with chronic obstructive pulmonary disease and is most commonly seen in males (58). It is a sign of lung hyperinflation (59). Characterized by a reduced transverse diameter of the intrathoracic portion of the trachea, the diagnosis is made if the ratio of the anteroposterior to transverse tracheal diameters is greater than 2:1 (28). On CT the trachea has a smooth inner margin and a normal wall thickness. There is frequent calcification of the cartilage rings (15,31). Inward bowing of the cartilage rings may occur, and weakening of the cartilage may lead to tracheomalacia (17).

FOCAL FOREIGN BODY

Foreign body aspiration is most common in children under the age of 10 years. Alcohol, sedation, increased age, and poor dentition increase the risk of foreign body aspiration in adults. Aspirated material is most likely to enter the lower lobes, more often on the right because the right main bronchus is of larger caliber and has a more direct line from the trachea. Most aspirated material is of vegetable origin, which can calcify over time (33). Chest radiographs may show acute air trapping, accentuated on an expiratory view, or atelectasis. Unless very radiopaque, the foreign body is rarely seen on conventional radiographs; fluoroscopy may demonstrate air trapping. CT can show the site of bronchial obstruction and associated air trapping or atelectasis. Radiolucent foreign bodies such as denture base material may be identified (60). In chronic obstruction, bronchial stenoses, bronchiectasis, and an endobronchial mass or granulation tissue may be identified. MRI has been used specifically to identify peanut aspiration; fat within the nut will produce a high signal on T1-weighted imaging (61,62). Mucus is usually of low attenuation on CT, has a bubbly appearance, and occupies the dependent portion of the airway. If there is diagnostic doubt, CT can be repeated after vigorous coughing (63).

BRONCHOLITHIASIS

Broncholithiasis is calcified material within a bronchus. It is secondary to calcified lymph nodes compressing the adjacent airway or eroding into it, leading to bronchial obstruction. Lymph node calcification is usually secondary to histoplasmosis, tuberculosis or fungal infection, sarcoidosis or silicosis. It is more common on the right. Endobronchial calcific material may be seen at bronchoscopy. CT is often useful for evaluation of peribronchial disease (33,64). Patients may develop broncholithoptysis (coughing up of broncholiths).

TRACHEAL DIVERTICULA

Tracheal diverticula are often associated with chronic obstructive pulmonary disease (65). They are mostly located on the posterolateral tracheal wall, near the thoracic inlet, and are usually right sided. The diverticulum protrudes between the cartilage and the muscular portion of the tracheal wall. On CT, they may appear as isolated air cysts or may demonstrate a connection with the trachea (17).

TRACHEOBRONCHIAL NEOPLASMS

Tracheal masses often remain undiagnosed and only produce symptoms when more than three-fourths of the tracheal lumen is occluded (66). Standard frontal and lateral chest radiographs diagnose only 23% to 45% of tracheal intraluminal masses (67–69). CT generally demonstrates the mass but cannot differentiate between mucosal or submucosal neoplasm or assess the presence of submucosal spread.

BENIGN NEOPLASMS

Benign neoplasms account for less than 10% of trachea and main bronchus tumors. Stridor is the most common presenting symptom. CT appearances are nonspecific, but generally the mass is smooth, well circumscribed, of soft tissue attenuation, and measures less than 2 cm (31,63). The neoplasm may be polypoid or sessile and does not breach the tracheal wall (70).

Squamous cell papilloma is the most common benign tracheal tumor. It consists of a proliferation of stratified squamous cell epithelium and grows in a papillary or sessile fashion around a fibrovascular core. More often found in the larynx than the trachea, it is more common in males and probably associated with smoking. Squamous cell papilloma has a wide age of presentation but generally occurs in adulthood (70) (Fig. 16.17).

Tracheobronchial papillomatosis is caused by the human papilloma virus and is usually acquired at birth from an infected mother. Children aged between 2 and 5 years are

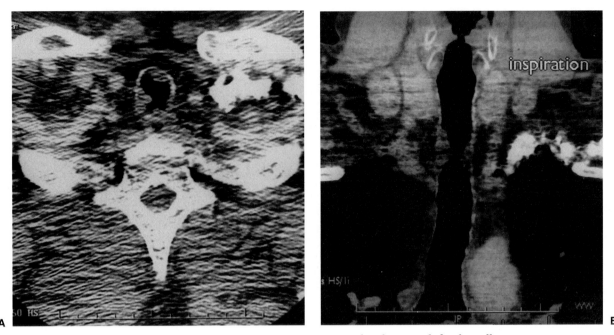

Figure 16.17 Squamous cell papillomas. *A.* Axial computed tomography shows multifocal small masses within the tracheal lumen. *B.* Coronal multiplanar reformat shows narrowing of the tracheal lumen by the multifocal papillomas.

most commonly affected. Papillomas tend to be multiple and usually spontaneously resolve; however, they can recur and have the potential to undergo malignant transformation into squamous cell carcinoma (63,71). Rarely, tracheobronchial dissemination can occur (less than 5%); less than 1% disseminate to the lung parenchyma. Pathology consists of small sessile or pedunculated masses with flattened squamous epithelium and a fibrovascular core. CT demonstrates the intraluminal masses that may carpet the airways. Lung lesions consist of nodules, air-filled cysts or thick-walled cavities, predominantly in the caudal aspects of the chest (70).

Although there are many other benign tumors affecting the tracheobronchial tree, all are rare and often do not possess specific imaging characteristics. Hamartomas are the most common benign lung tumor; however, just 3% occur within bronchi. They are slow growing and are seen in large bronchi. Endobronchial hamartomas contain the same cartilage, fat, fibrous, and epithelial components as pulmonary hamartomas (33). Pleomorphic adenomas are rare, there is a wide age range, and they are more common in males. They arise in the upper and middle thirds of the trachea (70).

Hemangiomas are seen in adults as a cavernous hemangioma of the larynx. Children present with capillary hemangiomas involving the subglottic trachea. They are a submucosal lesion, covered with respiratory epithelium, and appear as a rounded soft tissue mass on CT. Over 90% of infants will develop symptoms in the first 6 months of life and present with stridor (70). Granular cell tumors are of neurogenic origin and are more common in the bronchi than the trachea. They are most common in the fourth decade and in black females. They may be multiple and can be aggressive with local invasion. Most are seen at the level of the cervical trachea (70).

Chondromas are benign cartilaginous tumors rarely found in the trachea. They contain either hyaline or elastic cartilage and arise from the tracheal rings; therefore, growth may be intra- or extraluminal. Foci of calcification are seen in 75% of these tumors on CT. They have the potential to undergo malignant transformation (70). Leiomyomas are benign tumors of smooth muscle. They arise from the membranous portion of the trachea, usually in the lower third (Fig. 8.12). There is a wide age range and males and females are equally affected. They have a tendency to bleed, so biopsy is a relative risk (70). Schwannomas and neurofibromas are very rare and usually present in the fourth decade. They affect the lower third of the trachea (70).

PRIMARY MALIGNANT NEOPLASMS

Primary malignant neoplasms account for over 90% of tracheobronchial tumors. The most common is squamous cell carcinoma, followed by adenoid cystic carcinoma, bronchial carcinoid, mucoepidermoid tumor, and rare tumors such as chondrosarcoma (Fig. 16.18) and leiomyosarcoma (63). Squamous cell carcinoma accounts for 55% of tracheobronchial tumors. These tumors are seen generally seen in middle-aged male smokers, often with a history of alcohol abuse. About one-third of patients have other malignancies of the respiratory tract. About 10% are multifocal, often in the bronchi. The lesion may extend into the esophagus, leading to a fistula. Usually these cancers manifest as a large irregular mass on CT (Fig. 16.19) (63), although they can rarely grow circumferentially in the tracheal wall. If the entire tumor can be resected, surgical resected is usually advised, often followed by postoperative therapy. Generally, up to 6 cm of tracheal length can be resected successfully. One study reported median survival after surgery of 34 months.

Adenoid cystic carcinomas can arise from mucous glands in the trachea and bronchi. There is no smoking relationship, although males appear to be more often affected, usually in the third to fifth decades. They are slow-growing polypoidal masses that thicken the mucosa and can spread submucosally. Typically they arise in the middle or lower trachea on the posterolateral wall, and extraluminal growth is common (Fig. 16.20) (33,63,72). Adenoid cystic tumors used to be called cylindromas and classified with bronchial adenomas; however, this name and classification were discarded due to their misleading nature, erroneously suggesting a benign process. The best treatment is generally surgical resection with tracheal anastomosis, whenever possible. Postoperative radiation is often given. Patient survival is excellent (10-year median survival after surgery in one study), although late recurrences or metastases (e.g., 15 to 30 years after diagnosis) have been reported. Metastases tend to occur in lung, liver, bone, and brain.

Carcinoid tumors are of neuroendocrine origin (73), originating from Kulchitsky cells, which can secrete serotonin, corticotropin, and bradykinin. They are divided into two types. The first type, typical carcinoids, accounts for 75% to 90% (63). They present in the fifth and sixth decades, often with hemoptysis or obstructive atelectasis. They mostly arise in central bronchi; however, 10% may be peripheral. They are typically well defined and smooth and may be lobular, round, or ovoid (Fig. 16.21). They are slow growing and rarely metastasize (33). Stromal ossification or calcification may be demonstrated

---

The most common primary malignant tracheal tumor is squamous cell carcinoma.

Adenoid cystic carcinomas arise from the posterolateral tracheal wall, which is the location of the mucous glands from which they arise.

Eighty percent to 90% of carcinoid tumors are endobronchial; the remainder are pulmonary nodules.

A markedly enhancing endobronchial mass should suggest carcinoid tumor.

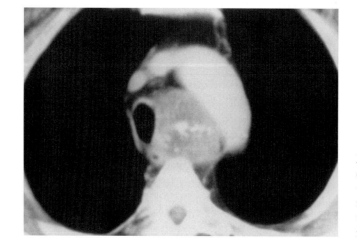

Figure 16.18 Tracheal chondrosarcoma. Axial computed tomography shows an exophytic mass arising from the wall of the trachea, deviating and narrowing the lumen.

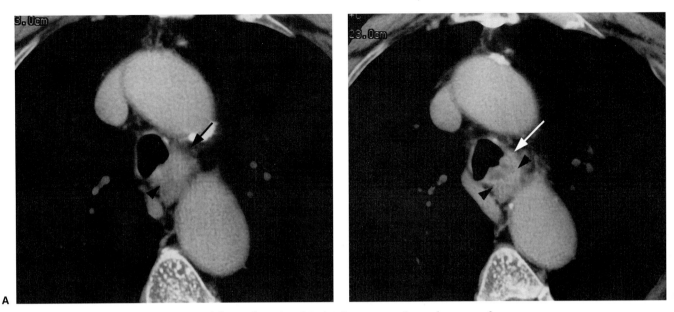

Figure 16.19 Squamous cell carcinoma of the trachea. *A and B.* Axial contrast-enhanced computed tomography demonstrates a focal irregular mass (*arrows*) arising from the tracheal wall. There is ill definition of the fat plane between the tracheal wall and the esophagus (*arrowheads*), suggesting local invasion.

on CT and there is marked contrast enhancement with iodinated contrast (74–76). MRI characteristics include high signal intensity on T2-weighted images and marked enhancement with gadolinium (63). The second type, atypical carcinoids, are less common, accounting for 10% to 25% of cases (63). They arise in a slightly older population (55 to 60 years). They may be central or peripheral, tend to be larger, and are more aggressive with an increased incidence of nodal metastases (33).

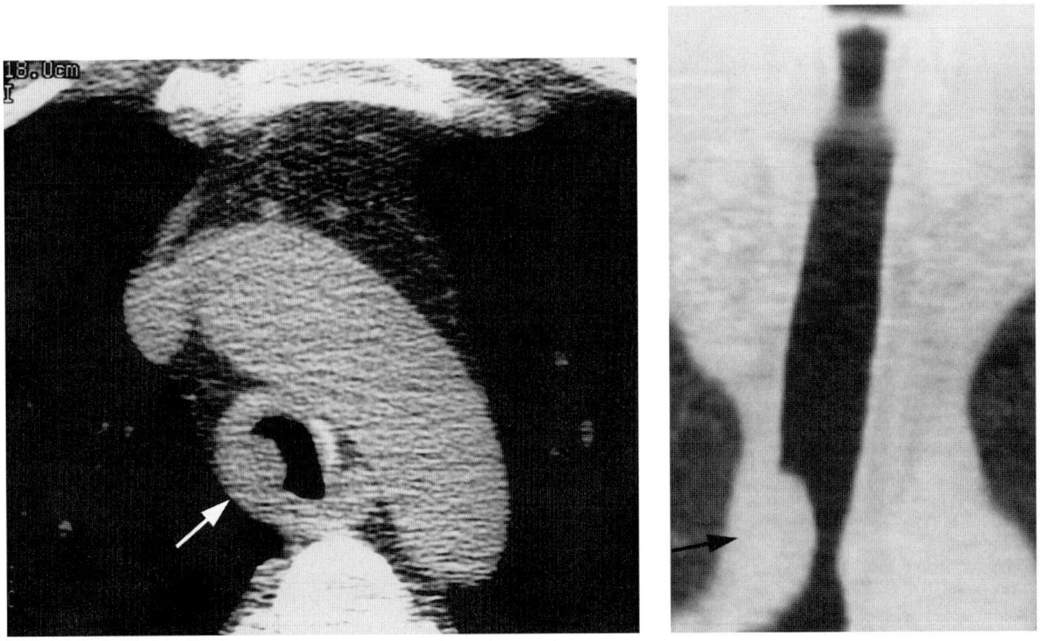

Figure 16.20 Adenoid cystic carcinoma. *A.* Axial computed tomography demonstrates a polypoid mass (*arrows*) arising from the posterolateral wall of the trachea. No extraluminal growth demonstrated. *B.* Multiplanar reformats help assess the craniocaudal extent of the mass.

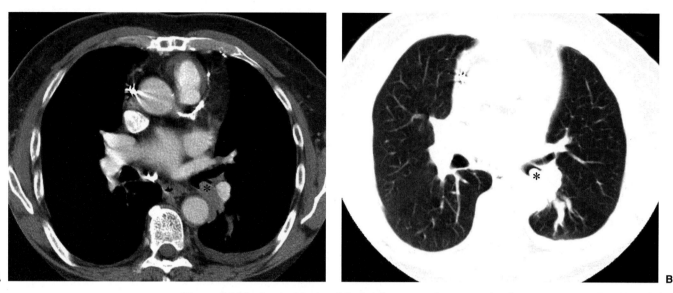

Figure 16.21 Carcinoid. *A and B.* Axial computed tomography demonstrates a polypoid endoluminal mass (*asterisks*) within the superior segmental bronchus of the left lower lobe, protruding into the left lower lobe bronchus lumen.

Mucoepidermoid tumors account for 1% to 5% of bronchial neoplasms. Males and females are equally affected, and there is a wide age range, with an average of 37 years (77). There is no association with smoking. They usually present with a focal endobronchial mass within a large central airway (33).

METASTASES

Metastatic tracheobronchial tumors arise either by local invasion or hematogenous spread. Common locally invading tumors include thyroid, esophageal, laryngeal, and lung carcinoma (Fig. 16.22). Hematogenous spread of tumor has been described with melanoma, breast, colon, genitourinary, and renal tumors. They produce an endoluminal, polypoidal,

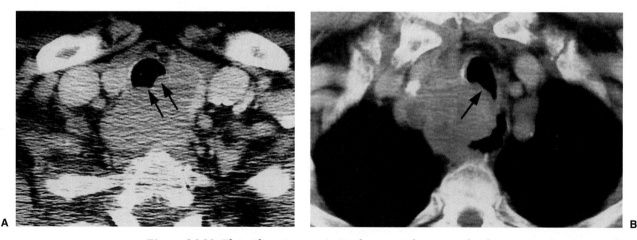

Figure 16.22 Thyroid carcinoma. *A.* Axial computed tomography demonstrates carcinoma of the thyroid invading the adjacent mediastinal structures, including the left posterolateral wall of the trachea (*arrows*). *B.* Esophageal carcinoma. Axial computed tomography demonstrates direct invasion of the adjacent trachea (*arrow*).

soft tissue mass (31,78). CT can demonstrate local invasion and endobronchial masses and complications such as distal atelectasis.

REFERENCES

1. Holbert JM, Strollo DC. Imaging of the normal trachea. *J Thorac Imaging* 1995;10:171–179.
2. Shih JY, Lee LN, Wu HD, et al. Sonographic imaging of the trachea. *J Ultrasound Med* 1997;16:783–790.
3. Callanan V, Gillmore K, Field S, Beaumont A, et al. The use of magnetic resonance imaging to assess tracheal stenosis following percutaneous dilatational tracheostomy. *J Laryngol Otol* 1997;111:953–957.
4. Salvolini L, Bichi Secchi E, Costarelli L, DeNicola M. Clinical applications of 2D and 3D CT imaging of the airways—a review. *Eur J Radiol* 2000;34:9–25.
5. Remy-Jardin M, Remy J, Artaud D, et al. Volume rendering of the tracheobronchial tree: clinical evaluation of bronchographic images. *Radiology* 1998;208:761–770.
6. Remy-Jardin M, Remy J, Artaud D, et al. Tracheobronchial tree: assessment with volume rendering—technical aspects. *Radiology* 1998;208:393–398.
7. Ferretti GR, Thony F, Bosson JL, et al. Benign abnormalities and carcinoid tumors of the central airways: diagnostic impact of CT bronchography. *AJR Am J Roentgenol* 2000;174:1307–1313.
8. Remy-Jardin M, Remy J, Deschildre F, et al. Obstructive lesions of the central airways: evaluation by using spiral CT with multiplanar and three-dimensional reformations. *Eur Radiol* 1996;6:807–816.
9. Quint LE, Whyte RI, Kazerooni EA, et al. Stenosis of the central airways: evaluation by using helical CT with multiplanar reconstructions. *Radiology* 1995;194:871–877.
10. Naidich DP, Lee JJ, Garay SM, et al. Comparison of CT and fiberoptic bronchoscopy in the evaluation of bronchial disease. *AJR Am J Roentgenol* 1987;148:1–7.
11. Mayr B, Ingrisch H, Haussinger K, et al. Tumors of the bronchi: role of evaluation with CT. *Radiology* 1989;172:647–652.
12. Henschke CI, Davis SD, Auh Y, et al. Detection of bronchial abnormalities: comparison of CT and bronchoscopy. *J Comput Assist Tomogr* 1987;11:432–435.
13. Perhomaa M, Lahde S, Rossi O, Suramo I. Helical CT in evaluation of the bronchial tree. *Acta Radiol* 1997;38:83–91.
14. Kittredge RD. Computed tomography of the trachea: a review. *J Comput Tomogr* 1981;5:44–50.
15. Gamsu G, Webb WR. Computed tomography of the trachea: normal and abnormal. *AJR Am J Roentgenol* 1982;139:321–326.
16. Breatnach E, Abbott GC, Fraser RG. Dimensions of the normal human trachea. *AJR Am J Roentgenol* 1984;142:903–906.
17. Webb EM, Elicker BM, Webb WR. Using CT to diagnose nonneoplastic tracheal abnormalities: appearance of the tracheal wall. *AJR Am J Roentgenol* 2000;174:1315–1321.
18. Fraser RG. Measurements of the calibre of human bronchi in three phases of respiration by cinebronchography. *J Can Assoc Radiol* 1961;12:102.
19. Jesseph JE, Merendino KA. The dimensional interrelationships of the major components of the human tracheobronchial tree. *Surg Gynecol Obstet* 1957;105:210.
20. Merendino KA, Kiriluk LB. Human measurements involved in tracheobronchial resection and reconstruction procedures: report of case of bronchial adenoma. *Surgery* 1954;35:590.
21. Alper H, Sener RN. Pulmonary aplasia: MR angiography findings. *Eur Radiol* 1996;6:89–91.
22. Kinsella D, Sissons G, Williams MP. The radiological imaging of bronchial atresia. *Br J Radiol* 1992;65:681–685.
23. Beigelman C, Howarth NR, Chartrand-Lefebrier, Grenier P. Congenital anomalies of tracheobronchial branching patterns: spiral CT aspects in adults. *Eur Radiol* 1998;8:79–85.
24. Rappaport DC, Herman SJ, Weisbrod GL. Congenital bronchopulmonary diseases in adults: CT findings. *AJR Am J Roentgenol* 1994;162:1295–1299.
25. Remy J, Smith M, Marache P, Nuyts JP. La bronche "tracheale" gauche pathogene. Revue de la litterature a propos de 4 observations. *J Radiol Electrol* 1977;58:621–630.
26. McGuinness, G, Naidich DP, Garay SM, et al. Accessory cardiac bronchus: CT features and clinical significance. *Radiology* 1993;189:563–566.
27. Stark P. Imaging of tracheobronchial injuries. *J Thorac Imaging* 1995;10:206–219.
28. Marom EM, Goodman PC, McAdams HP. Diffuse abnormalities of the trachea and main bronchi. *AJR Am J Roentgenol* 2001;176:713–717.

29. Ferretti GR, Bricault I, Coulomb M. Helical CT with multiplanar and three-dimensional reconstruction of nonneoplastic abnormalities of the trachea. *J Comput Assist Tomogr* 2001;25:400–406.

30. Brichet A, Verkindre C, Dupont J, et al. Multidisciplinary approach to management of postintubation tracheal stenoses. *Eur Respir J* 1999;13:888–893.

31. Kwong JS, Muller NL, Miller RR. Diseases of the trachea and main-stem bronchi: correlation of CT with pathologic findings. *Radiographics* 1992;12:645–657.

32. Palombini BC, Villanova CA, Araujo E, et al. A pathogenic triad in chronic cough: asthma, postnasal drip syndrome, and gastroesophageal reflux disease. *Chest* 1999;116:279–284.

33. Shepard JA. The bronchi: an imaging perspective. *J Thorac Imaging* 1995;10:236–254.

34. McAdam LP, O'Hanlan MA, Bluestone R, Pearson CM. Relapsing polychondritis: prospective study of 23 patients and a review of the literature. *Medicine (Baltimore)* 1976;55:193–215.

35. Dolan DL, Lemmon GB Jr, Teitelbaum SL. Relapsing polychondritis. Analytical literature review and studies on pathogenesis. *Am J Med* 1966;41:285–299.

36. Stern EJ, Graham CM, Webb WR, Gamsu G. Normal trachea during forced expiration: dynamic CT measurements. *Radiology* 1993;187:27–31.

37. Gilkeson RC, Ciancibello LM, Hejal RB, Montenegna H, Lange P. Tracheobronchomalacia: dynamic airway evaluation with multidetector CT. *AJR Am J Roentgenol* 2001;176:205–210.

38. Webb WR, Stern EJ, Kanth N, Gamsu G. Dynamic pulmonary CT: findings in healthy adult men. *Radiology* 1993;186:117–124.

39. Aquino SL, Shepard JA, Ginns LC, et al. Acquired tracheomalacia: detection by expiratory CT scan. *J Comput Assist Tomogr* 2001;25:394–399.

40. Daum TE, Specks U, Colby TV, et al. Tracheobronchial involvement in Wegener's granulomatosis. *Am J Respir Crit Care Med* 1995;151(2 Pt 1):522–526.

41. Maskell GF, Lockwood CM, Flower CD. Computed tomography of the lung in Wegener's granulomatosis. *Clin Radiol* 1993;48:377–380.

42. Screaton NJ, Sivasothy P, Flower CD, Lockwood CM. Tracheal involvement in Wegener's granulomatosis: evaluation using spiral CT. *Clin Radiol* 1998;53:809–815.

43. Case records of the Massachusetts General Hospital. Weekly clinicopathological exercises. Case 1-1995. An elderly man with a questionable bronchial carcinoid tumor of long duration and recently increasing tracheal obstructions. *N Engl J Med* 1995;332:110–115.

44. Urban BA, Fishman EK, Goldman SM, et al. CT evaluation of amyloidosis: spectrum of disease. *Radiographics* 1993;13:1295–1308.

45. Armstrong P, Wilson AG, DeeP, Hansell DM, et al. *Imaging diseases of the chest*, 3rd ed. St. Louis: Mosby, 2000.

46. Choe KO, Jeong HJ, Sohn HY. Tuberculous bronchial stenosis: CT findings in 28 cases. *AJR Am J Roentgenol* 1990;155:971–976.

47. Jokinen K, Palva T, Nuutinen J. Bronchial findings in pulmonary tuberculosis. *Clin Otolaryngol* 1977;2:139–148.

48. Feldman F, Seaman WB, Baker DC Jr. The roentgen manifestations of scleroma. *Am J Roentgenol Radium Ther Nucl Med* 1967;101:807–813.

49. Miller RH, Shulman JB, Canalis RF, Ward PH. Klebsiella rhinoscleromatis: a clinical and pathogenic enigma. *Otolaryngol Head Neck Surg* 1979;87:212–221.

50. Harvey-Smith W, Bush W, Northrop C. Traumatic bronchial rupture. *AJR Am J Roentgenol* 1980;134:1189–1193.

51. Semenkovich JW, Glazer HS, Anderson DC, et al. Bronchial dehiscence in lung transplantation: CT evaluation. *Radiology* 1995;194:205–208.

52. McAdams HP, Murray JG, Erasmus JJ, et al. Telescoping bronchial anastomoses for unilateral or bilateral sequential lung transplantation: CT appearance. *Radiology* 1997;203:202–206.

53. Lehman JD, Gordon RL, Kerlan RK Jr, et al. Expandable metallic stents in benign tracheobronchial obstruction. *J Thorac Imaging* 1998;13:105–115.

54. Katz L, Levine M, Herman P. Tracheobronchomegaly: the Mounier-Kuhn syndrome. *AJR Am J Roentgenol* 1962;88:1084–1094.

55. Aaby G. Tracheobronchomegaly. *Ann Thorac Surg* 1966;2:64–70.

56. Shin MS, Jackson RM, Ho KJ. Tracheobronchomegaly (Mounier-Kuhn syndrome): CT diagnosis. *AJR Am J Roentgenol* 1988;150:777–779.

57. Doyle AJ. Demonstration on computed tomography of tracheomalacia in tracheobronchomegaly (Mounier-Kuhn syndrome). *Br J Radiol* 1989;62:176–177.

58. Greene R. "Saber-sheath" trachea: relation to chronic obstructive pulmonary disease. *AJR Am J Roentgenol* 1978;130:441–445.

59. Trigaux JP, Hermes G, Dubois P, et al. CT of saber-sheath trachea. Correlation with clinical, chest radiographic and functional findings. *Acta Radiol* 1994;35:247–250.

60. Newton JP, Abel RW, Lloyd CH, Yemm R. The use of computed tomography in the detection of radiolucent denture base material in the chest. *J Oral Rehabil* 1987;14:193–202.

61. Imaizumi H, Kaneko M, Nara S, Saito H, Asakura K, Akiba H. Definitive diagnosis and location of peanuts in the airways using magnetic resonance imaging techniques. *Ann Emerg Med* 1994;23:1379–1382.

62. O'Uchi T, Tokumaru A, Mikami I, Yamasoba T, Kikuchi S. Value of MR imaging in detecting a peanut causing bronchial obstruction. *AJR Am J Roentgenol* 1992;159:481–482.

63. Marom EM, Goodman PC, McAdams HP. Focal abnormalities of the trachea and main bronchi. *AJR Am J Roentgenol* 2001;176:707–711.

64. Conces DJ Jr, Tarver RD, Vix VA. Broncholithiasis: CT features in 15 patients. *AJR Am J Roentgenol* 1991;157:249–253.

65. Goo JM, Im JG, Ahn JM, et al. Right paratracheal air cysts in the thoracic inlet: clinical and radiologic significance. *AJR Am J Roentgenol* 1999;173:65–70.

66. Weber AL, Grillo HC. Tracheal tumors. A radiological, clinical, and pathological evaluation of 84 cases. *Radiol Clin North Am* 1978;16:227–246.

67. Hajdu SI, Huvos AG, Goodner JT, Foote FW Jr, Beattie EJ Jr. Carcinoma of the trachea. Clinicopathologic study of 41 cases. *Cancer* 1970;25:1448–1456.

68. Houston HE, Payne WS, Harrison EG Jr, Olsen AM. Primary cancers of the trachea. *Arch Surg* 1969;99:132–140.

69. Manninen MP, Paakkala TA, Pukander JS, Karma PH. Diagnosis of tracheal carcinoma at chest radiography. *Acta Radiol* 1992;33:546–547.

70. McCarthy MJ, Rosado-de-Christenson ML. Tumors of the trachea. *J Thorac Imaging* 1995;10: 180–198.

71. Gruden JF, Webb WR, Sides DM. Adult-onset disseminated tracheobronchial papillomatosis: CT features. *J Comput Assist Tomogr* 1994;18:640–642.

72. Spizarny DL, Shepard JA, McLoud TC, Grillo HC, Dedrick CG. CT of adenoid cystic carcinoma of the trachea. *AJR Am J Roentgenol* 1986;146:1129–1132.

73. Müller NL, Miller RR. Neuroendocrine carcinomas of the lung. *Semin Roentgenol* 1990;25: 96–104.

74. Rosado de Christenson ML, Abbott GF, Kirejczyk WM, Galvin JR, Travis WD. Thoracic carcinoids: radiologic-pathologic correlation. *Radiographics* 1999;19:707–736.

75. Zwiebel BR, Austin JH, Grimes MM. Bronchial carcinoid tumors: assessment with CT of location and intratumoral calcification in 31 patients. *Radiology* 1991;179:483–486.

76. Shin MS, Berland LL, Myers JL, Clary G, Zorn GL. CT demonstration of an ossifying bronchial carcinoid simulating broncholithiasis. *AJR Am J Roentgenol* 1989;153:51–52.

77. Heitmiller RF, et al. Mucoepidermoid lung tumors. *Ann Thorac Surg* 1989;47:394–399.

78. Aberle DR, Brown K, Young DA, Batra P, Steckel RJ. Imaging techniques in the evaluation of tracheobronchial neoplasms. *Chest* 1991;99:211–215.

RADIOLOGY OF THE PLEURA

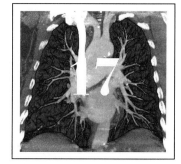

- Pleural Abnormalities
- Selected Topics in Radiology of the Pleura and Chest Wall

Evaluation of the pleura is in several important ways the evil twin of evaluation of the mediastinum. Whereas plain film assessment of the mediastinum is extremely limited, chest radiograph (CXR) evaluation of the pleura is generally efficacious. Although computed tomography (CT) is a phenomenal tool for assessing mediastinal anatomy and abnormality, pleural CT is often requested for indications of questionable validity. In this chapter we discuss typical pleural abnormalities, their differential diagnosis, and applications of CT.

PLEURAL ABNORMALITIES

The major pleural findings of abnormality are effusion, pneumothorax, focal or multifocal pleural implants or plaques, and solitary or multiple pleural masses.

PLEURAL EFFUSION

As discussed in Chapter 3, pleural effusion is typically gravity dependent. It accumulates in the most dependent portion of the chest, varying with changes in patient position. In the presence of pleural adhesions or scars, loculated effusion may occur. Pleural fluid may track into pleural fissures, even when not loculated. Although this is often easily recognizable based on its tapering cigar-shaped appearance (Fig. 17.1), it sometimes results in confusing appearances.

On standard frontal and lateral radiographs, the posterior costophrenic sulcus is the place to look for small pleural effusions. As effusion enlarges, it may blunt the lateral costophrenic angles, or it may accumulate in a subpulmonic location. Neophyte interpreters of radiographs seem to overcall pleural effusions on frontal radiographs more than any other finding. They are quick to assume that any basilar opacity on a portable radiograph indicates effusion. Most such "effusions" actually represent basilar atelectasis or epicardial fat or cardiomegaly on a hypoventilatory anteroposterior CXR. Our advice is to suggest pleural effusion if there are findings of effusion but to recognize that we cannot expect to diagnose everything with 100% accuracy on limited portable radiographs. In other words, try not to envision something simply because you are afraid of missing it.

Generally, the biggest challenge in the diagnosis of pleural effusion is to recognize its presence on supine or semisupine radiographs. In that situation, fluid layers posterior to

As pleural effusions are usually gravity-dependent, the posterior costophrenic sulcus is the place to look for small effusions.

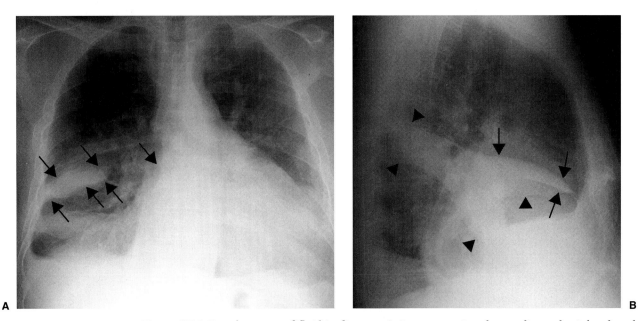

Figure 17.1 Pseudotumors of fluid in fissures. *A.* Posteroanterior chest radiograph: right pleural effusion tracks into major and minor fissures, with typical cigar-shaped appearance of fluid in minor fissure *(arrows)*. *B.* Lateral chest radiograph: similar cigar-shaped appearance of fluid in major fissure *(arrowheads)* is better appreciated *(arrows* indicate fluid in minor fissure).

the lung. Because it is visualized *en face*, there is no sharp edge to outline the margin of effusion against normal pleura or lung. As a consequence, vague opacity is present, typically worst at the bases of the hemithoraces and becoming gradually less obvious as the eye travels cephalad. In the presence of large supine effusion, fluid will typically "cap" over the apex of the hemithorax (Fig. 17.2).

If it is important to know whether there really is pleural effusion in such a patient, solutions are available. As previously discussed in Chapter 3, the first step is to obtain lateral decubitus radiography; the side of suspected effusion should be the down side. Pleural

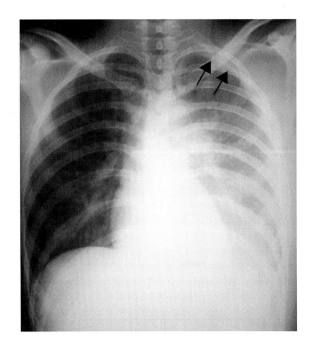

Figure 17.2 Supine left pleural effusion. Increased opacity throughout the left hemithorax with continued visualization of left lung vessels. Note fluid capping left apex *(arrows)*.

ultrasonography is an alternative, particularly when a small effusion is suspected, because ultrasonography can be used to guide thoracentesis as well. CT is *not* a reasonable alternative simply for detection of pleural effusion.

A potentially important effect of large pleural effusions is diaphragmatic inversion. In the presence of diaphragmatic inversion, the two hemidiaphragms move in opposite directions during respiration. As a consequence, air may move back and forth between the two lungs (pendelluft, or pendulum respiration) (1). The net effect is markedly increased dead space and significant dyspnea. Thoracentesis with removal of enough fluid to restore the affected hemidiaphragm to its normal position may result in marked relief of symptoms. Left hemidiaphragmatic inversion is more easily diagnosed because it results in mass effect in the left upper quadrant, displacing the gas-filled stomach (Fig. 17.3).

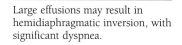
Large effusions may result in hemidiaphragmatic inversion, with significant dyspnea.

The other potentially important effect of diaphragmatic inversion is that it changes expected anatomic relationships that assist localization of peridiaphragmatic fluid at CT (2). In a patient with a normal convex-upward hemidiaphragm, fluid visualized outside the diaphragmatic outline is supradiaphragmatic (pleural) and fluid visualized inside the diaphragmatic outline is subdiaphragmatic (peritoneal) (2). In the presence of diaphragmatic inversion, these relationships are reversed.

In hospitalized patients, pleural effusions are most commonly seen with congestive heart failure or as a consequence of surgery. The stigmata of recent adjacent surgery (in the chest or in the upper abdomen) will usually be evident or might (rarely) be indicated in the provided clinical history for performance of the radiograph. If effusions are a result of congestive heart failure, they are typically bilateral and reasonably symmetric. Congestive heart failure effusions are occasionally unilateral and not infrequently somewhat asymmetric; in most such patients, right pleural effusion is larger.

When there is unilateral left pleural effusion (or left effusion is significantly larger than right effusion) in a nonsurgical patient, other etiologies should at least be considered (Box 17.1). For differential diagnostic purposes, in this situation you might run through categories of disease. First, because it is the category you do not want to forget, is neoplasm. Pleural metastases are far more common than pleural primary neoplasms. Many

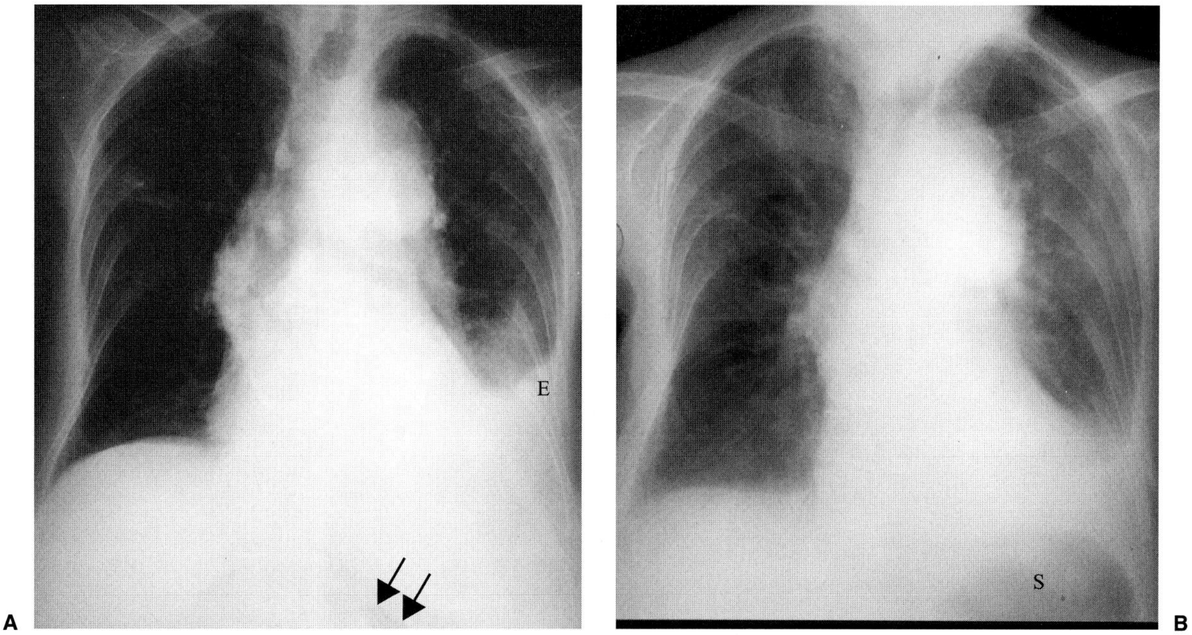

Figure 17.3 Effusion inverting left hemidiaphragm. *A.* Posteroanterior chest radiograph: typical left pleural effusion (E) with apparent left upper quadrant abdominal mass displacing stomach inferomedially *(arrows). B.* Posteroanterior chest radiograph after thoracentesis: stomach (S) in a more normal position, with no left upper quadrant mass.

Box 17.1: Causes of Pleural Effusion

Congestive heart failure
Surgery
Neoplasm—metastatic, primary
Inflammatory disease—infection, autoimmune
Abdominal disease—trauma, infection, inflammation, liver failure
Vascular—pulmonary embolus
Trauma—motor vehicle accident, stab or bullet wound, iatrogenic (catheter or feeding
  tube malposition)

---

primary neoplasms metastasize to the pleura. Those closest to the pleura (particularly lung and breast cancers) are especially likely, but in a given patient the most likely source of pleural metastases is that patient's neoplasm. In other words, even a primary neoplasm that is not frequently associated with pleural metastases deserves serious consideration if a patient with that neoplasm develops pleural effusion. Lymphoma is also in the differential diagnosis, especially if there are multiple enlarged thoracic lymph nodes.

Among abdominopelvic neoplasms, ovarian carcinoma deserves special mention. It frequently spreads to the peritoneum, and pleural effusion in a patient with malignant ascites sometimes reflects leakage of fluid through the diaphragm. Pleural metastases from ovarian carcinoma do occur; they are commonly referred to as Meig syndrome. In fact, the original description of Meig syndrome referred to the association of pleural effusion with benign ovarian fibroma (Fig. 17.4). Over time, this term has become less precise and is now usually applied to any combination of pleural effusion and ovarian mass. Patients with pleural metastases from any primary may have unilateral or bilateral effusions.

Malignant mesothelioma is the most common pleural primary neoplasm associated with pleural effusion, and most patients with malignant mesothelioma have pleural effusion (Fig. 17.5). Effusion is not usually an isolated finding in this setting. Instead, there is usually also

> Most patients with malignant mesothelioma have pleural effusion.

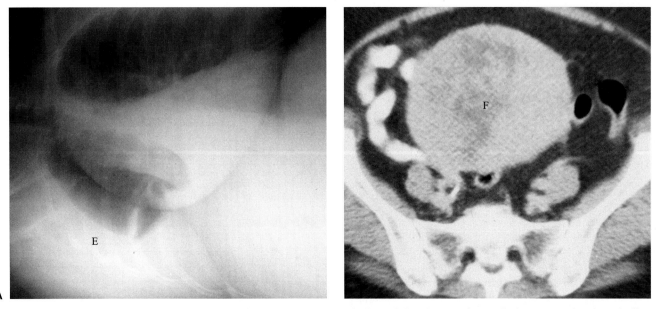

A   **B**

Figure 17.4 Meig syndrome. *A.* Right lateral decubitus radiograph: layering right pleural effusion (E). *B.* Pelvic computed tomography: large solid pelvic mass (F) represents an ovarian fibrothecoma.

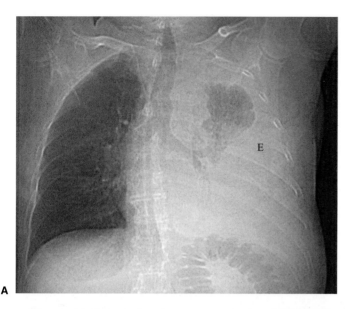

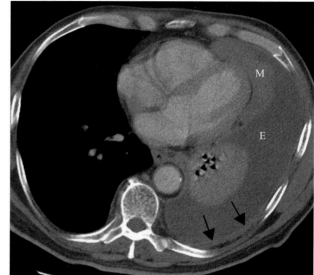

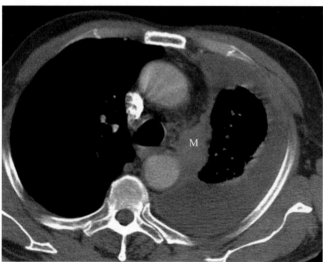

Figure 17.5 Malignant mesothelioma. *A.* Scout chest radiograph: large left pleural effusion (E) without right shift of the mediastinum. *B.* Computed tomography: effusion (E) is accompanied by solid pleural mass (M) and implants *(arrows). C.* Computed tomography more cephalad than *B*: additional pleural mass (M) adjacent to aortopulmonary window.

lobulated pleural mass. A history of asbestos exposure can be a helpful clue, but well-documented asbestos exposure is only established in about half of patients with malignant mesothelioma. In some patients lack of mediastinal shift away from the side of extensive pleural abnormality is a clue to the diagnosis of malignant mesothelioma (Fig. 17.6). Metastatic adenocarcinoma may closely mimic the appearance of malignant mesothelioma. Pleural effusions in patients with malignant mesothelioma are often unilateral.

Inflammatory disease is the next category to consider. Under this heading, infection is an important consideration. Empyema can occur as a consequence of any pneumonia. Some organisms, such as *M. tuberculosis* and fungi, have a particular predilection for the pleural space (Fig. 17.7). The differentiation of empyema from lung abscess can generally be accomplished by CXR alone. Empyema typically has right or obtuse angles with the adjacent chest wall, whereas lung abscess usually demonstrates acute angles. Empyema is usually lenticular in shape and therefore is much larger on one of two right-angle projections, whereas lung abscess is more spherical in shape and more similar in size on right-angle projections. In selected instances, CT can aid in this distinction by demonstrating that empyema is more mass-like, deflecting vessels and bronchi in its path, whereas lung abscess is more destructive of lung structures but less mass-like. Smoother margins of

CT signs of empyema include mass-effect on adjacent lung structures, smooth margins, lenticular shape, obtuse or right angles with lung parenchyma, and the "split pleura sign."

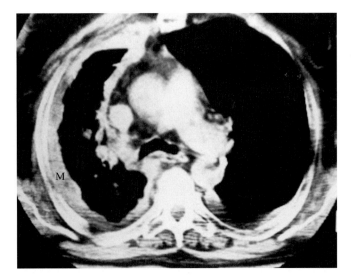

Figure 17.6 Malignant mesothelioma. Despite extensive right pleural abnormality (M), mediastinum is actually shifted to the right.

Thoracentesis is often required to establish an etiology for pleural effusion, whether effusion is benign or malignant.

pleural abnormality and the CT "split pleura sign" of enhancing visceral and parietal pleura around an empyema can also aid in the differential diagnosis (3) (Fig. 17.8).

However, CXR and CT alone cannot establish the presence or absence of infection in the lung or pleural space. Clinical findings (such as fever and elevated white blood cell count) are important in raising the possibility of infection. The role of imaging is to localize the infection to lung or pleura. The final etiology of pleural effusion is sometimes established on clinical grounds alone. In difficult cases, diagnosis generally relies on thoracentesis and analysis of pleural fluid; patients with lung infection commonly have uninfected pleural fluid (a so-called sympathetic effusion). The need for thoracentesis applies equally well to pleural neoplasm and to most other etiologies of pleural effusion.

Inflammatory pleural effusion also includes a variety of autoimmune and related disorders. Among collagen vascular diseases, pleural effusion is particularly likely in systemic

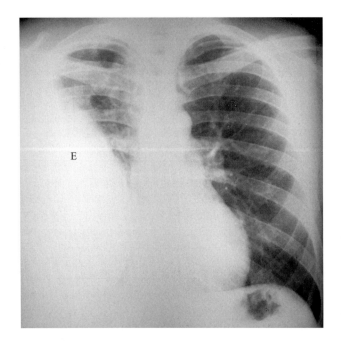

Figure   17.7 Tuberculous empyema (E).

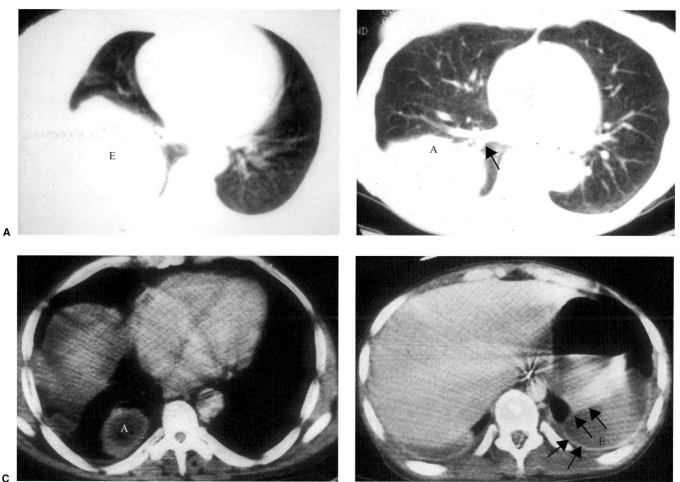

Figure 17.8 Empyema or lung abscess? *A.* Abnormality (E) is compressing and displacing vessels and bronchi in the right lung, typical of empyema. *B.* Abnormality (A) extends right up to undeviated vessels *(arrows)*, typical of abscess. *C.* Abnormality (A) has thick irregular wall, typical of abscess. *D.* Bilateral abnormalities (E) with smooth thin walls and separation of enhancing visceral and parietal pleura ("split pleura sign") *(arrows)*, typical of empyemas.

lupus erythematosus (Fig. 17.9) and rheumatoid arthritis. In fact, pleural effusion is the most common thoracic manifestation of rheumatoid arthritis. As with all extraarticular manifestations of rheumatoid arthritis, pleural effusion is far more common in men than in women. Effusion is also seen in patients with an autoimmune response after myocardial infarction (Dressler syndrome) or cardiac surgery. Pleural effusions in this category may be unilateral or bilateral, symmetric or asymmetric.

Next for consideration are abdominal etiologies of pleural effusion. Adjacent upper abdominal abnormalities can cause effusion. Common etiologies in this category are splenic trauma, subdiaphragmatic abscess (Fig. 17.10), pancreatitis, and ascites. History is obviously very helpful, and thoracentesis can be very revealing (e.g., if there is elevated pleural fluid amylase in a patient with pancreatitis). Patients with ascites, such as those with liver failure, develop pleural effusions for several reasons, including leak of ascitic fluid through the diaphragm and anasarca as a result of decreased serum albumin. When right subdiaphragmatic abscess is an important concern, ultrasound can be very helpful. Because referring clinicians remain uninformed about ultrasound's capabilities even at this relatively late date, they instead virtually always order CT, which is in fact better than ultrasound for left upper quadrant fluid collections. Most effusions resulting from abdominal disease are unilateral.

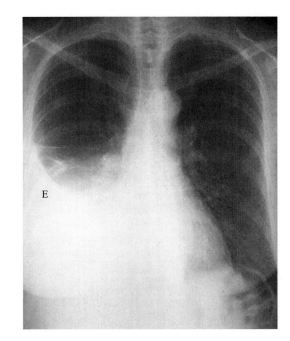

Figure 17.9 Systemic lupus erythematosus with right pleural effusion (E).

Another category to consider is vascular disease. In particular, pulmonary embolus is extremely difficult to diagnose via CXR. Most patients with pulmonary embolus have a normal CXR. When abnormality is present, it is often nonspecific; pleural effusion and atelectasis are the most common findings. Pleural effusion in pulmonary embolus can be unilateral or bilateral, because emboli are commonly multiple.

Trauma can result in pleural effusion. There may be obvious trauma, as in patients with multiple rib fractures. A somewhat less obvious example of trauma would be a patient with aortic laceration in the absence of fractures. An even less obvious example would be a malpositioned vascular catheter or feeding tube (4) (Fig. 17.11). Inadvertent placement of a feeding tube into the lung is usually benign as long as it is discovered before a feeding is administered. However, pleural placement is not similarly benign. Tension pneumothorax and empyema are among its important consequences. Traumatic pleural effusion is more commonly unilateral than bilateral.

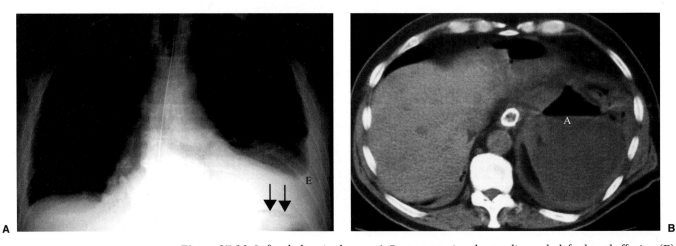

Figure 17.10 Left subphrenic abscess. *A.* Posteroanterior chest radiograph: left pleural effusion (E) with extraintestinal left upper quadrant gas (*arrows*). *B.* Computed tomography: large subdiaphragmatic gas and fluid collection is subphrenic abscess (A).

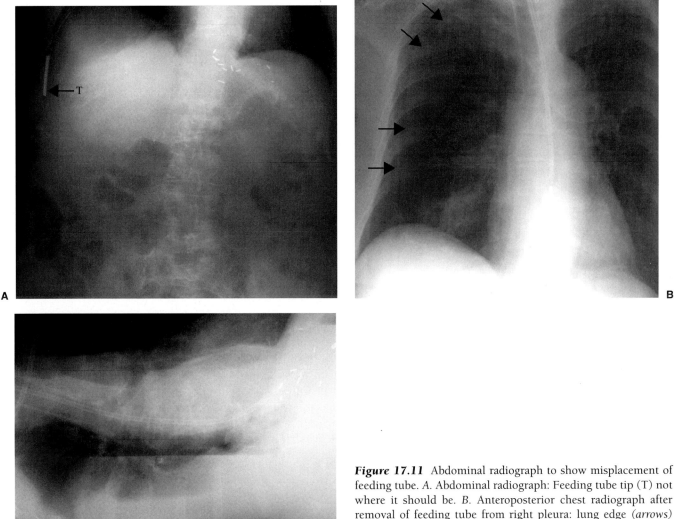

Figure 17.11 Abdominal radiograph to show misplacement of feeding tube. *A.* Abdominal radiograph: Feeding tube tip (T) not where it should be. *B.* Anteroposterior chest radiograph after removal of feeding tube from right pleura: lung edge (*arrows*) displaced by large pneumothorax. *C.* Right lateral decubitus radiograph: air and fluid in right pleura, indicating hydropneumothorax.

Congenital and miscellaneous causes probably account for some pleural effusions (such as in lymphangiectasia and in lymphangiomyomatosis). They are sufficiently uncommon causes of pleural effusion that they are not discussed further here.

PNEUMOTHORAX

Pleural air tends to accumulate in the nondependent portion of the pleural space. Upright frontal radiography is generally the preferred technique for detecting pneumothorax. As discussed in Chapter 3, lateral decubitus radiography with the suspected side of pneumothorax up is a perfectly acceptable alternative; in experiments with cadavers (5) it was even sometimes better than upright views for detecting pleural air.

The diagnosis of pneumothorax is best made by visualization of the lung edge outlined by pleural air (Fig. 17.12). Apical lucency and absence of vessels are far less reliable criteria that can be produced by bullae, for example. As with diagnosis of pleural effusion, detection of pneumothorax becomes trickier when the patient is supine. In that setting the

Because air accumulates in the non-dependent pleural space, upright or lateral decubitus radiographs are preferred for demonstration of pneumothorax.

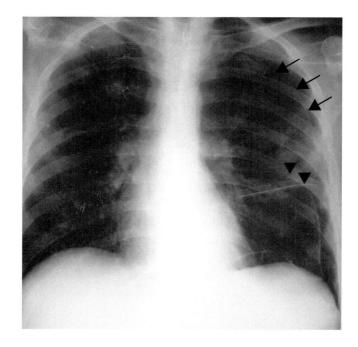

Figure 17.12 Moderate left pneumothorax. Lung edge is visualized *(arrows)*, and gas extends into the major fissure *(arrowheads)*.

nondependent portion of the pleural space is near the hemidiaphragm. Lucency near the lung bases raises concern for pneumothorax, particularly in the presence of the deep sulcus sign (Fig. 17.13), even when no lung edge is visualized. Air in the minor fissure has been reported as another sign of supine pneumothorax (Fig. 17.14). Just as pleural effusion can track into fissures, pneumothorax can be visualized in the major fissure (Fig. 17.12) or even in accessory fissures (Fig. 17.15).

The differential diagnosis for pneumothorax is far less extensive than that for pleural effusion (Box 17.2). Most cases are clearly related to some form of trauma or else occur

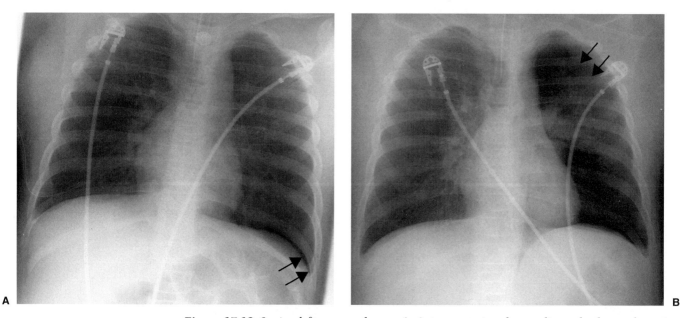

A   B

Figure 17.13 Supine left pneumothorax. *A.* Anteroposterior chest radiograph: deep sulcus sign *(arrows)*. *B.* Anteroposterior chest radiograph the next day: larger left pneumothorax outlines lung edge *(arrows)*.

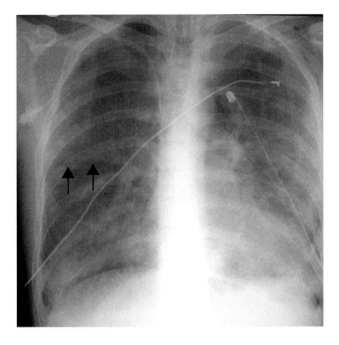

Figure 17.14 Supine right pneumothorax. Air tracks into minor fissure (*arrows*).

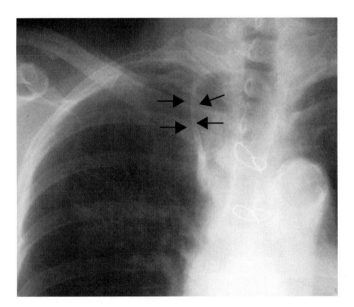

Figure 17.15 Right pneumothorax with air in azygos fissure (*arrows*).

Box 17.2: Causes of Pneumothorax

Ruptured bleb or bulla
Trauma (penetrating or with rib fracture)
Interstitial lung disease
Tuberculosis
Cavitary metastases (squamous, sarcomas)
Increased intrathoracic pressure

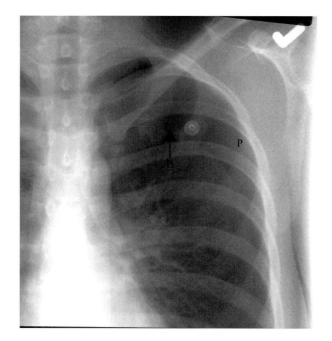

Figure 17.16 Ruptured bleb (B) outlined by resultant pneumothorax (P).

Pneumothorax can develop in any patient with chronic interstitial lung disease, but is particularly likely in males with eosinophilic granuloma and in females with lymphangiomyomatosis.

secondary to ruptured blebs (Fig. 17.16). The latter is the usual explanation for most spontaneous pneumothoraces and typically occurs in asthenic young males. Interstitial lung disease is another potential explanation for the development of pneumothorax. Any patient with honeycombing or lung cysts is at risk for the development of pneumothorax, but it is particularly likely in males with eosinophilic granuloma (Fig. 17.17) and in females with lymphangiomyomatosis.

In patients without interstitial lung disease, trauma, or ruptured blebs, there are other potential causes to consider, many with normal or nearly normal CXRs. Subpleural abnormalities that tend to cavitate are one group of causes, including tuberculosis and cavitary metastases. Overall, squamous primary neoplasms account for most cavitary metastases, but sarcomas actually have a higher predilection to cavitate (Fig. 17.18). Increased

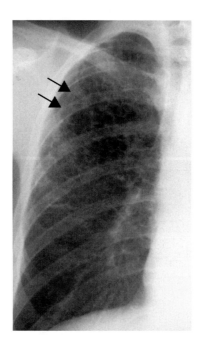

Figure 17.17 Eosinophilic granuloma with upper lobe honeycombing causing right apical pneumothorax. Lung edge outlined by *arrows*.

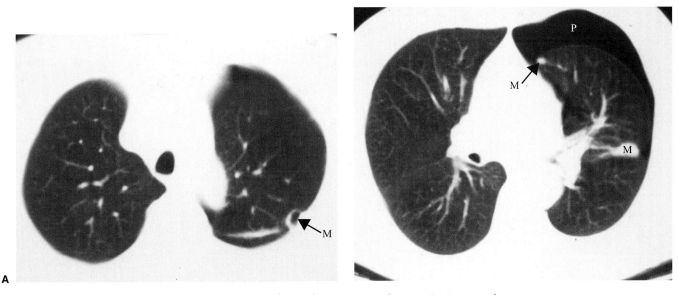

Figure 17.18 Cavitary metastatic osteosarcoma with resultant pneumothorax. *A.* Computed tomography of cavitary left upper lobe nodule (M). *B.* Computed tomography more caudal than *A:* other lung nodules (M) and moderate left pneumothorax (P).

intrathoracic pressure (such as in asthmatics and in pregnant patients) is another potential explanation for pneumothorax with an otherwise normal or nearly normal CXR. A rare cause is pleural endometriosis, which may explain cyclical pneumothoraces or hemothoraces. Knowledge of this rare entity may allow the enlightened visiting professor to score a major coup when presented with an unknown radiograph; sometimes things do not work out quite as well (Fig. 17.19).

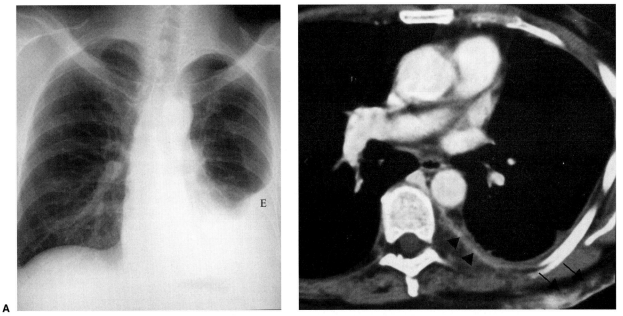

Figure 17.19 Cyclical hemothorax. Based on the history I immediately suggested pleural endometriosis. *A.* Posteroanterior chest radiograph: moderate left pleural effusion (E). *B.* Computed tomography: abnormal left posterior chest wall vessels (*arrows*) with pleural extension (*arrowheads*), indicating chest wall hemangioma as cause of hemothoraces.

Clinicians are frequently interested in knowing the percentage of the hemithorax occupied by a pneumothorax. It is hard to imagine that anyone can estimate such a percentage accurately. The chest is a complex three-dimensional structure, and many patients with suspected pneumothorax only have frontal radiographic evaluation. Instead, it is preferable to measure the displacement of the lung edge from the inner margin of the adjacent rib, often (but not always) at the lung apex. For persistent clinicians, a gestalt of small, moderate, or large pneumothorax may be helpful. Serial CXR assessment to determine whether pneumothorax is stable, resolving, or increasing is probably of even greater value.

PLEURAL IMPLANTS OR PLAQUES

CT is seldom necessary to demonstrate pleural fluid or air. Small amounts of fluid or air may be better detected by CT when positional views cannot be obtained, but this is an unusual circumstance. However, pleural implants or plaques are often far better seen with CT than on CXR. Rarely, the situation is reversed. In one memorable instance, a pleural

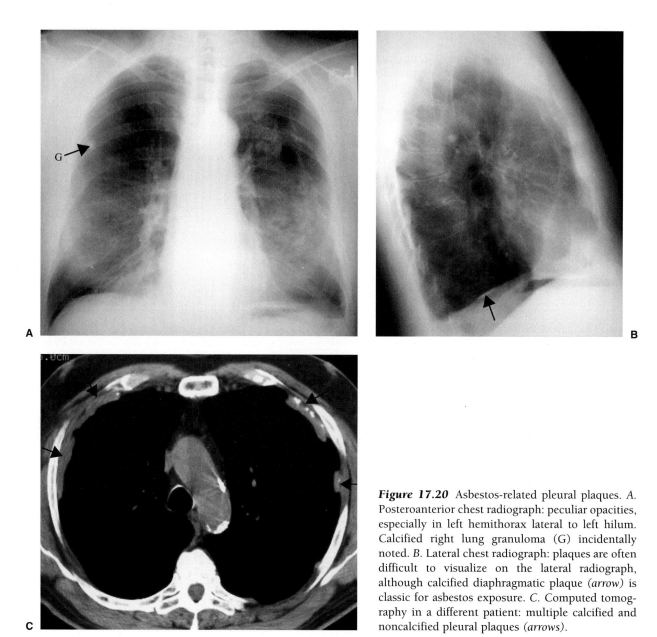

Figure 17.20 Asbestos-related pleural plaques. *A.* Posteroanterior chest radiograph: peculiar opacities, especially in left hemithorax lateral to left hilum. Calcified right lung granuloma (G) incidentally noted. *B.* Lateral chest radiograph: plaques are often difficult to visualize on the lateral radiograph, although calcified diaphragmatic plaque *(arrow)* is classic for asbestos exposure. *C.* Computed tomography in a different patient: multiple calcified and noncalcified pleural plaques *(arrows)*.

metastasis from malignant thymoma was questioned twice from CXRs and overlooked twice on resultant CTs. The pleural implant was finally seen by the interpreter of the patient's third CT, and it was also present in retrospect on the previous scans.

Pleural plaques are common in patients exposed to asbestos (Fig. 17.20). The skilled interpreter knows not to refer to this as asbestosis. Diagnosis of asbestosis implies the presence of interstitial lung disease; pleural plaques alone only indicate asbestos exposure. Plaques are usually bilateral and are sometimes visibly calcified. In fact, a very characteristic appearance of asbestos exposure is calcified plaques along the diaphragmatic pleura (Fig. 17.20B). Because many plaques are visualized *en face*, the resultant radiographic appearance is often that of irregularly shaped opacities that are poorly marginated. One of our pulmonologists who was a surprisingly skilled interpreter of chest radiographs used to say that the more bizarre the CXR appearance, the more likely it indicated pleural plaques.

Unilateral pleural plaques can also be seen with asbestos exposure. However, in this setting the alternative possibilities of old empyema and old hemothorax should be raised. Tuberculosis in particular may create a characteristic appearance of a small hemithorax with extensive pleural calcification, a so-called fibrothorax (Fig. 17.21).

The more bizarre the CXR appearance, the more likely it represents pleural disease, especially pleural plaques.

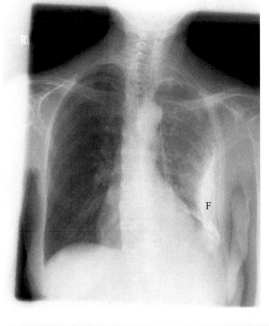

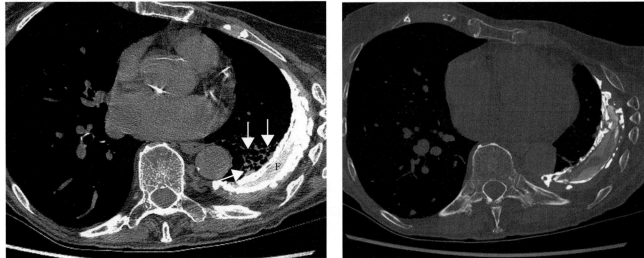

Figure 17.21 Fibrothorax resulting from tuberculosis. *A*. Posteroanterior chest radiograph: small left hemithorax with calcified pleural abnormality (F). *B*. Computed tomography viewed at soft tissue window settings: heavily calcified pleural abnormality (F) with adjacent left lung bronchiectasis (*arrows*). *C*. Bone window photography of *B*: better demonstration of internal composition of pleural abnormality.

Pleural implants may be seen with metastatic disease. More commonly, metastatic disease causes pleural effusion. However, even in that case CT may reveal soft tissue implants, suggesting the malignant nature of the effusion. Pleural hematoma may simulate the CT appearance of malignant effusion. Malignant thymoma often causes unilateral multifocal pleural implants, generally not associated with effusion.

An unusual cause of left pleural implants (except at the Radiological Society of North America [RSNA] film panel, where it is surprisingly common) is splenosis (Fig. 17.22). After left upper quadrant trauma, pieces of spleen may implant along the left pleural surface. In such a situation, surgical clips in the left upper quadrant and evidence of old left lower rib fractures constitute important diagnostic clues. Radionuclide scanning with damaged red blood cells may clinch the diagnosis.

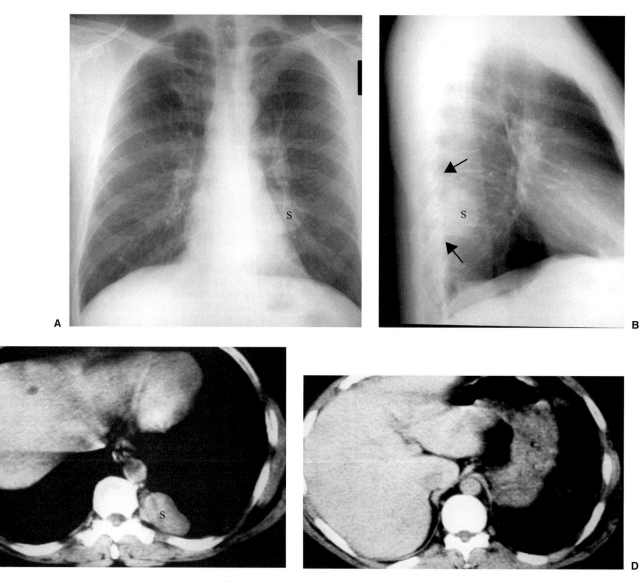

Figure 17.22 Thoracic splenosis. *A.* Posteroanterior chest radiograph: left infrahilar mass (S). *B.* Lateral chest radiograph: mass (S) is extraparenchymal, with right angles at the chest wall (*arrows*). *C.* Computed tomography: extraparenchymal shape of mass (S) confirmed. *D.* Computed tomography of upper abdomen: key additional finding is absence of spleen after trauma.

PLEURAL MASS(ES)

Many pleural masses are obscured on the CXR (and even at CT) by surrounding pleural effusion. CT is generally better able to distinguish solid elements of extensive pleural mass from effusion (Fig. 17.5), as in a typical malignant mesothelioma. However, not all pleural masses are accompanied by effusion.

Benign fibrous tumor of the pleura (previously known as benign mesothelioma) often presents as a single pleural mass. Tumor size runs the gamut from small to enormous. Lesions may be pedunculated, and as a consequence the tumor may change position in the thorax by twisting around the pedicle (Fig. 17.23). Even quite large benign fibrous tumors are generally distinct from malignant mesothelioma in their focal nature (malignant mesothelioma is typically relatively widespread in the pleura) and in the lack of associated pleural effusion. Clinical clues are sometimes also useful in diagnosing benign fibrous tumor. Lesions may present with associated hypertrophic pulmonary osteoarthropathy, and hypoglycemia is also sometimes associated with these tumors.

Benign fibrous tumors are generally easily recognized as pleural lesions by their shape. The situation is more confusing when a benign fibrous tumor occurs in a pleural fissure (6) (Fig. 17.24). In that circumstance the lesion will often appear to be round and will be sharply marginated on all sides. Such a lesion will appear to be a noncalcified lung nodule, in which case malignancy would be a significant concern. CT localization of the "nodule" to the pleural fissure makes benign fibrous tumor the overwhelmingly likely diagnosis.

Another benign etiology is pleural lipoma (Fig. 17.25). Intuitively, it would seem that a fatty lesion would obviously be less opaque on the CXR than a solid lesion. Except with enormous lesions, this turns out not to be true. Only at CT is the fatty nature of such a lesion usually evident.

Multiple pleural masses may reflect growth of any of the lesions described above in multiple implants. In addition, it may be very difficult to distinguish pleural from

> Benign fibrous tumor of pleura is generally easily recognizable as a pleural mass, but intrafissural fibrous tumors may closely simulate lung nodules.

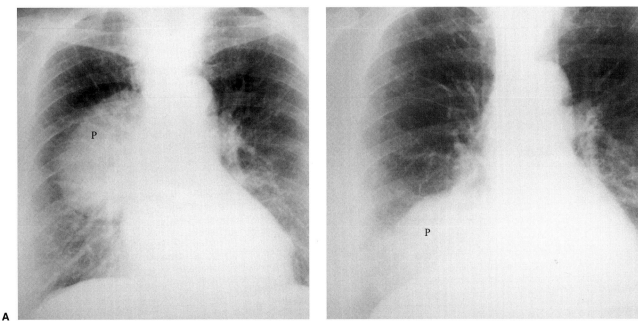

A   **B**

Figure 17.23 Mobile benign fibrous tumor of pleura. *A.* Posteroanterior chest radiograph in 1985: large mass (P) in upper right hemithorax. *B.* Posteroanterior chest radiograph in 1986: even larger mass (P) is now in lower right hemithorax. Lung torsion is another uncommon cause of thoracic lesions that change position. (Courtesy of Dr. Phil Templeton, Baltimore, MD.)

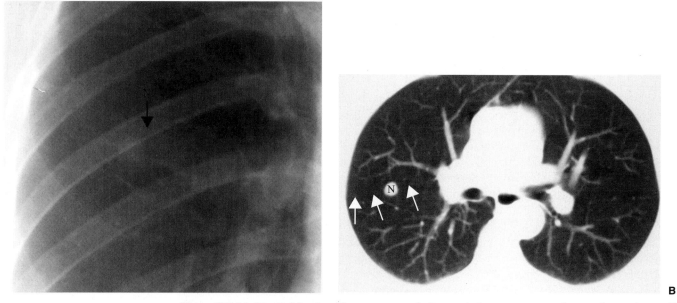

A   B

Figure 17.24 Fissural benign fibrous tumor of pleura. *A.* Posteroanterior chest radiograph: small right upper thoracic nodule (N). *B.* Computed tomography: lesion (N) appears to be round and smooth, suggesting that it is in the lung, but closer inspection shows that it is centered at the avascular plane of the major fissure *(arrows)*.

extrapleural masses (Box 17.3). A mass in either location often demonstrates sharp margination but only for part of its circumference (Figs. 17.26 and 17.27). The shape of the lesion is not always conclusive in the determination of its location. Demonstrable bone destruction indicates extrapleural masses, but otherwise they should be lumped together as extraparenchymal lesions. Common causes of extrapleural masses include metastatic disease, multiple myeloma, and trauma. This brief list is far from exhaustive (Fig. 17.28).

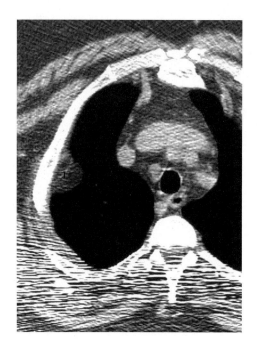

Figure 17.25 Pleural lipoma (L).

Box 17.3:. *Common Extrapleural Abnormalities*

Metastases
Multiple myeloma
Trauma
Fibrous dysplasia
Primary neoplasm (especially sarcoma)

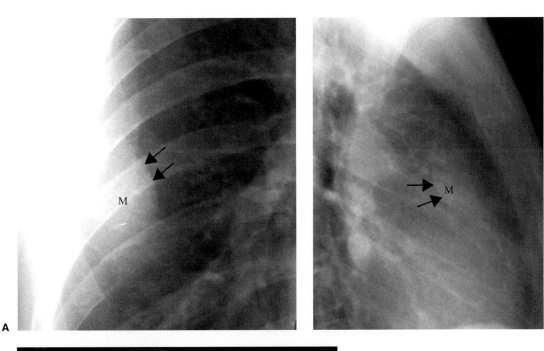

A

B

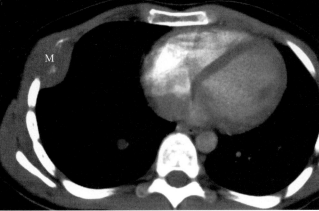

C

***Figure* 17.26** Extrapleural metastatic melanoma. *A.* Posteroanterior chest radiograph: mass (M) with sharp super-omedial border (*arrows*) that fades inferiorly. *B.* Lateral chest radiograph: mass (M) with sharp posterior border (*arrows*) but less distinct margin elsewhere. *C.* Computed tomography: lesion is a destructive rib metastasis (M).

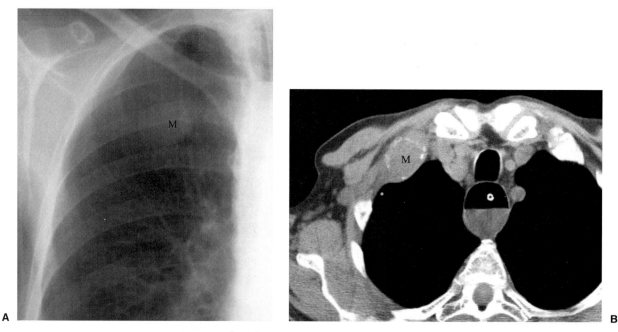

Figure 17.27 Extrapleural metastatic esophageal carcinoma. *A.* Posteroanterior chest radiograph: mass (M) with sharp inferior border but otherwise indistinct margins. *B.* Computed tomography: metastasis (M) to right first rib.

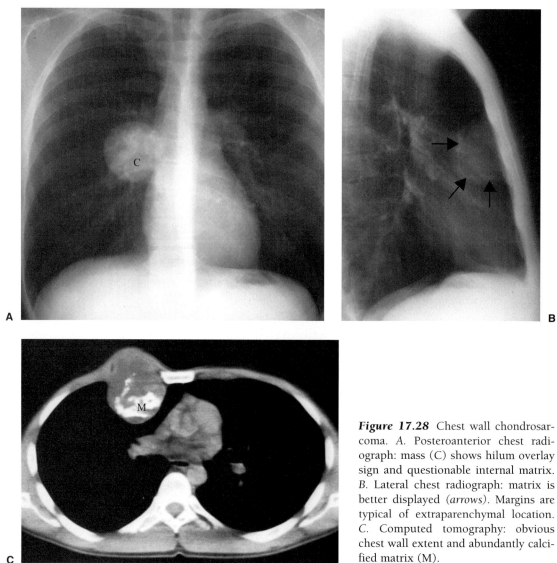

Figure 17.28 Chest wall chondrosarcoma. *A.* Posteroanterior chest radiograph: mass (C) shows hilum overlay sign and questionable internal matrix. *B.* Lateral chest radiograph: matrix is better displayed (*arrows*). Margins are typical of extraparenchymal location. *C.* Computed tomography: obvious chest wall extent and abundantly calcified matrix (M).

SELECTED TOPICS IN RADIOLOGY OF THE PLEURA AND CHEST WALL

CT has been used to image a wide variety of pleural and chest wall abnormalities. Because of its superior contrast resolution and the advantages of cross-sectional display of anatomy, it is quite clear that CT *can* image such lesions. The more important issue of whether CT *should* image various pleural and chest wall abnormalities is generally not addressed. In unselected cases CT makes little or no real contribution to the diagnostic workup. The CT appearance is often not specific for a given abnormality. Pleural abnormalities are often well seen on conventional radiographs (throughout this chapter) and are frequently diagnosed via thoracentesis or pleural biopsy. Chest wall abnormalities are often easily accessible to physical examination and, if necessary, biopsy.

In this section we discuss normal anatomy of the pleura and chest wall and address specific issues in pleural and chest wall CT. In particular, areas where CT is especially useful are highlighted, as well as those where it does not make a major contribution.

NORMAL ANATOMY AND ANATOMIC VARIANTS

Major, Minor, and Variant Fissures

CT identifies the major fissures with a frequency approaching 100%. Detection of the minor fissure is variable, ranging from 50% to 100% (7,8). More correctly, it is the parafissural lung that allows localization of the fissures with routine CT. Subpleural lung is composed primarily of secondary pulmonary lobules containing sparse and small-caliber vasculature. This relatively avascular lung is imaged at CT as a lucent band, which is the most common CT fissural appearance (Fig. 17.24B). When imaged perpendicular to the scan plane, the fissure is a thin line. Visualization as a line, which occurs more commonly on the left because that major fissure is more vertical, is frequent with thin section CT, where there is less volume averaging. Occasionally, the fissure appears as a dense band, probably because of partial volume effect or respiratory motion. A double fissure occurs with motion artifact, particularly cardiac motion at the left lung base.

The minor fissure is horizontal between the right upper and middle lobes, about 3 to 4 cm below the origin of bronchus intermedius. Given a parallel minor fissure and axial scanning plane, this fissure is seldom a line, even with thin section CT. Most often the minor fissure is a triangular avascular area, with its apex at the hilum. When the superior right middle lobe is convex, the superior minor fissure appears as a round or oval avascular zone. On scans through a convex superior middle lobe, lung anterior to the fissure is anterior segment of right upper lobe, and lung posterior to the fissure is superior segment of lower lobe. Bronchopulmonary segmental anatomy aids the differentiation of right upper and middle lobes. The upper lobe bronchi course lateral to their arteries, whereas the middle lobe bronchi course medial to their arteries (9). This relationship is constant even with volume loss.

Accessory fissures are more commonly visualized anatomically than radiographically. They can be demonstrated on CXR and CT. Most common are the superior and inferior accessory fissures. Other variants include azygos, hemiazygos, and left minor fissures.

The superior accessory fissure is between the superior segment of a lower lobe and the remaining lower lobe segments. It is more common on the right and is found in 5% to 30% of autopsy specimens (10). Because it is usually horizontal, the superior accessory fissure appears to be similar to minor fissure on frontal CXR, except that it is more caudal. On the lateral projection, this fissure extends posteriorly from the major fissure (Fig. 17.29). It was recognized by Proto and Speckman (11) in 6% of lateral radiographs. On CT, the superior accessory fissure is more caudal and posterior than the minor fissure. This appearance can be simulated by a horizontal major fissure, resulting from lower lobe volume loss (10). When slightly oblique, the superior accessory fissure can resemble the major fissure.

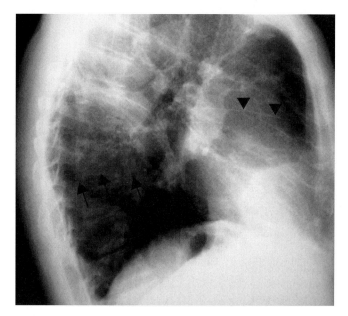

Figure 17.29 Superior accessory fissure (*arrows*) is posterior and caudal to minor fissure (*arrowheads*).

The inferior accessory fissure is present in 30%-50% of autopsy specimens, but is demonstrable radiographically in only 5%-10% of patients.

The inferior accessory fissure separates the medial basal segment from the remaining lower lobe basilar segments. It also occurs more commonly on the right. Although this fissure is present in 30% to 50% of autopsy specimens, it is radiographically demonstrable in only 5% to 10% of patients (10). The inferior accessory fissure appears on frontal and lateral radiographs as a thin vertical linear opacity that originates near the medial diaphragm, is posterior to the major fissure, and courses obliquely toward the hilum. The CT appearance depends on whether routine or thin sections are obtained, but when visible the fissure extends from the inferior pulmonary ligament to the major fissure (10).

A left minor fissure, which is found in 8% to 18% of anatomic specimens, separates the lingula from the remaining left upper lobe (12). Radiographs demonstrate the left minor fissure in less than 2% of patients (Fig. 17.30). Its CT appearance is analogous to the right minor fissure, although it occasionally occurs more cephalad (11).

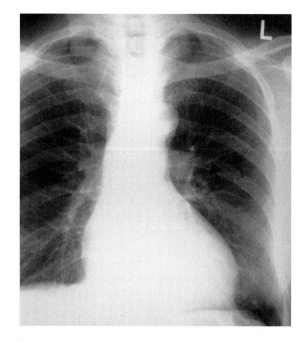

Figure 17.30 Left minor fissure (*arrows*).

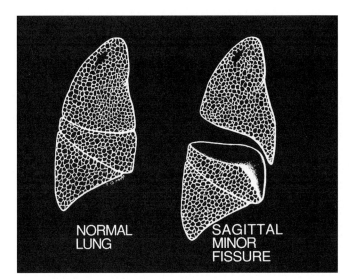

Figure 17.31 Drawing of typical and sagittal minor fissures. (From Gross BH, Spizarny DL, Granke DS. Sagittal orientation of the anterior minor fissure: radiography and computed tomography. *Radiology* 1988; 166:717–719, with permission.)

The azygos fissure is formed by four layers of pleura invaginating into the lung apex and extending to a laterally displaced azygos vein. It occurs in 1% of anatomic specimens and is demonstrated radiographically (Fig. 17.15) in 0.5% of patients (13). Almost all cases occur on the right, with a few reports of left hemiazygos fissures connecting to left superior intercostal vein. Given its vertical orientation, this fissure is often recognized on CT as an arcuate linear opacity extending from the posterolateral aspect of an upper thoracic vertebral body to the superior vena cava or right brachiocephalic vein. A nodular posterior azygos fissure can occur secondary to an intraparenchymal azygos vein.

A sagittal anterior minor fissure is a normal variant that can result in misleading appearances of right upper and middle lobe disease (14). Occurring as an oblique vertical linear opacity in the inferomedial right lung, the sagittal minor fissure results in inferomedial extension of right upper lobe (Fig. 17.31). As a result, the anterior segment of upper lobe occupies a paracardiac location and can border the diaphragm (14). Right upper lobe disease with a sagittal minor fissure can silhouette the heart (Fig. 17.32), whereas medial segment right middle lobe disease can spare the cardiac border. In either event, erroneous localization of disease may occur.

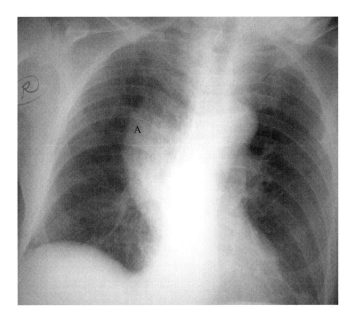

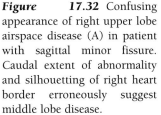

Figure 17.32 Confusing appearance of right upper lobe airspace disease (A) in patient with sagittal minor fissure. Caudal extent of abnormality and silhouetting of right heart border erroneously suggest middle lobe disease.

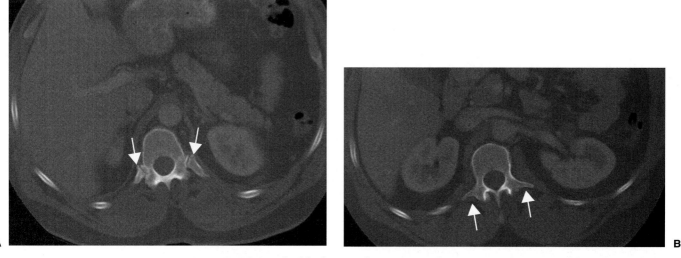

Figure 17.33 Vertebral body types for counting ribs. *A.* Lowest thoracic vertebra, characterized by medial ribs *(arrows)*. *B.* Highest lumbar vertebra, with transverse processes *(arrows)* rather than ribs.

Counting Ribs

Counting ribs (15) seems like a trivial subject until a CT is presented for evaluation of a bone scan abnormality of the eighth rib in a patient with normal rib radiographs. The value of precise anatomic localization of that rib becomes readily apparent. A step-by-step approach is as follows:

Step 1: The first rib is located on image with mid-clavicles.
Step 2: The next two or three ribs are counted on same slice.
Step 3: Progressively lower ribs are located at the costovertebral junctions.
Step 4: With bilateral lesions, each side is counted separately.

For lesions in the lower ribs, an alternative is to find the first lumbar-type vertebra (Fig. 17.33) and then count upward at the costovertebral junctions.

ISSUES IN PLEURAL AND CHEST WALL COMPUTED TOMOGRAPHY

Chest Wall Invasion in Lung Cancer

CT evaluation of chest wall invasion by lung masses is not very accurate. CT in 33 patients with peripheral pulmonary malignancies contiguous with a pleural surface was reviewed for useful signs in diagnosing chest wall invasion (16). Criteria that were evaluated included pleural thickening adjacent to the tumor, encroached upon or high attenuation extrapleural fat, asymmetric extrapleural soft tissues, apparent mass invading chest wall, and rib destruction. Individual CT criteria were either very sensitive but not specific (local pleural thickening) or very specific but not sensitive (all other criteria). Overall sensitivity was 38%, with a specificity of 40%. In one series (17), focal chest pain was much more specific than any CT signs. Magnetic resonance imaging may be more accurate than CT (18).

It should be noted that preoperative staging of chest wall involvement in lung cancer is not as important as assessment of mediastinal involvement. Local chest wall invasion does not contraindicate surgical resection, although it does necessitate *en bloc* resection of the contiguous chest wall. In light of the high morbidity of this procedure, we suggest chest wall invasion whenever we see local pleural thickening, thereby alerting the surgeon that *en bloc* resection may be necessary.

> CT evaluation of chest wall invasion by lung masses is not very accurate; focal chest pain may be more specific than any CT signs.

Lung Cancer Crossing Fissures

The double layer of fissural pleura creates a barrier to the spread of inflammation and neoplasm. This is especially true when lobar separation by fissures is complete. However, anatomic studies demonstrate fusion across part of right major fissure in approximately 70% of specimens, across minor fissure in more than 90% of specimens, and across left major fissure in 40% to 50% of specimens (19). Lobar fusion allows for disease spread that would otherwise be confined to one lobe or segment. When non-neoplastic disease crosses an intact fissure, it is commonly an atypical infection. Actinomycosis is especially likely to ignore anatomic barriers (Fig. 17.34), but blastomycosis, nocardiosis, and other fungal infections are also possible. Neoplasm is less likely to cross an intact fissure, but lymphoma has a predilection for crossing anatomic barriers (20).

In lung cancer patients who are candidates for lobectomy, extension of neoplasm anywhere across the left major fissure or across the right major fissure cephalad to the minor fissure necessitates pneumonectomy. CT assessment of transfissural crossing is up to 100% specific when correlated with pathologic findings but only 50% sensitive when standard scanning is performed (21). Thin section CT probably increases sensitivity.

Thin section CT scanning increases sensitivity for detecting extension of lung cancer across fissures, a finding that requires more extensive surgery if curative resection is attempted.

Malignant Effusion and Mesothelioma

The CT findings of malignant mesothelioma are well known. The typical diffuse, multifocal, irregular pleural mass is generally also well demonstrated by CXR. Final diagnosis typically requires biopsy of the lesion. Therefore, CT is not crucial for diagnosis in most patients. As for staging, the prognosis remains so poor for patients with malignant mesothelioma and for those with pleural metastases that the usefulness of CT staging remains doubtful. In fact, extent of pleural mesothelioma may be underestimated at CT because portions of tumor may be difficult to distinguish from pleural effusion.

Miscellaneous

Clinicians will often request chest CT in patients with a large pleural effusion of unknown etiology. CT is unfortunately as limited in value as CXR in this setting. Although clinicians believe that CT will better evaluate the compressed underlying lung for lung cancer, this is seldom true. Clinicians occasionally offer to perform thoracentesis to improve the yield

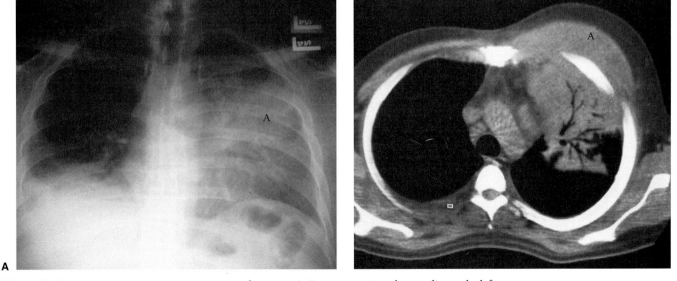

Figure 17.34 Actinomycosis crossing anatomic barriers. *A.* Posteroanterior chest radiograph: left upper lobe airspace disease (A) silhouettes left heart border. *B.* Computed tomography: gross extension of abnormality into left anterior chest wall (A), with underlying air bronchograms.

of CT; they should be reminded that CXR after thoracentesis may be more than enough for diagnostic purposes.

The important bottom line in this setting, as in many others, is how this study will change the patient's workup and management. In many circumstances it is clear that the proposed study (often CT) is superfluous. If that is the case, an alternative approach should be considered.

It is still possible (and preferable) to conclude on a positive note. Pleural abnormality is sometimes responsible for unusual radiographic appearances. CXR alone may be confusing in some such patients. In that setting, CT often renders a final diagnosis (or at least explains the reason for CXR confusion) with startling clarity. It is a helpful problem-solving tool in appropriately selected patients, even in occasional patients with findings that do not typically necessitate CT.

REFERENCES

1. Felson B. *Chest roentgenology*. Philadelphia: WB Saunders, 1973.
2. Alexander ES, Proto AV, Clark RA. CT differentiation of subphrenic abscess and pleural effusion. *AJR Am J Roentgenol* 1983;140:47–51.
3. Stark DD, Federle MP, Goodman PC, et al. Differentiating lung abscess and empyema: radiography and computed tomography. *AJR Am J Roentgenol* 1983;141:163–167.
4. Sheffner SE, Gross BH, Birnberg FA, et al. Iatrogenic bronchopleural fistula caused by feeding tube insertion. *J Can Assoc Radiol* 1985;36:52–55.
5. Carr JJ, Reed JC, Choplin RH, et al. Plain and computed radiography for detecting experimentally induced pneumothorax in cadavers: implications for detection in patients. *Radiology* 1992;183:193–199.
6. Spizarny DL, Gross BH, Shepard JO. CT findings in localized fibrous mesothelioma of the pleural fissure. *J Comput Assist Tomogr* 1986;10:942–944.
7. Frija J, Schmit P, Katz M, et al. Computed tomography of the pulmonary fissures: normal anatomy. *J Comput Assist Tomogr* 1982;6:1069–1074.
8. Proto AV, Ball JB. Computed tomography of the major and minor fissures. *AJR Am J Roentgenol* 1983;140:439–448.
9. Otsuji H, Hatakeyama M, Kitamura I. Right upper lobe versus right middle lobe. Differentiation with thin-section, high-resolution CT. *Radiology* 1989;172:653–656.
10. Godwin JD, Tarver RD. Accessory fissures of the lung. *AJR Am J Roentgenol* 1985;144:39–47.
11. Proto AV, Speckman JM. The left lateral radiograph of the chest. *Med Radiogr Photogr* 1979;55:30–74.
12. Austin JH. The left minor fissure. *Radiology* 1986;161:433–436.
13. Speckman JM, Gamsu G, Webb WR. Alterations in CT mediastinal anatomy produced by an azygous lobe. *AJR Am J Roentgenol* 1981;137:47–50.
14. Gross BH, Spizarny DL, Granke DS. Sagittal orientation of the anterior minor fissure: radiography and CT. *Radiology* 1988;166:717–719.
15. Bhalla M, McCauley DI, Golimbu C, et al. Counting ribs on chest CT. *J Comput Assist Tomogr* 1990;14:590–594.
16. Pennes DR, Glazer GM, Wimbish KJ, et al. Chest wall invasion by lung cancer: limitations of CT evaluation. *AJR Am J Roentgenol* 1985;144:507–511.
17. Glazer HS, Duncan-Meyer J, Aronberg DJ, et al. Pleural and chest wall invasion in bronchogenic carcinoma: CT evaluation. *Radiology* 1985;157:191–194.
18. Haggar AM, Pearlberg JL, Froelich JW, et al. Chest-wall invasion by carcinoma of the lung: detection by MR imaging. *AJR Am J Roentgenol* 1987;148:1075–1078.
19. Raasch BN, Carsky EW, Lane EJ. Radiographic anatomy of the interlobar fissures: a study of 100 specimens. *AJR Am J Roentgenol* 1982;138:1043–1049.
20. Shuman LS, Libshitz HI. Solid pleural manifestations of lymphoma. *AJR Am J Roentgenol* 1984;142:269–273.
21. Quint LE, Glazer GM, Orringer MB. Central lung masses: prediction with CT of need for pneumonectomy versus lobectomy. *Radiology* 1987;165:735–738.

THE THORACIC AORTA

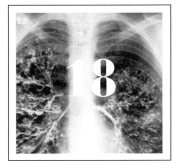

■ Aortic Dissection
■ Intramural Hematoma
■ Penetrating Atherosclerotic Ulcer
■ Coarctation
■ Pseudocoarctation
■ Aortic Aneurysm
■ The Repaired Aorta

Many articles and books have been written about the aorta. However, there is still confusion regarding the aorta and aortic diseases among radiologists. Specifically, confusion exists regarding the various terms used to describe acquired aortic diseases, progression of disease, and the postoperative aortic imaging features. In this chapter we discuss the congenital aorta, coarctation, and pseudocoarctation. Acquired aortic diseases are discussed, such as aortic dissection, intramural hematoma, penetrating ulcers, aneurysms, and rare tumors. Finally, the imaging features of the aorta after surgical intervention are described. The goal of this chapter is to clarify the terminology and provide a better understanding of the aorta and the diseases that affect it.

AORTIC DISSECTION

Acute aortic dissection is the most dramatic and common thoracic aortic emergency. Untreated dissections have a mortality of 36% to 72% within the first 48 hours and 62% to 91% within the first week. Dissections are classified as acute if the diagnosis occurs within 2 weeks or less of the first symptoms. Dissections detected after 2 weeks are classified as chronic. Acute aortic dissection usually occurs in patients between the ages of 30 and 85 years, with a peak incidence in the sixth and seventh decades of life. It is more common in men than women, at a ratio of 3:1 (1,2).

There are many conditions that increase a patient's risk of aortic dissection, as described in Table 18.1. These include systemic hypertension (90%) and connective tissue disorders such as Marfan syndrome, cystic medial necrosis, Ehlers-Danlos syndrome, and Turner syndrome. Aortic dissection noted in women younger than 40 years old is often associated with pregnancy. Congenital cardiovascular diseases, such as aortic stenosis, bicuspid aortic valve, and aortic isthmic coarctation, are all risk factors. Aortic dissection can also be induced by trauma, either blunt or iatrogenic during aortic cannulation or bypass surgery. A history of aortic surgery also increases the risk of subsequent dissection.

PRESENTING SYMPTOMS

The classic clinical presentation of aortic dissection is the acute onset of severe tearing or ripping substernal chest pain with radiation to the back. This occurs in up to 70% of patients. Aortic valvular murmur due to creation of aortic valve insufficiency occurs in up to 65% of patients. Asymmetric pulses, as well as absent femoral pulses (25%), may occur in the upper extremities if the aortic arch is involved. Unfortunately, 15% to 20% of

The classic presentation of aortic dissection is acute tearing substernal pain radiating to the back. However, atypical presentations are common and often result in delayed diagnosis.

Table 18.1: Risk Factors for Aortic Dissection

Hypertension	Aortic stenosis
Marfan syndrome	Bicuspid aortic valve
Ehlers-Danlos syndrome	Aortic coarctation
Cystic medial necrosis	Trauma
Pregnancy	Prior aortic surgery
Turner syndrome	

patients have no chest pain, making the diagnosis difficult. These patients usually present with symptoms related to secondary involvement of aortic branch vessels. Such presentations include myocardial infarction and congestive heart failure, abdominal pain due to mesenteric ischemia, stroke, confusion, coma, or syncope with involvement of the cranial or spinal arteries (25%) (1).

PATHOGENESIS

All aortic dissections have blood (hematoma) within the media of the aortic wall.

Aortic dissection is a tear of the aortic wall intima, followed by separation of the tunica media, thereby creating two channels for passage of blood. The true lumen is surrounded by intima, and the false lumen is surrounded by media. This is seen in approximately 70% of cases. The tear in the intima allows blood to enter the aortic wall and extend longitudinally along the wall, thus separating the media and forming true and false lumens. The entry point most commonly arises in the ascending aorta within several centimeters of the aortic root or in the descending aorta between the origin of the left subclavian artery and ligamentum arteriosum. Iatrogenically induced aortic dissections arise at sites of aortic cannulation, bypass grafting and cross-clamping, or during catheterization.

The exact etiology of dissection is still debated. The entry tear may come first, leading to hematoma in the aortic wall, or may arise after the hematoma has already developed. In some cases a tear is never found.

CLASSIFICATION

There are two widely used systems for the classification of aortic dissections: the Stanford classification and the DeBakey classification.

Stanford Classification

Stanford type A dissections involve the ascending aorta. Stanford type B do not.

Stanford A dissections involve the ascending aorta, regardless of the site of tear or distal extent. These dissections usually begin approximately 2 cm cephalad to the sinotubular junction. These comprise approximately 60% of all aortic dissections. Stanford B dissections involve only the descending aorta distal to the left subclavian artery and comprise approximately 40% of all dissections (3).

DeBakey Classification

DeBakey type I dissections involve ascending and descending thoracic aorta. Type II involves only the ascending aorta and type III, only the descending aorta.

A DeBakey I dissection involves both the ascending and descending aorta. DeBakey II involves only the ascending aorta, and DeBakey III involves only the descending aorta distal to the left subclavian artery. These occur as 30%, 20%, and 50% of dissections, respectively (4).

Ascending aortic dissection is a surgical emergency, because rupture into the pericardium, aortic valve failure, and coronary artery involvement are causes of mortality.

Dissections involving the ascending aorta are treated emergently and surgically because of the high mortality if not treated. Complications if untreated include acute aortic insufficiency in approximately 90% of patients due to destruction of aortic valve, acute heart failure, occlusion of coronary or supraortic branch vessels, rupture into the pleural space, or rupture into the pericardium with acute cardiac tamponade (1). Dissections involving only the descending aorta are associated with a lower complication rate and are treated medically when possible. However, risk of descending thoracic aorta ruptures increases at a greater than 6 cm diameter. This is accompanied by altered branch vessel perfusion or occlusion or pseudocoarctation syndrome with uncontrollable hypertension;

surgical intervention or therapeutic percutaneous stent grafting is required (1,5). Branch vessel occlusions, such as hepatic, mesenteric, or renal artery involvement, are associated with increased morbidity and mortality.

IMAGING

The methods used for the diagnosis of aortic dissection include catheter aortography (the traditional gold standard) and bedside transesophageal echocardiography. More commonly, noninvasive techniques, such as computed tomography (CT) and magnetic resonance imaging (MRI), are used both to establish the diagnosis of dissection and to evaluate the extent of dissection in the aorta and branch vessels.

Chest radiographs are the most commonly used radiologic examination in all acute thoracic conditions. Although findings can indicate the presence of aortic dissection (Table 18.2), a normal chest radiograph does not exclude the presence of an aortic dissection (Fig. 18.1).

> A normal chest radiograph does not exclude the diagnosis of aortic dissection.

CT is probably the most commonly used radiologic examination to diagnose and evaluate aortic dissection. Often, the extent is sufficiently well presented as to avert the need for catheter angiography before surgery and to plan for aortic stent grafting. Fast helical CT scanners accurately and consistently display the aorta and branch vessels (Fig. 18.1), and advanced multiplanar and three-dimensional reconstructions are important to do this. The CT findings of aortic dissection are listed in Table 18.3. The most characteristic finding is the intimal flap. The typical configuration of the flap is a linear filling defect within the aorta. The intimal flap may also have an atypical configuration: dissection of the entire intima creates a circumferential intimal flap, filiform (extremely narrow) true lumen, a three-channel aorta (Mercedes-Benz sign), and several false channels (Fig. 18.2). The dissection flap is more likely to be curved in an acute dissection and flat in a chronic dissection. CT findings that indicate a ruptured type B dissection include irregularity of the aortic wall, extravasation of vascular contrast material, mediastinal or pericardial hematoma, and hemothorax (1) (Fig.18.3).

> Helical CT with multiplanar reconstructions and magnetic resonance angiography are used for both diagnosis of dissection and surgical or stent-graft planning.

Once the diagnosis of aortic dissection is made, the key information needed by the surgeon is the extent of the dissection and whether branch vessels originate from the true lumen or false lumen. Key features that can be used to distinguish between the true and false lumens are listed in Table 18.4 (Fig. 18.4) (6,7).

> The false lumen is often larger than the true lumen, contains cobwebs (strands of media), and is filled with blood that may have slow flow or be thrombosed.

A limitation of CT is the use of intravenous contrast, for which some patients are known to be allergic and which must be avoided in other patients with acute renal failure secondary to dissection or preexisting renal insufficiency. In such settings, MRI is recommended (Table 18.5).

> The true lumen gives rise to the coronary arteries and aortic valve and may be surrounded by intimal calcification.

MRI features are similar to those seen on CT. The intensity of signaling of the false lumen is variable and dependent on the blood flow, as well as the age and composition of thrombus. Standard MRI techniques demonstrate pleural and pericardial effusions, mediastinal hemorrhage, and aortic wall thickening (Fig. 18.5).

Table 18.2: Chest Radiograph Findings of Aortic Dissection

Widening of the mediastinum
Diffuse enlargement of aorta ± irregular contour
Progressive aortic enlargement on serial examinations
Change in arch configuration on serial examinations
Inward displacement of intimal classification by ≥ 6 mm
Double aortic contour
Tracheal displacement to the right
Pleural effusion (especially on the left)
Pericardial effusion

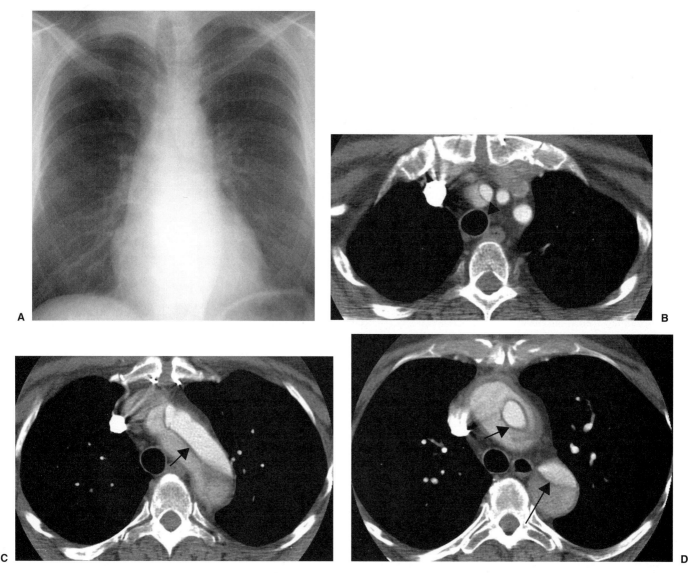

Figure 18.1 Stanford type A aortic dissection. *A.* Chest radiograph demonstrates abnormal aortic contour. *B–D.* Axial computed tomographies demonstrate perfusion of the true and false lumens with slower flow in the false lumen. *B.* Extension of dissection into right brachiocephalic artery (*arrowhead*) and into the aortic arch (*C*) (*arrow*). *D.* Dissection flap in ascending aorta (*small arrow*). Dissection flap in descending aorta (*long arrow*).

Table 18.3: Computed Tomographic Findings of Aortic Dissection

Intimal flap (approximately 70%)
Inward displacement of intimal calcifications
Hyperattenuating intima
Increased aortic diameter
Delayed enhancement of false lumen
Increased attenuation of acutely thrombosed false lumen (noncontrast computed tomography)
Mediastinal, pleural, or pericardial hematoma
Enlargement of the false lumen with compression of true lumen

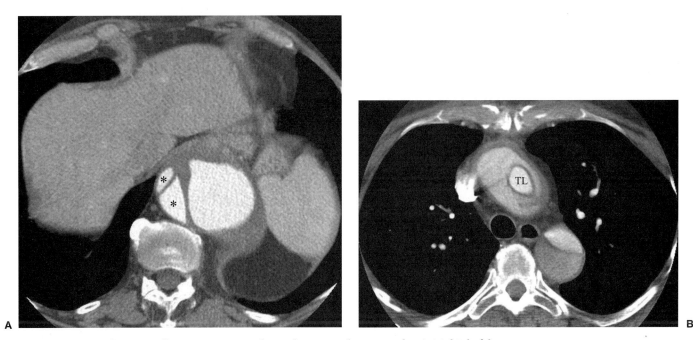

Figure 18.2 Aortic dissection flaps on contrast enhanced computed tomography. *A.* Multiple false lumens *(asterisks)*. *B.* Circumferential intimal flap in the ascending thoracic aorta. *TL,* true lumen.

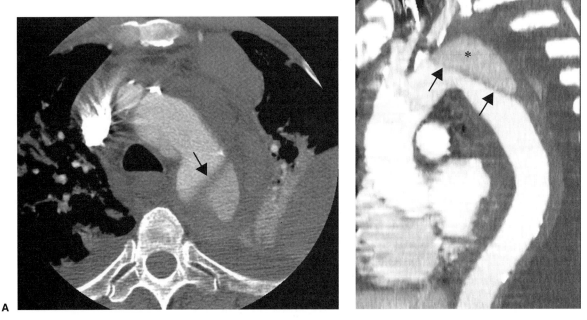

Figure 18.3 Stanford type B aortic dissection with ruptured false lumen. *A.* Contrast enhanced axial computed tomography demonstrates intimal flap *(arrow)* within the descending aorta. Note extensive hemomediastinum and bilateral pleural effusions. *B.* Oblique sagittal reconstruction demonstrates intimal flap *(arrows)* and false lumen *(asterisk)*.

Table 18.4: Features to Distinguish True and False Lumens on Computed Tomography

Acute Dissection
- True lumen
  - Surrounded by intimal calcification
  - Eccentric flap calcification
  - Continuous with undissected portion of aorta
  - In cases in the aortic arch with one lumen wrapping around the other, the inner lumen is the true lumen
- False lumen
  - Presence of cobwebs that are band or cords of media that bridge the junction of the dissection flap with the outer wall of the false lumen
  - Larger cross-sectional area than the true lumen
  - Presence of the break sign, which is an acute angle between the dissection flap and outer wall
  - Filled with contrast-enhanced slowly flowing blood or hematoma

Chronic dissection
- True lumen
  - Eccentric flap calcification
- False lumen
  - Outer wall calcification
  - Intraluminal thrombus within false lumen (Fig. 18.4)

Table 18.5: MR Imaging Findings of Aortic Dissection

Intimal flap.
Variable false lumen signal.
Intimal calcification is usually not seen. However, at times an intimal flap is seen as an intervening stripe of soft tissue signal intensity.
Signal flow voids in true lumen and false lumen depending on luminal flow rate (spin-echo MR).

MR, magnetic resonance.

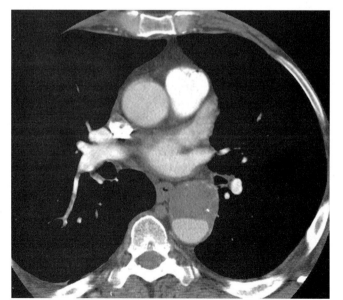

Figure 18.4 Chronic Stanford type B aortic dissection on axial computed tomography with calcification along the peripheral (outer wall) of the thrombosed false lumen.

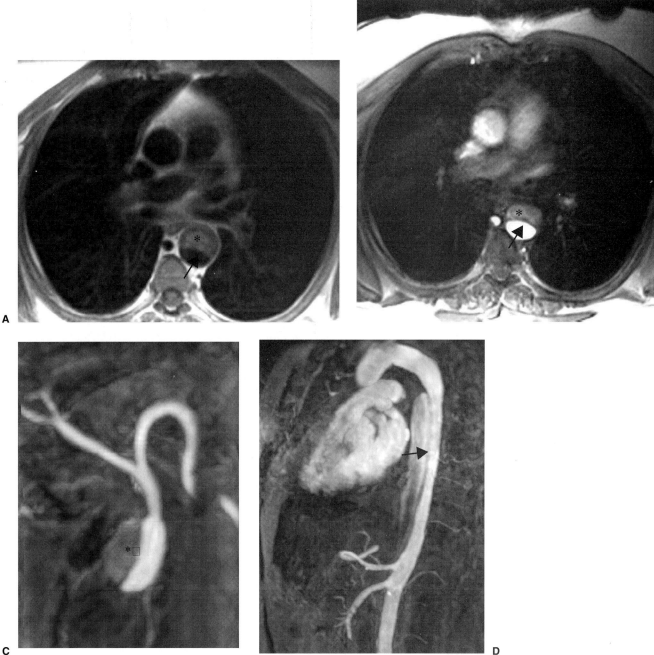

Figure 18.5 Stanford type B acute aortic dissection. *A.* Axial T1-weighted inversion recovery, *(B)* axial reconstruction three-dimensional gadolinium-enhanced magnetic resonance imaging, *(C)* coronal reconstruction from subvolume MIP gadolinium-enhanced magnetic resonance imaging of the aortic arch, and *(D)* sagittal three-dimensional gadolinium magnetic resonance imaging. Aortic dissection with intimal flap in descending aorta *(arrow)* and thrombosed false lumen. *Asterisk,* false lumen.

AORTOGRAPHY

At aortography dissection appears as an intimal flap or multiple lumens, with opacification of double channels. Linear radial lucency may be seen secondary to the torn or separated intima, with entry and reentry points. Additional findings include a true lumen compressed by the false lumen, a thick aortic wall greater than 5 mm, ulcer-like contrast projections beyond the true lumen, abnormal catheter position away from the lateral aortic border, and arterial branch occlusion.

A thin thrombosed false lumen can result in a normal-appearing aortogram.

Transesophageal Echocardiography

Acutely, transesophageal echocardiography can be used for diagnosis at the bedside but is insufficient for surgical planning.

This method can image the entire thoracic aorta, with the exception of the distal transverse arch that is partially obscured by the trachea. Transesophageal echocardiography has the advantage of being performed at the bedside in acutely ill or unstable patients. At transesophageal echocardiography, dissection appears as a mobile linear echo within the aortic lumen. Transesophageal echocardiography also provides information regarding ventricular and aortic valve function, both important in surgical decision making.

Management

Aortic dissection that involves branch vessels and compromises blood flow is treated based on the mechanism of occlusion. When the dissection flap extends into the lumen of the branch vessel and statically narrows it, treatment is usually angioplasty, with or without the deployment of an intravascular stent. When the dissection flap does not enter the branch vessel but dynamically occludes the vessel by prolapse of the intimal flap into the vessel origin, this obstructs the true lumen above the branch vessel origin and is usually treated with balloon fenestration of the dissection flap, intraaortic endoluminal stent in the true lumen, or both. Additionally, the compressed true lumen may be enlarged, by using an uncovered intraaortic stent (5,8).

Surgical treatment of type A dissection consist of replacing the ascending aorta, aortic root, and aortic valve, reconstructing the aortic root to restore aortic valve competence, and directing blood flow to the true lumen. The coronary arteries are reimplanted into the graft. Mortality rates for surgical treatment range from 10% to 35% (9). Type B dissections are usually treated medically with aggressive antihypertensive control and pain control. For type B dissections treated surgically, a graft is usually placed in the proximal descending thoracic aorta. Early postoperative complications of dissection include myocardial infarction, stroke, respiratory insufficiency, pulmonary embolism, aortic rupture, pseudoaneurysm, and graft infection. Late complications are noted 10 years or more after surgery in 15% to 30% of patients and require reoperation for dilatation of the dissected region to avoid rupture. Reoperation may be required for progressive reduction of myocardial perfusion due to aortic insufficiency (1).

Aortic Dissection Follow-Up

After the diagnosis or repair of an aortic dissection, follow-up imaging is usually performed annually. Complications that may be noted include an aneurysm of the false lumen, with continuous dilatation of the aorta that may result in aortic rupture. An aneurysm of the true lumen may develop, particularly in older hypertensive patients with advanced atherosclerosis. Obstruction or aneurysm of aortic branch vessels may also occur. Postoperatively, pseudoaneurysms may develop at the anastomosis of the graft to the native aorta, further weakening the aorta and usually requiring additional surgery.

Intramural Hematoma

Intramural hematoma was first described by Krutenberg in 1920 as bleeding into the outer layers of the aortic media due to rupture of the vasa vasorum without primary intimal tear, leading to subintimal hemorrhage (10). Intramural hematoma is a variant of aortic dissection, characterized by the absence of both the intimal tear and the direct flow communication between the true and false lumens. It has been postulated that a proximal intramural hematoma may be a precursor or early stage of classic aortic dissection. Acute intramural hematoma has a mortality of 21% (10). Intramural hematoma may progress to a classic aortic dissection, with rupture rates ranging from 32% to 40% for intramural hematoma confined to the descending aorta and 50% to 100% when it involves the ascending aorta. Hence, emergent surgical repair is usually recommended for intramural hematoma involving the ascending aorta.

Successful patient outcome with medical therapy has been shown similar to the treatment of type B classic aortic dissection. These patients can be frequently followed with annual noninvasive imaging studies, either CT or MRI. Surgery is performed if a classic aortic dissection or aortic rupture develops (11,12).

CLINICAL PRESENTATION

Initial presenting symptoms include chest pain (50% to 74%), intrascapular back pain (44% to 84%), and neurologic or vascular complications such as syncope, transient ischemic attack, hoarse voice, paraplegia, mesenteric ischemia, and acute renal failure (13). Patients are usually older than those with classic aortic dissection, with a mean age of 66 years versus 55 years for classic aortic dissection. There is an equal male-to-female ratio for intramural hematoma, compared with the 3:1 ratio for classic aortic dissection. Risk factors for intramural hematoma include hypertension or previous trauma.

IMAGING

Intramural hematoma can be diagnosed by CT, MRI, and transesophageal echocardiography. At aortography, it may not be detected due to the inability to opacify a false lumen with contrast in the absence of an entrance tear. This often occurs when the intramural hematoma is thin and does not deform the true lumen.

On nonintravenous contrast-enhanced CT, a continuous high attenuation crescent along the aortic wall representing hematoma is usually found without mass effect on the true lumen (Fig. 18.6). As in classic dissection, internally displaced intimal calcification may be seen. At intravenous contrast-enhanced CT, the crescentic area along the aortic wall appears as low attenuation thrombus. There is no intimal flap. The intramural hematoma usually maintains a constant circumferential relationship with the aortic wall. Associated features include pericardial effusion, hemothorax, pleural effusion, and hemomediastinum. Distinguishing an intramural hematoma from classic aortic dissection with a thrombosed false lumen is still problematic.

At MRI, focal crescentic wall thickening, without mass effect on the aortic lumen and an absence of intimal flap, is seen. In reference to true spin echo (SE) sequences, the signal characteristics of the intramural hematoma depend on the age of the hematoma. If acute, it appears high signal on T2-weighted images and isointense or hypointense to muscle on T1-weighted images due to oxyhemoglobin. When subacute, it is high signal on both T1- and T2-weighted images due to methemoglobin. When chronic, it appears low signal on T1- and T2-weighted images due to organization of the blood (14). At transesophageal echocardiography, intramural hematoma appears as localized circular or crescentic thickening of the aortic wall, greater than or equal to 5 mm, and again, no intimal tear is seen.

Acute intramural hematoma is a aortic dissection with no entry tear and appears as a thrombosed false lumen.

MANAGEMENT

Treatment consists of intensive care unit monitoring, aggressive medical treatment with antihypertensive therapy, and frequent serial follow-up noninvasive imaging studies. Surgery is performed in patients with coexistent aneurysmal dilatation or when the intramural hematoma progresses on serial studies. Evaluation of intramural hematoma on serial noninvasive imaging has shown that intramural hematomas may decrease in size and partially or completely resolve, particularly if the aortic diameter is less than 5 cm (12,15). Sometimes ulcer-like projections into the intramural hematoma develop, which can progress to saccular aneurysm. Fusiform aneurysms without ulcer-like projections and even overt aortic dissection can develop (12). Risk factors for overt aortic dissection

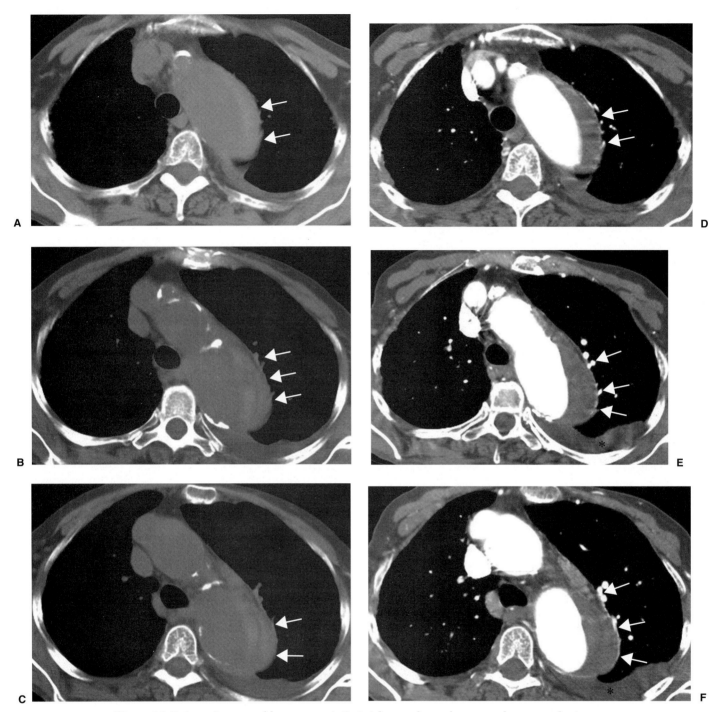

Figure 18.6 Acute intramural hematoma. *A–C.* Axial nonenhanced computed tomography images demonstrate a crescent of high attenuation blood (*arrows*) involving the arch and descending thoracic aorta. *D–F.* Contrast enhanced helical computed tomography images at the same three levels depict hypodense hematoma (*arrows*) when compared with the contrast enhanced true lumen. There is a left pleural effusion (*asterisk*).

include intramural hematoma involving the ascending aorta that had a maximum thickness of 16 mm, compression of the true lumen, and the presence of pericardial or pleural effusion (16).

PENETRATING ATHEROSCLEROTIC ULCER

Penetrating atherosclerotic ulcer is characterized by ulcerating atherosclerotic plaque that penetrates into the internal elastic lamina and media, resulting in hematoma formation within the media of the aortic wall (17,18). Penetrating atherosclerotic ulcer is most often seen in hypertensive elderly patients with a mean age of 70 years. There is a high prevalence of diffuse systemic atherosclerosis and hyperlipidemia. Clinical presentation includes chest or back pain. Less frequently, embolization of atheromatous debris or overlying thrombus results in ischemia and infarction of downstream tissues.

PATHOPHYSIOLOGY

Atheromatous ulcers develop in patients with advanced atherosclerosis. At this stage, lesions are usually asymptomatic and confined to the intimal layer. As the lesion progresses and a deep atheromatous ulcer penetrates through the elastic lamina into the media, an intramural hematoma is formed. The hematoma can extend through the adventitia, forming a false aneurysm. Rarely, it may progress to complete transmural aortic rupture (19).

In penetrating atherosclerotic ulcer, an ulcerated plaque erodes into the media, allowing the entry of blood into the aortic wall.

NATURAL HISTORY

Penetrating atherosclerotic ulcers can heal spontaneously. The aorta and penetrating atherosclerotic ulcer may remain stable. The intramural hematoma associated with the ulcer may become smaller or it can enlarge. In 25% to 30% of patients the ulcer extends through the media but not yet through the adventitia, resulting in saccular or fusiform false aneurysm or pseudoaneurysm. Transmural penetration or aortic wall rupture rarely occurs, approximately 8%. The aortic diameter itself may enlarge, sometimes as the result of incorporation of the ulcer crater (20).

In contrast to "classic" dissection, penetrating ulcers are associated with atherosclerotic disease in older individuals and are usually focal.

CHEST RADIOGRAPHY AND PHOTOGRAPHY

Chest radiographic findings include diffuse or focal enlargement of descending thoracic aorta, widening of the mediastinum indicative of hematoma, pleural fluid, left apical mass adjacent to the aortic arch, and deviation of the trachea. At aortography, findings include presence of an aortic ulcer similar in appearance to gastric ulcers on barium examinations. The ulcer is only seen if it projects tangentially from the aortic wall. Depression of aortic wall due to adjacent intramural hematoma and aortic wall thickening may also be seen (21).

COMPUTED TOMOGRAPHY

A focal contrast material–filled outpouching or focal ulcer is seen in the setting of extensive atherosclerosis, surrounding by localized subintimal hematoma. It most commonly occurs in the middle or distal thirds of the descending thoracic aorta, although any portion of the thoracic or abdominal aorta may be involved. Other findings include displacement of the calcified intima, pleural, extrapleural, and/or mediastinal fluid; a thick aortic wall associated with or without enhancement; contained perforation; or pseudoaneurysm (Fig. 18.7) (19).

On imaging tests, a penetrating ulcer extends beyond the expected location of the aortic wall.

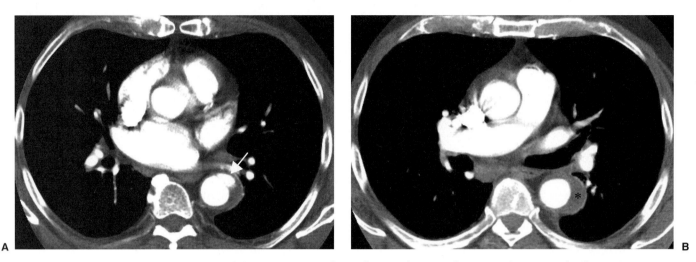

Figure 18.7 Penetrating atherosclerotic ulcer. Axial computed tomography depicts a penetrating ulcer of the left lateral wall of the descending aorta *(arrow)* (A) and intramural thrombus *(asterisk)* (B).

MAGNETIC RESONANCE

MRI demonstrates localized areas of high signal intensity on T1- and T2-weighting in the aortic wall representing localized subacute intramural hematoma. Signals are due to presence of methemoglobin. Ectasia, atherosclerotic disease, and focal aortic wall ulceration are found similar to CT (22,23).

MANAGEMENT

Critical complications of penetrating atherosclerotic ulcers may not be identified on initial imaging studies. Careful noninvasive follow-up with CT and MRI is mandatory to monitor the status of the ulcer and both the lumen diameter and wall thickness. Penetrating atherosclerotic ulcers are initially treated medically, with emphasis on aggressive hypertension control. If symptoms such as chest or back pain persist after medical therapy or signs of intramural hematoma expansion or impending rupture develop, surgical intervention is undertaken. Surgery entails local incision of the ulcerated portion of the aorta and replacement with an interposition graft. For patients who are not surgical candidates, endovascular stent graft placement or percutaneous embolization of the ulcer and associated pseudoaneurysm are used (24).

COARCTATION

Most patients with coarctation have a bicuspid aortic valve.

A coarctation is a congenital narrowing of the thoracic aortic lumen, characterized by eccentric narrowing of the proximal descending thoracic aorta, usually in the region of the ligamentum arteriosum. Coarctation is more common in males than females, with a ratio of 4:1. Manifestations of the anomaly range from minimal narrowing to complete luminal atresia. Coarctation is associated with complex obstructive lesions, such as tubular hypoplasia of the aortic arch, left ventricular outflow tract obstruction, and hypoplastic left heart syndrome. It is also associated with congenital intracardiac defects, such as ventricular septal defect, patent ductus arteriosus, aortic stenosis, and mitral stenosis (Table 18.6). Approximately 80% of patients have a bicuspid aortic valve, with or without aortic stenosis. Patients with Turner syndrome have an increased incidence of coarctation. Intracranial berry aneurysms involving the circle of Willis may be observed in patients with coarctation.

Table 18.6: Coarctation Associations

Ventricular septal defect
Patent ductus arteriosus
Aortic stenosis
Mitral stenosis
Bicuspid aortic valve
Turner syndrome
Vasculitis
Intracranial aneurysms

PATHOGENESIS

Congenital coarctation is a developmental anomaly of the paired primitive dorsal aorta. In contrast, an acquired coarctation may be idiopathic or may occur because of an inflammatory condition or postradiation vasculitis.

The older child or adult type is the more common than the infantile type. It is characterized by a localized, short, juxtaductal narrowing, creating an abrupt stenosis produced by a diaphragm-like ridge extending into the aortic lumen. This narrowing occurs near the ligamentum arteriosum, usually distal to the left subclavian artery. In addition to thoracic aortic coarctation, rarely is the abdominal aorta involved (0.5% to 2%). This may present as smooth diffuse or segmental narrowing of the abdominal aorta extending anywhere from the celiac axis to below the renal arteries (25). Patients present with severe hypertension caused by increased renin levels secondary to renal artery stenosis or decreased blood flow to renal arteries.

Coarctation of the aorta has a distinct appearance depending on the patient's age at the time of detection. The infantile type is characterized by a long segment of hypoplastic narrowing involving the aorta distal to origin of the innominate artery. It is associated with tubular hypoplasia of the aortic arch or descending thoracic aorta and has a high incidence of intracardiac abnormalities, especially bicuspid valve (Fig. 18.8).

Infantile coarctation usually involves a long segment of the aorta and presents with heart failure early in life.

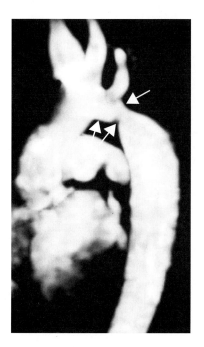

Figure 18.8 Coarctation of the aorta. Sagittal three-dimensional time-of-flight magnetic resonance image depicts bovine aortic arch and "diffuse" type coarctation distal to the innominate artery (*white arrows*).

CLINICAL PRESENTATION

Most coarctations are focal and may be asymptomatic, until hypertension or abnormal pulses prompt diagnosis.

Infants with aortic coarctation are usually symptomatic, presenting with congestive heart failure in the neonatal period. Lower extremity cyanosis, left ventricular failure, cardiomegaly, increased pulmonary vascularity (left-to-right shunt through patent ductus arteriosus/ventricular septal defect), and pulmonary venous hypertension may be seen. In contrast, most adults are asymptomatic. Physical examination demonstrates higher systolic blood pressure in the arms than in the legs, with similar diastolic pressures, thereby creating widened pulse pressure in the arms. This may be associated with weak and delayed femoral arterial pulses. Left ventricular enlargement and systolic ejection click occur. When symptomatic, patients usually suffer from hypertension, headache, epistaxis, dizziness, palpitations, and possibly claudication. The complications of aortic coarctation include aortic dissection, aneurysm, cerebrovascular accidents caused by rupture of berry aneurysm, and infective endocarditis.

CHEST RADIOGRAPH

Unilateral notching may occur if the coarctation is located between the right-sided circulation (innominate artery) and the left-sided circulation (left subclavian artery).

Symmetric, smooth, bilateral, inferior surface rib notching of the third to ninth posterior ribs is classic. Rib notching is caused by tortuous and dilated intercostal arteries that occur as collateral blood flow. On occasion, unilateral rib notching may occur. Left-sided rib notching occurs if the coarctation is located between the normal left subclavian artery and an aberrant right subclavian artery or if there is atresia or stenosis at the origin of the right subclavian artery. Right-sided rib notching occurs when the coarctation is located proximal to the left subclavian artery or if the origin of the left subclavian artery is stenotic or atretic (Fig. 18.9).

Bilateral rib notching and a "figure 3" aortic knob are the chest radiographic hallmarks of coarctation.

A "figure 3" sign is formed on the chest radiograph by the indentation in the contour of the descending aorta, with poststenotic dilatation. A "reverse 3" sign is seen on esophagram, creating an indentation on the esophagus at the level of the aortic arch at the site of poststenotic dilatation of the descending thoracic aorta. Additional findings include left ventricular hypertrophy, prestenotic ascending aorta dilatation if there is an associated stenotic bicuspid aortic valve, linear retrosternal aortic soft tissue opacity created by enlarged internal mammary arteries, and dilated brachiocephalic vessels (4).

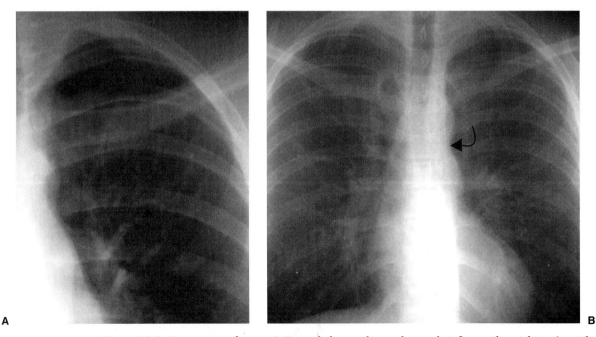

A   B

Figure 18.9 Coarctation of aorta. *A.* Frontal chest radiograph reveals inferior rib notching (*straight arrows*) and (*B*) "figure 3" sign (*curved arrow*).

ANGIOGRAPHY

In neonates, a discrete area of narrowing adjacent to ductus or ligamentum arteriosum is seen. In infants, a focal narrowing of the aorta is seen with or without aortic arch hypoplasia. In adults, the maximum stenosis is usually short and often resembles a diaphragm. The left subclavian artery may be stenotic at its origin or dilated. This dilatation accounts for the soft tissue widening seen in the left superior mediastinum on radiographs. Poststenotic dilatation, ascending aorta dilatation, and collateral vessels are seen (26).

COMPUTED TOMOGRAPHY AND MAGNETIC RESONANCE

Noninvasive imaging assessment of the aorta with CT or MRI can detect the coarctation, postoperative residual coarctation, or recurrent coarctation, as well as complications such as aneurysms and dissections (26,27).

Currently, MRI is the imaging modality of choice. MRI techniques performed in the axial and sagittal oblique plane can evaluate the entire ascending and descending aorta, defining the site and extent of stenosis and the concurrent collateral vessels (Fig. 18.10) (28). Cine MR and phase contrast imaging estimate hemodynamic information such as flow and pressure gradient measurements, thereby precluding the need for angiography (29). MRI is also used to noninvasively evaluate the postoperative aorta and potential complications.

> MRI is the test of choice for evaluating coarctation providing both anatomic and hemodynamic information.

MANAGEMENT

Surgical repair of coarctation entails resection and end-to-end anastomosis, patch angioplasty, subclavian flap aortoplasty (Waldhausen technique), Dacron patch, or Dacron

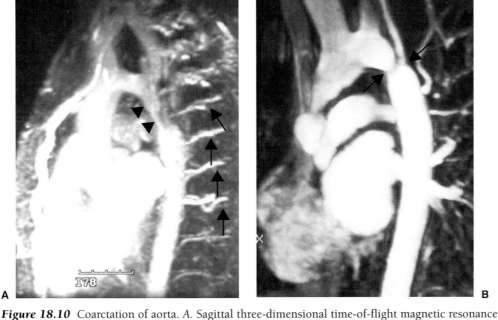

Figure 18.10 Coarctation of aorta. *A.* Sagittal three-dimensional time-of-flight magnetic resonance image demonstrates coarctation (*arrowheads*). Note internal mammary and thoracic intercostal collaterals (*arrows*). *B.* Subvolume maximum intensity projection along long axis aortic arch from three-dimensional gadolinium magnetic resonance imaging depicts coarctation (*arrows*) and collateral vessels. (From Gaba R, Carlos R, Weadock W, et al. Cardiac magnetic resonance imaging: technique, optimization and detection in pathology in clinical practice. Accepted pending revision to Radiographics, with permission.)

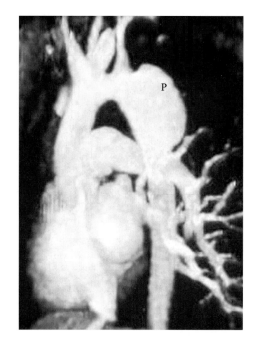

Figure 18.11 Pseudoaneurysm after repair. Oblique sag maximum intensity projection of three-dimensional gadolinium enhanced magnetic resonance imaging reveals pseudoaneurysm at site of Gore-Tex graft repair. (From Gaba R, Carlos R, Weadock W, et al. Cardiac magnetic resonance imaging: technique, optimization and detection in pathology in clinical practice. Accepted pending revision to Radiographics, with permission.)

bypass conduit. Balloon dilatation angioplasty has been successful with discrete juxtaductal type coarctation, for neonatal coarctation, and persistent pressure gradients after surgery. (30) Postoperative complications of aortic coarctation include restenosis at site of repair, pseudoaneurysm formation, intramural hematoma, dissection, and systolic paradoxical hypertension (31) (Fig. 18.11).

PSEUDOCOARCTATION

Pseudocoarctation is a redundant kinked aortic arch, usually with no pressure gradient across the "kink."

Pseudocoarctation is a congenital anomaly of the aorta characterized by redundancy and kinking of the descending aortic arch, just distal to the left subclavian artery at the ligamentum arteriosum (32). This kink usually creates little or no blood flow obstruction; therefore, there is usually no significant pressure gradient across the kink, and no collateral blood flow through collateral vessels is seen. Pseudocoarctation is associated with bicuspid aortic valve, patent ductus arteriosus, ventricular septal defect, aortic and subaortic stenosis, and anomalies of aortic arch branches.

PATHOGENESIS AND CLINICAL FEATURES

Pseudocoarctation develops because of the failure of the third to seventh dorsal aortic segments to properly condense and form a normal aortic arch. Patients are usually asymptomatic. Hypertension may be seen, particularly in middle-aged men. A systolic ejection murmur near the cardiac base may be detected on physical examination (33). In contrast to coarctation, the femoral pulses are present and either a small (less than 25 mm Hg) or absent arterial pressure gradient exists between the arms and legs.

CHEST RADIOGRAPHY

A smooth round to ovoid left superior mediastinal mass is seen, deforming the mediastinal contour. Below the mass, a denser round opacity is seen in the usual position of the aortic knob. The opacity represents the superimposed buckled aortic arch and descending aortic segments. The widened mediastinum is secondary to elongation of the ascending aorta and aortic arch, with a high-riding or cervical aortic arch (Fig. 18.12) (33).

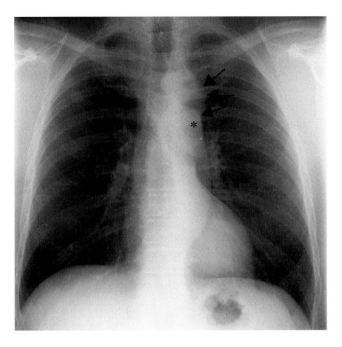

Figure 18.12 Pseudocoarctation of the aorta. Chest radiograph depicts a left superior mediastinal mass manifested by a bulge *(arrows)* above what appears to be the aortic knob *(asterisk)*. No rib notching is apparent.

COMPUTED TOMOGRAPHY, MAGNETIC RESONANCE IMAGING, AND ANGIOGRAPHY

CT delineates the solid mass identified on chest radiograph as vascular, with its continuity to the aorta. The ascending aorta is normal in caliber. The narrowed segment of the descending aorta distal to the kink is often dilated and then gradually narrows to normal caliber. The aortic arch is abnormally high in position. An aneurysm or dissection below the kink rarely occurs. There is an increased distance between the left common carotid and left subclavian artery, anterior displacement of the esophagus, and anteromedial descending aorta (Fig. 18.13). CT cannot assess whether there is a pressure gradient across the

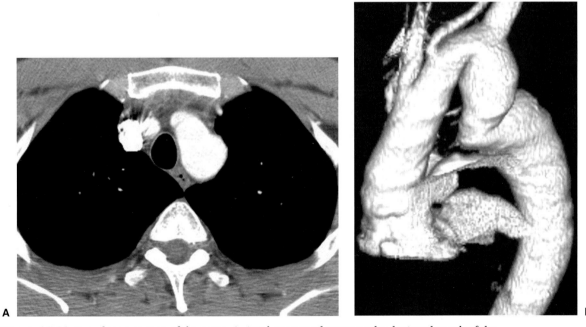

Figure 18.13 Pseudocoarctation of the aorta. *A.* Axial computed tomography depicts the arch of the pseudocoarcted aorta high in the mediastinum. *B.* Sagittal three dimensional shaded surface display computed tomography of reconstruction.

kink, unless collateral vessels are seen, in which case a gradient is by definition present, but the severity of the gradient remains unmeasured. At angiography the pressure gradient is measured; however, this generally has been relatively replaced by the use of MRI for the diagnosis of pseudocoarctation, allowing both anatomic definition and measurement of any pressure gradient by MRI.

The angiographic findings of a high position of the aortic arch, presence of a kink without stenosis, and collateral vessels or impediment of blood flow can be evaluated noninvasively with MRI. Cine phase contrast MRI can estimate physiologic flow information, such as flow or pressure gradient measurements (29). Although pseudocoarctation is not treated surgically, close attention with noninvasive imaging may be performed for the early detection of aneurysm or dissection. Monitoring and early surgical intervention is undertaken to prevent the increase risk of aortic rupture (34).

AORTIC ANEURYSM

Thoracic aortic aneurysm is defined as abnormal irreversible dilatation of the aortic lumen, generally greater than 4 cm in diameter. It is degeneration of the aortic media, specifically weakening and destruction of the elastic fibers that results in aneurysm formation (35). The aortic aneurysm may be classified according to location, morphology, integrity of aortic wall, and etiology. Causes of aortic aneurysm are listed in Table 18.7.

CLASSIFICATION ACCORDING TO LOCATION

Aneurysm locations may be summarized as follows:

1. Ascending thoracic aorta, between aortic annulus and origin innominate artery;
2. Transverse aortic arch, in conjunction with brachiocephalic vessels;
3. Descending aorta, originating distal to origin of the left subclavian artery;
4. Thoracoabdominal, which originates in the descending thoracic aortic and extends below the diaphragm to involve a variable extent of the abdominal aorta.

Aneurysms that classically involve the ascending aorta are due to cystic medial necrosis, connective tissue disorders such as Marfan and Ehlers-Danlos syndromes, and syphilis, the latter now rare. Aneurysms involving the descending aorta are usually atherosclerotic, posttraumatic, infectious (mycotic), or inflammatory (rheumatoid arthritis and ankylosing spondylitis) (36).

CLASSIFICATION ACCORDING TO MORPHOLOGY

Morphology may be characterized as either fusiform or saccular. Fusiform aneurysms involve the entire aortic circumference, thus appearing cylindrical or spindle-shaped. Saccular aneurysms are sharply delineated and usually involve a localized segment of the aorta. They can present as an eccentric outpouching from one side of the aortic wall.

Table 18.7: Etiologies of Aortic Aneurysms

Atherosclerosis
Infection (mycotic)
Cystic medial necrosis
Connective tissue disorders (Marfan and Ehlers-Danlos syndromes)
Syphilis
Trauma
Inflammatory (rheumatoid arthritis, ankylosing spondylitis)

CLASSIFICATION ACCORDING TO AORTIC WALL INTEGRITY

Aneurysms can be classified as true aneurysms or false aneurysms depending on the integrity of aortic wall. True aneurysms are characterized by an intact aortic wall, composed of all three layers: intima, media, adventitia. Atherosclerotic and connective tissue disorder–related aneurysms are true aneurysms. False aneurysms or pseudoaneurysms are characterized by a disrupted aortic wall contained by the adventitia, perivascular connective tissue, and organized blood clot (37). Posttraumatic and infectious (mycotic) aneurysms are usually false aneurysms.

CLASSIFICATION ACCORDING TO ETIOLOGY

Atherosclerosis

Thoracic aortic aneurysms are most commonly caused by atherosclerosis. These occur in elderly hypertensive patients with a mean age of 69 years (range, 42 to 94 years) (38). Three-fourths of atherosclerotic aneurysms occur in men, and smokers are at increased risk. There is a high incidence of other cardiovascular diseases in patients with thoracic aortic aneurysms, including coronary artery disease, cerebrovascular disease, and aneurysms of abdominal aorta and iliac arteries (39). The basis for aneurysm formation is degeneration and fibrous replacement of the media underlying the atherosclerotic intimal lesions. Once dilatation occurs, the aneurysm wall is exposed to increased mechanical stress; poor nutrition leads to further degeneration and progressive enlargement of the aneurysm. Atherosclerotic aneurysms are usually fusiform because of the long segments of the aorta they affect. However, they can be saccular in up to 20% of patients. They most commonly involve the aortic arch and descending thoracic aorta, usually distal to the left subclavian artery. They are relatively uncommon in the ascending aorta (37).

> Most thoracic aortic aneurysms are fusiform in morphology and secondary to atherosclerosis.

Cystic Medial Degeneration

Cystic medial degeneration is the most common cause of an ascending aorta aneurysm (37). It may be associated with disorders such as Marfan or Ehlers-Danlos syndromes or acquired weakness or a defect in the aortic media. The cause of cystic medial degeneration is unknown. It is postulated to be the result of ongoing repetitive aortic injury and repair that occurs in the aging aorta. This process eventually leads to aortic wall weakening and dilatation.

> The most common case of an ascending aortic aneurysm is cystic medial degeneration.

Marfan Syndrome

Marfan syndrome is characterized by musculoskeletal deformities, ocular abnormalities, generalized defect of connective tissue, and cardiovascular lesions. Cardiovascular manifestations are present in 98% of patients and may cause death in more than 90%. Manifestations include aortic root dilatation complicated by aortic dissection or rupture, usually extending into sinuses of Valsalva, and valve regurgitation. Aortic regurgitation is present in up to 81% of patients with an aortic root diameter greater than 5 cm and in 100% of patients with an aortic diameter greater than 6 cm. Aneurysmal dilatation generally diminishes higher up in the ascending aorta, and the aortic arch is usually normal. Aortic lesions in patients with Marfan syndrome are identical to idiopathic medial cystic degeneration; however, the onset of degeneration occurs earlier in life and progresses more rapidly. Because of the risk of aortic emergency, patients with Marfan syndrome are usually followed with serial annual imaging, such as CT, MRI, and/or echocardiography (Fig. 18.14).

> Because of the high risk of aortic abnormality, patients with Marfan syndrome usually undergo regular surveillance with echocardiography and CT or MRI.

Annuloaortic Ectasia

Annuloaortic ectasia is a pathoanatomic description for the combined lesions of aortic root aneurysm and aortic valve regurgitation due to dilatation of the aortic annulus. This is

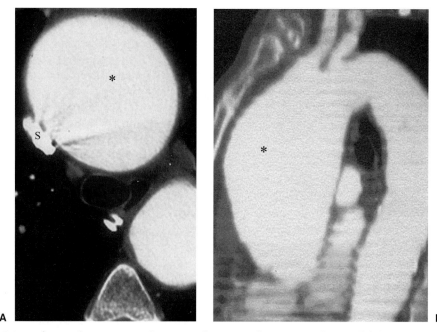

Figure 18.14 Marfan syndrome. A. Axial computed tomography image and sagittal (B) reconstruction of ascending aortic aneurysm (*asterisk*). Compressed superior vena cavas (S).

associated with degenerative changes in the aortic media even in the absence of Marfan syndrome. Aortic rupture and to lesser extent aortic dissection are frequent complications.

Posttraumatic Aneurysms

Posttraumatic aneurysms are usually the result of rapid deceleration injury and most commonly secondary to motor vehicle accident injury. They may also result from penetrating trauma. The two most common sites of aortic tears are at points of relative aortic fixation, the aortic knob and at the level of the ligamentum arteriosum just distal to the origin of the left subclavian artery. The proximal tears usually result in sudden death. The proximal descending tears arise from a circumferential tear of the intima and media and are often contained by the adventitia. Posttraumatic aneurysms are classified as false aneurysms and are an acute surgical emergency. A focal aneurysm presenting in the proximal descending aorta distant from the time of surgery should raise suspicion for delayed pseudoaneurysm (Fig. 12.1).

> Saccular aneurysms should raise suspicion of a posttraumatic aneurysm (especially if at the ligamentum arteriosum) or mycotic aneurysm.

Syphilis

Syphilis, once the most common cause of a thoracic aneurysm, is rare today. Approximately 12% of patients with untreated syphilis develop cardiovascular disease. Symptoms usually occur 10 to 30 years after primary infection and are usually confined to the thoracic aorta, with the ascending aorta and transverse arch as the most common sites. Manifestations include aortic aneurysm, aortic insufficiency, and asymmetric enlargement of the sinuses of Valsalva. Most of the aneurysms are saccular, with about one-fourth fusiform. The prognosis for untreated syphilitics (luetic) aneurysm is poor, with death occurring within months of symptom onset. In 40% of cases, death is due to aortic rupture.

Mycotic Aneurysm

The term was first used by William Osler in 1885 to describe aneurysms from septic emboli in patients with bacterial endocarditis. Today this term is used for any infected aneurysm. Predisposing factors include immunocompetent states such as malignancy, alcoholism, steroid use or chemotherapy, drug abuse, and aortic trauma caused by accidents, surgical manipulation, or arterial catheterization (37).

The pathogenesis of mycotic aneurysm includes the embolization of infected material directly to diseased intima or vasa vasorum; direct extension from inflammatory process (such as osteomyelitis or abscess); and invasion of the aortic wall from intravascular sources or lymphangitic spread. Infectious agents usually responsible for these aneurysms include *Staphylococcus aureus*, *Salmonella* species, *Pneumococcus*, and non-hemolytic *Streptococcus*. These are classified as false aneurysms (pseudoaneurysms) and are typically saccular (Fig. 18.15). Unlike noninfected aneurysms, mycotic aneurysms are usually symptomatic. Patients present with thoracic or back pain, fever, and laboratory changes indicating infection.

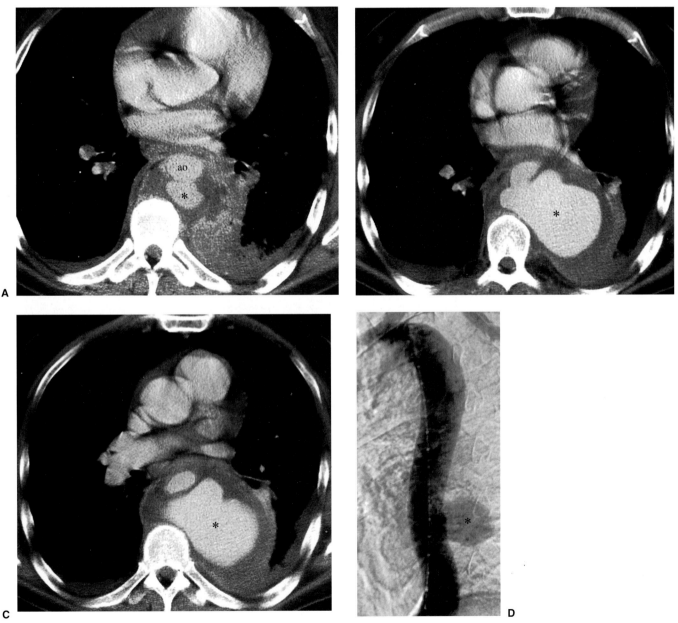

Figure 18.15 Mycotic aneurysm. *A.* Axial computed tomography when the patient was first seen with contrast material–filled ulcer (*asterisk*) in descending thoracic aorta (ao), intramural hematoma, and bilateral pleural fluid collections. *B and C.* Six weeks later, images at same level and at the level of the descending right pulmonary artery demonstrate interval growth of the pseudoaneurysm (*asterisk*). *D.* Angiogram depicts the pseudoaneurysm.

CLINICAL MANIFESTATIONS

Most patients with atherosclerotic aneurysms are asymptomatic and are first diagnosed by routine chest radiograph or during evaluation for some other disease (40). Symptoms are produced by the enlarging space-occupying nature of the aneurysm, which compresses adjacent mediastinal structures. Symptoms include chest pain, hoarseness due to compression of recurrent laryngeal nerve, postobstructive atelectasis due to compression of bronchus, and dysphagia secondary to esophageal compression. Physical signs are rare; on occasion a large aneurysm can be palpated in the suprasternal notch. Additional physical signs include venous distension due to obstruction of the superior vena cava or innominate vein, vocal cord paralysis, abnormal pulsations in the upper anterior chest wall, tracheal deviation or "tug," and Horner syndrome (36). Patients with impending or actual rupture and aneurysm larger than 5 cm experience severe chest pain.

CHEST RADIOGRAPHS

Many thoracic aneurysms are detected as an incidental finding on a chest radiograph performed for another purpose, because they are clinically silent.

A mediastinal mass immediately adjacent to and indistinguishable from the aortic contours should raise the suspicion of aortic aneurysm. Other findings include mediastinal widening, particularly of the aorta; aortopulmonary window and left paraspinal stripe; and displacement and/or compression of the trachea and esophagus. Leaking or ruptured aneurysms are associated with hemothorax and mediastinal widening. Ascending aortic aneurysms produce abnormal convex opacity of the right superior mediastinum and fill the retrosternal clear space on the lateral view. Aortic arch aneurysms produce diffuse aortic enlargement or superimposed localized mass (Fig. 18.16).

COMPUTED TOMOGRAPHY

CT is an extremely valuable noninvasive modality to confirm the diagnosis and delineate the extent of thoracic aortic aneurysms. The findings of aortic aneurysm on CT are listed in Table 18.8. It allows detection of not just the contrast-filled lumen as seen in aortograms, but also the intraluminal thrombus. Characteristic CT findings include focal or diffuse aortic dilatation and deformity, peripheral curvilinear and plaque-like intimal calcification at the edge of the aorta or near the aortic margin, thickened aortic wall, filling of the patent portion of lumen by contrast media, and intraluminal thrombus that may be

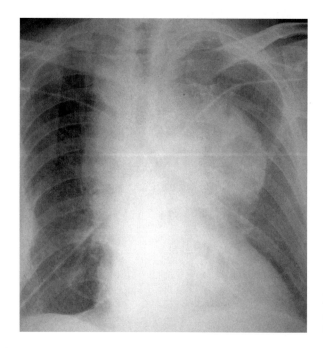

Figure 18.16 Ruptured aneurysm. Anteroposterior chest radiograph reveals a widened mediastinum.

Table 18.8: Computed Tomographic Imaging Findings of Aortic Aneurysm

Focal or diffuse aortic dilatation
Peripheral curvilinear intimal calcification
Thickened aortic wall
Intraluminal thrombus
Displacement of mediastinal structures
Periaortic hematoma
Pleural fluid collections

circumferential or crescentic. The intraluminal thrombus may have internal calcification with linear or curvilinear pattern when longstanding (41). Displacement of mediastinal structures, bone erosions, and presence of periaortic hematoma or pleural fluid collections may be seen (36,42). CT may also detect impending or actual aortic rupture and dissection, particularly when the aneurysm is greater than 5 cm in diameter. Other complications include aortobronchial fistula, compression of the right pulmonary artery, aortoesophageal fistula, and distal embolization, the latter leading to ischemia or infarction of bowel and abdominal organs. The aorta may rupture into the mediastinum, pericardium, pleural sac, or extrapleural space (Fig. 18.17). The presence of pleural or extrapleural blood on the left, and rarely across the posterior mediastinum into the right side of the chest, and contained aortic leak "draped aorta" are all signs of impending or actual rupture. A contained leak can be found when the aneurysm is in close contact with the spine, with lateral draping of the aneurysm around the vertebral body with a deficient posterior aortic wall (43,44).

> Hemoptysis in a patient with an aortic aneurysm or prior aortic graft should raise the suspicion of an aortobronchial fistula.

Previous authors have advocated the use of angiography for the evaluation of aneurysms involving the aortic arch. As CT has evolved with angiographic features and multiplanar reconstruction, it has become the first line of imaging, even when the aneurysm involves the aortic arch (45). Quint et al. (45) showed that CT can accurately determine the need for intraoperative hypothermic circulatory arrest during repair.

MAGNETIC RESONANCE IMAGING

MRI can accurately detect and assess aortic aneurysms. Multiplanar capability allows for precise measurement of ascending aortic aneurysm. MRI can accurately identify effacement of the sinotubular junction by aortic root aneurysm.

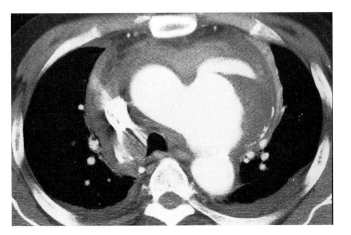

Figure 18.17 Computed tomography depicts a ruptured aortic arch aneurysm, hemomediastinum (high attenuation material indicative of blood), and small bilateral pleural effusions.

THE REPAIRED AORTA

Thoracic surgery and endoscopic procedures of the aorta change its normal appearance. Evaluation of the postprocedural aorta with noninvasive imaging provides monitoring and early detection of complications, allowing intervention before aortic rupture occurs. Knowledge of the postoperative appearance enables one to distinguish the postoperative structures that may mimic pathology from complications that require prompt surgical intervention.

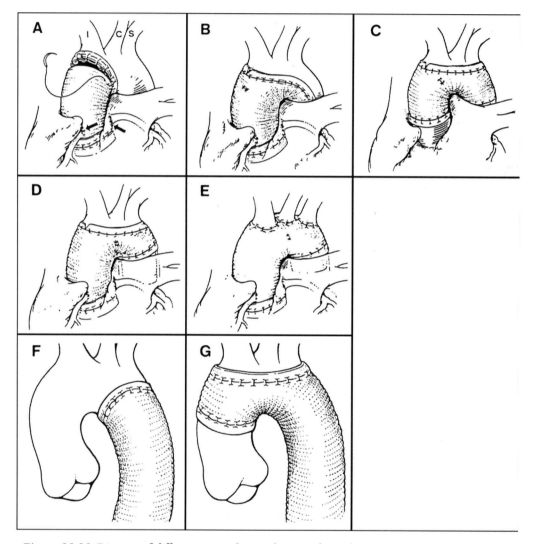

Figure 18.18 Diagram of different surgical procedures performed. *A.* Root replacement with distal anastomosis at the level of the brachiocephalic (innominate) artery (I). *Arrows,* coronary artery anastomoses; *C,* left common carotid artery; *S,* left subclavian artery. *B.* Root, ascending aorta, and partial arch replacement. *C.* Complete arch replacement with reimplantation of the arch vessels as a single island. *D.* Complete root and arch replacement with the elephant trunk technique used as a staged procedure for complete replacement of the aorta. *E.* Same as *D* except each arch vessel is implanted separately. *F.* Descending aortic graft. *G.* Descending aortic graft with complete arch replacement and reimplantation of the arch vessels as a single island. Coronary arteries are anastomosed to the root graft in parts *A, B, D,* and *E* (frontal view); heart removed in *F* and *G.* (A–E from Deeb GM, Jenkins E, Bolling SF, et al. Retrograde cerebral perfusion during hypothermic circulatory arrest reduces neurologic morbidity. *J Thorac Cardiovasc Surg* 1995;109:259–268; Quint LE, Francis IR, Williams DM, et al. Synthetic interposition grafts of the thoracic aorta: postoperative appearance on serial CT studies. *Radiology* 1999;211:317–324, with permission.)

Surgical procedures are complex. Portions of the aorta may be resected or opened, grafts may be sewn end to end or end to side, branch vessels may be reimplanted or grafted using synthetic interposition grafts (Fig. 18.18), or an inclusion graft technique may be used (46). The continuous suture graft inclusion technique (Fig. 18.19) entails aortotomy, graft inclusion, and enclosure of the graft within the native aorta. This technique creates a potential space between the graft and native aorta that may contain fluid, blood, thrombus, or contrast media in the setting of partial suture dehiscence. The potential space between the graft and native aorta may contain small amount of blood and gas normally in the immediate postoperative period. Blood may leak into the space if the suture dehiscences, either proximally or distally. This is evident on CT with contrast material in the space (Fig. 18.20). Aortic enlargement or pseudoaneurysm formation may occur. In chronic cases, thrombus may occupy the space. Although rare, aortic graft infection may occur. Fluid between the graft and native aorta 6 weeks after surgery is highly suspicious. The presence of gas in the space 2 weeks after surgery is virtually pathognomonic of infection (37). Other complications include perigraft blood flow and perigraft thickening (47).

When repaired using synthetic interposition grafts, the aorta has a characteristic appearance on CT. Early postoperative findings include pleural or pericardial effusion, mediastinal lymph node enlargement, and/or left lower lobe atelectasis.

During aortic reconstruction felt pledgets and strips are used to reinforce sutures. On CT, these present as high-attenuation material bordering the aortic wall or graft. The felt pledgets are also used to repair bypass cannulation sites in the native aorta or air evacuation needle sites in the graft. Felt strips are used to reinforce the graft to aorta anastomosis (Figs. 18.21 and 18.22). The felt may be mistaken for contrast material secondary to a leaking graft (Fig. 18.23). There is often circumferential low attenuation and/or soft tissue attenuation material surrounding or adjacent to the aortic graft. This may diminish over time or remain unchanged. This can be mistaken for an infected surgical site or a leaking aorta. The normal appearance of the reconstructed aorta should not be mistaken for pathology. These include a collapsed native aorta adjacent to the graft (Fig. 18.24), reinforcement of the graft with bovine pericardium (Fig. 18.25), and

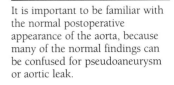

It is important to be familiar with the normal postoperative appearance of the aorta, because many of the normal findings can be confused for pseudoaneurysm or aortic leak.

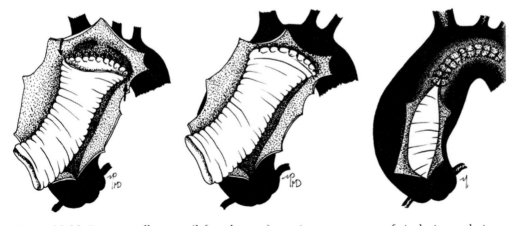

Figure 18.19 Diagrams illustrate (*left and center*) continuous suture graft inclusion technique. After aortotomy, graft material is placed within the native aorta. The distal anastomosis is created first, followed by the proximal anastomosis, both with continuous-suture technique. In these illustration, the hemiarch technique is shown, with a tongue of graft material extending along the inferior surface of the aortic arch, beyond the origins of the great vessels (*straight arrow in left*). The superior edge of the graft material does not extend beyond the origin of the brachiocephalic artery (*curved arrow in left*). *Right.* The native aortic sac is wrapped around the prothesis, and its cut edges are sutured together. (From Rofsky NM, Weinreb JC, Grossi EA, et al. Aortic aneurysm and dissection: normal MR imaging and CT findings after surgical repair with the continuous-suture graft-inclusion technique. *Radiology* 1993;186:195–201, with permission.)

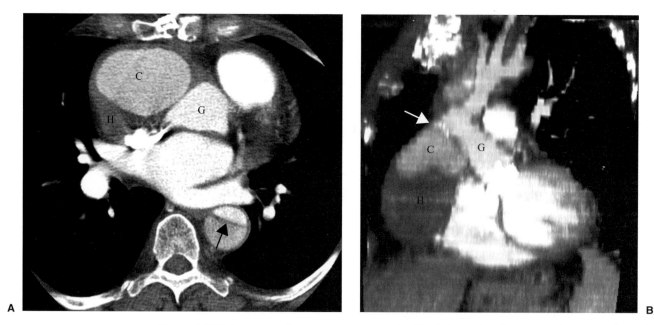

Figure 18.20 Large pseudoaneurysm and contained leak 4 months after composite root grafting. *A.* Axial computed tomography and (*B*) parasagittal reconstruction demonstrate low attenuation material, hematoma (H) and extravasated contrast material (C) adjacent to the distal anastomosis (*white arrow in B*). *Black arrow in A*, dissection flap in descending aorta.

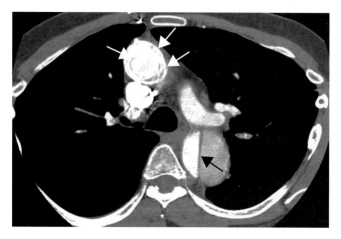

Figure 18.21 Felt reinforcing ring. Axial computed tomography depicts felt reinforcing ring (*white arrows*) at anastomosis of an ascending aortic interposition graft. *Black arrow*, dissection flap in descending aorta.

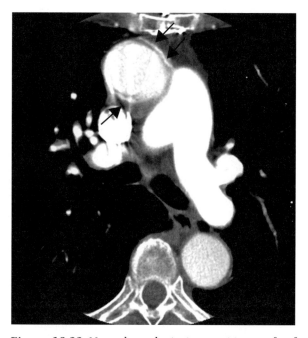

Figure 18.22 Normal synthetic interposition graft of ascending aorta 14 months after surgery. Computed tomographic image demonstrates circumferential high attenuation felt reinforcing ring (*arrows*) around the ascending aortic graft.

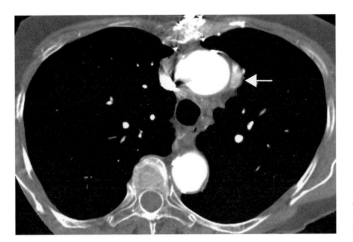

Figure 18.23 Synthetic interposition graft demonstrates felt (*arrow*) reinforcing ring at distal anastomosis, which can mimic a pseudoaneurysm

the presence of a coronary button. In the latter, a small portion of the native aorta around the coronary artery ostium (coronary button) is implanted onto the graft. On occasion, a button may be mistaken for a pseudoaneurysm (Fig. 18.26) (48). At times, surgical intervention is not undertaken because of the poor condition of the patient. In such cases, percutaneous endovascular stent grafts are the procedure of choice (Fig. 18.27).

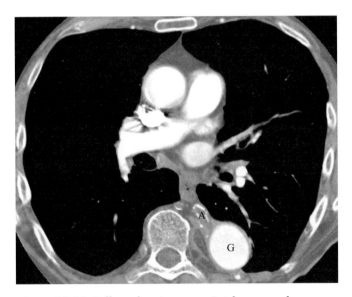

Figure 18.24 Collapsed native aorta. Axial computed tomography 27 months after reconstruction of descending thoracic aorta demonstrates the collapsed native aorta (A) medial to graft (G).

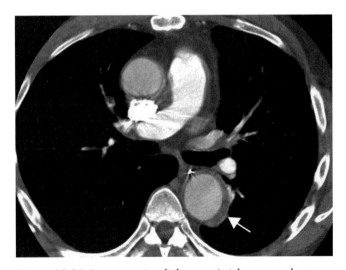

Figure 18.25 Bovine pericardial wrap. Axial computed tomography 29 months after reconstruction of the descending thoracic aorta demonstrates low attenuation material along the left of the aorta (*arrow*) representing the bovine pericardial wrap.

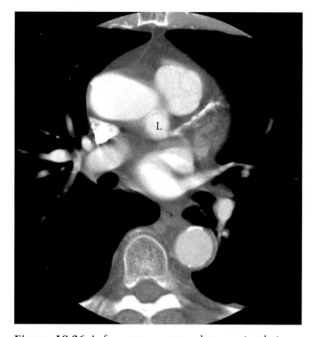

Figure 18.26 Left coronary artery button simulating a pseudoaneurysm. Computed tomographic image demonstrates an outpouching from the ascending thoracic aortic graft. L, left coronary artery button. This may simulate a pseudoaneurysm.

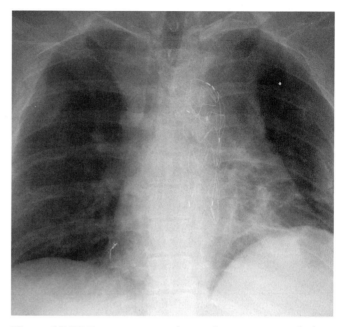

Figure 18.27 Percutaneous endovascular stent. Frontal chest radiograph reveals an endovascular stent in the descending thoracic aorta after traumatic injury.

REFERENCES

1. Sebastia C, Pallisa E, Quiroga S, et al. Aortic dissection: diagnosis and follow-up with helical CT. *Radiographics* 1999;19:45–60; quiz 149–150.
2. Fisher ER, Stern EJ, Godwin JD, 2nd, et al. Acute aortic dissection: typical and atypical imaging features. *Radiographics* 1994;14:1263–1271; discussion 1271–1264.
3. Roberts WC. Aortic dissection: anatomy, consequences, and causes. *Am Heart J* 1981;101:195–214.
4. Williams J. *The great vessels in fundamentals of diagnostic radiology*. Baltimore: Williams & Wilkens, 1994:605–625.
5. Williams DM, Lee DY, Hamilton BH, et al. The dissected aorta. Part III. Anatomy and radiologic diagnosis of branch-vessel compromise. *Radiology* 1997;203:37–44.
6. Williams DM, LePage MA, Lee DY. The dissected aorta. Part I. Early anatomic changes in an in vitro model. *Radiology* 1997;203:23–31.
7. LePage MA, Quint LE, Sonnad SS, et al. Aortic dissection: CT features that distinguish true lumen from false lumen. *AJR Am J Roentgenol* 2001;177:207–211.
8. Heiberg E, Wolverson M, Sundaram M, et al. CT findings in thoracic aortic dissection. *AJR Am J Roentgenol* 1981;136:13–17.
9. Williams DM, Joshi A, Dake MD, et al. Aortic cobwebs: an anatomic marker identifying the false lumen in aortic dissection—imaging and pathologic correlation. *Radiology* 1994;190:167–174.
10. Ledbetter S, Stuk JL, Kaufman JA. Helical (spiral) CT in the evaluation of emergent thoracic aortic syndromes. Traumatic aortic rupture, aortic aneurysm, aortic dissection, intramural hematoma, and penetrating atherosclerotic ulcer. *Radiol Clin North Am* 1999;37:575–589.
11. Sueyoshi E, Matsuoka Y, Sakamoto I, et al. Fate of intramural hematoma of the aorta: CT evaluation. *J Comput Assist Tomogr* 1997;21:931–938.
12. Song JK, Kim HS, Kang DH, et al. Different clinical features of aortic intramural hematoma versus dissection involving the ascending aorta. *J Am Coll Cardiol* 2001;37:1604–1610.
13. Kim JK, Park SW, Jeong JO, et al. Clinical features and prognosis of acute aortic intramural hem-

orrhage compared with those of acute aortic dissection: a single center experience. *Jpn Heart J* 2001;42:91–100.

14. Yamada T, Tada S, Harada J. Aortic dissection without intimal rupture: diagnosis with MR imaging and CT. *Radiology* 1988;168:347–352.

15. Sawhney NS, DeMaria AN, Blanchard DG. Aortic intramural hematoma: an increasingly recognized and potentially fatal entity. *Chest* 2001;120:1340–1346.

16. Choi SH, Choi SJ, Kim JH, et al. Useful CT findings for predicting the progression of aortic intramural hematoma to overt aortic dissection. *J Comput Assist Tomogr* 2001;25:295–299.

17. Hayashi H, Matsuoka Y, Sakamoto I, et al. Penetrating atherosclerotic ulcer of the aorta: imaging features and disease concept. *Radiographics* 2000;20:995–1005.

18. Welch TJ, Stanson AW, Sheedy PF 2nd, et al. Radiologic evaluation of penetrating aortic atherosclerotic ulcer. *Radiographics* 1990;10:675–685.

19. Kazerooni EA, Bree RL, Williams DM. Penetrating atherosclerotic ulcers of the descending thoracic aorta: evaluation with CT and distinction from aortic dissection. *Radiology* 1992;183: 759–765.

20. Quint LE, Williams DM, Francis IR, et al. Ulcerlike lesions of the aorta: imaging features and natural history. *Radiology* 2001;218:719–723.

21. Troxler M, Mavor AI, Homer-Vanniasinkam S. Penetrating atherosclerotic ulcers of the aorta. *Br J Surg* 2001;88:1169–1177.

22. Harris JA, Bis KG, Glover JL, et al. Penetrating atherosclerotic ulcers of the aorta. *J Vasc Surg* 1994;19:90–98; discussion 98–99.

23. Yucel EK, Steinberg FL, Egglin TK, et al. Penetrating aortic ulcers: diagnosis with MR imaging. *Radiology* 1990;177:779–781.

24. Williams DM, Lee DY, Hamilton BH, et al. The dissected aorta: percutaneous treatment of ischemic complications—principles and results. *J Vasc Intervent Radiol* 1997;8:605–625.

25. Hallett JW Jr, Brewster DC, Darling RC, et al. Coarctation of the abdominal aorta: current options in surgical management. *Ann Surg* 1980;191:430–437.

26. Phillips R, Culham J. Coarctation of the aorta. In: Braum, ed. *Abrams' angiography,* 4th ed. Philadelphia, 1997:434–463.

27. Godwin JD, Herfkens RJ, Brundage BH, et al. Evaluation of coarctation of the aorta by computed tomography. *J Comput Assist Tomogr* 1981;5:153–156.

28. Gaba R, Carlos R, Weadock W, et al. Cardiac MR imaging: technique, optimization and detection in pathology in clinical practice. Accepted pending revision to Radiographics.

29. Nayler GL, Firmin DN, Longmore DB. Blood flow imaging by cine magnetic resonance. *J Comput Assist Tomogr* 1986;10:715–722.

30. Bank ER, Aisen AM, Rocchini AP, et al. Coarctation of the aorta in children undergoing angioplasty: pretreatment and posttreatment MR imaging. *Radiology* 1987;162:235–240.

31. Rees S, Somerville J, Ward C, et al. Coarctation of the aorta: MR imaging in late postoperative assessment. *Radiology* 1989;173:499–502.

32. Soler R, Pombo F, Bargiela A, et al. MRI of pseudocoarctation of the aorta: morphological and cine-MRI findings. *Comput Med Imag Graph* 1995;19:431–434.

33. Gaupp RJ, Fagan CJ, Davis M, et al. Pseudocoarctation of the aorta. *J Comput Assist Tomogr* 1981;5:571–573.

34. Gay WA Jr, Young WG Jr. Pseudocoarctation of the aorta. A reappraisal. *J Thorac Cardiovasc Surg* 1969;58:739–745.

35. Mistovich JJ, Griffiths B. Aortic dissection and aortic aneurysm: pathophysiology, assessment and management. *Emerg Med Serv* 2001;30:49–55, 60.

36. Frist WH, Miller DC. Aneurysms of ascending thoracic aorta and transverse aortic arch. *Cardiovasc Clin* 1987;17:263–287.

37. Posniak HV, Demos TC, Marsan RE. Computed tomography of the normal aorta and thoracic aneurysms. *Semin Roentgenol* 1989;24:7–21.

38. Pressler V, McNamara JJ. Thoracic aortic aneurysm: natural history and treatment. *J Thorac Cardiovasc Surg* 1980;79:489–498.

39. McNamara JJ, Pressler VM. Natural history of arteriosclerotic thoracic aortic aneurysms. *Ann Thorac Surg* 1978;26:468–473.

40. Pressler V, McNamara JJ. Aneurysm of the thoracic aorta. Review of 260 cases. *J Thorac Cardiovasc Surg* 1985;89:50–54.

41. Torres WE, Maurer DE, Steinberg HV, et al. CT of aortic aneurysms: the distinction between mural and thrombus calcification. *AJR Am J Roentgenol* 1988;150:1317–1319.

42. Godwin JD. Conventional CT of the aorta. *J Thorac Imag* 1990;5:18–31.
43. Halliday KE, al-Kutoubi A. Draped aorta: CT sign of contained leak of aortic aneurysms. *Radiology* 1996;199:41–43.
44. Kucich VA, Vogelzang RL, Hartz RS, et al. Ruptured thoracic aneurysm: unusual manifestation and early diagnosis using CT. *Radiology* 1986;160:87–89.
45. Quint LE, Francis IR, Williams DM, et al. Evaluation of thoracic aortic disease with the use of helical CT and multiplanar reconstructions: comparison with surgical findings. *Radiology* 1996; 201:37–41.
46. Deeb GM, Jenkins E, Bolling SF, et al. Retrograde cerebral perfusion during hypothermic circulatory arrest reduces neurologic morbidity. *J Thorac Cardiovasc Surg* 1995;109:259–268.
47. Rofsky NM, Weinreb JC, Grossi EA, et al. Aortic aneurysm and dissection: normal MR imaging and CT findings after surgical repair with the continuous-suture graft-inclusion technique. *Radiology* 1993;186:195–201.
48. Quint LE, Francis IR, Williams DM, et al. Synthetic interposition grafts of the thoracic aorta: postoperative appearance on serial CT studies. *Radiology* 1999;211:317–324.

ADULT CONGENITAL HEART DISEASE

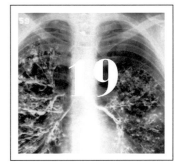

■ Noncyanotic Congenital Heart Disease
■ Cyanotic Congenital Heart Disease

Advances in the treatment of congenital heart disease over the past five decades have led to significant growth in the number of surviving patients. Accurate statistics are lacking, but estimates of adult patients with congenital heart disease in the United States in the year 2000 were more than 750,000 (1). Most adult cases consist of simple defects such as bicuspid aortic valve, right aortic arch, and atrial septal defect. However, patients with more severe forms of congenital disease, such as pulmonary atresia, Ebstein anomaly, and transposition of the great arteries, can also survive into adulthood. For this reason, radiologists should have a broad understanding of the anatomic and physiologic aspects of congenital heart disease. In this chapter we provide a broad overview of adult congenital heart disease, with an emphasis on chest radiography, computed tomography (CT), and magnetic resonance imaging (MRI). The discussion focuses on patients who have not had prior surgical corrective procedures, cases where radiologists can be the first to provide clues for early diagnosis.

The chapter is divided into two sections (Table 19.1). The first section is a discussion of congenital defects that do not produce cyanosis, such as anomalies of the aorta, left-to-right intracardiac shunts, and other miscellaneous conditions. The second section addresses the more complex cyanotic defects.

NONCYANOTIC CONGENITAL HEART DISEASE

BICUSPID AORTIC VALVE

The congenitally bicuspid aortic valve, after mitral valve prolapse, is the second most common major cardiac malformation (2). The malformation occurs as frequently as 2 in every 100 births (3). The finding sometimes remains clinically silent throughout life, found incidentally at autopsy. However, the tendency is to have progressive thickening and fibrosis of the valve with aging. Valve stenosis is the most common complication of this malformation. When stenosis occurs, virtually all adult patients will have calcification of the valve found at pathologic tissue examination. Abundant aortic valve calcification found on chest radiographs in a patient under the age of 50 should be mentioned in reports as a possible diagnosis of valve stenosis, especially if associated with dilatation of

Bicuspid aortic valve is the second most common major cardiac malformation after mitral valve prolapse.

Table 19.1: Outline of Congenital Heart Disease

Acyanotic Conditions	Cyanotic Conditions
Bicuspid aortic valve	Eisenmenger physiology
Aortic arch anomalies	Tetralogy of Fallot
Anomalous coronary artery origins	Ebstein anomaly
Left-to-right cardiac shunts	Rare adult conditions
Pulmonary valve stenosis	Abnormal situs
Absent pulmonary valve	
Cor triatriatum	
Corrected transposition	
Left superior vena cava	
Azygos continuation of the inferior vena cava	

Aortic valve calcification, particularly in individuals less than 50 years of age, has a high association with aortic valve stenosis.

the ascending aortic outline (Fig. 19.1). Incidental identification of abundant aortic valve calcification on chest CT in patients under the age of 55 should also be reported as a possible case of aortic valve stenosis (Fig. 19.2) (4). Congenital subaortic and supraaortic valve stenoses are uncommon conditions in adults shown on occasion on imaging studies (Fig. 19.3).

Table 19.2: Common Anomalies of the Aortic Arch

Left aortic arch with aberrant right subclavian artery
Right aortic arch with aberrant left subclavian artery
Mirror image right aortic arch
Double aortic arch
Cervical aortic arch

ANOMALIES OF THE THORACIC AORTA

The nature of the embryologic development of the aortic arch and its branches leads to rather common malformations that can be clinically silent or can lead to clinical symptoms. Some of the anomalies are common, and others are quite rare (5,6). Table 19.2 outlines some of the common arch anomalies.

The *left aortic arch with aberrant right subclavian artery* is the most common major arterial anomaly, affecting 0.4% to 2% of the population. In this anomaly, the right subclavian artery takes off as the final branch of the aorta, not as the first branch. Patients with this anomaly are usually asymptomatic or have symptoms of dysphagia. There is no increase in the incidence of other associated congenital defects. Over half of these patients will show an abnormal mediastinal contour at the aortic arch level on frontal chest radiographs representing dilatation of the proximal portion of the aberrant artery, the so-called diverticulum of Kommerell (Fig. 19.4A). Lateral chest radiographs can show the abnormality as opacity projecting in the mediastinum behind the trachea, anterior to the spine, and above the aortic arch (the Raider triangle) (Fig. 19.4B) (7). The retrotracheal opacity represents the subclavian artery as it passes behind the esophagus and trachea through the mediastinum. If desired clinically, CT can prove the diagnosis of the aberrant artery (Fig. 19.4C). On occasion, the aberrant right subclavian artery can be seen as an oblique edge coming off the aorta and as an opacity projecting through the trachea extending to the right on the frontal view (Fig. 19.5) (8).

A right aortic arch identified incidentally in an adult almost always has an aberrant left subclavian artery.

Right aortic arch with mirror image branching has a very high (95%) association with severe congenital heart disease, including truncus arteriosus and tetralogy of Fallot.

The *right aortic arch with aberrant left subclavian artery* origin is an anomaly that is also generally an incidental finding on chest radiographs. However, there is a small association with other congenital heart defects. Chest radiographs show a right aortic arch

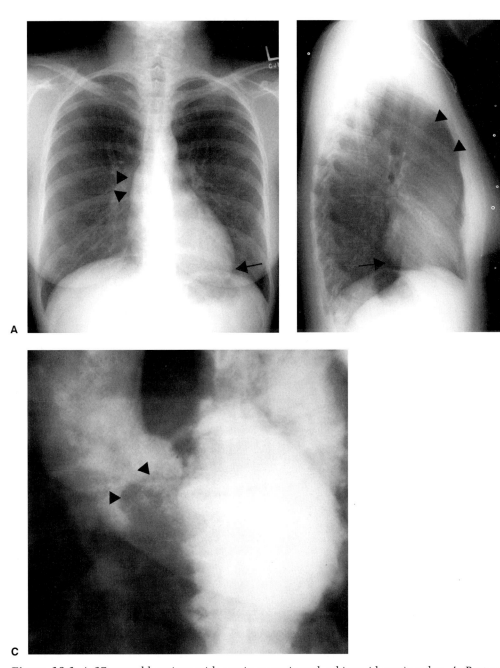

Figure 19.1 A 37-year-old patient with aortic stenosis and a bicuspid aortic valve. *A.* Postero-anterior chest radiograph shows a convex opacity along the right side of the mediastinum (*arrow-heads*) representing poststenotic dilatation of the ascending aorta. In this case the left ventricle is enlarged, showing elongation of the heart and pointing of the cardiac apex toward the left costophrenic angle (*arrow*). *B.* Lateral chest radiograph demonstrates the dilated ascending aorta (*arrowheads*) and posterior displacement of the left ventricle at the posterior-inferior cardiac margin (*arrow*). *C.* Frame from a cineangiogram of the aortic root shows "doming" (*arrowheads*) of the stenotic bicuspid aortic valve.

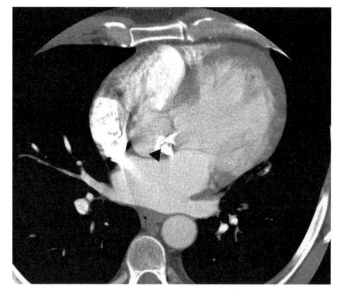

Figure 19.2 A 45-year-old woman with a bicuspid aortic valve and valve stenosis. Computed tomography image at the aortic valve level shows abundant calcification of the valve (*arrowhead*).

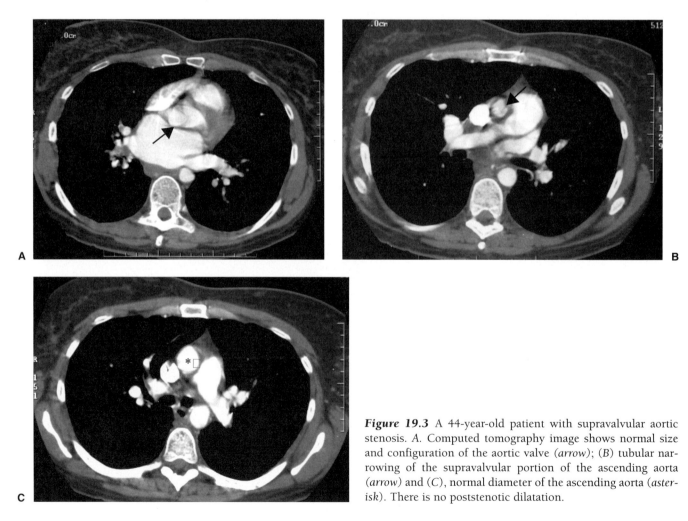

Figure 19.3 A 44-year-old patient with supravalvular aortic stenosis. *A.* Computed tomography image shows normal size and configuration of the aortic valve (*arrow*); (*B*) tubular narrowing of the supravalvular portion of the ascending aorta (*arrow*) and (*C*), normal diameter of the ascending aorta (*asterisk*). There is no poststenotic dilatation.

with opacity in the Raider triangle on the lateral view representing the aberrant artery (Fig. 19.6).

The *mirror image right aortic arch* (no aberrant subclavian artery) has a high rate (95%) of association with severe congenital heart disease, usually of the cyanotic type such as tetralogy of Fallot, truncus arteriosus, or pulmonary atresia. However, the anomaly can be seen as an incidental finding on chest radiographs and CT studies. The *double aortic arch* forms a complete vascular ring, usually presenting in childhood with symptoms of compression of mediastinal structures. On occasion, the double arch first presents in adulthood (Fig. 19.7). The *cervical aortic arch* anomaly is relatively rare, usually presenting as an incidental finding (Fig. 19.8).

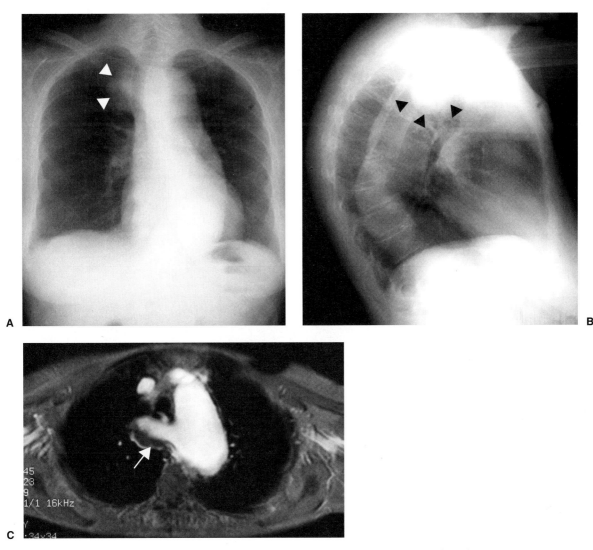

Figure 19.4 A 77-year-old patient with aneurysmal dilatation of the thoracic aorta and an aberrant right subclavian artery. *A.* Posterior anterior chest radiograph shows a left aortic arch. A mass-like protuberance projecting to the right of the superior mediastinum (*arrowheads*) represents an aneurysm of an aberrant right subclavian artery. *B.* The lateral chest radiograph shows an opacity posterior to the tracheal air column (*arrowheads*) in Raider's triangle representing the aberrant subclavian artery shown on end. *C.* A computed tomography image of the arch demonstrates an aneurysm of the aberrant right subclavian artery. Thrombus is shown in the posterior portion of the aneurysm (*arrow*).

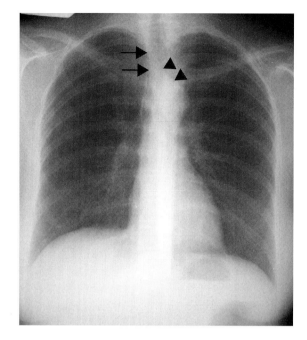

Figure 19.5 Posterior anterior chest radiograph shows an aberrant right subclavian artery as an oblique opacity (*arrowheads*) arising from the aortic arch, passing to the right. In this case the artery can be seen through the tracheal air column (*arrows*).

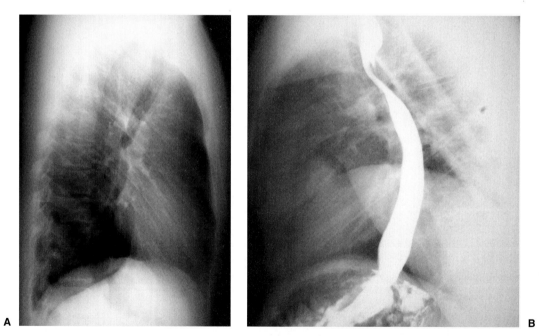

A   B

Figure 19.6 An adult patient with a right-sided aortic arch and an aberrant left subclavian artery. *A.* Lateral chest radiograph shows the aberrant left subclavian artery as a round opacity in Raider's triangle. *B.* Lateral view of an esophagram shows a posterior impression on the barium column caused by the aberrant left subclavian artery.

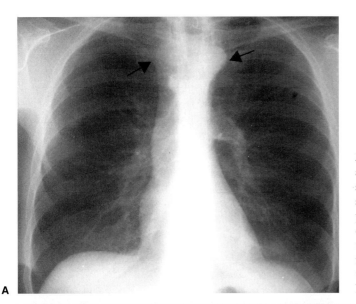

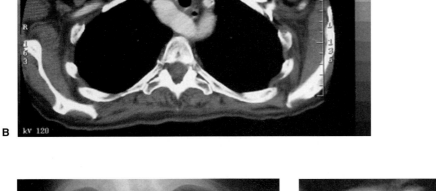

Figure 19.7 A 63-year-old patient with a double aortic arch. *A.* Posterior anterior chest radiograph shows a double aortic arch as opacities lying on both sides of the tracheal air column *(arrows)*. *B.* Computed tomography image shows the double arches coming together posteriorly as a single descending thoracic aorta. The arches arose from a single ascending aortic lumen below this axial section. In this case, the arches are of equal caliber. The left arch is hypoplastic in many cases.

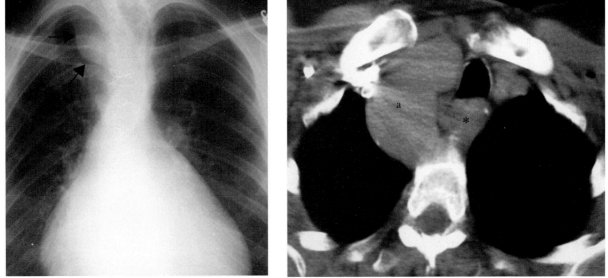

Figure 19.8 A 59-year-old patient with prior surgery for rheumatic heart disease and a right-sided cervical aortic arch. *A.* Posteroanterior view of the chest radiograph shows the high cervical right arch *(arrows)* at the thoracic inlet, displacing the trachea to the left. *B.* Computed tomography section shows the right cervical arch (a) at the thoracic inlet. There is an aberrant left subclavian artery *(asterisk)*.

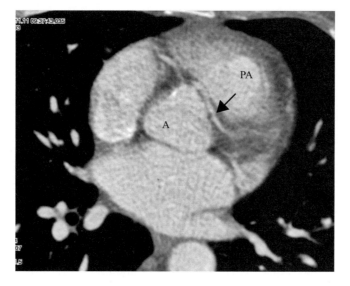

Figure 19.9 Computed tomography image shows an aberrant anterior descending coronary artery origin (*arrow*) arising from the right coronary sinus of Valsalva next to the right coronary artery. The left anterior descending artery passes between the aorta (A) and root of the pulmonary artery (PA). (Courtesy of James Mastromatteo, MD, Boston, MA.)

ANOMALOUS CORONARY ARTERY ORIGINS FROM THE AORTA

Anomalous origin of a coronary artery can occur from the pulmonary artery or aorta. Patients with ectopic origin of both coronary arteries from the pulmonary artery are discovered early in life because of severe myocardial ischemia. Origin of one main coronary from the pulmonary artery with the other from the aorta is also a serious malformation, but some patients do survive past childhood. Ectopic origin of one or both coronary arteries, or of individual branches, from the aorta is compatible with life, found in 0.6% to 0.9% of the population (9,10). On occasion, CT or MRI can show these aberrant origins as an incidental finding. At other times, patients with unexplained chest pain and abnormal stress tests or a familial history of sudden death at a young age are referred for echocardiography, CT or MRI to show the coronary artery origins. The course of the ectopic coronary arteries can proceed from the origin to its myocardial distribution by several possible routes (11). The artery can pass between the pulmonary artery and aortic root (Fig. 19.9) or can course anterior or posterior to these structures. When a major coronary artery such as the left main or left anterior descending artery passes between the pulmonary artery and the aorta, there is a small risk of sudden death.

Anomalous coronary artery origin may be a cause of unexplained chest pain, particularly in young adults in whom atherosclerotic disease is less likely.

LEFT-TO-RIGHT SHUNTS

Atrial Septal Defect

The isolated small patent foramen ovale or atrial septal secundum defect is the most common postchildhood left-to-right shunt (12), with an estimated prevalence of 0.6 per 1000 (1). Ventricular septal defects are more common in children, but most close spontaneously or are repaired. Large atrial septal defects such as sinus venosus and ostium primum defects or atrial septal defects associated with other anomalies are usually discovered in childhood. Chest radiographs of patients with atrial septal defect show increased pulmonary vascularity and enlarged pulmonary arteries (Fig. 19.10). The heart can be normal in size but can enlarge, particularly in patients who develop mitral and tricuspid valve regurgitation (Fig. 19.11). Right ventricular enlargement is usually evident on the lateral view (Fig. 19.12). The aortic arch is relatively small in many patients with atrial septal defect. Cardiac MRI (Fig. 19.13) and CT (Fig. 19.14) can show the defect, although echocardiography is the primary modality used to confirm the diagnosis. Table 19.3 lists the common differential diagnosis for noncyanotic cardiac shunts.

An isolated arterial septal defect is the most common postchildhood left-to-right cardiac shunt.

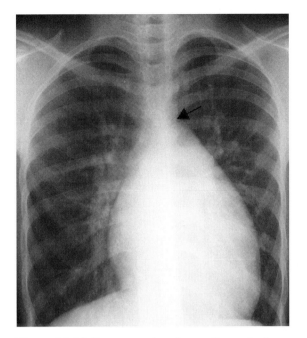

Figure 19.10 Posteroanterior chest radiograph shows increased pulmonary vascularity. The central pulmonary arteries are dilated. The rounded right heart border represents right atrial dilatation, and the round left heart margin is secondary to right ventricular enlargement. Many patients, like this one with atrial septal defect, have an associated small aortic arch *(arrow)*.

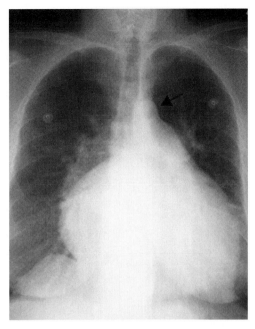

Figure 19.11 Posteroanterior chest radiograph shows markedly dilated chambers in this 76-year-old patient with an atrial septal defect. Echocardiography revealed tricuspid and mitral valve regurgitation. The aortic arch *(arrow)* shows atheromatous calcification but remains small in diameter.

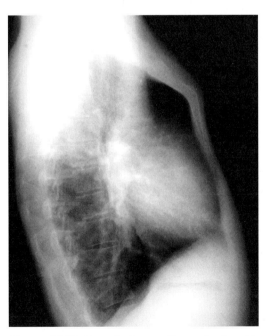

Figure 19.12 Lateral chest radiograph of a 49-year-old patient with an atrial septal defect shows fullness posterior to the sternum, representing right ventricular dilatation. There is pectus carinatum deformity of the sternum, an anomaly with known association with septal defects.

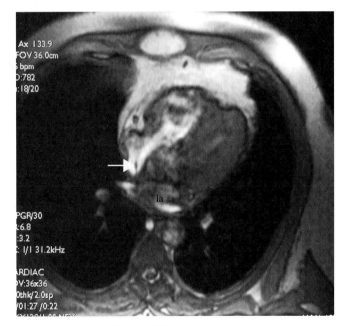

Figure 19.13 A 28-year-old patient with a patent foramen ovale. Frame from a cine-magnetic resonance imaging study in the four-chamber view shows a small dark jet of blood *(arrow)* crossing the interatrial septum from the left atrium (la) to the right atrium through the patent foramen ovale.

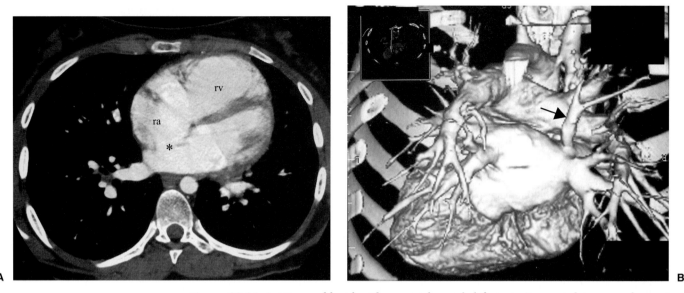

A

B

Figure 19.14 A 17-year-old girl with an atrial septal defect. *A.* Computed tomography section through all four cardiac chambers shows the atrial septal defect (*asterisk*) as interruption of the septum between the two atria. The right atrium (ra) and right ventricle (rv) are dilated, and the ventricular septum is flattened because of high pressure and volume in the right ventricle. *B.* Reconstructed three-dimensional image of the left atrium and pulmonary veins shows an anomalous course of a vertical vein emptying the posterior segment of the right upper lobe into the left atrium (*arrow*). Anomalies of pulmonary veins occur frequently in association with atrial septal defect, often emptying into the right atrium or vena cava.

Ventricular Septal Defect

> Ventricular septal defects are uncommon in adults, usually either closing spontaneously (the majority) or having been closed surgically during childhood.

> Eisenmenger physiology with pulmonary hypertension develops secondary to chronically elevated pulmonary blood flow with elevated right ventricular pressure creating a bidirectional shunt and leading to cyanosis.

Isolated ventricular septal defects are relatively common congenital malformations in children. Many of these shunts close spontaneously. The estimated prevalence in adults is 0.3 per 1000 (1). Adults presenting with ventricular septal defects for the first time can be asymptomatic or can present with pulmonary hypertension and Eisenmenger physiology (13). Eisenmenger physiology occurs when there is pulmonary hypertension secondary to chronic increases in pulmonary blood flow and elevated right ventricular pressure.

The elevated right ventricular pressure stifles left ventricular shunting and eventually leads to bidirectional flow across the septum, which in turn leads to cyanosis. Patients with small ventricular septal defects can have normal pulmonary vascularity and heart size. In these cases the diagnosis is made on physical examination and echocardiography. In patients with large shunts or Eisenmenger physiology, chest radiographs show increased pulmonary vascularity, enlargement of the central pulmonary arteries, right ventricular enlargement, and a normal aortic arch (Fig. 19.15). Left atrial enlargement is commonly seen in children but is usually absent in adults unless there is mitral valve regurgitation (14). MRI can show these defects in detail (Fig. 19.16).

Table 19.3: Congenital Noncyanotic Cardiac Shunts
Atrial septal defect
Ventricular septal defect
Patent ductus arteriosus
Partial anomalous pulmonary venous return
Coronary artery fistula
Ruptured sinus of Valsalva aneurysm

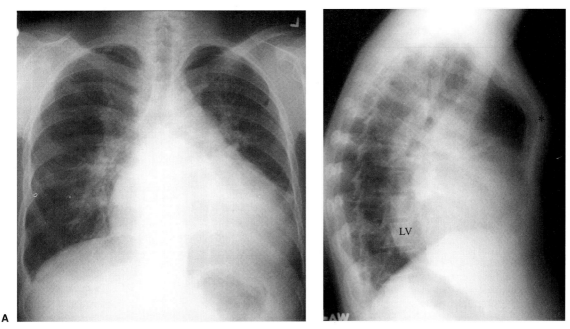

A   B

Figure 19.15 A 38-year-old patient with a 2:1 left-to-right shunt through a ventricular septal defect. *A.* A posteroanterior chest radiograph shows shunt vascularity, cardiomegaly, dilated central pulmonary arteries, and normal size of the aortic arch. *B.* A lateral chest radiograph on the same patient shows dilatation of the left ventricle (LV) posterior to the inferior vena cava. The dilated right ventricle is shown as fullness behind the sternum. This patient shows pectus carinatum deformity of the sternum (*asterisk*).

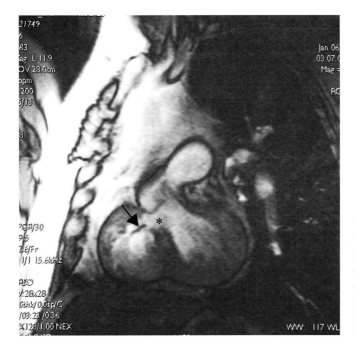

Figure 19.16 A 48-year-old patient with a ventricular septal defect. Image from cine magnetic resonance imaging in the double-oblique short-axis view shows blood flow as a black jet (*arrow*) across the interventricular septum through a high septal defect (*asterisk*).

Patent Ductus Arteriosus

Most patent ductus arteriosi close spontaneously or are repaired during childhood. For this reason, patients rarely first present with patent ductus as adults. McManus (15) summarized the pathologic findings of 46 patients 50 years of age or older. In this summary, patients generally had cardiomegaly, and calcification was frequently present in the arch and ductus. Pulmonary hypertension was severe. Chest radiographs in adults with patent ductus look much like chronic ventricular septal defect, showing increased pulmonary vascularity, dilated central pulmonary arteries, and dilated cardiac chambers (Fig. 19.17). However, many patients with patent ductus will have a dilated aortic arch (16). The diagnosis of patent ductus can also be suspected when chest radiographs show shunt vascularity and calcification of the ductus (Fig. 19.18). MRI and CT (Fig. 19.19) can confirm the diagnosis.

> Ductus calcification (in the aortopulmonary window) with shunt vascularity should raise suspicion for a patent ductus arteriosus in adults.

Partial Anomalous Pulmonary Venous Return

Partial anomalous pulmonary venous return occurs in 0.4% to 0.7% of postmortem studies (17). The condition can be an isolated anomaly or can be associated with the congenital pulmonary venolobar syndrome, a spectrum of anomalies of the lung, cardiovascular structures, and chest wall (18,19). Associated atrial septal defects are common. The anomaly produces physiologic left-to-right shunting of oxygenated blood into the right heart circulation. The "scimitar syndrome" describes the anatomic course of an anomalous pulmonary vein of the right lung that curves inferiorly, disappearing at the diaphragm (Fig. 19.20) as it drains into the inferior vena cava or other nearby venous structures. Atrial septal defects can coexist. This syndrome almost always occurs in association with hypogenetic lung. Anomalous pulmonary veins are more often found as isolated abnormalities, most of the time without significant clinical implication. These venous drainage anomalies can involve either lung (Figs. 19.21, 19.22, and 19.23).

> Partial anomalous pulmonary venous return is commonly associated with an atrial septal defect.

> In scimitar syndrome, the "scimitar" (Turkish word for *sword-like*) vein drains into a vein below the diaphragm, such as an hepatic vein or the inferior vena cava.

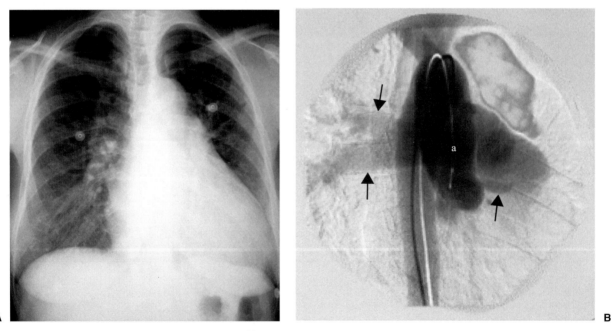

A **B**

Figure 19.17 A 44-year-old patient with 3:1 shunt to the pulmonary arteries through a patent ductus arteriosus. *A.* Posteroanterior chest radiograph shows shunt vascularity in the lungs, cardiac enlargement, and dilated central pulmonary arteries reflecting increased flow and pulmonary hypertension. The aorta is enlarged, a common finding in patients with this anomaly. *B.* Digital angiogram in the frontal view after injection of contrast material in the aortic root. The contrast fills the proximal aorta (a), with early filling of the pulmonary arteries (*arrows*) through the patent ductus. The ductus is not shown directly in this view.

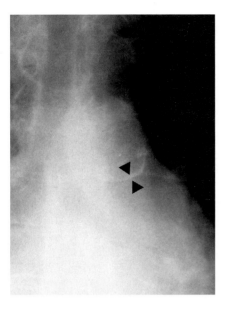

Figure 19.18 Posteroanterior chest radiograph in a 72-year-old patient with a calcified patent ductus arteriosus. The ductus is shown as a calcified tubular structure *(arrowheads)* projecting between the aortic arch and the pulmonary artery.

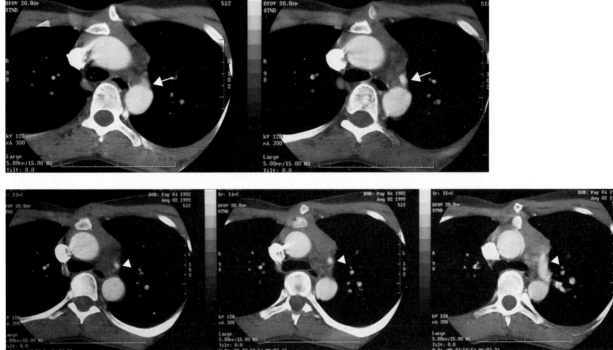

Figure 19.19 Images from a computed tomography in a 17-year-old patient who had previous repair of an ascending aortic aneurysm demonstrate incidental finding of a small patent ductus arteriosus. A. The patent ductus *(arrows)* arises from the junction of the aortic arch and descending thoracic aorta. B. The ductus *(arrowheads)* extends anteriorly and inferiorly to the top of the pulmonary artery.

Ruptured Sinus of Valsalva Aneurysm

The three sinuses of Valsalva dilate naturally as a consequence of aging. The sinuses also dilate in disease states, such as Marfan syndrome and ankylosing spondylitis. Congenital dilatation of one sinus is a rare condition, probably related to a defect in the media of the aortic wall behind a sinus of Valsalva (20). Seventy percent of these aneurysms involve the right anterior cusp and 29% the posterior cusp. Less than 1% of these aneurysms involve the left cusp. Most ruptured aneurysms empty into the right ventricle and less commonly into the right atrium. A left-to-right shunt is suddenly created with new communication

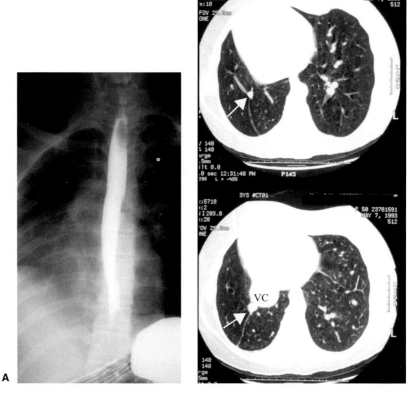

Figure 19.20 A 50-year-old patient with the "scimitar" syndrome. *A.* A posteroanterior chest radiograph demonstrates a small right lung and hemithorax with mediastinal shift to the right. The pulmonary vessels in the right lung are hypoplastic. The anomalous right pulmonary vein is hidden behind the heart in this case. Blood flow to the right lung is increased because of the presence of atrial and ventricular septal defects, as well as a patent ductus arteriosus. *B.* Computed tomography images show the anomalous vein *(arrows)* extending inferiorly to its point of entry into the inferior vena cava (VC).

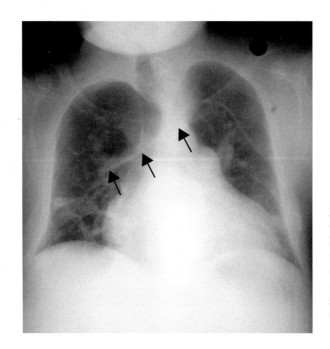

Figure 19.21 A 28-year-old patient with sickle cell disease. The patient has an anomalous draining vein from the right upper lobe. Posteroanterior chest radiograph demonstrates a catheter that extends from the left subclavian vein, into the superior vena cava, into the anomalous vein *(arrows)*.

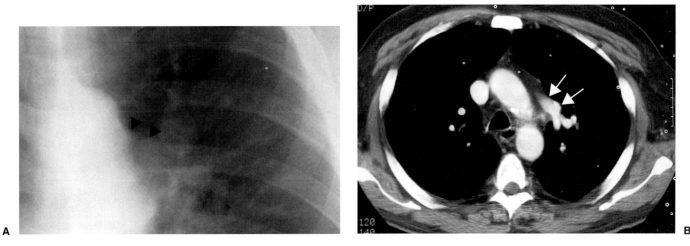

Figure 19.22 A 62-year-old patient with anomalous venous drainage of the left upper lobe. *A.* A posteroanterior chest radiograph shows an oblique opacity (*arrowheads*) at the aortopulmonary window representing an anomalous left upper lobe vein. *B.* A computed tomography shows the anomalous left upper lobe vein (*arrows*) that drains into the left brachiocephalic vein.

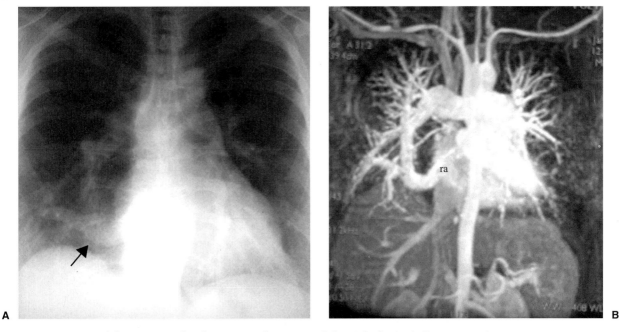

Figure 19.23 An adult patient with a large anomalous vein of the right lung. *A.* Posteroanterior chest radiograph shows a large anomalous draining vein (*arrow*) of the right lung. *B.* Reconstructed contrast-enhanced coronal magnetic resonance image shows the anomalous right pulmonary vein emptying into the right atrium (ra).

between the aorta and right-sided cardiac chamber. Chest radiographic changes depend on the size of the aneurysm and corresponding shunt. The aneurysm, if large, can be seen as a bulge near the aortic root. Two of our four patients with sinus of Valsalva aneurysm had cardiomegaly on radiographs, and shunt vascularity was shown in one (Fig. 19.24). MRI can be a valuable tool to show the anatomy before surgery (Fig. 19.25).

PULMONIC VALVE STENOSIS

Congenital stenosis of the pulmonic valve is a common anomaly, comprising about 6% to 10% of all congenital heart disease. There are several different types of stenosis, including the typical domed valve, the dysplastic valve, and the bicuspid valve (21). Pulmonic valve stenosis can go undetected until adulthood, when the defect is an isolated finding and when the degree of stenosis is not severe. The diagnosis is made if right heart failure occurs, if a murmur is found on physical examination, or on occasion when a radiologist discovers the diagnosis as an incidental finding. The chest radiographs of these patients show dilatation of the main and left pulmonary arteries and normal heart size until right heart failure intervenes (Fig. 19.26). Poststenotic turbulent blood flow causes dilatation of the main pulmonary artery and the directly aligned left pulmonary artery. The nondilated right pulmonary artery is protected from the effect of turbulent flow as it extends perpendicular to the flow through the main pulmonary artery.

> Isolated dilation of the main and left pulmonary arteries, sparing the right pulmonary artery, should raise suspicion of pulmonic valve stenosis.

ABSENT PULMONIC VALVE

Congenital absence of the pulmonic valve is a rare anomaly, found in a small percentage of patients with tetralogy of Fallot. It is even more unusual to see absence of the valve as an isolated defect. In this condition, a ring of thickened tissue is present at the expected location of the valve leaflets (21). Patients have wide-open pulmonic regurgitation with a dilated right ventricle and atrium (Fig. 19.27).

COR TRIATRIATUM

In this condition, the common pulmonary vein fails to incorporate into the upper posterior portion of the left atrium during fetal development of the heart chambers. As a consequence, the left atrium is subdivided into two portions by a septum with a perforation

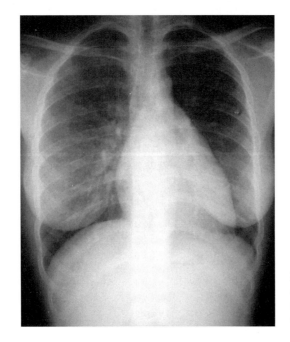

Figure 19.24 Posteroanterior chest radiograph in a 20-year-old patient with sudden rupture of a sinus of Valsalva shows shunt vascularity and upper normal heart size.

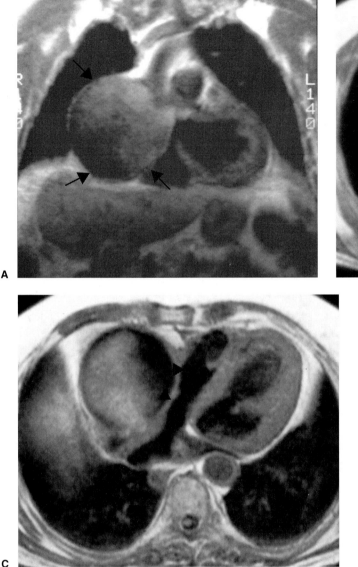

A

B

C

Figure 19.25 Magnetic resonance images of a 74-year-old patient with a huge, nonruptured, sinus of Valsalva aneurysm. *A.* Coronal view shows the large sinus of Valsalva aneurysm (*arrows*) occupying the entire right margin of the mediastinum adjacent to the heart. *B.* Axial view shows the aneurysm (*arrowheads*) arising from the right side of the aortic root. The origin of the aneurysm could arise from either the right or noncoronary sinus. *C.* Axial view shows the aneurysm compressing the right atrial and ventricular chambers (*arrowheads*).

(Fig. 19.28). The upper "chamber" receives the pulmonary veins, whereas the lower "chamber" communicates with the left atrial appendage and empties through the mitral valve. If the opening of the septation is small, pulmonary venous and capillary pressures are elevated. Most cases are discovered in infancy or childhood, but adult patients can present with chronic and recurrent heart failure (22).

CORRECTED TRANSPOSITION OF THE GREAT VESSELS

Patients with congenitally corrected transposition of the great vessels, unassociated with other cardiac defects, can survive into adulthood without detection. Patients with this anomaly have atrioventricular and ventriculoarterial discordance. In other words, the right atrium empties deoxygenated blood into the left ventricle, which in turn pumps blood into the transposed pulmonary artery. Oxygenated blood returns from the lungs though the pulmonary veins into the left atrium, which empties into the right ventricle, which in turn pumps the blood into the transposed aorta. Thus, blood is oxygenated and pumped to the systemic circulation in a normal sequence. With advancing age, the systemic ventricle (anatomic right ventricle) begins to fail.

In corrected transposition, deoxygenated blood from the systemic venous circulation flows in the lungs, is oxygenated, and flows into the aorta without a shunt lesion; however, the order of the chambers it passes through is abnormal (right atrium → left ventricle → pulmonary artery → left atrium → right ventricle → aorta).

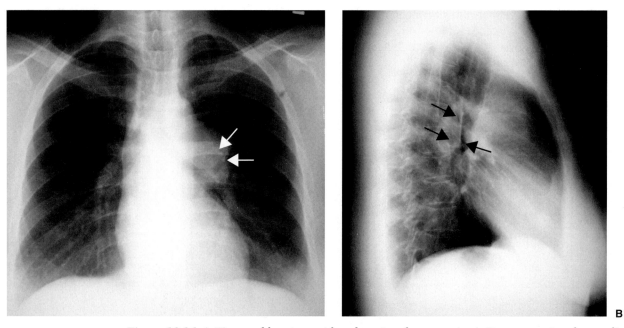

Figure 19.26 A 51-year-old patient with pulmonic valve stenosis. *A.* Posteroanterior chest radiograph shows a dilated left pulmonary artery *(arrows)* projecting above the left main bronchus. Heart size and pulmonary vascularity are normal. *B.* Lateral radiograph shows dilatation of the left pulmonary artery *(arrows)*.

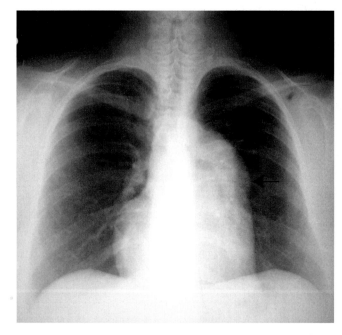

Figure 19.27 Posteroanterior chest radiograph of a 28-year-old patient with absence of the pulmonic valve. The outflow portion of the right ventricle *(arrow)* and the main and left pulmonary arteries are markedly dilated. The right pulmonary artery has a normal diameter.

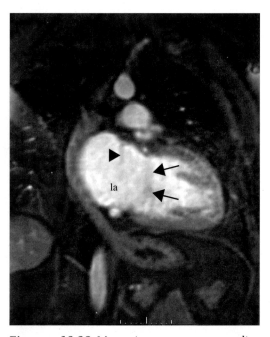

Figure 19.28 Magnetic resonance cardiac angiogram in the coronal view of a 68-year-old patient with cor triatriatum. A web *(arrowhead)* projects within the left atrium (la), above the mitral valve *(arrows)*.

The onset of failure of the systemic ventricle can be attributed to myocardial ischemia in the hypertrophied right ventricular myocardium during periods of high oxygen demand such as stress or exercise (23). Incompetence of the left atrioventricular valve and conduction disturbances also contribute to the development of heart failure. Detection of an abnormally configured cardiovascular outline could be the first clinical clue in making this diagnosis. The classic configuration of the cardiovascular outline was described in 1978, with further description in 1985 (24,25). Many patients will show a convex outward configuration of the left cardiovascular margin caused by levopositioning of the ascending aorta (Fig. 19.29).

With age, the morphologic right ventricle that pumps blood into the aorta, thereby pumping against higher systemic arterial pressure (versus lower pulmonary artery pressure), begins to fail.

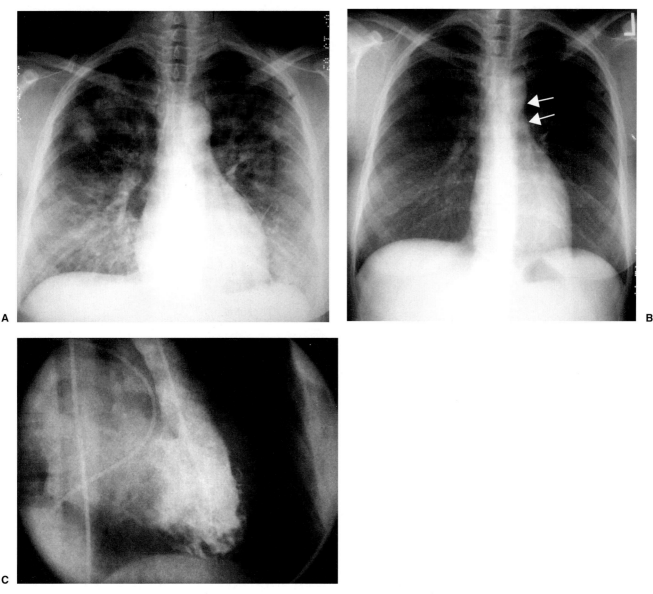

Figure 19.29 A 30-year-old patient with congenitally corrected transposition of the great arteries. *A.* Posteroanterior chest radiograph shows widespread pulmonary edema. *B.* Follow-up frontal chest radiograph after treatment demonstrates a convex left cardiac margin *(arrows)* representing the levopositioned ascending aorta. *C.* Frame from a cine-angiogram shows levopostioning of the ascending aorta that exits from a trabeculated ventricle, with the configuration of an anatomic "right ventricle."

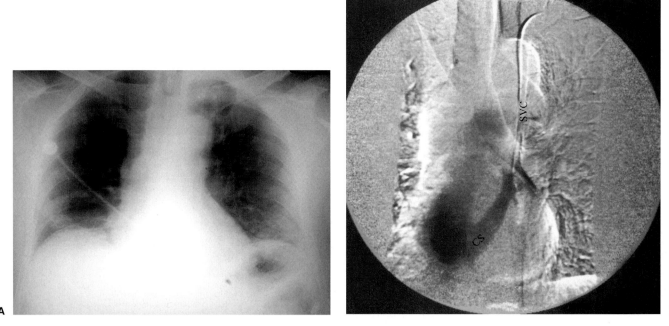

Figure 19.30 An adult patient with passage of a left subclavian catheter into a left superior vena cava. *A.* Posteroanterior chest radiograph shows a left subclavian catheter extending down the left side of the mediastinum. *B.* Digital subtraction angiogram shows the connection of the superior vena cava (SVC) and the coronary sinus (CS).

PERSISTENT LEFT SUPERIOR VENA CAVA

Cases of persistent left superior vena cava are usually discovered incidentally at chest CT or as a result of an abnormal catheter position on a chest radiograph (Fig. 19.30). This anomaly is the most common congenital abnormality of the thoracic veins, occurring in about 0.3% of the population. The left vena cava extends down the left side of the mediastinum and empties into the coronary sinus. Thus, a left paramediastinal position of a catheter is seen on chest radiographs (26). The differential of left-sided catheters on chest radiographs is shown on Table 19.4.

A duplicated superior vena cava is more common than an isolated left superior vena cava.

Table 19.4: *Left Paramediastinal Catheter Position*

Left superior vena cava
Left superior intercostal vein
Left pericardiophrenic vein
Left internal thoracic vein
Left subclavian artery to descending thoracic aorta

AZYGOS CONTINUATION OF THE INFERIOR VENA CAVA

If the right subcardinal vein fails to form the suprarenal segment of the inferior vena cava, the result is congenital absence and azygos continuation of the inferior vena cava (27). In these patients, the azygos and hemiazygos veins dilate in response to increased venous blood flow. This anomaly is often associated with abnormalities of situs. Chest radiographs show dilatation of the azygos vein, and problems such as situs inversus can be observed in some patients (Fig. 19.31).

With azygos continuation of the inferior vena cava, the azygos vein is dilated, and the inferior vena cava opacity on the lateral view of the chest radiograph may be absent.

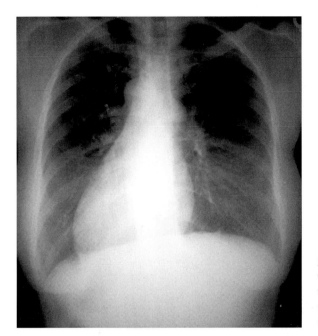

Figure 19.31 A 37-year-old patient with azygos continuation of the inferior vena cava. Posteroanterior chest radiograph shows situs inversus and a dilated azygos vein.

Cyanotic Congenital Heart Disease

No data are available that describe the numbers of and frequency of occurrence of complex congenital heart disease in adults. It is estimated that about 117,000 of these patients were alive in the United States in the year 2000 (1). Cyanotic congenital heart disease can be categorized by the presence or absence of shunt vascularity. This type of classification aids radiologists in deriving lists of differential diagnosis (Tables 19.5 and 19.6). The most common forms of adult congenital cyanotic disease are left-to-right high volume shunts resulting in Eisenmenger physiology, tetralogy of Fallot, and Ebstein anomaly. Rarely, adults with other forms of severe cyanotic disease without prior surgical treatment present for treatment and diagnosis.

Eisenmenger Physiology

Many adults presenting with cyanotic congenital heart disease suffer from chronic uncorrected left-to-right shunts, resulting in Eisenmenger physiology. In these cases, patients have severe pulmonary hypertension with markedly elevated right heart pressures. The pulmonary hypertension is caused by chronic exposure of the pulmonary vessels to marked increases in blood flow, resulting in pulmonary vascular obstructive disease (28). The systemic type pressure in the right chambers causes admixture shunting of desaturated blood to the systemic circulation, producing clinical cyanosis. Chest radiographs of these patients show marked dilatation of the central pulmonary arteries, associated with enlargement of the right ventricle and right atrium (Figs. 19.32 and

Table 19.5: Cyanosis with Shunt Vascularity

Eisenmenger physiology of left-to-right shunts
Transposition of the great vessels
Truncus arteriosus
Total anomalous venous return
Single ventricle
Tricuspid valve atresia with transposition

Table 19.6: Cyanosis without Shunt Vascularity

- Tetralogy of Fallot
- Hypoplastic right heart syndrome
  - Tricuspid valve atresia
  - Pulmonic valve atresia
  - Hypoplastic right ventricle
- Ebstein anomaly

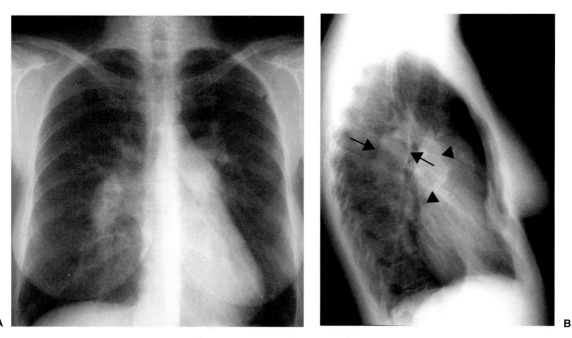

A   B

Figure 19.32 A 42-year-old patient with atrial septal defect and gradual onset of cyanosis secondary to Eisenmenger physiology. *A.* Posteroanterior chest radiograph shows marked dilatation of the central pulmonary arteries. The aortic arch is small, a common finding in patients with atrial septal defect. *B.* Lateral view of the chest shows dilated right *(arrowheads)* and left *(arrows)* pulmonary arteries. Pectus deformity of the sternum obscures the enlarged right ventricle.

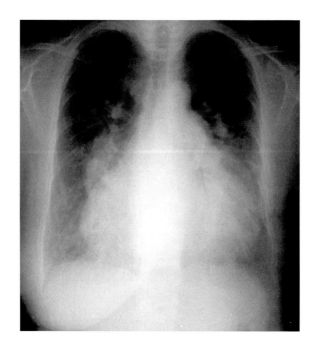

Figure 19.33 Posteroanterior chest radiograph of a 63-year-old patient with an atrial septal primum defect and Eisenmenger physiology. The central pulmonary arteries and all cardiac chambers are dilated.

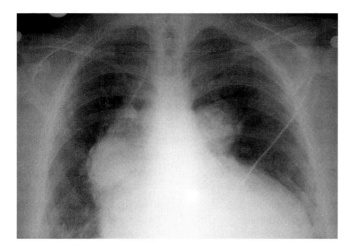

Figure 19.34 Anteroposterior bedside chest radiograph of a 58-year-old patient with marked pulmonary arterial hypertension and Eisenmenger physiology. The patient had an uncorrected 4-cm ventricular septal defect and an atrial septal defect. The markedly dilated central pulmonary arteries have curvilinear peripheral calcification.

19.33). On occasion, the central pulmonary arteries show peripheral calcification (Fig. 19.34). The pulmonary vessels in the mid-lungs are enlarged, reflecting the chronic increase in pulmonary blood flow and pressure.

Signs of Eisenmenger physiology are a large right atrium, right ventricle, and central pulmonary arteries (as a manifestation of pulmonary hypertension) and increased pulmonary blood flow (a manifestation of the shunt lesion).

TETRALOGY OF FALLOT

Another common congenital cause of cyanosis in adults is tetralogy of Fallot. The four components of the malformation are pulmonary stenosis, ventricular septal defect, positioning of the aorta over the interventricular septum, and hypertrophy of the right ventricular myocardium. Adult cases differ from cases appearing in childhood because the ventricular septal defects are smaller, and/or right ventricular outflow obstruction is less severe (29). These cases with a milder form of malformation are sometimes referred to as "pink tetralogy." The radiographic appearance in adults can be similar to that shown in children, showing decreased pulmonary vascularity and a boot-shaped heart due to right ventricular enlargement (Fig. 19.35). However, the configuration is usually not boot shaped in adults, as it often is in infants. In addition, in many instances, adults show normal heart size and pulmonary vascularity because of the milder form of outflow obstruc-

Adults presenting with tetralogy of Fallot usually have smaller septal defects than children and may therefore have normal heart size and normal pulmonary vascularity. The classic "boot-shaped" heart may be absent.

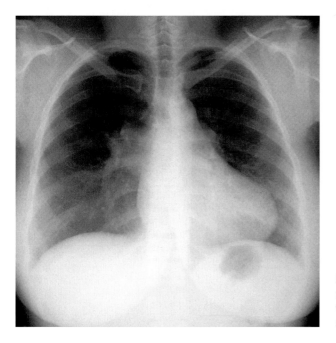

Figure 19.35 Posteroanterior chest radiograph of a 28-year-old patient with tetralogy of Fallot and a boot-shaped heart.

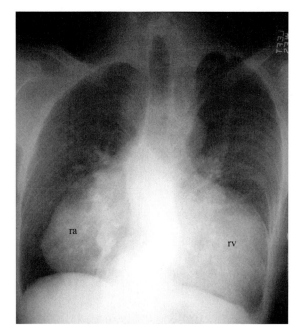

Figure 19.36 Posteroanterior chest radiograph of a 61-year-old patient with untreated tetralogy of Fallot. The right atrium (ra) and right ventricle (rv) are markedly dilated.

tion. In unusual instances the heart can be markedly enlarged (Fig. 19.36). A collateral blood flow pattern due to systemic-to-pulmonary artery anastomoses is sometimes observed (Fig. 19.37).

EBSTEIN ANOMALY

Ebstein anomaly consists of displaced septal and posterior tricuspid valve leaflets into the right ventricle, associated with abnormalities of the wall of the inlet portion of the ventri-

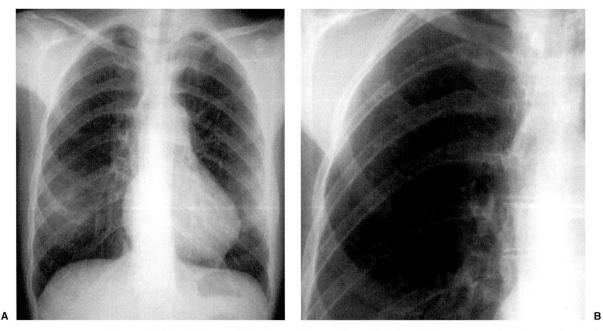

Figure 19.37 A 40-year-old patient with tetralogy of Fallot. *A.* Posteroanterior chest radiograph shows rounding of the cardiac apex because of right ventricular enlargement. *B.* Magnified view shows an abnormal branching pattern of the pulmonary vasculature, representing systemic-to-pulmonary artery collateral vessels.

cle. Only the anterior valve leaflet remains attached to the tricuspid annulus. Blood flow through the right atrium and ventricle is impaired by severe tricuspid regurgitation and by the reduced size of the contracting portion of the ventricular chamber. A right-to-left shunt is produced through a patent foramen of ovale or atrial septal defect. The most severe form of the disease shows extensive thinning of the wall ("atrialization") of the right ventricle with little remaining functional component of the myocardium. The mildest forms of the malformation have displaced leaflets but little thinning and encroachment into the functional portion of the right ventricle. Patients can present at any age depending on the severity of the malformation. Although cyanosis is common in neonates and infants, adults present more commonly with arrhythmia (30).

Associated electrocardiographic abnormalities include right axis deviation, right bundle branch block, and a high incidence of Wolff-Parkinson-White syndrome. The imaging characteristics of the anomaly vary according to the degree of malformation. Standard radiographs usually show cardiomegaly, with marked enlargement in many cases. The degree of cardiac enlargement can be mild in adults (Fig. 19.38). Radiologic images show right-sided chamber dilatation. MRI is an excellent imaging modality, particularly when surgical correction is contemplated (31). However, MR images can be difficult to obtain if there are conduction abnormalities and arrhythmias because of electrocardiographic gating problems during image acquisition (Fig. 19.39).

> Adults with Ebstein anomaly most commonly present with arrhythmias due to conducting system abnormalities.

RARE CYANOTIC HEART DISEASE IN ADULTS

On rare occasions, clinicians request imaging examinations for patients with severe cyanotic malformations that have not had prior surgical correction.

In *complete transposition of the great vessels*, the atria and ventricles have a normal configuration but the pulmonary artery and aorta switch positions. The pulmonary artery arises from the left ventricle and the aorta from the right ventricle. Thus, oxygenated blood returns from the lungs through the pulmonary veins, through the left atrium and left ventricle, only to be pumped back out of the pulmonary arteries to the lungs once

> Rarely, a patient with a large shunt lesion (atrial or ventricular septal defect, patent ductus arteriosus) can present in adulthood with complete transposition of the great arteries.

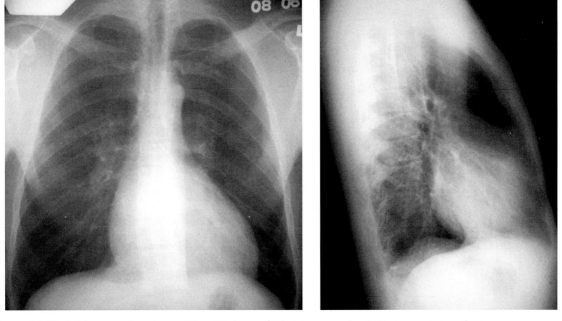

Figure 19.38 A 35-year-old patient with mild form of Ebstein anomaly. *A.* Posteroanterior chest radiograph shows rounding and increased circumference of the right heart margin secondary to right atrial dilatation. The pulmonary blood flow pattern is normal to decreased. *B.* Lateral view of the chest shows retrosternal fullness because of right ventricular dilatation.

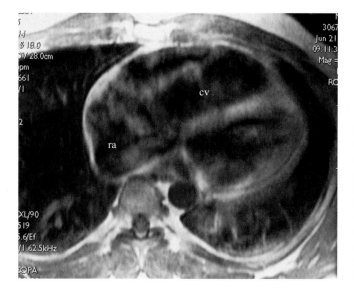

Figure 19.39 Axial magnetic resonance image of a 39-year-old patient with Ebstein anomaly. Anatomic detail is obscured because of difficulty in electro-cardiographic capture because of arrhythmia. The right atrium (ra) and ventricle (rv) are dilated. The abnormal tricuspid valve leaflets cannot be identified because of motion artifact.

again. This configuration is incompatible with life unless there is shunting of oxygenated blood to the systemic circulation through atrial and/or ventricular septal defects or when there is a single ventricle and/or patent ductus arteriosus. On rare occasion, when the shunt is large, a patient can survive naturally into adulthood without having a corrective procedure (32). Chest radiographs show increased pulmonary vascularity, dilated central pulmonary arteries, and cardiac enlargement with an elongated heart and narrow pedicle, the so-called egg-on-a-string appearance (Fig. 19.40). Pulmonary blood flow can appear decreased if the condition is associated with pulmonic stenosis. Cross-sectional imaging can be used to visualize the arrangement of the pulmonary arteries, aorta, and cardiac chamber configuration (Fig. 19.41).

Truncus arteriosus is a cyanotic condition characterized by the presence of a single arterial trunk exiting the heart, overriding a high membranous ventricular septal defect. The truncus gives rise to the pulmonary and coronary arteries. Chest radiographs most commonly show shunt vascularity because of the preferential flow to the lower resistance pulmonary vasculature compared with the systemic circulation. The truncus is right-sided

The "egg-on-a-string" configuration is classic for complete transposition.

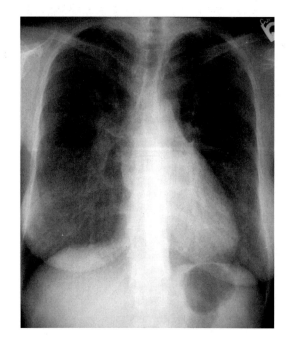

Figure 19.40 Posteroanterior chest radiograph of a 38-year-old patient with untreated transposition of the great arteries. The heart is enlarged and elongated with a relatively narrow pedicle, the so-called "egg-on-a-string" configuration.

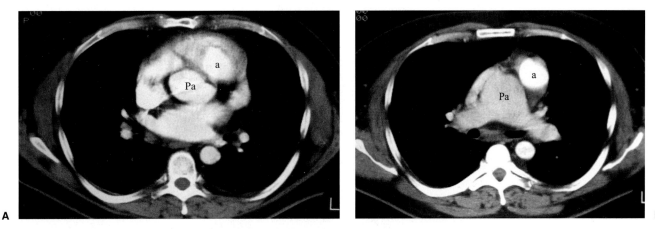

Figure 19.41 Computed tomography images of a middle-aged patient with transposition of the great arteries. *A.* The pulmonary artery (Pa) arises from the posterior left ventricle, and the aorta (a) arises from the anterior right ventricle. *B.* The pulmonary artery (Pa) lies to the right of the aorta (a). The pulmonary artery (Pa) is dilated because of increased pressure and flow from the systemic left ventricle.

in about 25% of cases. Truncus arteriosus can be associated with pulmonic stenosis, in which case the pulmonary vascularity can be normal or decreased (Fig. 19.42). The truncus is dilated, and the heart is usually enlarged with a right ventricular configuration (rounded and uplifted cardiac apex).

Pulmonary atresia can occur as an isolated defect with an intact ventricular septum or can be associated with a ventricular septal defect with or without an overriding aorta. When a ventricular defect is present, the cases can be considered clinically as an extreme form of tetralogy of Fallot. Chest radiographs usually show decreased pulmonary vascularity. However, pulmonary flow can be normal or increased when augmented by flow from a large ductus arteriosus or systemic-to-pulmonary artery collateral vessels (Fig. 19.43). The heart may be normal in size or enlarged. The aorta is usually dilated and left sided. Right arch position is unusual, and if present other diagnoses should be considered (33). MRI can be useful in depicting the pulmonary arteries beyond the point of atresia for planning purposes before surgical bypass (Fig. 19.44).

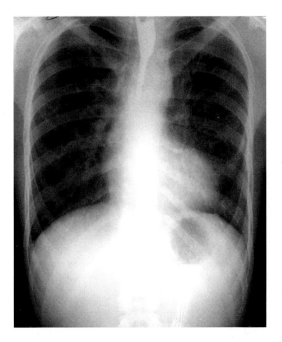

Figure 19.42 Posteroanterior chest radiograph of an 18-year-old patient with truncus arteriosus. The coronary arteries and pulmonary arteries arose from the proximal truncus in this rare case, and the pulmonary arteries were stenotic. The pulmonary arterial stenosis protected the lungs by allowing adequate, not excessive, pulmonary blood flow. The cardiac apex is rounded, indicating right ventricular dilatation, and the enlarged truncus appears in the usual position of the aortic arch.

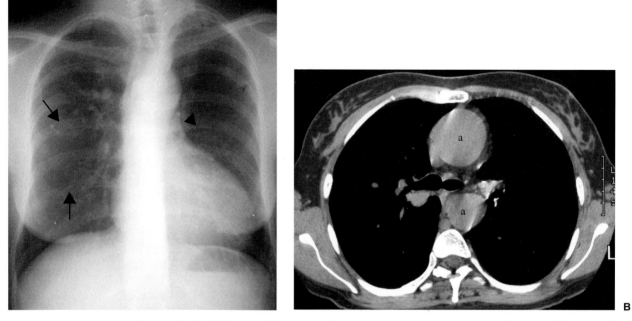

A   B

Figure 19.43 A 39-year-old patient with pulmonary atresia and a ventricular septal defect. *A.* Posteroanterior chest radiograph shows cardiomegaly and a dilated aortic arch. The central pulmonary arteries are small as shown, by example, at the left hilum *(arrowhead)*. Systemic-to-pulmonary artery collateral vessels are shown bilaterally *(arrows)*. *B.* Non–contrast-enhanced computed tomography image at the aortopulmonary window shows dilated ascending and descending aortic segments (a). There are no central pulmonary arteries.

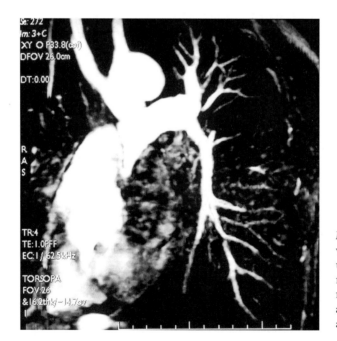

Figure 19.44 A 47-year-old patient with pulmonary atresia and ventricular septal defect. Three-dimensional reconstructed contrast-enhanced magnetic resonance image shows atresia of the main pulmonary artery.

Table 19.7: Situs and Associated Congenital Defects

Situs solitus with:
    Levoversion—no associated defects
    Mesoversion—often no associated defects
    Dextroversion—associated with severe defects
Situs inversus with:
    Dextroversion—associated with less complex defects
    Levoversion—associated with severe defects
    Mesoversion—associated with less complex defects

ABNORMAL SITUS

Abnormalities of situs are encountered on occasion in adult patients. Many cases show situs inversus, a mirror image of the normal arrangement of the viscera or situs solitus. Situs inversus is associated with a normal incidence of other cardiac anomalies. In situs solitus the cardiac apex is usually on the left (levoversion), and in situs inversus the apex is usually on the right (dextroversion). Either situs solitus or inversus can have a midline heart (mesoversion). The terms dextrocardia, levocardia, and mesocardia usually refer to the cardiac position in the thorax, unrelated to the visceral situs. Other cardiac apex locations are associated with an increase in congenital heart defects (Table 19.7). Situs solitus with dextroversion of the heart has a high incidence of associated complex cyanotic defects such as pulmonary atresia or tricuspid atresia. Similarly, situs inversus with levoversion of the heart is associated with complex defects (34). Situs ambiguous, or heterotaxy syndrome, applies to patients with discordant thoracic and abdominal situs (35,36). Heterotaxy syndrome can be discovered in adults without any associated cardiac malformation. However, cardiac anomalies are common (Fig. 19.45).

Patients with situs inversus totalis have no increased incidence of cardiac anomalies.

Dextro-, levo- and mesocardia refer to cardiac position, not situs.

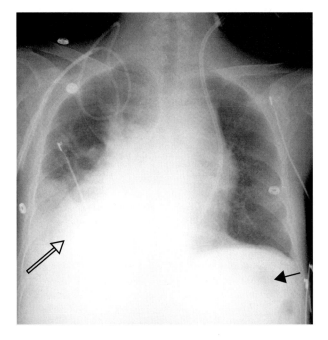

Figure 19.45 Anteroposterior chest radiograph of a 35-year-old patient with heterotaxy syndrome. Cardiac anomalies include a single common atrium and a ventricular septal defect. The cardiac apex *(long, open arrow)* is on the right (dextroversion), whereas the stomach bubble *(arrow)* and splenic flexure lie on the left side.

REFERENCES

1. Warnes CA, Liberthson R, Danielson GK, et al. Task Force 1: The changing profile of congenital heart disease in adult life. *J Am Coll Cardiol* 2001;37:1170–1175.
2. Roberts WC. The 2 most common congenital heart diseases. *Am J Cardiol* 1984;53:1198.
3. Spindola-Franco H, Fish BG. *Radiology of the heart: cardiac imaging in infants, children, and adults.* New York: Springer-Verlag, 1985:190.
4. Lippert JA, White CS, Mason AC, et al. Calcification of aortic valve detected incidentally on CT scans: prevalence and clinical significance. *AJR Am J Roentgenol* 1995;164:73–77.
5. Spindola-Franco H, Fish BG. *Radiology of the heart: cardiac imaging in infants, children, and adults.* New York: Springer-Verlag, 1985:584–608.
6. Stewart JR, Kincaid OW, Edwards JE. *An atlas of vascular rings and related malformations of the aortic arch system.* Springfield, IL: Charles C Thomas 1964.
7. Raider LR, Landry BA, Brogdon BG. The retrotracheal triangle. *Radiographics* 1990;10: 1055–1079.
8. Proto AV, Cuthbert NW, Raider L. Aberrant right subclavian artery: further observations. *AJR Am J Roentgenol* 1987;148:253–257.
9. Kimbiris D, Iskandrian AS, Segal BL, et al. Anomalous aortic origin of coronary arteries. *Circulation* 1978;58:606–615.
10. Baltaxe H, Wixson D. The incidence of congenital anomalies of the coronary arteries in the adult population. *Radiology* 1977;122:47–52.
11. Roberts WC. Major anomalies of coronary arterial origin seen in adulthood. *Am Heart J* 1986; 111:941–963.
12. Steiner RM, Gross GW, Flicker S, et al. Congenital heart disease in the adult patient: the value of plain film chest radiology. *J Thorac Imaging* 1995;10:1–25.
13. Perloff JK. Congenital heart disease in the adult: clinical approach. *J Thorac Imaging* 1994;9: 260–268.
14. Elliott LP. *Cardiac imaging in infants, children, and adults.* Philadelphia: J.B. Lippincott, 1991:573.
15. McManus BM. Patent ductus arteriosus. In: Roberts WC, ed. *Adult congenital heart disease.* Philadelphia: F.A. Davis, 1987:455–476.
16. Swischuk LE. Patent ductus arteriosus. *Semin Roentgenol* 1985;20:236–243.
17. Spindola-Franco H, Fish BG. *Radiology of the heart: cardiac imaging in infants, children, and adults.* New York: Springer-Verlag, 1985:317.
18. Felson B. *Chest roentgenology.* Philadelphia: W.B. Saunders, 1973:81–92.
19. Woodring JH, Howard TA, Kanga JF. Congenital pulmonary venolobar syndrome revisited. *Radiographics* 1994;14:349-369.
20. Roberts WC. *Adult congenital heart disease.* Philadelphia: F.A. Davis, 1987:670–675.
21. Jeffery RF, Moller JH, Amplatz K. The dysplastic pulmonary valve: a new roentgenographic entity: with a discussion of the anatomy and radiology of other types of valvular pulmonary stenosis. *AJR Am J Roentgenol* 1972;114:322–339.
22. Van Son JAM, Danielson GK, Schaff HV, et al. Cor triatriatum: diagnosis, operative approach, and late results. *Mayo Clin Proc* 1993;68:854–859.
23. Graham TP Jr, Bernard YD, Mellen BG, et al. Long-term outcome in congenitally corrected transposition of the great arteries: a multi-institutional study. *J Am Coll Cardiol* 2000;36:255–261.
24. Bream PR, Elliott LP, Bargeron LM Jr. Plain film findings of anatomically corrected malposition: its association with juxtaposition of the atrial appendages and right aortic arch. *Radiology* 1978; 126:589–595.
25. Guit GL, Kroon HM, van Voorthuisen AE, et al. Congenitally corrected transposition in adults with left atrioventricular valve incompetence. *Radiology* 1985;155:567–570.
26. Godwin JD, Chen JTT. Thoracic venous anatomy. *AJR Am J Roentgenol* 1986;147:674–684.
27. Bass JE, Redwine MD, Kramer LA, et al. Spectrum of congenital anomalies of the inferior vena cava: cross-sectional imaging findings. *Radiographics* 2000;20:639–652.
28. Brickner ME, Hillis LD, Lange RA. Congenital heart disease in adults. *N Engl J Med* 2000;342: 334–342.
29. Swischuk LE, Sapire DW. *Basic imaging in congenital heart disease*, 3rd ed. Baltimore: Williams & Wilkins, 1986:164–175.

30. Celermajer DS, Bull C, Till JA, et al. Ebstein's anomaly: presentation and outcome from fetus to adult. *J Am Coll Cardiol* 1994;23:170–176.
31. Choi YH, Park JH, Choe YH, et al. MR imaging of Ebstein's anomaly of the tricuspid valve. *AJR Am J Roentgenol* 1994;163:539–543.
32. Kidd L, O'Neal Humphries J. Complete and congenitally corrected transposition of the great arteries. In: Roberts WC, ed. *Adult congenital heart disease*. Philadelphia: F.A. Davis, 1987: 521–540.
33. Spindola-Franco H, Fish BG. *Radiology of the heart: cardiac imaging in infants, children, and adults*. New York: Springer-Verlag, 1985:519.
34. Spindola-Franco H, Fish BG. *Radiology of the heart: cardiac imaging in infants, children, and adults*. New York: Springer-Verlag, 1985:620–621.
35. Van Praagh R. The importance of segmental situs in the diagnosis of congenital heart disease. *Semin Roentgenol* 1985;20:254–271.
36. Winer-Muram HT, Tonkin ILD. The spectrum of heterotaxic syndromes. *Radiol Clin North Am* 1989;27:1147–1170.

ACQUIRED CARDIAC DISEASE

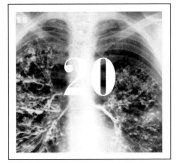

- Cardiac Valve Disease
- Myocardial Disease
- Pericardial Disease
- Ischemic Heart Disease
- Neoplastic Disease

Heart disease is the leading cause of death in the United States. Patients with acquired heart disease can present with classic clinical syndromes, such as angina and myocardial infarction or with vague symptoms such as fatigue or shortness of breath. However, many patients with heart disease present with atypical clinical signs and symptoms or are entirely free of any sign of disease. Radiologists play a key role in making the initial diagnosis of heart disease in many cardiac patients. Imaging is also one of the most important tools used to assess the effectiveness of treatment of cardiovascular disease. In this chapter we cover the basic imaging features of adult acquired heart disease, with an emphasis on chest radiography. Table 20.1 provides an outline of topics covered.

CARDIAC VALVE DISEASE

MITRAL VALVE DISEASE

According to the American Heart Association 2000 statistical update (1), there were 40,000 hospital discharges secondary to mitral valve disease in the year 2000. Approximately 2,500 U.S. citizens died, and 6,100 other deaths involved mitral disease as a contributing factor. Pure mitral stenosis comprises 25% of all cases of mitral disease, pure insufficiency 37%, and combined mitral stenosis and insufficiency 39% (2). Postinflammatory disease (chronic fibrosis) commonly causes mitral stenosis, whereas floppy valve and inflammatory disease are the most common causes of mitral insufficiency.

Combined mitral stenosis and insufficiency is more common than isolated stenosis or isolated insufficiency.

The radiographic diagnosis of mitral valve disease centers on detection of a dilated left atrial chamber (Table 20.2). It should be mentioned, however, that the left atrial volume must increase more than 200% to be detected on radiography (3). The "double density" sign occurs in the frontal projection when the left atrial opacity projects through the right atrial outline (Fig. 20.1). The left atrium can be seen normally through the right atrium but should be considered enlarged when the distance between the right lateral margin of the left atrium and the bottom of the mid-point of the left main bronchus measures more than 7 cm (4). Focal enlargement of the left atrial appendage in the frontal view is an additional important sign of mitral disease (Fig. 20.2). The enlarged atrial appendage projects as a local bump along the left heart outline, below the level of the left main bronchus. This

Left atrial volume must be twice that of normal to be detectable radiographically.

Table 20.1: Outline of Topics: Imaging of Adult Acquired Heart Disease

Valve disease
   Mitral
   Aortic
   Pulmonic and tricuspid
Myocardial disease
   Cardiomyopathy
   Myocarditis
Neoplastic disease
Pericardial disease
   Pericardial effusion
   Constrictive pericarditis
Coronary artery disease
   Coronary calcification
   Myocardial infarction

Table 20.1: Chest Radiograph Signs of Left Atrial Enlargement

Double density
Fourth mogul
Displaced left main and lower lobe bronchi
Posterior bulge of upper posterior cardiac outline
Displaced barium-filled esophagus

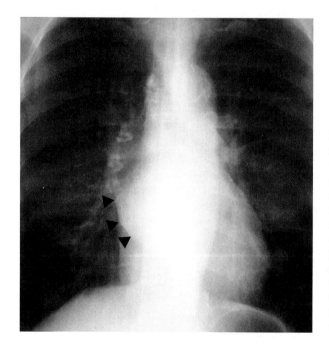

Figure 20.1 Posteroanterior chest radiograph of a 66-year-old patient with mitral valve stenosis. The left atrium can be seen as a hemispherical opacity (*arrowheads*) projecting through the right atrium, the so-called "*double density*" sign. The normal left atrium can be seen in some patients as a "*double density*." To be called enlarged, the distance from the right lateral margin of the left atrium to the mid-point of the left main bronchus should measure more than 7 cm in most patients.

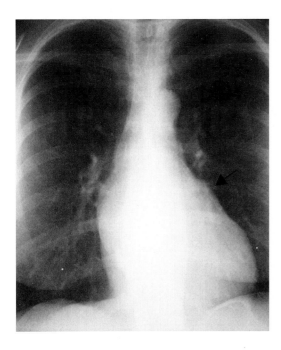

Figure 20.2 Posteroanterior chest radiograph of a 42-year-old patient with mitral valve stenosis. The left atrial appendage is enlarged, producing a localized bump *(arrow)* along the left heart margin, below the level of the left main bronchus. This bump is sometimes referred to as the *"fourth mogul."* The other moguls represent the aortic arch, left pulmonary artery, and lateral margin of the left ventricle. The enlarged left atrium casts a double density behind the right atrium.

bump is often called the *"fourth mogul,"* because the enlarged appendage opacity is in addition to the normally found opacities of the aortic arch, left pulmonary artery, and lateral margin of the left ventricle. However, enlargement of the appendage is sometimes absent in left atrial dilatation. This lack of enlargement of the left atrial appendage sometimes indicates thrombosis of the appendage (5). The appendage is most commonly enlarged when the valve disease is rheumatic in origin and is less likely enlarged when the cause is nonrheumatic (6). In some patients the left main bronchus is displaced upward and backward, although this is not a very reliable sign (7). Posterior displacement of the upper posterior cardiac margin and carina or left lower lobe bronchus can also be seen in the lateral view (Fig. 20.3). Focal displacement of a barium-filled esophagus was used in the past, before introduction of echocardiography, to show left atrial enlargement (Fig. 20.4).

Focal left atrial appendage enlargement (the *"fourth mogul"* on a posteroanterior chest radiograph) should raise suspicion of mitral valve disease.

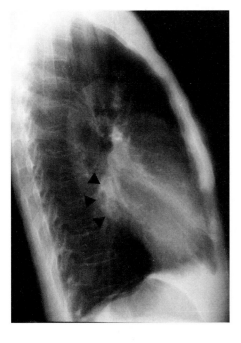

Figure 20.3 Lateral chest radiograph on the same patient with mitral stenosis shown in Fig. 20.1. The upper portion of the posterior margin of the heart, formed by the posterior wall of the enlarged left atrium, bulges posteriorly *(arrowheads)*.

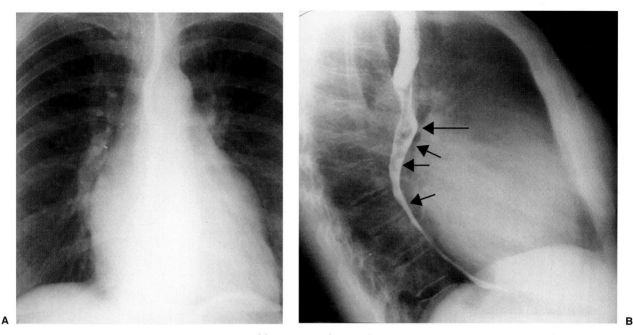

Figure 20.4 51-year-old patient with mitral regurgitation. *A.* Posteroanterior chest radiograph shows the double density and fourth mogul signs of left atrial enlargement. *B.* Lateral radiograph shows posterior displacement *(arrows)* of the barium-filled esophagus by the enlarged left atrium. The carina is also displaced posteriorly *(long arrow)*.

Mitral Valve Stenosis

The underlying functional abnormality in mitral valve stenosis relates to obstruction at the valve with a pressure gradient between the atrium and left ventricle. As a result of the obstruction left atrial pressure elevates, with corresponding elevation of the pulmonary venous, capillary, and arterial pressures. As capillary pressure rises, blood flow can redistribute from the bases into the upper portions of the lungs ("cephalization" or "redistribution") (Fig. 20.5). Increased blood flow in the upper portions of the lungs produces increased diameters of arteries and veins in the upper lungs, with corresponding decreased

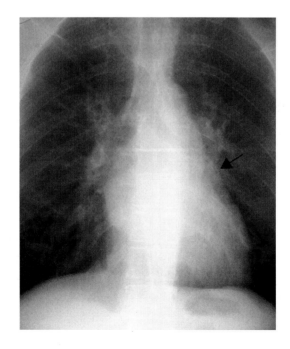

Figure 20.5 Posteroanterior chest radiograph of a 36-year-old patient with mitral stenosis. Pulmonary vessels in the upper portions of the lungs are relatively dilated compared with the lower portions of the lungs. This "redistribution" or "cephalization" of pulmonary blood flow indicates pulmonary venous hypertension secondary to elevated left atrial pressure. The enlarged left atrium is shown as a double density behind the right atrium, and there is a subtle convexity *(arrow)* along the left heart margin reflecting dilatation of the left atrial appendage.

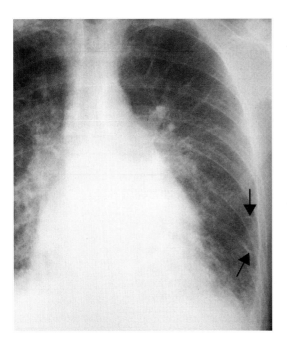

Figure 20.6 Posteroanterior chest radiograph of a 45-year-old patient with severe mitral stenosis. View of the left lung shows Kerley B lines (*arrows*) and perihilar haze indicative of interstitial edema.

sized vessels in the lung bases. This sign can be seen on occasion in upright patients, where blood flow ordinarily dominates in the dependent portions of the lungs. Cephalization of pulmonary blood flow can only be diagnosed in upright patients who have clear lungs at full inspiration. When pulmonary capillary pressure rises further, hydrostatic pressure in the capillary bed overcomes colloid osmotic pressure. Thus, fluid extravasates into the interstitium of the lungs, creating Kerley lines, linear opacities representing fluid in interlobular septa (Fig. 20.6). The left ventricle maintains a normal size in mitral stenosis.

Right-sided chambers can enlarge secondary to chronic pulmonary arterial hypertension. Identification of mitral valve leaflet calcification can be helpful in diagnosing mitral valve stenosis, although large amounts of valve leaflet calcification are necessary for the calcific opacity to become visible on the lateral chest radiograph (Fig. 20.7). Most patients do not have enough calcification to be detected on radiographs. Valve calcification should be distinguished from the commonly seen "C-shaped" calcification of the mitral annulus

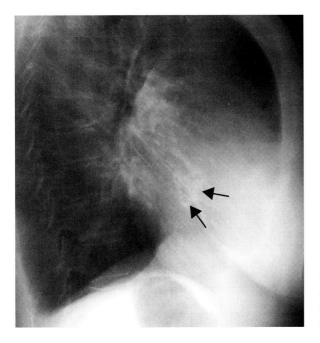

Figure 20.7 Lateral chest radiograph of a 73-year-old patient with mitral stenosis. There is heavy calcification in the mitral valve (*arrows*).

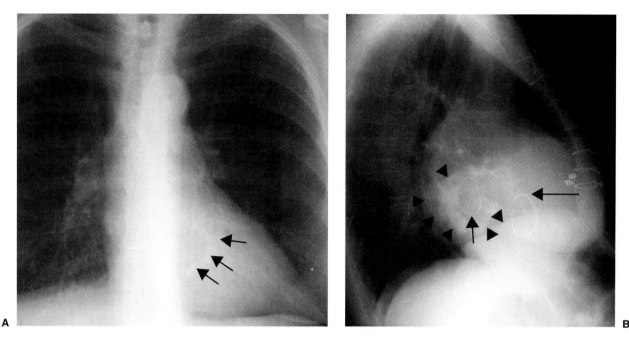

Figure 20.8 *A.* Posteroanterior chest radiograph of a 44-year-old patient with chronic renal failure, without valve disease, shows typical curvilinear calcification of the mitral annulus *(arrows)*. *B.* 75-year-old patient with previous history of mitral and tricuspid valve repair. Lateral chest radiograph shows the prosthetic valve ring at the mitral position *(arrow)* surrounded by dense calcification *(arrowheads)* of the mitral annulus. A tricuspid valve ring is also shown *(long arrow)*.

Mitral annulus calcification may be an indication of atherosclerosis but is not an indicator of mitral valve stenosis or insufficiency.

A calcified left atrial wall should raise suspicion of rheumatic mitral valvular disease.

(Figs. 20.8A and B). Calcification of the annulus is common in the elderly, possibly related to systemic atherosclerosis (8). Uncommonly, calcific deposits in the wall of the left atrium are shown on chest radiographs (Fig. 20.9) or computed tomography (CT) (Fig. 20.10). Left atrial wall calcification is often associated with a history of rheumatic fever, and the calcification is therefore likely due to rheumatic carditis (9). Mural thrombi in the left atrium can also calcify.

Mitral Valve Insufficiency
Incompetence of the mitral valve can be due to a variety of pathologic conditions. Postinflammatory disease (usually rheumatic), floppy valve, ischemic heart disease, endocardi-

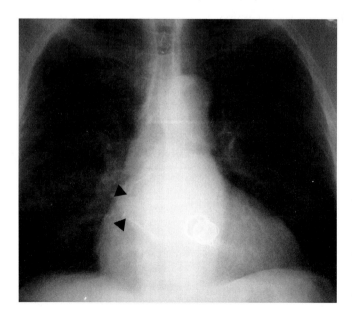

Figure 20.9 Posteroanterior chest radiograph of a 66-year-old patient with a Starr-Edwards valve placed for rheumatic mitral valve disease. Note the curvilinear calcification *(arrowheads)* outlining the lateral wall of the left atrium.

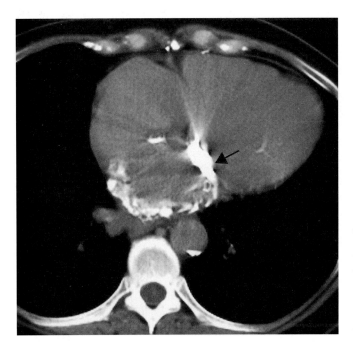

Figure 20.10 Computed tomography image of a 56-year-old patient who has had mitral valve replacement for mitral stenosis. Note the mural calcifications of the left atrium. An arrow points to the prosthetic valve.

tis, idiopathic rupture of chordae, and cardiomyopathy are etiologic possibilities. Chest radiographs show left atrial dilatation, and the degree of enlargement can be quite marked. In contrast with mitral stenosis, the left ventricle also dilates (Fig. 20.11). Left ventricular dilatation is due to the demand for increased left ventricular stroke volume in light of the regurgitant flow fraction. Redistribution of blood flow is uncommon in pure chronic mitral regurgitation, as is pulmonary edema, because left atria can be compliant with nor-

In mitral insufficiency, the left atrium and left ventricle are enlarged because of increased blood volume from the "regurgitated" blood. In contrast, only the left atrium is enlarged with mitral stenosis.

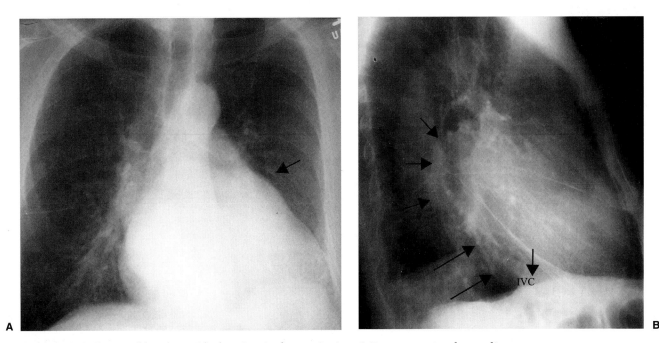

Figure 20.11 A 78-year-old patient with chronic mitral regurgitation. *A.* Posteroanterior chest radiograph shows marked left atrial enlargement. The left atrial opacity behind the right atrium (double density) has a large diameter, and the left atrial appendage is also very large *(arrow). B.* Lateral chest radiograph shows enlargement of the upper posterior heart margin *(arrows),* representing the dilated left atrium. The inferior posterior margin of the heart, representing a dilated left ventricle *(long arrows),* is displaced posterior relative to the inferior vena cava (IVC).

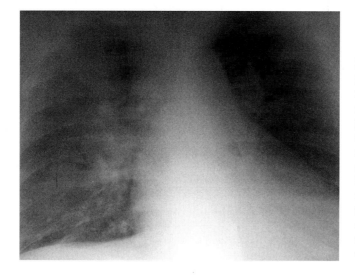

Figure 20.12 Bedside antero-posterior chest radiograph of a 59-year-old patient with acute myocardial infarction. The patient had acute pulmonary edema secondary to papillary muscle rupture. The pulmonary edema predominates in the right lung, especially the upper portion of the right lung. This distribution of edema in the correct clinical setting should suggest the diagnosis of acute mitral valve regurgitation.

mal left atrial pressures (10). If heart failure occurs, redistribution and pulmonary edema can be seen on chest radiographs. Pulmonary edema is more apt to occur in acute mitral regurgitation due to ruptured chordae and acute ischemia of the papillary muscles, sometimes with atypical distribution of pulmonary edema predominating in the right upper lobe (Fig. 20.12) (11).

AORTIC VALVE DISEASE

The American Heart Association 2000 statistical update states that 11,600 patients died of aortic valve disease, with 24,000 having aortic valve disease mentioned as a contributing factor. There were 40,000 hospital discharges with this diagnosis. Most cases of aortic valve disease occur in conjunction with a congenital bicuspid valve or secondary to degenerative and postinflammatory diseases (12–14). As our population ages, the proportion of patients with a degenerative etiology is increasing (15,16).

Aortic Stenosis

Aortic stenosis with left ventricular failure is a poor prognostic sign.

The pathophysiology of aortic stenosis is based on outflow obstruction, left ventricular pressure overload, and increased myocardial wall thickness. Heart size remains normal until heart failure occurs, an ominous clinical sign. With concentric hypertrophy of the left ventricle, sometimes the left cardiac margin on the frontal view has a somewhat rounded configuration. However, the primary signs of aortic valve stenosis include poststenotic dilatation of the ascending aorta and aortic valve calcification (Fig. 20.13). Poststenotic dilation of the ascending aorta evolves with the chronic stress of a jet of blood flow that impacts the aortic wall. Calcification of the valve is common and increases with age. In fact, calcification in the aortic valve without any functional obstruction occurs in one in four or five patients over 65 years of age. The valve calcification is best seen on the lateral view, because the valve usually projects over the spine in the frontal projection. When calcification is observed on chest radiographs of younger individuals or is associated with signs and symptoms of heart failure, aortic stenosis should be suggested. Incidental observation of aortic valve calcification on chest CT occurs frequently and is usually clinically insignificant. However, abundant aortic valve calcification found on CT in patients less than 55 years of age should be considered possible aortic stenosis (17).

Aortic valve calcification is common in adults over 65 years of age. When seen in younger individuals, it should raise suspicion of aortic valvular stenosis.

Aortic Valve Insufficiency

Aortic valve insufficiency, or regurgitation, creates a volume load on the left ventricle. The causes of aortic insufficiency are listed in Table 20.3. Left ventricular stroke volume must

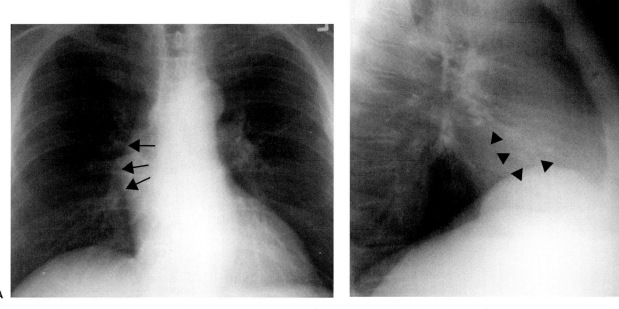

Figure 20.13 59-year-old patient with aortic valve stenosis. *A.* Posteroanterior chest radiograph shows abnormal protrusion of the right mediastinal outline *(arrows)* representing the margin of a dilated ascending aorta. Heart size is normal. The valve lies over the spine and valve calcification is obscured. *B.* Lateral chest radiograph shows dense calcification of the aortic valve *(arrowheads).*

increase to compensate for regurgitation to maintain normal forward cardiac output. By way of illustration, to maintain forward cardiac output of 5 L/min in a patient with 5 L/min of regurgitant flow, there would be a need for a left ventricular output of 10 L/min.

The left ventricle dilates in cases of aortic valve insufficiency, and the thoracic aorta can dilate. The degree of aortic dilatation varies on chest radiography, but identification of left ventricular dilatation is necessary for radiologists to make a diagnosis of aortic regurgitation. The cardiac outline enlarges, and the apex in the frontal view is often displaced laterally and inferiorly toward the costophrenic angle (Fig. 20.14). In the frontal view the dilated ascending aorta can displace the mid-mediastinal outline to the right and the aortic arch can enlarge. In the lateral view, the left ventricle lies inferior and posterior relative to the other cardiac chambers. When dilated, the left ventricle projects more than 18 mm posterior to the inferior vena cava, often intersecting the diaphragm behind the inferior vena cava (18).

> An enlarged left ventricle and ascending aorta should raise suspicion for aortic valvular insufficiency.

> Aortic and mitral valvular disease commonly coexist. The valve leaflets are in direct physical continuity, permitting an inflammatory process such as rheumatic disease to involve both valves. This is known as Lutembacher syndrome.

PULMONIC AND TRICUSPID VALVE DISEASE

The incidence of acquired disease confined to the pulmonic and tricuspid valves is low compared with mitral and aortic valve disease (Table 20.4). The American Heart Association 2000 statistical update reveals only 11 patient deaths due to primary disease of the

Table 20.3: Causes of Aortic Valve Insufficiency

Idiopathic valve degeneration
Bicuspid aortic valve
Postinflammatory valve disease including rheumatic fever
Aortic dissection
Atherosclerotic aneurysm
Infection (bacterial, mycotic and syphilitic)

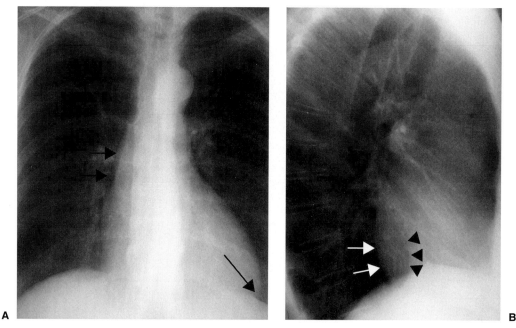

Figure 20.14 64-year-old patient with pure aortic valve insufficiency. *A.* Posteroanterior chest radiograph shows cardiac enlargement. The long axis of the heart *(long arrow)* elongates downwards toward the left costophrenic angle, a finding indicating left ventricular dilatation. The ascending aorta is dilated, presenting as a convex lateral border of the mid-right mediastinal contour *(small arrows)*. *B.* Lateral chest radiograph shows posterior displacement of the inferior cardiac margin *(arrows)*, projecting more than 18 mm behind the inferior vena cava (positive Rigler sign) *(arrowheads)*. This configuration indicates left ventricular dilatation.

right-sided cardiac valves (1). Most commonly, primary disease of the right-sided valves is due to rheumatic disease, almost always associated with disease also involving the left-sided cardiac valves. Carcinoid disease is uncommon and rarely recognized on radiographs (Fig. 20.15). Secondary disease of these valves due to pulmonary hypertension is more common (19).

Pulmonary Hypertension

Pulmonary hypertension results in right atrial and ventricular pressure and/or volume overload, with enlargement of these chambers (Fig. 20.16). Pulmonic and tricuspid valve insufficiency are common sequelae (Fig. 20.17). Frontal chest radiographs show rounded enlargement of the left cardiac margin with upward displacement of the cardiac apex, representing right ventricular enlargement. Right atrial dilatation causes increased circumference and lateral displacement of the right cardiac margin. The pulmonary arteries are enlarged. The dilated right ventricle can be detected in the lateral view as fullness behind the sternum, although this is not a reliable radiographic sign (20).

Table 20.4: Causes of Acquired Pulmonic and Tricuspid Valve Disease

Primary disease
   Rheumatic
   Carcinoid syndrome
   Bacterial endocarditis
   Traumatic rupture
Secondary cause
   Pulmonary hypertension

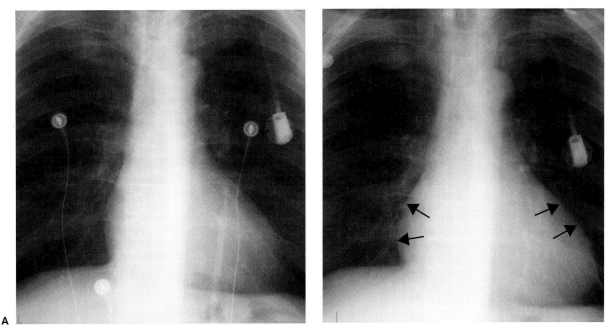

A   B

Figure 20.15 61-year-old patient with carcinoid heart disease and tricuspid valve insufficiency. *A.* Posteroanterior chest radiograph shows normal heart size and configuration. *B.* Posteroanterior chest radiograph 2 months later after development of tricuspid insufficiency shows enlargement of the right atrium *(arrows on left)* and ventricle *(arrow on right)*.

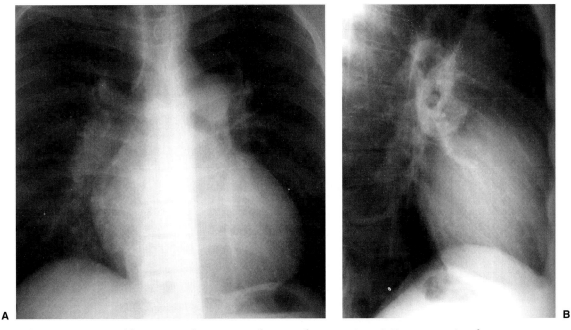

A   B

Figure 20.16 26-year-old patient with primary pulmonary hypertension. *A.* Posteroanterior chest radiograph shows rounding of the right heart margin representing a dilated right atrium. The cardiac apex is rounded and elevated secondary to right ventricular enlargement. The central pulmonary arteries are dilated. *B.* Lateral chest radiograph shows retrosternal fullness caused by the dilated right ventricle. The right atrium is not border forming in this view.

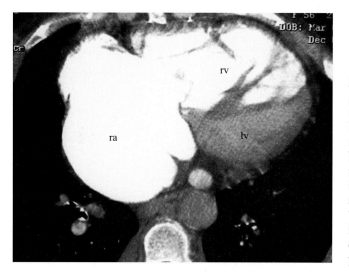

Figure 20.17 Computed tomography angiogram of a 56-year-old patient with pulmonary hypertension secondary to chronic pulmonary thromboembolism. The patient has pulmonic and tricuspid valve insufficiency. The right atrium (ra) and ventricle (rv) are dilated. The interventricular septum is flattened and left ventricle (lv) is displaced posteriorly because of pressure and volume overload.

MYOCARDIAL DISEASE

CARDIOMYOPATHY

The American Heart Association reports that 29,000 patients died because of cardiomyopathy in 2000 (1). The diagnosis of cardiomyopathy was mentioned in the deaths of 53,000 individuals. The cardiomyopathies can be categorized by etiologic or functional classification schemes (Table 20.5).

Dilated Cardiomyopathy

Idiopathic dilated cardiomyopathy is a disease characterized by dilatation of both ventricles or of the left ventricle alone. The true incidence of this disease is difficult to determine, because many cases are unrecognized. The annual incidence is reported to be 36 cases per 100,000 in the United States annually, with 10,000 deaths (21). Almost half of the cases are "idiopathic," although some investigators have implicated a viral-immune etiology in these cases. Secondary dilated cardiomyopathy can be caused by a variety of etiologies (22) (Table 20.6).

Table 20.5: Etiologic and Functional Classifications of the Cardiomyopathies

Etiologic classification
 Primary cardiomyopathy
  Pathologic process involving the myocardium, not affecting other organs
 Secondary cardiomyopathy
  Myocardial disease as one manifestation of systemic disease
Functional classification
 Dilated
  Characterized by dilated ventricles and systolic dysfunction
 Hypertrophic
  Inappropriate myocardial hypertrophy with preserved or enhanced contractile
   function
  Decreased wall compliance with resultant diastolic dysfunction
 Restrictive
  Infiltrative or noninfiltrative myocardial disease with normal systolic function
  Normal diastolic volumes but with stiff myocardium causing impaired ventricular
   filling

Table 20.6: Causes of Secondary Dilated Cardiomyopathy

Toxic
 Hydrocarbons (e.g., alcoholic)
 Drugs (e.g., chemotherapeutic agents, cocaine)
 Lead, cobalt, mercury
Inflammatory
 Connective tissue disease (e.g., scleroderma)
 Sarcoidosis
 Churg-Strauss
Neuromuscular
 Muscular dystrophy including Duchenne
 Friedrich ataxia
Metabolic
 Electrolyte abnormalities (e.g., hypocalcemia)
 Endocrine abnormalities (e.g., hypothyroidism)
 Nutritional deficiencies including thiamine
Miscellaneous causes
 Familial
 Hypertension
 Chronic ischemia
 Peripartum

Pathology shows dilated cardiac chambers with normal or decreased wall thickness. The valves can be scarred, and the annuli of the mitral and tricuspid valves are often dilated. Symptoms of heart failure are usually evident, although some patients are diagnosed based on the incidental finding of cardiomegaly on chest radiography. Ninety-five percent of patients have advanced disease with severe symptoms of left-sided heart failure. Dangerous ventricular arrhythmias commonly are the cause of death in these patients, and many require placement of defibrillating devices. Prognosis is poor, as 50% of patients die within 5 years of initial diagnosis.

Chest radiographs show generalized global cardiac enlargement (Fig. 20.18). Signs of heart failure are also commonly shown, including redistribution of pulmonary blood flow

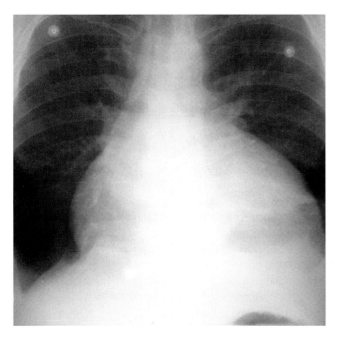

Figure *20.18* Posteroanterior chest radiograph of a 35-year-old patient with idiopathic dilated cardiomyopathy. The cardiac chambers are diffusely dilated.

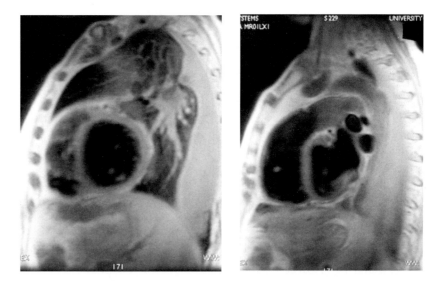

Figure 20.19 *A, B.* Sagittal black-blood proton-density magnetic resonance images of a 48-year-old patient with dilated cardiomyopathy. The ventricular chambers are dilated, and there is thinning of the myocardium.

Diffuse cardiac enlargement is the hallmark of dilated cardiomyopathy radiographically.

and interstitial pulmonary edema. Cross-sectional imaging can be used to characterize the morphology of the cardiac chambers and myocardium (Fig. 20.19). The diagnosis of dilated cardiomyopathy secondary to underlying disease such as sickle cell anemia can be suspected on chest radiographs (Chapter 13). The diagnosis is suspected on radiographs when there are typical osseous and cardiac abnormalities (Fig. 20.20).

Hypertrophic Cardiomyopathy

The heart may be normal size on radiographs in hypertrophic cardiomyopathy, because ventricular hypertrophy does not increase ventricle size (it decreases ventricular capacity).

Hypertrophic cardiomyopathy is characterized by biventricular myocardial hypertrophy without chamber dilatation or associated causal factors such as hypertension (23). Many patients have asymmetric hypertrophy, with pronounced involvement of the interventricular septum. The disease can cause sudden death, often in patients under the age of 40. Left ventricular hypercontractility and diastolic dysfunction create vigorous emptying but poor compliance and chamber filling during diastole. Chest radiographs of adults most commonly show normal heart size, although on occasion there can be enlargement. Cardiac magnetic resonance imaging (MRI) can be helpful in diagnosis (24) (Fig. 20.21).

Restrictive Cardiomyopathy

Restrictive cardiomyopathy and constrictive pericarditis are difficult to separate based on physiology and clinical presentation.

Restrictive cardiomyopathy results in diastolic dysfunction, with impaired filling of noncompliant ventricles. On cardiac catheterization, the physiologic changes are indistinguishable from constrictive pericarditis. Clinical symptoms can be due to right or left ventricular failure, and often signs and symptoms of right heart failure predominate. Left-sided failure produces symptoms of pulmonary edema, whereas right-sided heart failure can manifest as soft tissue edema and ascites. Restrictive cardiomyopathy occurs with less frequency compared with the other types of cardiomyopathy and is uncommon in the United States. The disease is much more common elsewhere in the world (e.g., equatorial Africa). The causes are multifactorial (Table 20.7) (25).

The cardiac size and configuration are usually normal on chest radiography. However, CT, echocardiography, radionuclide imaging, and cardiac MRI have been used in the diagnosis of restrictive cardiomyopathy, often to exclude the diagnosis of constrictive pericarditis.

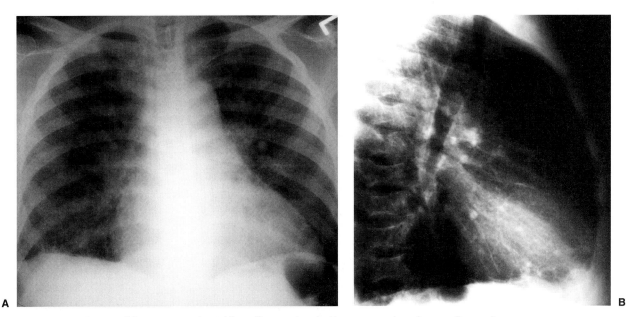

A   B

Figure 20.20 38-year-old patient with sickle cell anemia. *A.* Posteroanterior chest radiograph shows generalized cardiomegaly. The ribs are sclerotic with appearance compatible with bone infarcts. *B.* Lateral chest radiograph shows cardiac enlargement and typical changes of sickle cell disease involving the spine.

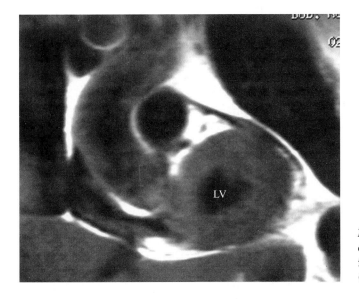

Figure 20.21 50-year-old man with hypertrophic cardiomyopathy. Coronal magnetic resonance black-blood image shows concentric hypertrophy of the left ventricle (LV).

Table 20.7: Causes of Restrictive Cardiomyopathy

Amyloidosis	Sarcoidosis
Familial	Idiopathic
Scleroderma	Gaucher
Endomyocardial fibrosis	Radiation
Carcinoid heart disease	

Cardiac amyloidosis is the most common form of restrictive cardiomyopathy found in the United States. Both primary and secondary amyloidosis can involve the heart, and amyloid deposits are common in the senile heart. When the disease becomes symptomatic, the myocardium is thickened with infiltrating amyloid deposition and is noncompliant. The chambers are often normal in volume but can be small or moderately dilated. The heart can dilate with the senile form of amyloid myocardial disease (Fig. 20.22). Echocardiography and technetium-99m pyrophosphate or indium-111 radionuclide imaging have been used to diagnose cardiac amyloidosis. Cardiac amyloidosis has also been diagnosed with MRI (26). Cardiac sarcoidosis can cause inflammation of the myocardium with subsequent fibrosis. Much of the time myocardial sarcoidosis is subclinical, but on occasion sarcoidosis can produce symptoms of functional impairment with diastolic dysfunction. Chest radiographs usually show a normal heart size, although the heart can enlarge when heart failure is severe (Fig. 20.23). Imaging with thallium-201 or gallium-67 can reveal abnormal uptake in cardiac sarcoidosis, and cardiac MRI can also be used (Fig. 20.24) (26).

MYOCARDITIS

Myocarditis, inflammation of heart muscle, is usually asymptomatic. On the other hand, myocarditis can cause sudden death. Our understanding of the epidemiology of myocarditis has been limited because of its insidious nature (27). The etiology of the disease is often unknown clinically, although there are many known causes, such as infectious, toxic, and immune-related etiologies (e.g., heart transplant rejection). Tables 20.8 and 20.9 list a sampling of types of infectious and toxic etiologies. Viral myocarditis is a major cause of myocarditis in the United States, and the diagnosis can be suspected in the acute phase by demonstration of rising antibody titers. Animal studies have implicated an infectious-immune etiology for myocarditis and idiopathic dilated cardiomyopathy (28).

The findings on chest radiography in patients with myocarditis vary according to the extent of disease. The findings can be normal in patients with subclinical disease. However, generalized global cardiac enlargement with pulmonary edema can be seen in patients with extensive disease. In acute myocarditis, often viral in origin, heart failure can be so severe and progressive that artificial circulatory support, and urgent heart transplantation may be necessary (Fig. 20.25).

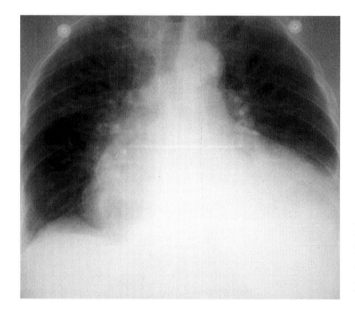

Figure **20.22** 78-year-old patient with senile cardiac amyloid disease. Posteroanterior chest radiograph shows generalized cardiac enlargement and heart failure.

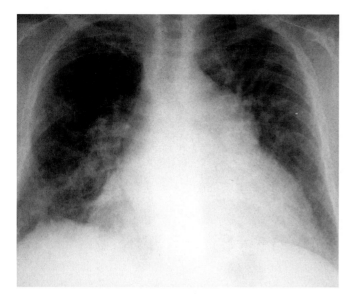

Figure 20.23 Posteroanterior chest radiograph of a 52-year-old patient with sarcoid heart disease shows generalized cardiomegaly. There is diffuse interstitial lung disease secondary to sarcoidosis.

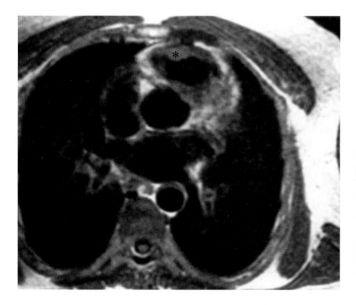

Figure 20.24 T1-weighted axial spin-echo image of a patient with known sarcoid heart disease demonstrates sarcoid infiltration of the myocardium *(asterisk)*, with signal intensity greater than normal myocardium, involving the anterior wall of the outflow portion of the right ventricle.

Table 20.8: Causes of Infectious Myocarditis

Bacterial: *Mycoplasma pneumoniae*
Protozoal: toxoplasmosis
Parasitic: echinococcus granulosus
Viral: coxsackievirus and human immunodeficiency virus
Others: fungus, spirochetes, and rickettsia

Table 20.9: Causes of Toxic Myocarditis

Drug induced: cocaine, ethanol
Heavy metals: iron
Miscellaneous: radiation

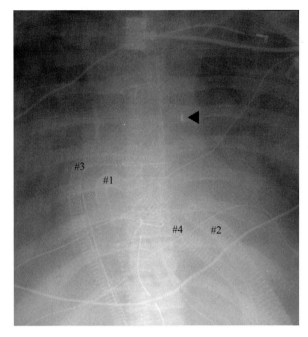

Figure 20.25 Supine bedside anteroposterior chest radiograph of a 25-year-old patient with acute viral myocarditis. There is widespread pulmonary edema despite the presence of biventricular circulatory support with two extracorporeal support devices and an intraaortic balloon pump *(arrowhead)*. Right heart support is achieved by removal of blood from the right atrium by one cannula (# 1) and return to the pulmonary artery through a separate cannula (# 2). Left-sided circulatory support is achieved by removal of blood from the left atrium through a cannula placed through the right superior pulmonary vein (# 3), with return of blood to the aorta under systemic pressure. The cannula (# 4) returning blood to the ascending aorta appears short because the distal portion of the cannula is radiolucent. The extracorporeal pumps produce constant pressure. The intraaortic balloon pump is placed to produce a more physiologic cyclical pressure waveform.

PERICARDIAL DISEASE

There are many forms of acquired pericardial disease. The disease can be acute or chronic, clinical and physiologic findings are variable, and there are many etiologies (29–30). Table 20.10 provides an outline of the types of pericardial effusion, with examples of a few of the many causes.

Pericardial disease with effusion can exist without physiologic abnormality and without clinical symptoms. However, abnormal physiology of acute tamponade and chronic constrictive pericarditis can produce severe and life-threatening conditions. With acute tamponade, the heart is compressed by fluid accumulation within the pericardial sac associated with elevated intrapericardial pressures. The high pressure within the pericardium inhibits diastolic filling of the ventricles, with subsequent decreased stroke volume and cardiac output. Acute tamponade is most commonly due to trauma, often iatrogenic after open cardiac surgery (Fig. 20.26). If uncorrected, death can occur. Tamponade can also occur in a subacute fashion (Fig. 20.27).

Fluid in the pericardium increases intrapericardial pressure, thereby decreasing diastolic filling of the ventricles and resulting in decreased cardiac output.

PERICARDIAL EFFUSION

The pericardium normally contains approximately 50 mL of fluid. When the volume of pericardial fluid exceeds 200 to 250 mL, chest radiographs can be helpful in making the diagnosis of abnormal pericardial fluid accumulation. However, chest radiography is not

Table 20.10: Types of Pericardial Effusion

Serous
   Hypoalbuminemia
   Viral pericarditis
   Heart failure
Chylous
   Idiopathic
   Postsurgical
Hemorrhagic
   Postsurgical
   Postinfarction
   Traumatic
   Neoplastic
   Infectious
   Postradiation
   Systemic disease (e.g., uremia)

particularly sensitive or specific in making a diagnosis of pericardial effusion (31). Chest radiographs of patients with large effusions can show typical features of the "water bottle" heart (Fig. 20.28). This configuration shows symmetric enlargement of the cardiopericardial outline, shaped somewhat like a chocolate candy kiss. The "*hilum overlay*" sign presents when fluid distension of the superior recesses of the pericardium obscures the outline of the left pulmonary artery. The epicardial "fat pad" sign is produced when the pericardial layers and fluid widen the space between the anterior epicardial fat and substernal fat stripes more than 4 mm (Fig. 20.29) (32). Echocardiography, CT (Fig. 20.30), and MRI (Fig. 20.31) can substantiate the radiographic diagnosis of pericardial effusion. In the past, before development of ultrasound, CT or MRI, carbon dioxide injection into the pericardial sac was used to make the diagnosis (Fig. 20.32). Air in the pericardial sac can be seen on chest radiographs of many patients after open-heart surgery; large hydropneumopericardium (Fig. 20.33) is rarely seen.

The radiographic epicardial "*fat pad*" sign is specific, but not sensitive, for pericardial effusion.

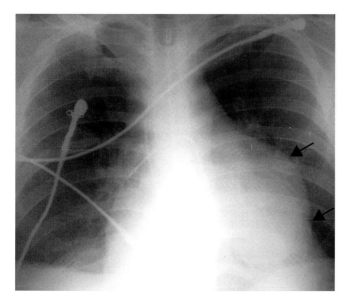

Figure 20.26 An anteroposterior supine bedside chest radiograph of a 55-year-old patient after mitral valve repair with sudden change in vital signs. The bulge of the left heart margin (*arrows*) was caused by a pericardial hematoma that compressed the right ventricle. The pulmonary vasculature is oligemic because of tamponade and reduced cardiac output.

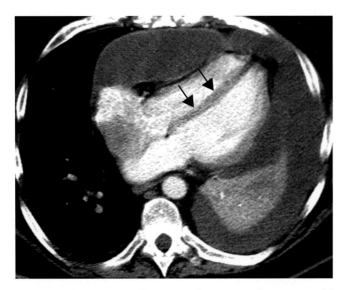

Figure 20.27 Computed tomography image of a 58-year-old patient with purulent pericarditis. A loculated anterior pericardial fluid collection compresses the right ventricle and reverses the usual curvature of the ventricular septum *(arrows)*.

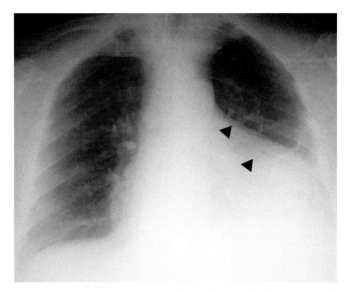

Figure 20.28 Anteroposterior chest radiograph of a 76-year-old patient with a large pericardial effusion of unknown etiology. Note the enlarged cardiac outline with a globular shape mimicking a chocolate *"candy kiss"* or *"water bottle."* The apparent heart outline overlies the left hilum including the left pulmonary artery opacity *(arrowheads)*; this is the so-called hilar overlay sign.

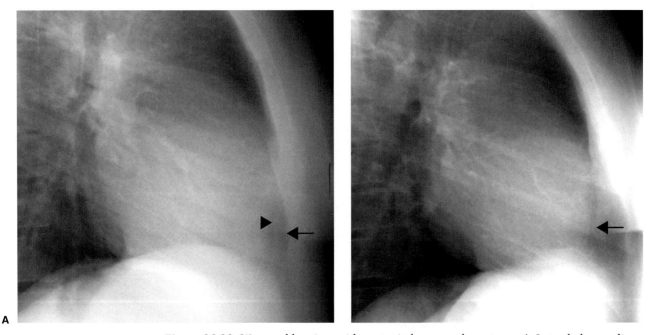

Figure 20.29 27-year-old patient with systemic lupus erythematosus. *A.* Lateral chest radiograph shows a positive *"fat pad"* sign. The lucency of the epicardial fat *(arrowhead)* is separated from the mediastinal fat lucency *(arrow)* by a distance of 9 mm, indicating the presence of a small pericardial effusion. *B.* Follow-up lateral chest radiograph after treatment shows a normal pericardial stripe *(arrow)*.

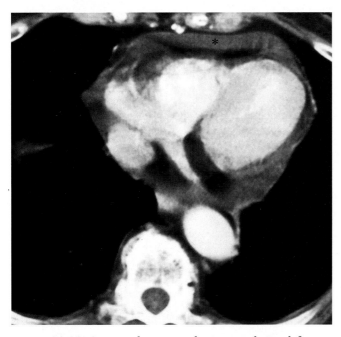

Figure 20.30 Computed tomography image obtained from a 74-year-old patient with chronic exudative pericardial effusion. The pericardial effusion *(asterisk)* is well demarcated by epicardial and mediastinal fat.

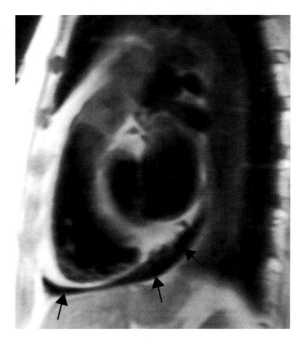

Figure 20.31 Sagittal proton-density, black-blood, magnetic resonance image of a 66-year-old patient with a simple pericardial effusion *(arrows)* located inferior to the heart.

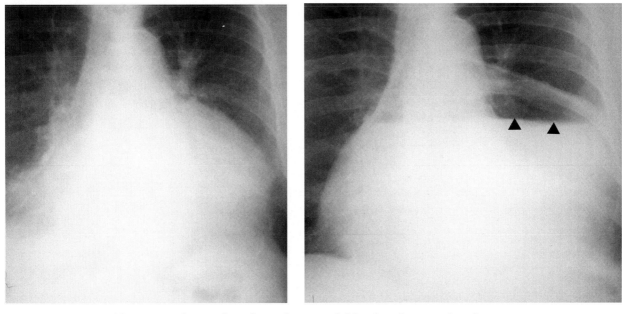

A B

Figure 20.32 84-year-old patient with myxedema heart disease and dilated cardiomyopathy. The patient was worked up in 1965, before the advent of cross-sectional imaging. *A.* Posteroanterior chest radiograph shows enlargement of the cardiac outline. The configuration is compatible with dilated cardiomyopathy with or without pericardial effusion. *B.* Posteroanterior chest radiograph obtained after injection of carbon dioxide into the pericardial sac. The air–fluid level *(arrowheads)* proves the diagnosis of pericardial effusion and shows the anatomy of the superior reflection of the pericardium.

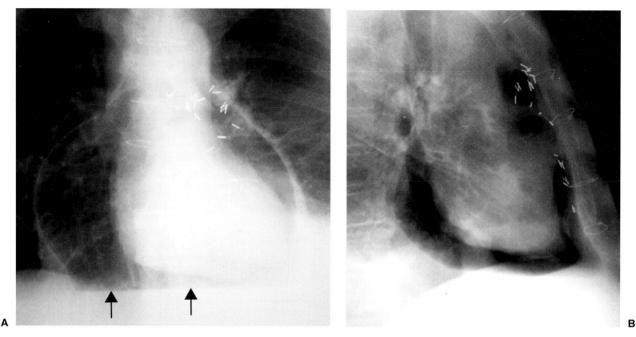

Figure 20.33 64-year-old patient with hydropneumopericardium thought to have accumulated by ball-valve mechanism through a sternal suture. The air was withdrawn by percutaneous catheter insertion and did not recur. *A.* A posteroanterior chest radiograph shows an air–fluid level (*arrows*) in the pericardial sac representing the hydropneumopericardium. Note the anatomic extent of the pericardial reflection. *B.* Lateral chest radiograph shows the extensive pericardial air collection.

CONSTRICTIVE PERICARDITIS

In chronic constrictive pericarditis (Fig. 20.34), ventricular filling is impeded by loss of compliance. The cardiac chambers are constricted by the thickened pericardium, and diastolic pressures are elevated. Elevated venous pressures, with inhibition of venous return, can lead to development of ascites and soft tissue edema. The two layers of normal pericardium measure 2 to 3 mm together (33). In constrictive pericarditis the pericardial lay-

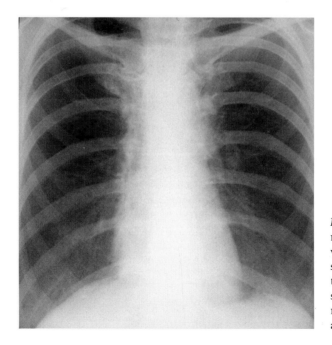

Figure 20.34 Posteroanterior chest radiograph of a 45-year-old patient with chronic constrictive pericarditis secondary to mediastinal radiation therapy. Heart size is normal, but somewhat small. Paramediastinal radiation fibrosis is present and there are small pleural effusions.

ers are fused and thickened, typically measuring more than 4 mm (Fig. 20.35). The cardiopericardial outline can appear normal or enlarged. Approximately half of the patients with constriction have calcification of the pericardium, although calcified pericardium occurs without constriction and constriction can occur without calcification. Calcification presents as curvilinear opacity, conforming to the anatomy of the pericardial sac (Fig. 20.36). Pericardial calcification is distinguished from myocardial calcification by its distribution and its amorphous and often thick appearance. Myocardial calcification is usually confined to the left ventricle, whereas pericardial calcification can be seen along the surfaces of the other chambers, particularly along the right ventricle and in the atrioventricular groove (34) (Fig. 20.37). MRI does not show calcification but demonstrates pericardial thickening and sometimes can be used to show impaired diastolic function. Table 20.11 lists CT and MRI signs of pericardial constriction.

Patients with constrictive pericarditis and restrictive cardiomyopathy can have similar clinical and physiologic findings. CT and MRI can be helpful in differentiating between the two diagnoses (35). The presence of pericardial thickening or other signs of constric-

> Pericardium at least 4 mm thick is abnormal.

> Myocardial calcification is usually confined anatomically to one chamber, whereas pericardial calcification crosses the anatomic location of cardiac chambers.

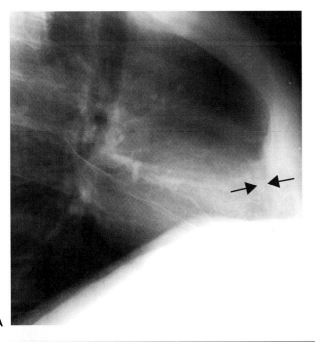

A

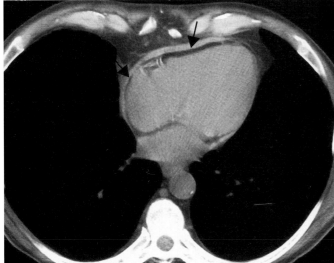

B

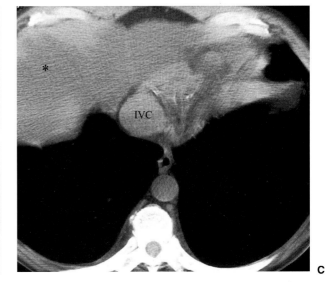

C

Figure 20.35 69-year-old patient with chronic constrictive pericarditis. *A.* A lateral chest radiograph shows a positive epicardial "*fat pad sign*" indicative of thickening of the pericardium (*arrows*). *B.* Computed tomography demonstrates thickening of the pericardium (*arrows*) anteriorly and laterally. *C.* Computed tomography at the level of the diaphragm shows dilatation of the inferior vena cava (IVC) and abdominal fluid (*asterisk*) above the dome of the right hemidiaphragm.

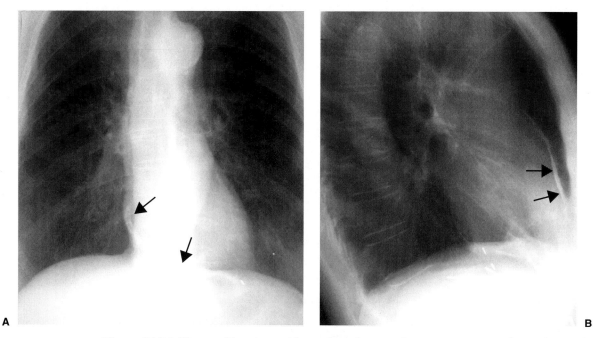

A   B

Figure 20.36 73-year-old patient without clinical signs of constrictive pericarditis. Chest radiographs show extensive pericardial calcification. The diffuse pattern of distribution distinguishes pericardial from myocardial calcification. *A.* Posteroanterior chest radiograph shows thick pericardial calcification *(arrows)* along the right and inferior heart margins. *B.* Lateral chest radiograph shows calcification *(arrows)* of the anterior portion of the pericardium.

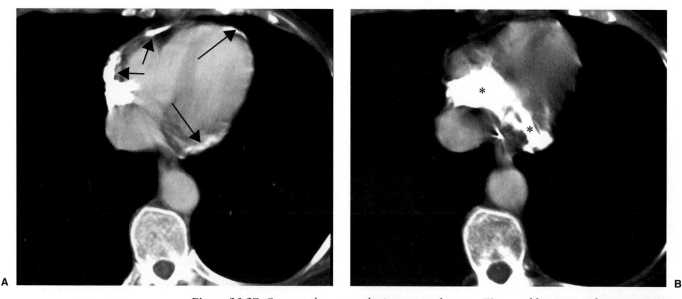

A   B

Figure 20.37 Computed tomography images on the same 73-year-old patient with nonconstrictive pericardial calcification shown in Fig. 20.36. *A.* Computed tomography image at the inferior portions of the ventricular chambers shows calcified pericardium adjacent to the right *(short arrows)* and left ventricles *(long arrows)*. *B.* More caudal image demonstrated abundant calcification at the inferior atrioventricular groove *(asterisks)*.

Table 20.11: Computed Tomography/Magnetic Resonance Imaging Signs of Constrictive Pericarditis

Pericardial thickening and/or calcification
Tubular deformity of one or both ventricles
Flattening of the interventricular septum
Dilatation of one or both atria
Dilatation of inferior and superior vena cava

tion suggests that the abnormality is pericardial in origin, and pericardiectomy can be done in an attempt to alleviate the clinical syndrome (36). A normal pericardium with thickening of the myocardium suggests cardiomyopathy as the diagnosis, a nonsurgical disease except for transplantation.

ISCHEMIC HEART DISEASE

The American Heart Association estimates that over 12 million Americans suffer from coronary heart disease. Almost 500,000 individuals died from coronary disease in 1998, the single leading cause of mortality. Chest radiography, echocardiography, and cardiac nuclear medicine play major roles in managing patients with coronary disease. MRI and CT methods of imaging coronary artery disease are rapidly improving.

Atherosclerotic cardiovascular disease is the leading cause of death in the United States.

IMAGING OF THE CORONARY ARTERIES

Coronary arteriography is the accepted method used to examine the coronary arteries. Noninvasive methods using MRI and CT are under development but have not yet achieved the accuracy necessary to replace the invasive and costly catheter procedure. There are circumstances where noninvasive imaging is useful in evaluating the coronary arteries. For example, CT and MRI can diagnose ectopic origin of the coronary arteries. Chest radiography and fluoroscopy often show calcification of the coronary arteries (Fig. 20.38) (37).

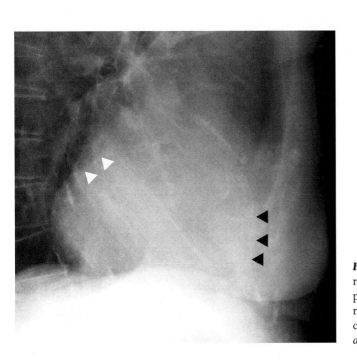

Figure 20.38 Lateral chest radiograph of an 88-year-old patient shows calcification of the right (*black arrowheads*) and left circumflex coronary (*white arrowheads*) arteries.

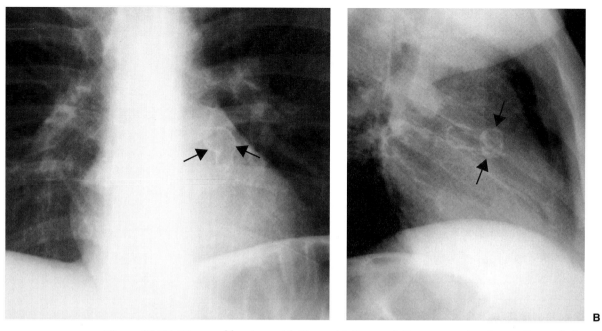

Figure 20.39 23-year-old patient with Kawasaki disease. *A.* Posteroanterior chest radiograph shows a calcified aneurysm *(arrows)* of the left anterior descending coronary artery. *B.* Lateral chest radiograph shows the same coronary artery aneurysm *(arrows)*.

This observation should not be considered clinically useful in older patients but should be mentioned if observed in young patients, under the age of 40. On occasion, a diagnosis of Kawasaki disease can be made by observation of calcified coronary aneurysms on chest radiographs (Fig. 20.39). Several authors have suggested that the incidental finding of extensive coronary arterial calcium with standard CT can have clinical implications (Fig. 20.40) (38,39). As with radiography, the standard CT finding of abundant coronary calcium in patients under the age of 40 should be mentioned on interpretation. Detection of

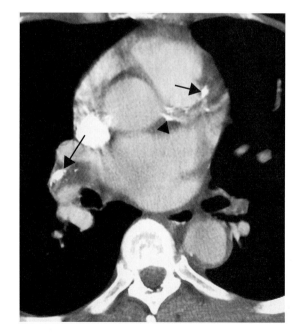

Figure 20.40 Computed tomography image of a 60-year-old patient obtained to evaluate chronic calcified pulmonary artery thromboembolism *(long arrow)* demonstrates the incidental finding of calcification in the left main *(arrowhead)* and left anterior descending *(small arrow)* coronary arteries. The coronary arterial calcification was of no clinical value in this patient.

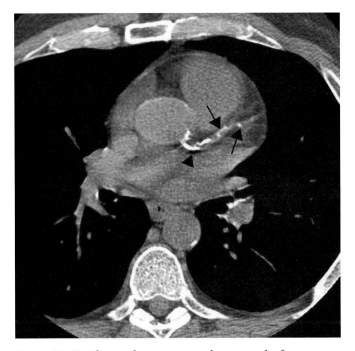

Figure 20.41 Electron beam computed tomography for coronary artery calcium of a 59-year-old man with angina demonstrates abundant calcium in the left main *(arrowhead)* and left anterior descending *(arrows)* coronary arteries.

calcium with standard CT in older patients is of doubtful clinical usefulness. Large groups of patients are now being screened for coronary artery disease by quantifying coronary calcium with electron beam or multidetector helical CT (Fig. 20.41). The resultant coronary calcium "score" is then compared with data normalized by sex and age. Abnormal increased calcium may be a signal of clinically significant disease (40).

The total coronary calcium score is a measure of total atherosclerotic burden (calcified and noncalcified plaque) and may be a useful predictor of the risk for future cardiac events, similar to the use of other risk factors such as hyperlipidemia, smoking, diabetes, and family history.

MYOCARDIAL MANIFESTATIONS OF CORONARY ARTERY DISEASE

Acute and/or chronic ischemia can damage the myocardium. Ischemic myocardial disease can present with a variety of findings on chest radiographs. Chest radiographs can be normal or demonstrates nonspecific findings of cardiomegaly and heart failure. For example, patients with ischemic cardiomyopathy (dilated cardiomyopathy associated with severe coronary artery disease) show nonspecific cardiomegaly indistinguishable from idiopathic cardiomyopathy. Some patients with acute ischemic disease have normal heart size and extensive pulmonary edema (Fig. 20.42). Specific radiographic abnormalities can occur with myocardial damage secondary to coronary artery disease (Table 20.12).

Myocardial infarction can result in formation of a ventricular aneurysm. As an infarct heals, fibrous tissue replaces cardiac muscle (Fig. 20.43). The scarred portion of the ventricular wall can be motionless (akinetic) or can move outward instead of inward during systole (dyskinesis). If the scarred region assumes the shape of a persistent outward bulge, it is considered a true aneurysm that can sometimes be shown on chest radiographs (Figs. 20.44 and 20.45). In some patients the infarct region can calcify without forming an aneurysm, presenting as a thin curvilinear opacity over the heart on chest radiographs. Most commonly, this occurs at the left ventricular apex or anterolateral wall (Figs. 20.46 and 20.47). Pathologically, true aneurysms have remnants of myocardial wall within regions of scarring. In contrast, pseudoaneurysms represent regions of transmural infarction with rupture constrained by overlying pericardium, with no remaining ele-

Focal calcification of the left ventricular apex indicates a calcified infarct and should raise suspicion of a ventricular aneurysm.

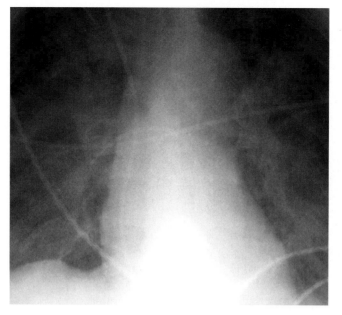

Figure 20.42 Bedside antero-posterior chest radiograph of a 69-year-old patient with acute myocardial infarction. There is extensive pulmonary edema with a normal heart size. In situations with acute ischemic disease the myocardium can be noncompliant, and cardiomegaly can take days to develop.

Table 20.12: Radiographic Signs of Myocardial Infarction

Calcified myocardial infarct
Left ventricular aneurysm
Left ventricular pseudoaneurysm
Ruptured interventricular septum

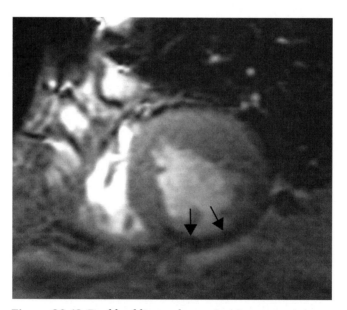

Figure 20.43 Double-oblique, short-axis, cine-magnetic resonance, contrast-enhanced image of a 76-year-old patient with an inferior wall left ventricular infarct. The inferior wall of the left ventricle (*arrows*) is thinned and demonstrates a magnetic resonance signal deficit compared with other portions of the left ventricular myocardium.

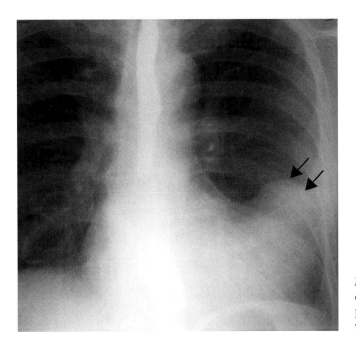

Figure 20.44 Posteroanterior chest radiograph of a 70-year-old patient with a large chronic left ventricular aneurysm *(arrows)*.

ments of the ventricular wall. Pseudoaneurysms typically occur in the posterior-basal segment of the left ventricle near the posterior interventricular groove (Fig. 20.48). It is important to recognize the possibility of pseudoaneurysm because they are susceptible to rupture (41). Imaging with contrast ventriculography, CT, or MRI can be helpful in distinguishing aneurysm from pseudoaneurysm by demonstrating a relative narrow orifice or "neck" leading from the ventricular chamber to a pseudoaneurysm (42) (Fig. 20.49).

Pseudoaneurysms are usually due to transmural infarction and are full-thickness wall ruptures contained by the pericardium.

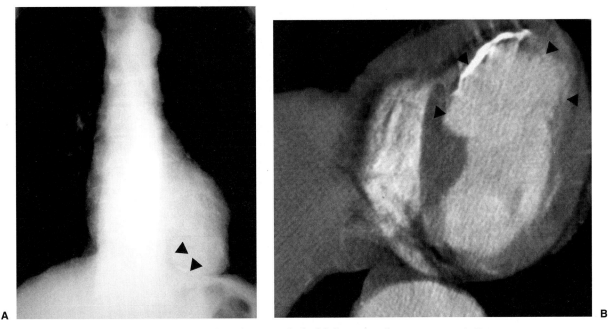

A

B

Figure 20.45 An 86-year-old patient with a chronic calcified left ventricular aneurysm. *A.* Posteroanterior chest radiograph shows a rounded calcification *(arrowheads)* at the inferior margin of the cardiac apex. *B.* Computed tomography image shows the apical calcification and a well-defined rounded aneurysm *(arrowheads)*.

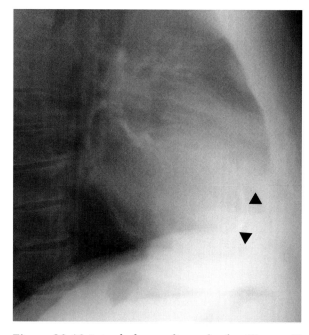

Figure 20.46 Lateral chest radiograph of a 68-year-old patient with an old calcified left ventricular apical infarct (*arrowheads*). In this case, the infarct healed as a calcified scar, without the outward bulge of a ventricular aneurysm.

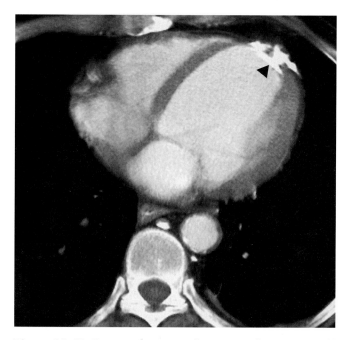

Figure 20.47 Computed tomography image of an 80-year-old patient with a calcified apical infarct. There is calcification in a region of marked myocardial thinning (*arrowhead*). The left ventricular chamber is dilated, but there is no well-defined aneurysm with a neck.

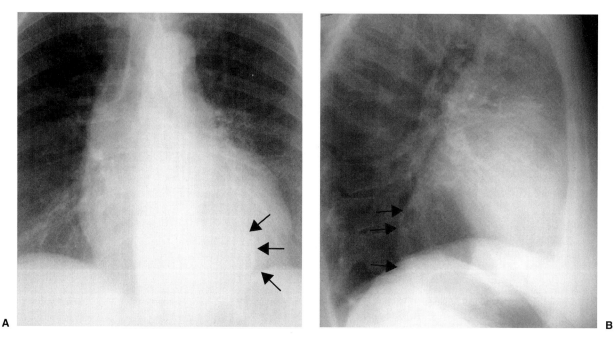

A

B

Figure 20.48 63-year-old patient with a history of inferior wall myocardial infarction. Left ventriculography demonstrated a posterior-inferior wall pseudoaneurysm. *A.* Posteroanterior chest radiograph shows the pseudoaneurysm presenting as a rounded opacity (*arrows*) projecting over the inferior portion of the cardiac outline. *B.* Lateral chest radiograph shows the typical posterior-inferior bulge of a pseudoaneurysm (*arrows*).

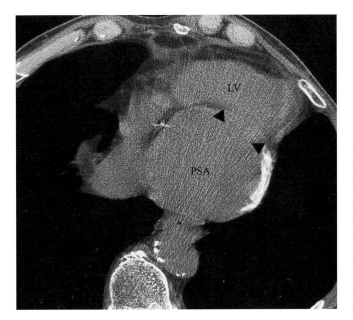

Figure 20.49 Computed tomography image of an 82-year-old patient shows an large rounded opacity representing a pseudoaneurysm (PSA) at the posterior-inferior aspect of the left ventricle (LV). The lateral margin of the pseudoaneurysm is calcified. A narrow neck *(arrowheads)* helps distinguish a pseudoaneurysm from a true aneurysm.

NEOPLASTIC DISEASE

Primary neoplasms of the heart and pericardium are rare, found at autopsy in 0.001% to 0.03% of cases (43). About three-fourths of these primary lesions are benign (Table 20.13), most commonly myxomas (44). CT and MRI are very helpful in making a diagnosis, assessing the extent of disease, and planning a surgical approach. Table 20.14 lists the most common primary malignant neoplasms of the heart and pericardium. Sarcomas are the most common primary malignant neoplasm and second most common overall, after myxoma (45). Metastatic disease is far more prevalent, perhaps 40 times more common than benign tumors (Table 20.15) (46).

Chest radiographs show cardiac enlargement in many cases of neoplasm, although some patients have normal heart and mediastinal contours (47). On occasion, neoplastic disease can present on chest radiographs as a mass-like contour abnormality of the cardiopericardial outline (Fig. 20.50). Benign pericardial cysts (Fig. 20.51), lipomas, and ventricular aneurysm (Fig. 20.52) can have the same appearance. Therefore, the diagnosis and extent of neoplastic disease can be better evaluated with CT (Figs. 20.53 to 20.56) or MRI (Figs. 20.57, 20.58, and 20.59) (48). MRI is superior to CT in many cases because of faster image acquisition, the ability to image in multiple planes, and superior contrast resolution (49). MRI relaxation characteristics allow for better soft tissue characterization of masses.

Cardiac malignancy is more commonly metastatic to the heart than primary to the heart.

Table 20.13: Benign Primary Cardiac and Pericardial Neoplasms
Myxoma
Papillary fibroelastoma
Fibroma
Paraganglioma
Lipoma
Hemangioma

Table 20.14: Malignant Primary Neoplasms of the Heart and Pericardium

Sarcoma of mesenchymal cell origin
    Angiosarcoma (most common)
    Rhabdomyosarcoma
    Fibrosarcoma
    Osteosarcoma
Lymphoma
Pericardial mesothelioma

Table 20.15: Common Sources of Metastatic Disease to the Heart

Breast
Bronchogenic
Renal cell
Melanoma
Leukemia

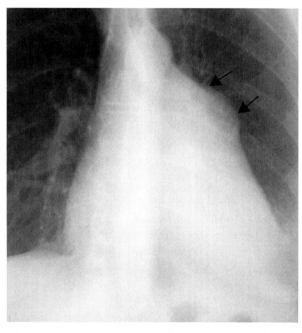

Figure 20.50 Posteroanterior chest radiograph of a 61-year-old patient with a primary leiomyosarcoma of the outflow portion of the right ventricle *(arrows)*.

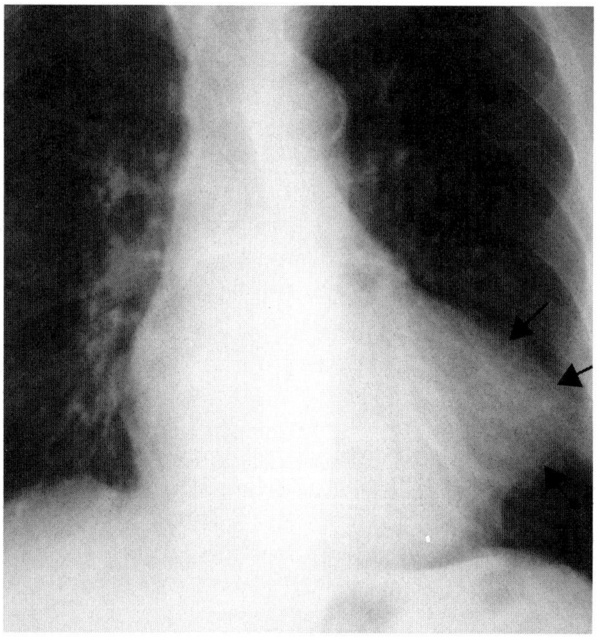

Figure 20.51 Posteroanterior chest radiograph of a 73-year-old patient with a pericardial cyst *(arrows)*.

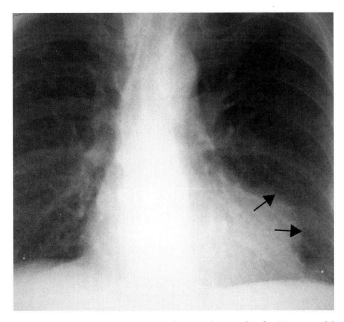

Figure 20.52 Posteroanterior chest radiograph of a 70-year-old patient with a left ventricular aneurysm *(arrows)*.

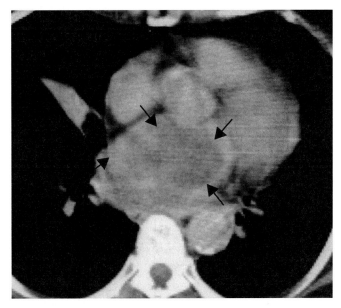

Figure 20.53 Computed tomography image of the heart of a middle-aged patient shows a filling defect in the left atrium *(arrows)*, representing an intraluminal myxoma.

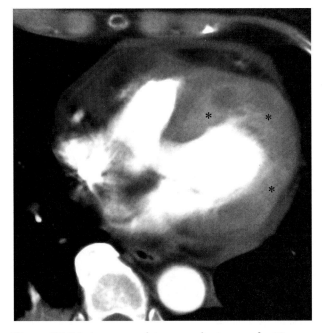

Figure 20.54 A computed tomography image of a 70-year-old patient with metastases to the myocardium *(asterisks)*.

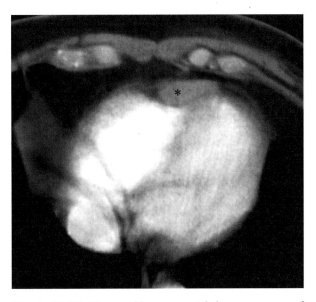

Figure 20.55 61-year-old woman with breast cancer and metastasis to the epicardium. A computed tomography image shows a solitary metastasis in the epicardial fat *(asterisk)* beneath the pericardium, compressing the apex of the right ventricle.

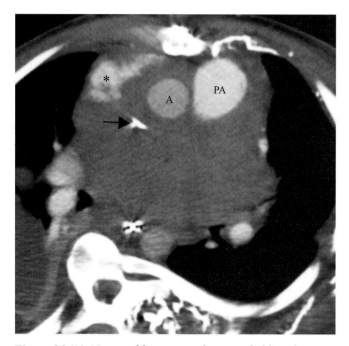

Figure 20.56 21-year-old patient with pericardial lymphoma. A computed tomography image shows extensive abnormal soft tissue infiltration at the superior aspect of the pericardial sac. The lymphomatous tissue surrounds the aorta (A) and pulmonary artery (PA). The superior vena cava is obliterated, and its position is shown by a venous catheter (*arrow*). Contrast is shown in the right atrial appendage (*arrowhead*).

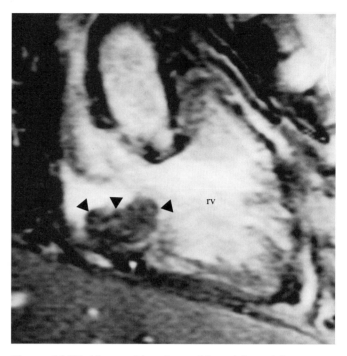

Figure 20.57 40-year-old patient with a right atrial myxoma. Fast-cine magnetic resonance image in the two-chamber view of the right atrium and ventricle (rv) shows a polypoid myxoma in the right atrium (*arrowheads*).

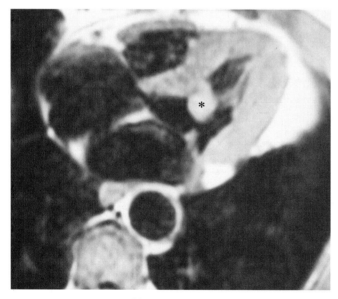

Figure 20.58 65-year-old patient with metastatic renal cell carcinoma. Spin-echo axial magnetic resonance study shows a left ventricular polypoid metastasis (*asterisk*) attached to the ventricular septum.

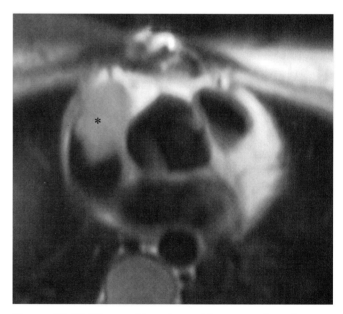

Figure 20.59 37-year-old patient with metastatic melanoma. Proton density-weighted axial magnetic resonance image shows a metastasis (*asterisk*) extending from the right atrial appendage into the right atrium.

REFERENCES

1. American Heart Association. *2001 Heart and stroke statistical update.* Dallas: American Heart Association, 2000.
2. Olson LJ, Subramanian R, Ackermann DM, et al. Surgical pathology of the mitral valve: a study of 712 cases spanning 21 years. *Mayo Clin Proc* 1987;22–34.
3. Levin AR, Frand M, Baltaxe HA. Left atrial enlargement. *Radiology* 1972;104:615–621.
4. Higgins CB, Reinke RT, Jones NE, et al. Left atrial dimension on the frontal thoracic radiograph: a method for assessing left atrial enlargement. *AJR Am J Roentgenol* 1978;130:251–255.
5. Matsuyama S, Watabe T, Kuribayashi S, et al. Plain radiographic diagnosis of thrombosis of left atrial appendage in mitral valve disease. *Radiology* 1983;146:15–20.
6. Green CE, Kelley MJ, Higgins CB. Etiologic significance of enlargement of the left atrial appendage in adults. *Radiology* 1982;142:21–27.
7. Murray JG, Brown AL, Anagnostou EA, et al. Widening of the tracheal bifurcation on chest radiographs: value as a sign of left atrial enlargement. *AJR Am J Roentgenol* 1995;164:1089–1092.
8. Roberts WC. Morphologic features of the normal and abnormal mitral valve. *Am J Cardiol* 1983; 51:1005–1028.
9. Chen JTT. *Essentials of cardiac roentgenology,* 1st ed. Boston: Little, Brown and Company, 1987: 107.
10. Carlsson E, Gross R, Holt RG. The radiological diagnosis of cardiac valvular insufficiencies. *Circulation* 1977;55:921–933.
11. Schnyder PA, Sarraj AM, Duvoisin BE, et al. Pulmonary edema associated with mitral regurgitation: prevalence of predominant involvement of the right upper lobe. *AJR Am J Roentgenol* 1993;161:33–36.
12. Subramanian R, Olson LJ, Edwards WD. Surgical pathology of pure aortic stenosis: a study of 374 cases. *Mayo Clin Proc* 1984;59:683–690.
13. Subramanian R, Olson LJ, Edwards WD. Surgical pathology of combined aortic stenosis and insufficiency: a study of 213 cases. *Mayo Clin Proc* 1985;60:247–254.
14. Lakier JB, Copans H, Rosman HS, et al. Idiopathic degeneration of the aortic valve: a common cause of isolated aortic regurgitation. *J Am Coll Cardiol* 1985;5:347–351.
15. Passik CS, Ackermann DM, Pluth JR, et al. Temporal changes in the causes of aortic stenosis: a surgical pathologic study of 646 cases. *Mayo Clin Proc* 62:119–123.
16. Lester SJ, Heilbron B, Gin K, et al. The natural history and rate of progression of aortic stenosis. *Chest* 1998;113:1109–1114.
17. Lippert JA, White CS, Mason AC, et al. Calcification of aortic valve detected incidentally on CT scans: prevalence and clinical significance. *AJR Am J Roentgenol* 1995;164:73–77.
18. Hoffman RB, Rigler LG. Evaluation of left ventricular enlargement in the lateral projection of the chest. *Radiology* 1965;85:93.
19. Altrichter PM, Olson LJ, Edwards WD, et al. Surgical pathology of the pulmonary valve: a study of 116 cases spanning 15 years. *Mayo Clin Proc* 1989;64:1352–1360.
20. Murphy ML, Blue LR, Ferris EJ, et al. Sensitivity and specificity of chest roentgenogram criteria of right ventricular hypertrophy. *Invest Radiol* 1988;23:853–856.
21. Dec GW, Fuster V. Idiopathic dilated cardiomyopathy. *N Engl J Med* 1994;331:1564–1575.
22. Kasper EK, Agema WRP, Hutchins GM, et al. The causes of dilated cardiomyopathy: a clinicopathologic review of 673 consecutive patients. *J Am Coll Cardiol* 1994;23:586–590.
23. Roberts WC. Morphologic aspects of the cardiomyopathies. In: Elliott LP, ed. *Cardiac imaging in infants, children, and adults.* Philadelphia: J.B. Lippincott, 1991:461–463.
24. Park JH, Kim YM, Chung JW, et al. MR imaging of hypertrophic cardiomyopathy. *Radiology* 1992;185:441–446.
25. Kushwaha SS, Fallon JT, Fuster V. Restrictive cardiomyopathy. *N Engl J Med* 1997;336:267–276.
26. Friedrich MG. Magnetic resonance imaging in cardiomyopathies. *J Cardiovasc Magn Res* 2000;2: 67–82.
27. Feldman AM, McNamara D. Myocarditis. *N Engl J Med* 2000;343:1388–1398.
28. Kawai C. From myocarditis to cardiomyopathy: mechanisms of inflammation and cell death: learning from the past for the future. *Circulation* 1999;99:1091–1100.
29. Elliott LP. *Cardiac imaging in infants, children, and adults.* Philadelphia: J.B. Lippincott, 1991: 371–378.
30. Spindola-Franco, Fish BG. *Radiology of the heart.* New York: Springer-Verlag, 1985:651–652.

31. Eisenberg MJ, Dunn MM, Kanth NK, et al. Diagnostic value of chest radiography for pericardial effusion. *J Am Coll Cardiol* 1993;22:588–593.

32. Carsky EW, Mauceri RA, Azimi F. The epicardial fat pad sign. *Radiology* 1980:137:303–308.

33. Silverman PM, Harell GS. Computed tomography of the normal pericardium. *Invest Radiol* 1983; 18:141–144.

34. MacGregor JH, Chen JTT, Chiles C, et al. The radiographic distinction between pericardial and myocardial calcifications. *AJR Am J Roentgenol* 1987;148:675–677.

35. Masui T, Finck S, Higgins CB. Constrictive pericarditis and restrictive cardiomyopathy: evaluation with MR imaging. *Radiology* 1992;182:359–373.

36. Rienmuller R, Gurgan M, Erdmann E, et al. CT and MR evaluation of pericardial constriction: a new diagnostic and therapeutic concept. *J Thorac Imaging* 1993;8:108–121.

37. Margolis JR, Chen JTT, Kong Y, et al. The diagnostic and prognostic significance of coronary artery calcification. *Radiology* 1980;137:609–616.

38. Timins ME, Pinsk R, Sider L, et al. The functional significance of calcification of the coronary arteries as detected on CT. *J Thorac Imaging* 1991;7:79–82.

39. Moore EH, Greenberg RW, Merrick SH, et al. Coronary artery calcifications: significance of incidental detection on CT scans. *Radiology* 1989:711–716.

40. Janowitz WR. CT imaging of coronary artery calcium as an indicator of atherosclerotic disease: an overview. *J Thorac Imaging* 2001;16:2–7.

41. Frances C, Romero A, Grady D. Left ventricular pseudoaneurysm. *J Am Coll Cardiol* 1998;32: 557–561.

42. Brown SL, Gropler RJ, Harris KM. Distinguishing left ventricular aneurysm from pseudoaneurysm. *Chest* 1997;111:1403–1409.

43. Burke A, Virmani R. Tumors of the heart and great vessels. In: *Atlas of tumor pathology*, 3rd series fasc 16. Washington, DC: Armed Forces Institute of Pathology, 1996.

44. Tazelaar HD, Locke TJ, McGregor CGA. Pathology of surgically excised primary cardiac tumors. *Mayo Clin Proc* 1992;67:957–965.

45. Grebenc ML, Rosado di Christenson ML, Burke AP, et al. Primary cardiac and pericardial neoplasms: radiologic-pathologic correlation. *Radiographics* 2000;20:1073–1103.

46. Strauss BL, Matthews MJ, Cohen MH, et al. Cardiac metastases in lung cancer. *Chest* 1977;71: 607–611.

47. Bear PA, Moodie DS. Malignant primary cardiac tumors: the Cleveland Clinic experience, 1956 to 1986. *Chest* 1987;92:860–862.

48. Aroaz PA, Mulvagh SL, Tazelaar HD, et al. CT and MR imaging of benign primary cardiac neoplasms with echocardiographic correlation. *Radiographics* 2000;20:1303–1319.

49. Mader MT, Poulton TB, White RD. Malignant tumors of the heart and great vessels: MR imaging appearance. *Radiographics* 1997;17:145–153.

PULMONARY VASCULAR DISEASE

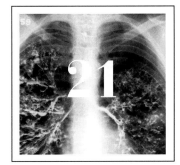

- Pulmonary Thromboembolic Disease
- Pulmonary Arterial Hypertension
- Pulmonary Tumor Embolism
- Pulmonary Arteriovenous Malformation
- Pulmonary Artery Stenosis
- Pulmonary Artery Aneurysms and Pseudoaneurysms
- Pulmonary Artery Aplasia and Hypoplasia

Pulmonary vascular disease is often overlooked as an etiology for chest pain and dyspnea. Conditions may be life threatening, in the case of acute pulmonary embolism (PE), or may be the cause of chronic symptoms, in the case of pulmonary hypertension and chronic PE. In this chapter we discuss acute and chronic PE, pulmonary arterial hypertension (PAH), and briefly touch on the congenital and acquired abnormalities of the pulmonary arteries, including pulmonary arteriovenous malformations (AVMs), tumor embolism, and stenosis, aneurysms, and tumors of the pulmonary arteries.

PULMONARY THROMBOEMBOLIC DISEASE

PE is the third most common acute cardiovascular disease after ischemic heart disease and stroke, and is an important cause of patient morbidity and mortality. The incidence of PE is 600,000 annually in the U.S., and the mortality of untreated PE approximately 30% (1). Hence, it is prudent to diagnose PE accurately and quickly, and to initiate treatment in a timely fashion. Accurate diagnosis is imperative, not only to decrease the morbidity and mortality after treatment, but to avoid the risks of hemorrhage associated with anticoagulation seen in up to 7% of patients, especially in the case of a false-positive test result for PE.

The diagnosis of acute PE continues to pose a challenge to clinicians and radiologists. Ancillary tests include the electrocardiogram, which may demonstrate a right heart strain pattern, and the blood test D-dimer, which when negative is useful to exclude venous thrombosis. However, the D-dimer test is nonspecific and may also be abnormal with myocardial infarction, pneumonia, heart failure, cancer, and recent surgery (2,3).

Venous thrombi form most commonly in veins of the lower extremities and pelvis and then dislodge, propagating cranially into the pulmonary arterial tree. Radiologic evaluation of the patient may include evaluation of the thorax with chest radiography, ventilation-perfusion (V/Q) scans, computed tomography (CT), and magnetic resonance imaging (MRI) and evaluation of the lower extremity veins with CT venography, MR venography, or ultrasound.

Radiology plays a major role in the diagnosis of PE, and the ubiquitous chest radiograph is the first investigation of choice. V/Q scintigraphy has played a major role in the diagnosis of PE. Though angiography is the standard of reference, it is infrequently used (4,5). The advent of newer helical scanners, electron beam scanners, and particularly multidetector helical scanners has significantly changed the way PE is diagnosed. Multidetector CT is now routinely used in the diagnosis of PE. Magnetic resonance angiography may also be used in the diagnosis of PE and is particularly useful in cases where there is a history of allergy to iodinated contrast media. Transthoracic and transesophageal echocardiography are useful in the diagnosis of large central PE in patients with acute right heart strain and right heart failure. Transesophageal echocardiography can be performed at the bedside and is particularly helpful in medically unstable patients.

Ultrasound venography is now used as the primary modality for the diagnosis of deep vein thrombosis (DVT) of the lower extremities and has virtually replaced the more invasive direct catheter venography. Magnetic resonance venography is useful, particularly in patients where ultrasound is difficult due to body habitus. Similarly, indirect CT venography is used for evaluating DVT in combination with a CT pulmonary angiogram (CTPA), giving CT the advantage of imaging both the thrombus burden in the extremities and pelvis and the pulmonary arterial tree in a single comprehensive examination. The goal in evaluating suspected venous thromboembolic disease is to have a cost-effective noninvasive test with high sensitivity and specificity.

ETIOLOGY AND PATHOPHYSIOLOGY

PE and DVT are a spectrum of the same disease process, best described as venous thromboembolic disease. PE is a consequence of thrombus, most commonly formed in the deep veins of the pelvis and lower extremities. Thrombus can also originate in the veins of the head, neck, upper extremities, inferior vena cava, right atrium, and right ventricle. Risk factors for DVT are listed in Table 21.1.

In most fatal PE, at autopsy the thrombus is localized proximal to the knee (6). After dislodgement, the venous thrombus propagates through the right heart and into the pulmonary arterial circulation, usually lodging in the main, lobar, or segmental pulmonary arteries, and as a shower of emboli into the subsegmental and smaller pulmonary arteries. In some cases, this leads to acute right ventricular failure. Fatal PE results as a consequence of central occlusive thrombus in patients with normal cardiopulmonary reserve but may also occur with smaller occlusive thrombi in patients with underlying cardiopulmonary compromise. In the uncommon event of a patent foramen ovale, atrial septal defect, or ventricular septal defect, paradoxical emboli may be seen resulting in stroke and mesenteric and renal ischemia.

Pulmonary emboli are more often multiple than solitary and occur more often in the right lung than the left lung. They are most frequently found in the lower lobes, probably due to the greater pulmonary blood flow to the lower lobes. Pulmonary hemorrhage, infarction, or atelectasis may occur as a consequence of PE. Acute PE is treated with either

Pulmonary emboli are usually multiple and located in areas of greatest pulmonary blood flow.

Table 21.1: Risk Factors for Pulmonary Thromboembolic Disease

Venous stasis
Immobilization
Surgery
Long airplane flights
Malignancy
Indwelling catheters
Abnormality of the wall of the veins (such as thrombophlebitis)
Hypercoagulable states
Pregnancy
Oral contraceptive pills
Antithrombin C
Protein C and S deficiency

anticoagulation or, if contraindicated, with an inferior vena cava filter. Treatment with anticoagulants prevents more clot forming while the body dissolves the clot. If this fails, intravenous thrombolysis with recombinant tissue plasminogen activator may be given over a period of 8 to 12 hours and occasionally up to 24 hours in hemodynamically stable patients. In hemodynamically unstable patients, intraarterial thrombolysis as a part of thrombectomy may be performed, with the thrombolytic agent directly injected into the thrombus. Surgical embolectomy may be required in large occlusive PE and carries a high mortality. If thrombolysis fails to resolve the emboli, chronic thromboembolic pulmonary hypertension (CTEPH) may ensue.

CLINICAL PRESENTATION

The clinical manifestations of PE are nonspecific and include dyspnea, chest pain that is often pleuritic in nature, hemoptysis, cough, syncope, or even death. Tachypnea, tachycardia, atrial fibrillation, hypotension, fever, and a pleural friction rub may be noted on physical examination (7). Because of the nonspecific nature of the signs and symptoms, the diagnosis is often overlooked or confused with other diagnoses. Arterial oxygen saturation is often low, especially in cases of significant PE. The electrocardiogram may demonstrate tachycardia, atrial fibrillation, or a right heart strain pattern with $S_1Q_3T_3$ pattern or a new right bundle branch block; more commonly the electrocardiogram is normal.

RADIOLOGY IN THE DIAGNOSIS OF ACUTE PULMONARY EMBOLISM

Chest Radiograph

Although the chest radiograph is usually the first imaging examination performed in patients with suspected PE, it may be completely normal even in the presence of near fatal PE. When abnormal, the findings are usually nonspecific. Chest radiographic findings are uncommon due to the dual blood supply from bronchial arteries. The main use of a chest radiograph is to exclude other disease processes that mimic the clinical signs and symptoms of PE, such as pneumonia, pneumothorax, rib fractures, aortic dissection, pleural effusions, pericardial effusion, tumor, and hiatal hernia (8). The radiograph is used in conjunction with the V/Q scan in the evaluation of PE, because it is used in the interpretation scheme for V/Q scans (9).

The chest radiograph findings are given in Table 21.2. Historical findings of PE on chest radiography are rarely encountered (Table 21.2), such as the *Westermark sign*, which is pulmonary oligemia distal to an obstructing embolus (Fig. 21.1), and the *Fleischner sign*, which is a large central pulmonary artery due to central thrombus with abrupt tapering, also known as the *knuckle sign*. These signs are mainly seen when there is PE without infarction. The *Hampton hump*, a wedge-shaped pleural based opacity with the apex pointing toward the hilum and the base abutting the pleura, particularly along the diaphragmatic pleura, is highly suggestive of pulmonary infarction. Pulmonary infarcts maintain their shape as they resolve, which may take several months. Occasionally, an infarct is mistaken for a solitary pulmonary nodule. Although most infarcts resolve completely, many leave an area of linear scar and occasionally a small nodule.

> Chest radiographs in patients with suspected PE are most useful to exclude other disease processes that may be causing symptoms, such as pneumonia or edema.

> No chest radiograph, normal or abnormal, can be used to exclude PE.

> Westermark sign, Fleischner sign, and Hampton hump are classic but very uncommon radiographic findings of PE.

Table 21.2: Chest Radiograph Findings of Acute Pulmonary Embolism

Specific Findings	Nonspecific Findings
Westermark sign	Atelectasis
Fleischner sign	Elevated hemidiaphragm
Hampton hump	Pleural effusion(s)
	Dilated central pulmonary arteries

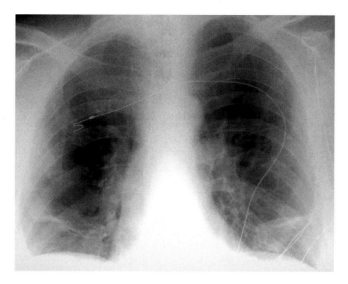

Figure 21.1 Westermark sign. Chest radiograph demonstrates pulmonary oligemia in the right mid-lung, secondary to central right pulmonary embolus.

The nonspecific radiograph findings in PE with infarction include an elevated hemidiaphragm, pleural effusion, and atelectasis. Pleural effusions are quite common and are often small and unilateral. These often occur early and are frequently hemorrhagic. Occasionally, they can be large or bilateral. Effusions may be an isolated finding in up to one-third of patients with PE and are seen in approximately two-thirds of patients when accompanied by pulmonary hemorrhage or infarction.

In the original Prospective Investigation of Pulmonary Embolism Diagnosis (PIOPED) study, the sensitivity and specificity of the V/Q lung scan was determined using pulmonary angiogram as the gold standard in the evaluation of suspected acute PE (10). The study concluded that clinical assessment combined with the V/Q scan established or excluded the diagnosis of acute PE in only a small number of patients. A normal chest radiograph was uncommon, found in 12% of patients. Radiographic signs poorly correlate with the diagnosis of PE and did not help to confirm or exclude the diagnosis of PE.

Radionuclide Imaging

The principle underlying V/Q scintigraphy in the diagnosis of PE is the detection of decreased or absent perfusion, with corresponding normal ventilation. *Perfusion scintigraphy* is performed by intravenous injection of technetium-99m–labeled albumin macroaggregates ranging from 10 to 100 μm in size. These microparticles lodge in the precapillary arterioles of the pulmonary vascular bed. Eight static views are obtained (anterior, posterior, both laterals, and both anterior and posterior obliques). *Ventilation scintigraphy* is most often obtained after inhalation of radiolabeled gas such as xenon-133 or aerosols such as technetium-99m diethylenetriaminepentaacetic acid or technetium-99m pyrophosphate. Again, eight images are obtained as above, preferably in the upright position and especially with xenon. A normal V/Q scan is illustrated in Fig. 21.2.

Although the diagnosis of PE is based on a mismatched perfusion defect (i.e., perfusion defect in an area that is normally ventilated), the test is not specific for the diagnosis of PE. Most V/Q scan interpretations require interpretation in conjunction with a current chest radiograph. The current criteria used in the diagnosis of PE are the revised PIOPED criteria (11,12) (Table 21.3). Using these criteria, a V/Q scan is labeled as normal, very low probability, low probability, intermediate/indeterminate probability (Fig. 21.3), and high probability (Fig. 21.4) for the diagnosis of PE. Although a normal V/Q scan virtually excludes a PE and a high probability scan confirms a PE, in the PIOPED study only 14% of patients had a normal V/Q scan and 13% of patients had a high probability V/Q scan. The other 73% of patients had an indeterminate V/Q scan, a nonconclusive result requiring further evaluation with other studies, such as pulmonary angiography.

Most chest radiographs in pulmonary embolism are nonspecific.

V/Q scans for PE are most specific when perfusion defects occur in areas of normal ventilation.

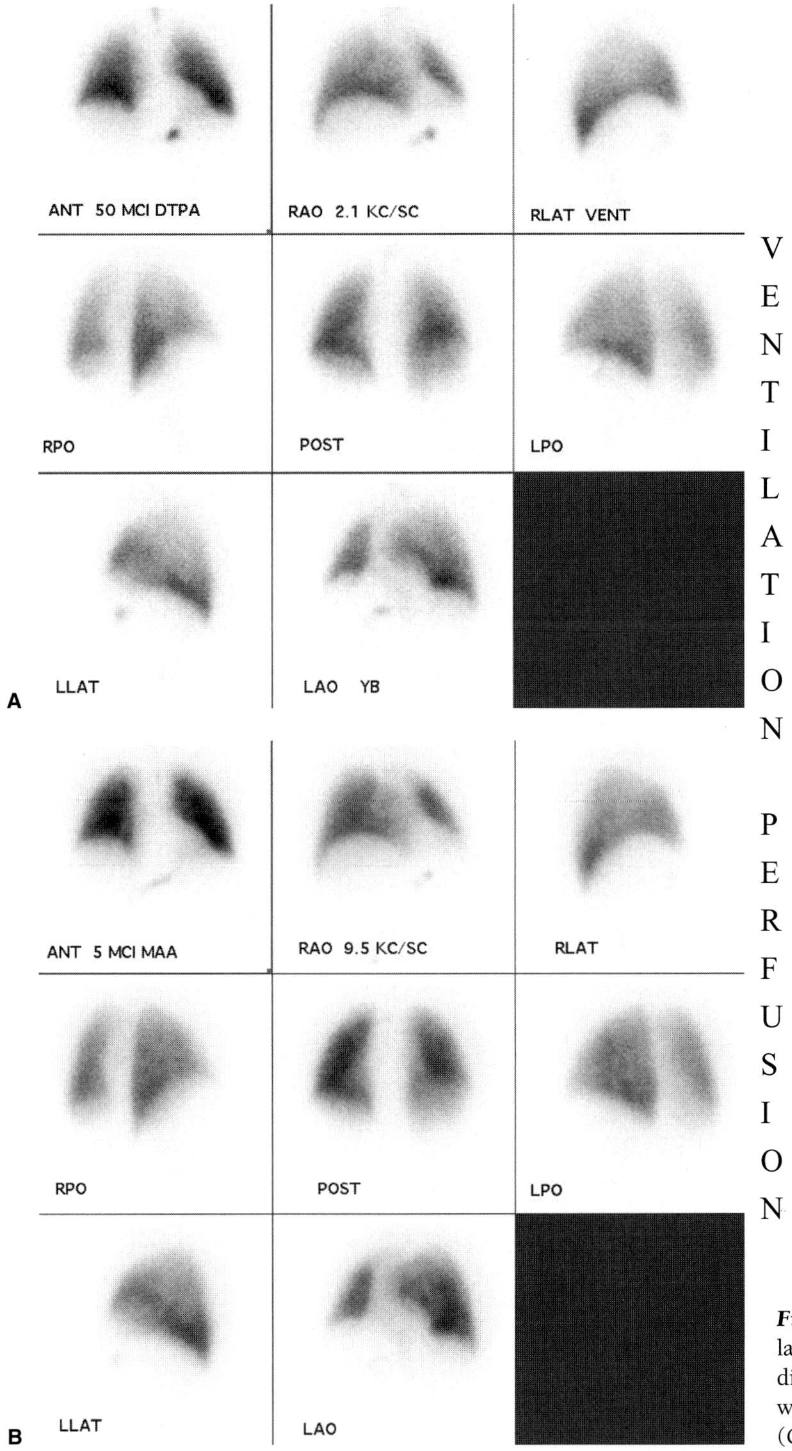

ANT 50 MCI DTPA   RAO 2.1 KC/SC   RLAT VENT

RPO   POST   LPO

LLAT   LAO YB

A

V E N T I L A T I O N

ANT 5 MCI MAA   RAO 9.5 KC/SC   RLAT

RPO   POST   LPO

LLAT   LAO

B

P E R F U S I O N

Figure 21.2 Normal ventilation-perfusion scan. *A*. Ventilation scan, with uniform uptake of technetium-99m diethylenetriaminepentaacetic acid. *B*. Perfusion scan, with uniform uptake of Tc microaggregates of albumin. (Courtesy of Dr. C. Bui, Ann Arbor, MI.)

Table 21.3: Revised PIOPED Ventilation Perfusion Interpretation Categories and Criteria

High probability	≥2 large (>75% of a segment) segmental equivalent perfusion defects substantially larger than corresponding ventilation or radiographic abnormalities or without any ventilation or radiograph abnormalities.
Intermediate/indeterminate probability	0.5 to 1.5 mismatched segmental equivalent perfusion defects. This may be 1 large plus 1 moderate mismatched perfusion defects, or 1 to 3 moderate.
	Solitary moderate or large segmental size triple match in lower lobe.
	Multiple opacities with associated perfusion defects.
Low probability	A single large or moderate size matched segmental defect.
	>3 small segmental perfusion defects (<25% of a segment) with a normal chest radiograph.
	Moderate sized pleural effusion with no other perfusion defect in either lung.
Very low probability	Nonsegmental lesion, linear atelectasis, costophrenic angle effusion with no other perfusion defect in either lung.
	>2 VQ matched defects with normal chest x-ray.
	1–3 small segmental perfusion defects.
	Solitary triple matched defect in the mid or upper lung zone.
Normal	No perfusion defects present.

VQ, ventilation perfusion.
From Gottschalk A, Stein PD, Henry JW, et al. Matched ventilation, perfusion and chest radiographic abnormalities in acute pulmonary embolism. *J Nuclear Med* 1996;37:1636–1638; Stein PD, Relyea B, Gottschalk A. Evaluation of individual criteria for low probability interpretation of ventilation-perfusion lung scans. *J Nuclear Med* 1996;37:577–581; and Gottschalk A, Sostman HD, Coleman RE, et al. Ventilation-perfusion scintigraphy in the PIOPED study. Part II. Evaluation of the scintigraphic criteria and interpretations. *J Nuclear Med* 1993;34:1119–1126, with permission.

Pulmonary Angiography

Pulmonary angiography is the reference test (gold standard) for the diagnosis of PE.

Pulmonary angiography is considered the reference test for the diagnosis of PE, against which all other tests are compared. Pulmonary angiography is recommended when there is an indeterminate V/Q scan, a discordance between the V/Q result (low probability, very low probability), and a high clinical suspicion for PE, indeterminate CTPA, or in cases of acute massive PE. It is particularly useful when catheter-guided thrombolysis or catheter-guided thrombectomy with direct injection of thrombolytic agent into the thrombus is to be performed. An invasive test, it requires a venous puncture usually at the groin and placement of a catheter through the right atrium and right ventricle into the main pulmonary artery, followed by selective placement in the right and left pulmonary arteries. Passage through the heart may induce an arrhythmia, including right bundle branch block. Therefore, patients with left bundle branch block should have a pacemaker in during the procedure. Contrast media is then injected and images obtained in the anteroposterior and oblique projections of each lung. It is a relatively safe invasive test, with a low mortality rate of 0.5% and morbidity rate of 3% to 5%, but is an extremely underused modality, used in only 12% to 14% of patients with nondiagnostic V/Q scans (4,13–15).

Pulmonary angiography is underused in the diagnosis of PE.

Pulmonary angiography allows direct visualization of the clot burden. The angiographic signs of PE are a filling defect within an opacified pulmonary artery (Fig. 21.5) or occlusion of a pulmonary arterial branch (16,17). Absent or reduced opacification of small arterial branches is sometimes seen, corresponding to a perfusion defect on perfusion scintigraphy. A good quality negative pulmonary angiogram virtually excludes PE. However, angiography has its limitations. It is an invasive test that is underused and not available at all centers.

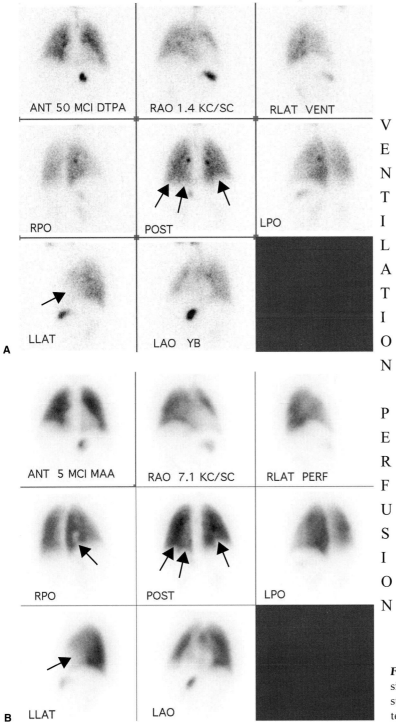

V
E
N
T
I
L
A
T
I
O
N

P
E
R
F
U
S
I
O
N

Figure 21.3 Intermediate probability ventilation-perfusion scan. (*A*) Ventilation and (*B*) perfusion scans demonstrate multiple small mismatched defects (*arrows*). (Courtesy of Dr. C. Bui, Ann Arbor, MI.)

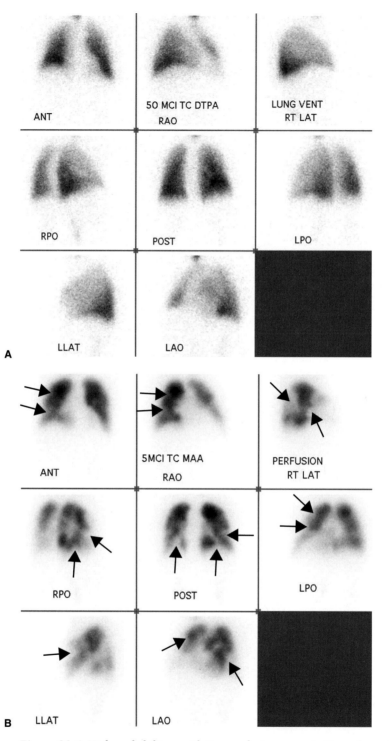

Figure 21.4 High probability ventilation-perfusion scan. *A.* Normal ventilation scan with uniform uptake of technetium-99m diethylenetriaminepentaacetic acid. *B.* Perfusion scan demonstrating multiple defects (*arrows*) that are mismatched, compatible with acute pulmonary embolism. (Courtesy of Dr. C. Bui, Ann Arbor, MI.)

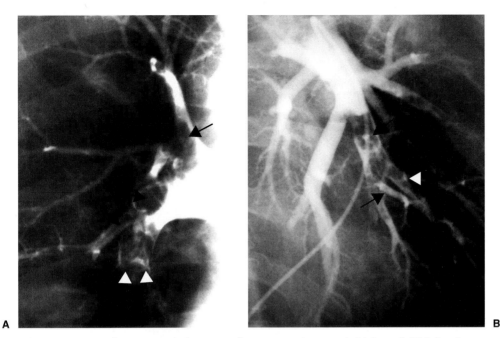

A   B

Figure 21.5 Acute pulmonary embolism on pulmonary angiogram. *A.* Right and (*B*) left pulmonary artery selective injections demonstrating multiple filling defects (*arrows*) and vessel cutoff sign (*arrowheads*). (Courtesy of Dr. K. Cho, Ann Arbor, MI.)

Computed Tomography

PE has incidentally been encountered on thoracic CT examinations as early as 1978. With the advent of new, faster, helical CT scanners, the ability of CT to detect PE as a primary test has received a great deal of interest (18,19). Techniques and scanners have evolved over the last decade; since the introduction of four-row multidetector and greater detector CT scanners, CT has taken on a more dominant role in the evaluation of suspected PE, right down to the subsegmental level (20). CTPA has been almost as reliable as pulmonary angiography in the detection of PE up to the segmental level; with multidetector CT, this reliability may also extend to the subsegmental level (21). Up to one-third of cases at the subsegmental level are misdiagnosed, even at pulmonary angiography (10). With thinner collimation, subsegmental emboli can be seen in 61% to 70% of cases (19,22). There is ongoing debate about the clinical significance of isolated subsegmental PE and whether these should be treated. Treatment may especially benefit patients with cardiopulmonary compromise; in patients with normal cardiopulmonary physiology there is more debate.

Helical Computed Tomography Pulmonary Angiogram

Iodinated contrast, 120 to 150 mL, is usually injected via the antecubital vein, at 4 to 5 mL/s. The timing of intravenous contrast bolus is crucial in obtaining diagnostic quality images. The technique has to be optimized for the CT scanner being used. Scanning is done from caudal to cranial direction to minimize streak artifact from the superior vena cava and to avoid breathing motion artifact from the diaphragm, during the latter part of the scan, if the patient cannot breath-hold.

Using single detector CT, the patient is scanned from the domes of the diaphragm to the top of the aortic arch in a single breath-hold following a scan delay of 25 seconds. Images are obtained at 2.5 mm to 3 mm collimation and reconstructed at 1.5 to 2 mm intervals. Using the 4 row multidetector CT scanner, because of the scanner speed, the entire chest can be scanned in 17 to 22 seconds, following a scan delay of 20 seconds at 1.25 mm collimation with images reconstructed at 0.625 mm intervals. Using 8-row detector multidetector CT the scan time is reduced again by half and on 16-row detector multidetector CT, to one-fourth, or approximately 5 seconds—of great benefit in patients with shortness of breath.

CTPA is interpreted on a workstation and read using a scrolling mode with altering of the window level and width dynamically for optimal evaluation of the pulmonary arteries. The scrolling mode is used to pan through the main, lobar, segmental, and subsegmental pulmonary arteries; hence, it is extremely important to be familiar with the pulmonary arterial anatomy.

Acute PE is principally diagnosed by visualizing a low attenuation filling defect within a well-opacified pulmonary artery (Figs. 21.6 and 21.7). Other CT findings of acute PE are listed in Table 21.4. Some of these signs include the "railway track" sign (Fig. 21.8D), the vessel cutoff sign, and the rim sign (Fig. 21.8C), where there is a filling defect due to thrombus with a rim of contrast around it. If there is occlusive thrombus, the corresponding artery may be larger and completely filled with low attenuation thrombus. In the case of nonocclusive thrombus, the rim sign may be seen or low attenuation thrombus can be seen in the center of the artery as a nonadherent thrombus or occasionally at the periphery. Ancillary signs of PE, although nonspecific by themselves, can be helpful in case of subtle thrombus. These can manifest as small pleural effusions, atelectasis, or pulmonary infarct distal to a PE (Fig. 21.8), oligemia or mosaic attenuation (Fig. 21.9) due to differential perfusion, and, in case of massive PE, signs of right heart strain with enlargement of the right ventricle and straightening of the interventricular septum.

The source of thrombus can occasionally be seen on the chest CT, such as in the superior vena cava, brachiocephalic veins, other neck veins, or the right atrium (Fig. 21.10). Pulmonary infarcts appear as triangular areas with a broad base in contact with the pleural surface and apex directed centrally, with a feeding vessel at the apex. Classic pulmonary infarcts do not enhance, whereas atelectasis or consolidation due to pneumonia often enhances. An advantage of CT is its capability of detecting thoracic abnormalities that mimic signs and symptoms of PE, aiding appropriate and immediate management of these patients (23). These abnormalities manifest as pleural, parenchymal, pericardial, or chest wall disease, seen in up to 40% to 70% of patients with suspected PE, such as pneumonia or abscess (Fig. 21.11), tumor (Fig. 21.12), septic emboli, malignant or nonmalignant pleural effusions, pericardial effusion (Fig. 21.13), pneumothorax, and chest wall tumors.

Pitfalls in the diagnosis of PE on CT are listed in Table 21.5. It is important to use the scrolling mode, so as not to mistake a vein for an artery, an adjacent perihilar node for an arterial filling defect, or mucoid-filled dilated bronchi for an arterial filling defect. Poor contrast bolus causing inadequate opacification of the pulmonary arteries, extensive breathing motion artifact, cardiac motion artifact, low signal-to-noise ratio due to large

Intraluminal filling defects on CT are very specific for the diagnosis of PE.

The neck, extremity, and mediastinal veins should all be examined on pulmonary embolism CTs for the source of emboli.

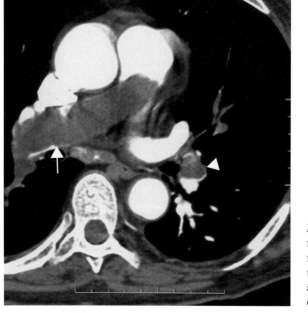

Figure 21.6 Acute massive pulmonary embolism. Computed tomography demonstrates a large central thrombus in right main pulmonary artery (*arrow*). Left lobar pulmonary embolism is also noted (*arrowheads*).

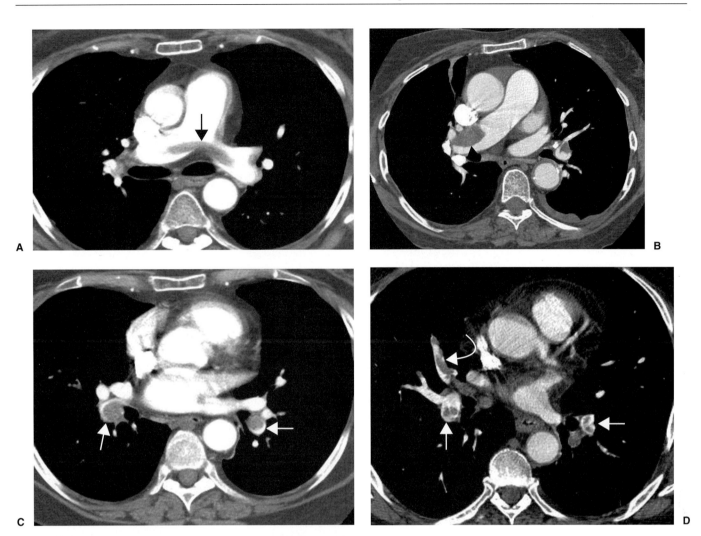

Figure 21.7 Acute pulmonary embolism. Computed tomography demonstrates *(A)* saddle embolus *(arrow)*, *(B)* central pulmonary embolism in right main pulmonary artery *(arrow)*, and *(C)* bilateral lobar pulmonary embolism, with rim sign demonstrated *(arrows)*. Note lobar pulmonary embolism in the left lower lobe *(arrowhead)* and *(D)* segmental pulmonary embolism *(arrows)*. Tram track sign is seen in the middle lobe pulmonary artery *(curved arrow)*. E. Subsegmental pulmonary emboli are also demonstrated *(arrows)*.

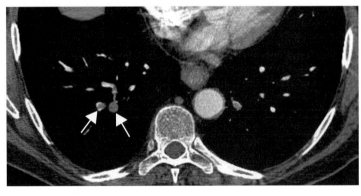

Table 21.4: Findings of Acute Pulmonary Embolism on Computed Tomography

Direct	Indirect
Clot	Pulmonary infarct
Railway track sign	Large pulmonary artery
Vessel cutoff	Pleural effusion
Rim sign	Atelectasis
	Mosaic attenuation

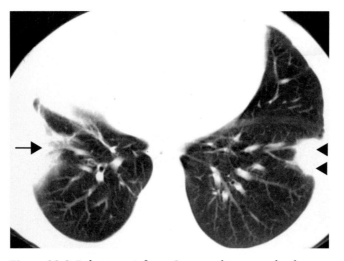

Figure 21.8 Pulmonary infarct. Computed tomography demonstrating right wedge-shaped peripheral pulmonary infarct (*arrow*) and somewhat rounded left lower lobe pulmonary infarct (*arrowheads*) secondary to pulmonary embolism.

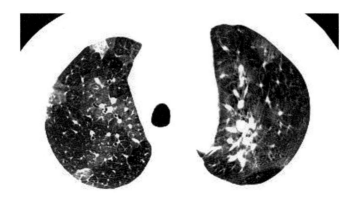

Figure 21.9 Mosaic attenuation. Computed tomography demonstrating hypo- and hyperattenuated lung parenchyma.

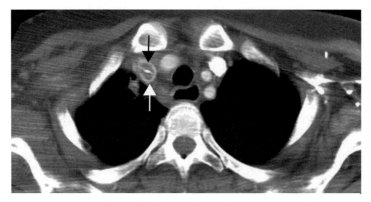

Figure 21.10 Brachiocephalic vein thrombosis. Computed tomography demonstrates a filling defect (*arrow*) representing thrombus in the right brachiocephalic vein surrounding a venous catheter.

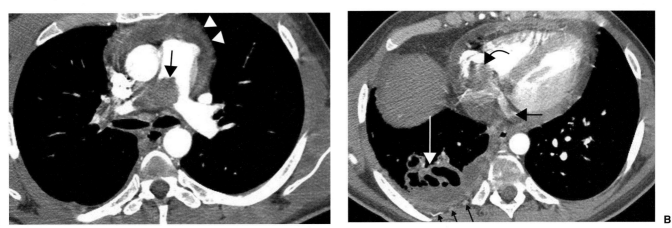

Figure 21.11 Conditions clinically mimicking acute pulmonary embolism. *A.* Computed tomography demonstrates an infected thrombus *(arrow)* (positive blood cultures), pericardial effusion *(arrowheads)* and *(B)* right lower lobe lung abscess *(white arrow)* with an adjacent empyema *(short arrows)*, and a right atrial myxoma *(curved arrow)*.

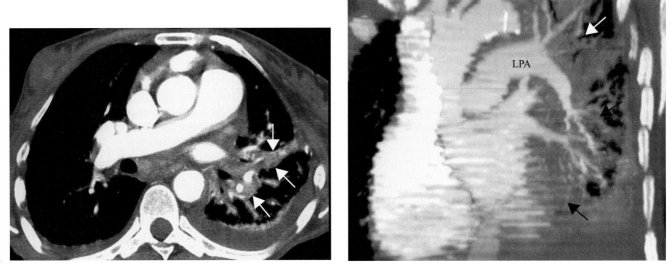

Figure 21.12 Conditions clinically mimicking acute pulmonary embolism. *A.* Axial computed tomography and *(B)* sagittal computed tomography reformat, demonstrate left hilar abnormal soft tissue *(arrows)* and enlarged nodes surrounding the left pulmonary artery (LPA) and its branches, secondary to bronchogenic carcinoma.

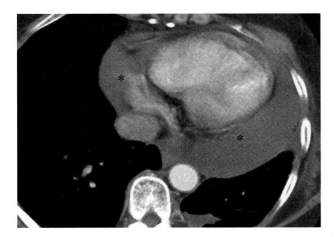

Figure 21.13 Conditions clinically mimicking acute pulmonary embolism. Computed tomography demonstrating a large pericardial effusion (asterisk) in a patient later diagnosed with systemic lupus erythematosus.

Table 21.5: Pitfalls in the Diagnosis of Acute Pulmonary Embolism on Computed Tomography

Pulmonary Embolism Mimics	Limitations in Accurate Diagnosis
Partial volume averaging	Image noise in large patients
Perihilar/bronchopulmonary lymph nodes	Respiratory motion artifact
Mucoid impacted bronchi	Cardiac motion artifact
Mistaking a pulmonary vein for an artery	Streak artifact from lines and tubes

patient size, and artifact from tubes and lines in critically ill patients can sometimes pose a challenge in the evaluation of PE in these patients (24–26).

Electron Beam Computed Tomography

Electron beam CT allows scanning during maximal opacification of vessels with the main advantage of very short aquisition times in the order of 14 to 17 seconds, with subsequent decreased respiratory and cardiac motion artifacts. Breath-holding is not mandatory, and a smaller amount of contrast material is administered peripherally (80 to 120 mL). Images are performed at 3 to 6 mm collimation and reconstructed at 3 to 1.5 mm collimation (27–29). Image interpretation is similar to that described for helical CT. With thin-section helical scanners there is no statistically significant difference in the number of analyzable pulmonary arteries; electron beam CT has a minor advantage in evaluation of the paracardiac arteries.

Computed Tomography Venography

With the advent of faster multidetector CT scanners, it has been possible to evaluate the pelvic and lower extremity veins, allowing evaluation of the pulmonary emboli and the cause thereof, DVT in the lower extremities, with a single study.

After a scan delay of 3 minutes from the intravenous injection given for CTPA, the patient is scanned from the caudad to cranial direction from the level of the tibial plateaus to the iliac crests at 7.5 mm collimation. Images are reconstructed at 3.75 mm collimation and are interpreted at the workstation, using a scrolling mode. DVT is diagnosed when there is an occlusive or nonocclusive filling defect (Figs. 21.14 and 21.15). Venous enhancement of more than 80 Hu is needed to identify DVT. Reasons that optimal venous enhancement may not be obtained include arterial inflow problems, particularly peripheral vascular occlusive disease, hypotension, and hemodilution. Orthopedic hardware may cause extensive artifact, limiting evaluation of segments of veins. Several investigators have demonstrated a high sensitivity and specificity in the detection of DVT, using venous sonography as the reference test; the accuracy for CT venography to detect DVT in the infrapopliteal vessels is not yet known (30,31). An advantage of CT is the ability to evaluate the iliac vessels and the inferior vena cava, which are difficult to evaluate with sonography particularly in large patients (Fig. 21.21).

Helical CT venography, combined with CTPA, is highly accurate for the diagnosis of DVT from the inferior vena cava through the popliteal veins.

Magnetic Resonance Imaging

MRI is useful in the evaluation of suspected PE, particularly in patients allergic to iodinated contrast medium, in children, and in pregnant women, because it does not involve ionizing radiation. Intravenous gadolinium is used as a contrast agent. With evolving scanners and techniques, there is no uniform single MRI protocol. PE is detected as a flow void, and the remainder of the normal signal from flowing blood is processed to obtain two-dimensional and three-dimensional images (Figs. 21.16 and 21.17) (32,33).

Multiplanar reformatting can help evaluation, as in CT. MRI, like CT, allows direct visualization of emboli. It is useful in the detection of central and segmental PE, whereas at the subsegmental level accuracy is less well evaluated. Newer and faster MR scanners and recirculating MR contrast agents may improve MRI accuracy. Furthermore, MRI per-

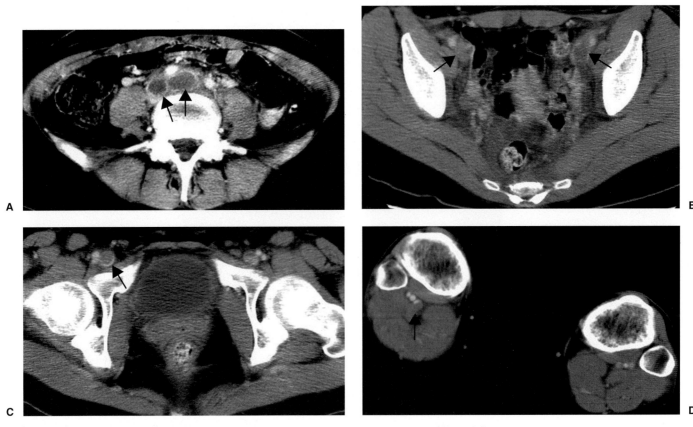

Figure 21.14 Acute deep venous thrombosis. Computed tomography demonstrates filling defects of acute deep vein thrombosis in (A) bilateral common iliac veins (*arrows*), (B) bilateral external iliac veins (*arrows*), (C) right common femoral vein (*arrow*), and (D) right calf vein (*arrow*).

fusion techniques may assist in the evaluation of PE, especially in the case of small acute emboli or in the evaluation of thromboembolic disease leading to pulmonary arterial hypertension (34). Defects in pulmonary perfusion are comparable with perfusion defects on V/Q scan in cases of PE. Ventilation scanning is also now possible with MRI (35).

MR venography has been shown to be comparable with or even better than ultrasound and conventional venography for the detection of DVT, and is particularly useful in the evaluation of patients in whom sonography is not possible. Like CT, it allows direct visualization of clot in the pelvis and lower extremity veins but without the administration of

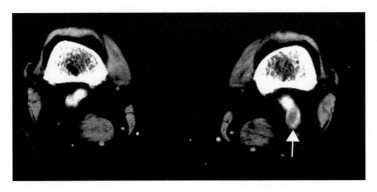

Figure 21.15 Acute popliteal venous thrombosis. Computed tomography demonstrates a filling defect in the left popliteal vein, with the rim sign (*arrow*).

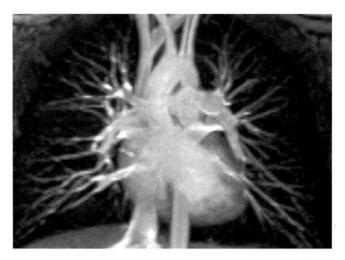

***Figure* 21.16** Normal magnetic resonance angiography of the pulmonary arteries (PA).

contrast. Gradient-echo and time-of-flight images demonstrate low signal clot occluding a vein or low signal clot surrounded by high signal flowing blood.

CHRONIC PULMONARY EMBOLISM

Chronic PE can be difficult to diagnose and can be a cause of pulmonary hypertension. The imaging findings of chronic PE represent recanalization of the arterial lumen previously occluded by an acute central clot. As such, it appears as webs, stenoses, or peripheral thrombi that may or may not be calcified. The most specific finding is low attenuation thrombus at the periphery of the vessel or adherent to the vessel wall, and it may be irregular and may contain calcium. Chronic PE can lead to pulmonary hypertension. Enlarged and tortuous central pulmonary arteries with pruning of the peripheral pulmonary arteries indicate pulmonary hypertension. Mosaic attenuation can also be seen.

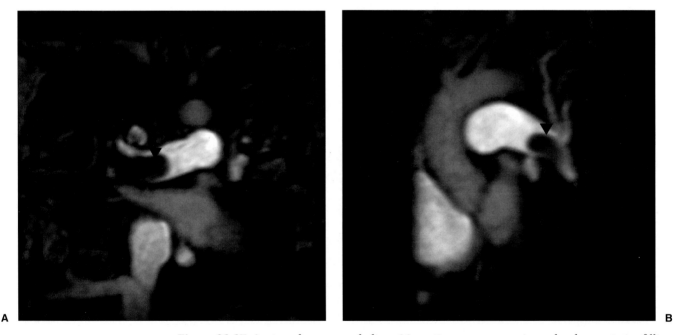

***Figure* 21.17** Acute pulmonary embolism. Magnetic resonance angiography demonstrates filling defect (*arrow*) compatible with pulmonary embolism in the (*A*) right and (*B*) left main pulmonary arteries. (Courtesy of Dr. Ruth Carlos, Ann Arbor, MI.)

RADIOLOGY IN THE DIAGNOSIS OF CHRONIC PULMONARY EMBOLISM

Chest Radiograph

The chest radiograph may be normal in early chronic thromboembolic disease. Enlarged central pulmonary arteries, with narrow caliber peripheral arteries, peripheral oligemia, and right ventricular enlargement, can result as a consequence of recurrent chronic PE (Fig. 21.18).

Ventilation-Perfusion Scanning

The findings are similar to those of acute PE. Multiple mismatched perfusion defects are diagnostic of multiple segmental emboli. A high proportion of indeterminate/intermediate probability V/Q scans occur in patients with chronic PE.

Pulmonary Angiography

Angiographic signs of chronic PE are the presence of eccentric mural thrombi, webs or bands, intimal irregularities, varying caliber of the vessels (Fig. 21.19), abrupt vessel narrowing, pouch defects, or complete obstruction of the vessels. Poststenotic dilation can be seen distal to a narrowing or web.

Computed Tomography

CT is the imaging modality of choice in the evaluation of patients with PAH and suspected CTEPH (36,37). CTPA may demonstrate eccentric thrombus adjacent to a vessel wall in the form of crescentic mural-adherent thrombus (Fig. 21.20). The thrombus may be retracted, or there may be recanalization of thrombus with contrast seen traversing the intraluminal filling defect. Arterial webs and narrowing (Figs. 21.21, 21.22, and 21.23), irregular caliber vessels with abrupt narrowing of the arteries, or complete occlusion at the level of the narrowing can also be seen (38,39). Calcification is seen in approximately 10% of chronic central thrombi (Figs. 21.18 and 21.24). Secondary signs include irregular or nodular arterial walls, abrupt narrowing of arteries, or abrupt cutoff of peripheral segmental arteries. A marked variation in size of segmental vessels is more specific for chronic pulmonary thromboembolism than mosaic attenuation.

Webs, wall thickening, and stenosis are the hallmarks of chronic PE on both CT and catheter angiography.

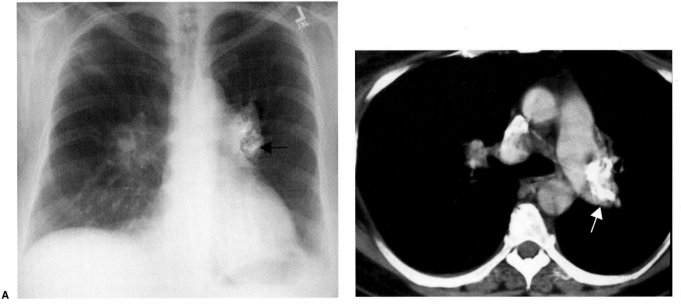

Figure 21.18 Calcified chronic pulmonary embolism. *A.* Chest radiograph and *(B)* computed tomography demonstrating calcification in the left pulmonary artery, compatible with calcified thrombus *(arrow)*.

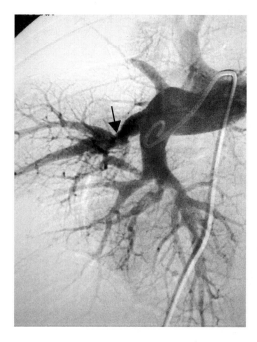

Figure 21.19 Chronic pulmonary embolism with stenosis. Selective right pulmonary angiogram demonstrating segmental stenosis of the right upper lobe pulmonary artery *(arrow)*. (Courtesy of Dr. K. Cho, Ann Arbor, MI.)

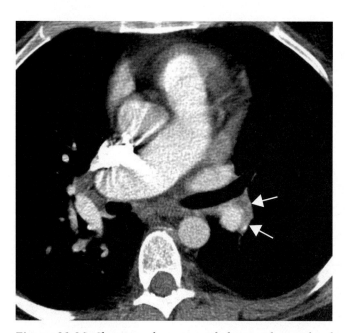

Figure 21.20 Chronic pulmonary embolism with peripheral filling defect. Computed tomography demonstrates a crescentic filling defect in left lower lobe pulmonary artery *(arrows)*.

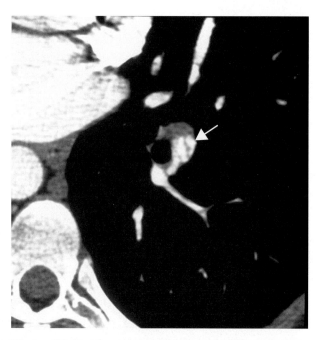

Figure 21.21 Chronic pulmonary embolism with web. Computed tomography demonstrates a linear filling defect in left lower lobe pulmonary artery *(arrow)*.

Mosaic perfusion is a lung finding of chronic PE on CT.

A mosaic perfusion pattern to the lungs on CT, described as patchy areas of decreased attenuation interspersed with areas of increased or normal attenuation due to regional differences in blood flow (Fig. 21.9), may occur with CTEPH (40). The areas of hypoattenuation represent decreased perfusion and areas of hyperattenuation represent perfused or hyperperfused lung. However, sometimes it is difficult to differentiate between primary vascular disease, small airways disease, and pulmonary parenchymal disease as the cause of mosaic pattern. The number and caliber of the vessels helps to distinguish between

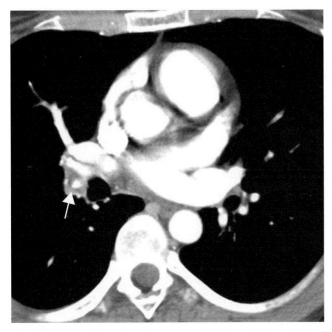

Figure 21.22 Chronic pulmonary embolism with recanalization of thrombus. Computed tomography demonstrates central contrast within thrombus (*arrow*) in the right descending pulmonary artery.

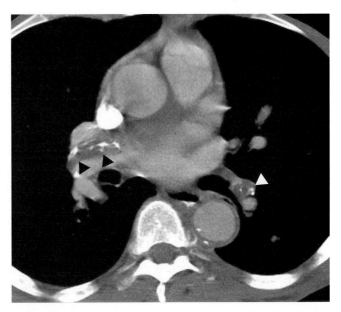

Figure 21.23 Chronic pulmonary embolism with calcified thrombus. Computed tomography demonstrates a low attenuation thrombus (*arrowheads*) with calcification.

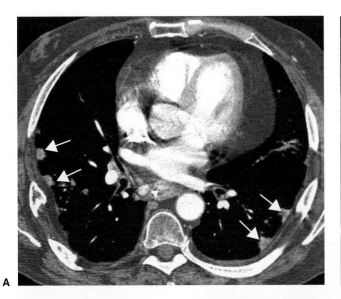

A

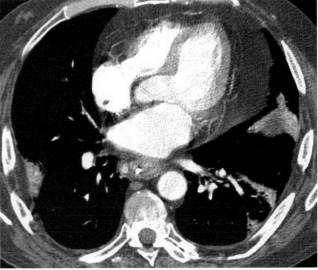

B

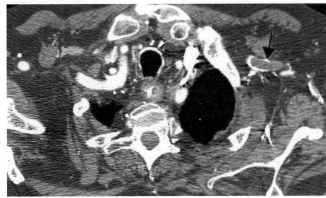

C

Figure 21.24 Septic emboli. Computed tomography demonstrates (A) bilateral peripheral nodules with peripheral enhancement (*arrows*), (B) bilateral peripheral wedge-shaped abnormalities, and (C) thrombus in the left subclavian vein (*arrow*) (infected porta catheter removed was the source of the septic emboli).

these etiologies. In pulmonary parenchymal disease, the vessel caliber is uniform throughout areas of varying attenuation, whereas in the other two the vessels are decreased in caliber in the hypoattenuated areas. Airway and primary vascular disease can be differentiated by air trapping found on expiratory images in patients with small airways disease but not in patients with vascular disease. High resolution CT may demonstrate cylindrical airway dilatation adjacent to stenotic or obstructed pulmonary arteries in up to two-thirds of patients (41).

Magnetic Resonance Imaging

MR angiographic features are similar to CT and conventional angiography (42). The peripheral arteries in patients with chronic PE are of varying caliber. MR images may be reconstructed in two or three dimensions, producing image quality similar to conventional angiography, now possible with multidetector CT. The main advantage of MRI is the ability to provide quantitative measurements of pulmonary perfusion, flow measurements in the pulmonary arteries, and quantitative analyses of the ejection fraction of the right ventricle before and after treatment. The disadvantages are poor spatial resolution, breathing motion artifacts, longer imaging times, and less availability. It is particularly useful in patients allergic to iodinated contrast media.

SEPTIC PULMONARY EMBOLISM

Septic emboli often arise from infected central venous catheters or occur in patients with intravenous drug abuse due to peripheral septic thrombophlebitis (Fig. 21.24) or tricuspid valve endocarditis (43). Occasionally, infection from the pharynx or parapharyngeal space can extend into the internal jugular vein, leading to septic emboli or Lemierre syndrome (Fig. 21.25). Other causes include infection in patients with immunologic deficiencies, skin infection, infected arm and pelvic veins, and infected arteriovenous fistulas. Blood cultures in these patients are often positive for *Staphylococcus aureus* and less commonly *Streptococcus*. Patients present with fever, cough, and hemoptysis.

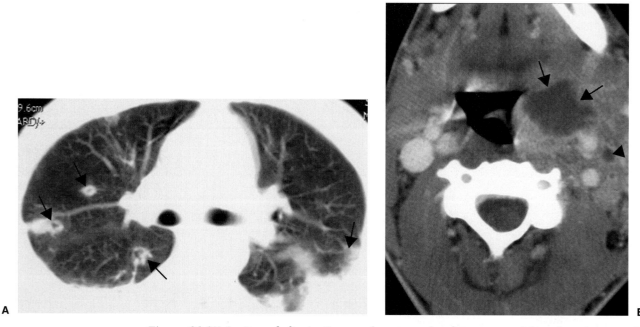

Figure 21.25 Septic emboli. *A.* Computed tomography demonstrates bilateral cavitary septic emboli *(arrows)*. *B.* Computed tomography of the neck in the same patient demonstrates a left parapharyngeal abscess *(arrow)*, the source of the septic emboli, and thrombus in the left internal jugular vein *(arrowhead)*.

Septic emboli on chest radiograph and CT manifest as multiple, ill-defined, wedge-shaped, or round peripheral nodules, which may be unilateral or bilateral and can be asymmetric (Figs. 21.24 and 21.25). They can come and go, with new lesions appearing and others resolving due to showering of infected foci into the pulmonary artery circulation over time. As they evolve, they may become better defined, smaller, and demonstrate cavitation (Fig. 21.25). Extension into the pleural space can occur, resulting in an empyema. On CT, vessels may be associated with the nodules. The *feeding vessel sign*, different stages of cavitation and intracavitary debris, and peripheral enhancement may be seen. Septic emboli can result in pulmonary infarction, seen as a triangular wedged-shaped opacity that demonstrates peripheral enhancement due to blood flow from bronchial arteries and central low attenuation or nonenhancement.

> Multiple, new, peripheral, ill-defined nodules, with or without cavitation, should raise suspicion for septic embolism.

PULMONARY ARTERIAL HYPERTENSION

Pulmonary arterial hypertension (PAH) is defined as systolic pulmonary artery pressure above 30 mm Hg or mean value of 18 mm Hg. The most common presenting feature of patients with pulmonary hypertension is dyspnea. Patients may have other symptoms, such as decreased exercise tolerance, fatigue, chest pain, syncope, cyanosis, and peripheral edema. The clinical diagnosis is based on a combination of physical signs, echocardiography, and radiology, with right heart catheterization being the definitive diagnostic test. The etiologies of pulmonary hypertension are listed in Table 21.6. Pulmonary hypertension may be either primary or secondary in etiology, with diseases grouped into a precapillary and postcapillary classification.

Primary pulmonary hypertension is rare and is idiopathic in etiology, occurring three times more commonly in young or middle-aged women than in men. It has an incidence of approximately one per million. Patients present with dyspnea, fatigue, angina, syncope, and cor pulmonale. Secondary precapillary causes of PAH include chronic thromboembolic disease, interstitial lung disease and obstructive pulmonary parenchymal disease, anorexigenic drugs, congenital heart disease (Fig. 21.26), and human immunodeficiency virus infection.

Table 21.6: Etiologies of Pulmonary Hypertension

Precapillary			Postcapillary	
Primary Vascular Disease	*Pleuropulmonary Disease*	*Alveolar Hypoventilation*	*Cardiac Disease*	*Pulmonary Venous Disease*
Primary pulmonary hypertension	Emphysema	Neuromuscular disease	Left ventricular failure	Pulmonary veno-occlusive disease
Pulmonary thromboembolic disease	Diffuse interstitial lung disease	Obesity	Left atrial myxoma/ thrombus	Anomalous pulmonary venous drainage
Multiple pulmonary artery stenoses	Bronchiectasis (cystic fibrosis)	Obstructive sleep apnea	Cor triatriatum	Fibrosing mediastinitis
Pulmonary vasculitis	Post-pneumonectomy	Chronic upper airways obstruction in children	Mitral valve disease	Congenital stenoses of pulmonary veins
Pulmonary capillary hemangiomatosis	Fibrothorax			Thrombosis
Immunologic (SLE, scleroderma)	Chest wall deformity			Neoplasms

SLE, systemic lupus erythematosus.

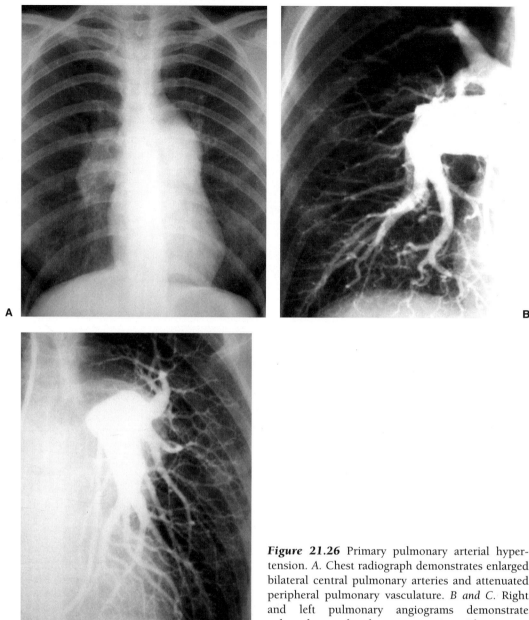

Figure 21.26 Primary pulmonary arterial hypertension. *A.* Chest radiograph demonstrates enlarged bilateral central pulmonary arteries and attenuated peripheral pulmonary vasculature. *B and C.* Right and left pulmonary angiograms demonstrate enlarged central pulmonary arteries with tortuous distal pulmonary arteries.

Pulmonary veno-occlusive disease is a rare postcapillary cause of PAH in which webs due to recanalized thrombus and intimal fibrosis are seen in the pulmonary veins. Before 1990, the diagnosis was often made postmortem but now is more frequently made antemortem by recognizing the various modes of presentation and with the help of high resolution CT. The diagnosis is usually made by excluding other causes of pulmonary hypertension, with the findings of interstitial edema and ground glass opacity on chest radiograph or high resolution CT. In capillary hemangiomatosis, nodular collections of thin-walled capillaries invade the pulmonary arteries, veins, and bronchioles; it is considered a subset of pulmonary veno-occlusive disease by some authors. Less than 1% of patients with chronic liver failure may also develop PAH, which may be secondary to circulating vasoactive substances that the liver fails to metabolize (44).

Pulmonary hypertension is a significant cause of morbidity and mortality but is a potentially treatable condition. Therapy ranges from medical treatment with vasodilators to surgical treatment with lung or combined heart–lung transplant. The treatment of choice for CTEPH is pulmonary endarterectomy. In cases of suspected CTEPH, pulmonary angiography or CT may be performed, as described earlier.

RADIOLOGY IN THE DIAGNOSIS OF PULMONARY HYPERTENSION

Chest Radiograph

The classic radiographic findings of advanced PAH are enlargement of the central pulmonary arteries that may be tortuous with pruning of the peripheral arteries, peripheral oligemia, and right ventricular enlargement (Fig. 21.27) (45). Calcification of the central pulmonary arteries can be seen in severe chronic PAH. A completely normal CXR film speaks against the diagnosis of primary pulmonary hypertension; the National Institutes of Health registry showed that only 6% of patients with primary PAH have a normal chest radiograph. There is controversy regarding the exact measurement of the vessel diameter and degree of PAH, because such measurements vary with magnification, patient positioning, and patient size. The upper limit of normal for the right interlobar pulmonary artery on the frontal chest radiograph is 15 mm or less in women and 16 mm or less in men. For the left descending pulmonary artery, the upper limit of normal on the lateral chest radiograph is 17 mm (46).

> The upper limit of normal for the right interlobar pulmonary artery is 15 mm in women and 16 mm in men on the frontal chest radiograph.

> The upper limit of normal for the right interlobar pulmonary artery on the lateral radiograph is 16 mm.

Echocardiography

PAH is usually evaluated noninvasively with echocardiography, allowing assessment of cardiac chamber size, valve function, wall thickness and function, the detection of intracardiac shunts, and an estimate of pulmonary arterial pressure. The latter is estimated from right ventricular peak systolic pressure. In addition to pulmonary arterial enlargement, the right atrium and ventricle may be enlarged, with accompanying tri-

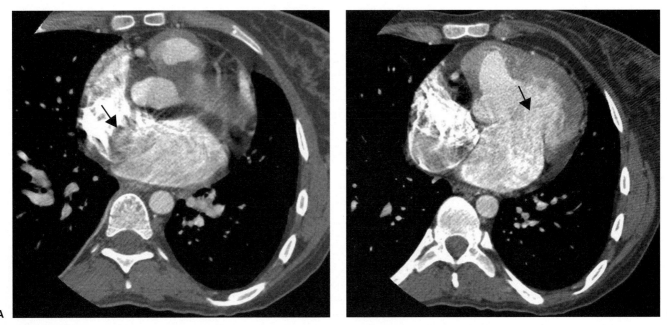

A   B

Figure 21.27 Congenital heart disease as a cause of pulmonary hypertension. A. Computed tomography demonstrates an atrial septal defect (*arrow*) and a (B) ventricular septal defect (*arrow*).

cuspid valve regurgitation. The superior and inferior vena cava may also be enlarged. The use of microbubbles in the form of an agitated saline bolus administered intravenously aids in the detection of intracardiac shunts. Stress echocardiography can be performed to evaluate the dynamic response of the heart to physical or pharmacologic stress (47).

Ventilation-Perfusion Scanning

The findings are similar to those of chronic thromboembolic disease causing PAH. Multiple mismatched perfusion defects are diagnostic of multiple segmental emboli; however, there are a high number of indeterminate/intermediate probability V/Q scans (48). In the absence of CTEPH, the V/Q scan may be normal or low probability in patients with PAH.

Computed Tomography

CT is the imaging modality of choice in the evaluation of patients with PAH and suspected CTEPH, evaluating both the lung parenchyma with high resolution CT technique and pulmonary artery with CTPA, discussed earlier in the chapter. Multidetector CT scanners are also useful in the evaluation of cardiac disease (Fig. 21.27). CT in primary pulmonary hypertension demonstrates marked dilatation of the central pulmonary arteries with abrupt tapering and small caliber peripheral vessels with resultant oligemia or hypoattenuation of the lungs. The upper limit of normal of the main pulmonary artery on CT is 29 mm, above which PAH should be suggested (49). Mosaic attenuation may be present. The CT findings of CTEPH were covered earlier in this chapter. Pericardial effusions are commonly seen in patients with PAH and are usually small to moderate in size. High resolution CT is useful in the evaluation of the lung parenchyma in patients undergoing intravenous prostacyclin therapy for pulmonary hypertension. Ground glass attenuation, centrilobular nodules, and septal lines may be associated with a high risk of treatment failure (50).

In pulmonary veno-occlusive disease, the imaging findings are those of pulmonary hypertension and edema. The central pulmonary veins may also be very small, and there is often gravity-dependent ground glass attenuation, thickened interlobular septa, pleural effusions, and a normal sized left atrium (51). Centrilobular nodules are often seen with pulmonary capillary hemangiomatosis.

Magnetic Resonance Imaging

MR angiographic features in primary pulmonary hypertension are similar to those on CT and conventional angiography. The peripheral vessels in primary pulmonary hypertension may be uniform in caliber, whereas those in patients with chronic PE are of varying caliber.

PULMONARY TUMOR EMBOLISM

Pulmonary tumor embolism is rare in clinical practice but is often seen at autopsy. Occasionally, it may be a presenting feature of malignancy. Patients may present with pleuritic chest pain, dyspnea, cough, hemoptysis, and weight loss. Primary tumors that are associated with pulmonary tumor embolism are bronchoalveolar cell carcinoma; carcinoma of the breast, kidney (Fig. 21.28), and stomach, hepatoma; and choriocarcinoma. Tumor emboli are clumps of malignant cells that can partially or completely occlude pulmonary arteries. On CT, MRI, and angiography they appear similar to acute venous thromboemboli. Dilated and beaded arteries are also seen (52,53). Because these are rarely diagnosed antemortem, the response to chemotherapy has not been tested. High mortality is noted in these patients.

Beaded and/or thick-walled pulmonary arteries should raise suspicion of pulmonary tumor embolism.

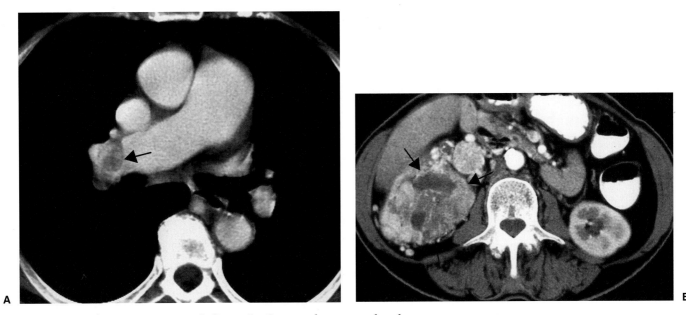

Figure 21.28 Pulmonary tumor embolism. *A.* Computed tomography demonstrates tumor embolism in the right pulmonary artery *(arrow)* from *(B)* right renal cell carcinoma *(arrows).*

PULMONARY ARTERIOVENOUS MALFORMATION

Pulmonary AVMs represent an abnormal vascular connection between the pulmonary arteries and pulmonary veins, with no intervening capillary network. They can range from microscopic communications to large malformations, with a large single feeding vessel and draining vein, or complex malformations, with multiple feeding vessels and draining veins. Pulmonary AVMs are right-to-left shunts that may manifest as cyanosis, polycythemia, stroke, brain abscess, or paradoxical emboli. More commonly they present as an incidental finding on a chest radiograph or CT. Hemoptysis or hemothorax are uncommon (9%). Pulmonary AVMs can be single or multiple. Approximately 60% of patients with multiple pulmonary AVMs have hereditary hemorrhagic telangiectasia, also known as Osler-Weber-Rendu syndrome (Chapter 13). Pulmonary AVMs are single in 60% to 70% of cases and multiple in 30%. They are more common in the lower lobes than in the upper lobes.

> Pulmonary AVMs are commonly part of Osler-Weber-Rendu syndrome.

On *chest radiography*, AVMs are often seen as well-defined nodules, which are somewhat lobulated and range from 1 cm to several centimeters in size. They are often associated with a feeding artery originating at the hilum and a draining vein coursing toward the left atrium. Although most AVMs have a single feeding artery and draining vein, approximately 20% have two or more feeding vessels. The characteristic appearance of lobulated enhancing nodules with a draining vein and a feeding artery or a serpiginous mass of vessels is diagnostic of AVMs on intravenous contrast-enhanced *CT* (Fig. 21.29) (54,55). Calcification is occasionally seen in a nodule due to the presence of a phlebolith. CT is especially useful for posttherapy follow-up and may demonstrate persistence of a lesion or enlarging lesions. Three-dimensional CT is particularly useful in delineating the number, size, and exact location of the AVM and has been found to be comparable with pulmonary angiography. Nonetheless, *pulmonary angiography* is the definitive diagnostic test and is often performed for absolute confirmation, exact delineation of the size, location, and number of AVMs, and the number of feeding arteries and draining veins. Pulmonary angiography also aids therapeutic intervention, such as embolization. Treatment of AVMs reduces the symptoms of hypoxemia and reduces the risks of paradoxical emboli which may present clinically as a brain abscess.

> Most pulmonary AVMs have a single feeding artery and a single draining vein.

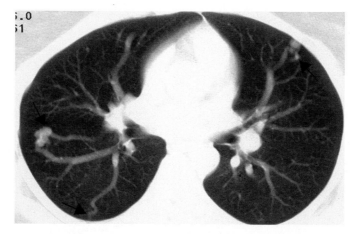

Figure 21.29 Arteriovenous malformations. Computed tomography demonstrating bilateral arteriovenous malformations *(arrows),* with feeding vessels and draining veins.

PULMONARY ARTERY STENOSIS

Stenosis of the pulmonary artery may be single or multiple (Table 21.7). Williams-Beuren syndrome is a rare congenital disorder with pulmonary artery stenosis, mental retardation, and peculiar facies. Central pulmonary artery stenosis is often associated with cardiovascular abnormalities and congenital heart disease; the latter is discussed in Chapter 19. Extrinsic pulmonary artery compression is usually secondary to an adjacent mediastinal or hilar neoplasm (Fig. 21.30) or fibrosing mediastinitis (Fig. 21.31). Patients may present with signs and symptoms of PE. Patients with peripheral pulmonary artery stenosis may demonstrate a loud second heart sound and a systolic murmur.

On *chest radiograph,* the pulmonary vasculature may be diminished distal to a pulmonary artery stenosis, or there may be poststenotic dilatation, especially if pulmonary artery stenosis is the only abnormality. *CT* readily demonstrates pulmonary artery stenosis, especially with the reconstruction capability of multidetector CT. CT is particularly useful in the evaluation of the causes of compression of the pulmonary arteries. Selective *pulmonary angiography* may be useful in the detailed evaluation of the stenosis and the distal vasculature.

PULMONARY ARTERY ANEURYSMS AND PSEUDOANEURYSMS

Aneurysms of the pulmonary artery are rare and may be idiopathic, congenital, or secondary, as listed in Table 21.8. Congenital aneurysms are commonly proximal and associated with pulmonary valve stenosis. Hughes-Stovin syndrome is a rare disorder in which small and large aneurysms of the pulmonary arteries are accompanied by thrombosis of the dural

Table 21.7: Etiologies of Pulmonary Artery Stenosis

Congenital	Extrinsic/Pulmonary Artery Compression
Associated with congenital heart disease	Ehlers-Danlos syndrome
William-Beuren syndrome	Fibrosing mediastinitis
Down syndrome	Sequela of radiation treatment
Ehlers-Danlos syndrome	

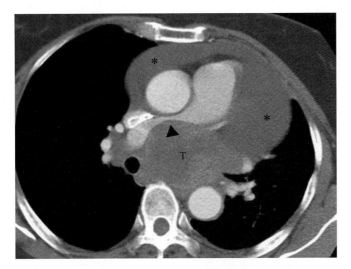

Figure 21.30 Pulmonary artery stenosis. Computed tomography demonstrates extrinsic compression of the right main pulmonary artery (*arrowheads*) from large central tumor (T) and an associated pericardial effusion (*arrows*).

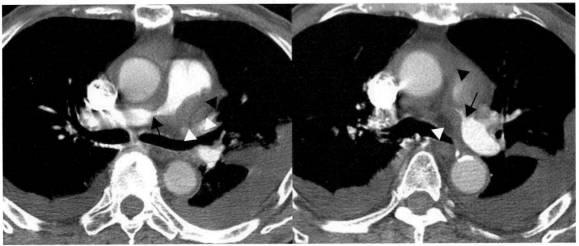

Figure 21.31 Pulmonary artery stenosis. Computed tomography demonstrates stenoses of the (A) right (*arrow*) and (B) left (*long arrow*) pulmonary arteries from surrounding abnormal soft tissue secondary to mediastinal fibrosis.

Table 21.8: Etiologies of Pulmonary Artery Aneurysms

Congenital	Idiopathic	Secondary
Associated with pulmonary valve stenosis and ASD	Hughes-Stovin syndrome Williams syndrome	Pulmonary hypertension Trauma Infection—syphilis, TB, mycosis Marfan syndrome Behçet disease Sequela of pulmonary parenchymal disease
ASD, atrial septal defect; TB, tuberculosis.		

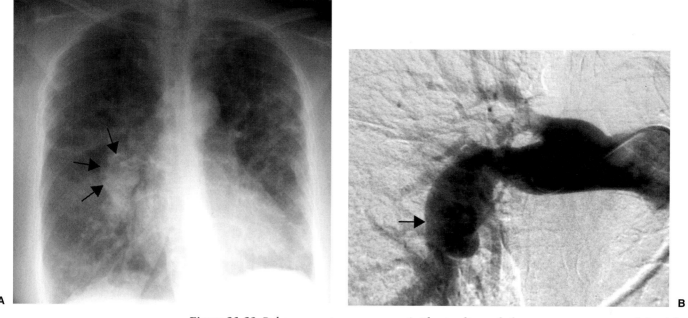

Figure 21.32 Pulmonary artery aneurysm. *A.* Chest radiograph demonstrates aneurysm of the right descending pulmonary artery *(arrows)* secondary to pulmonary hypertension from sarcoidosis. Note bilateral mid lung interstitial linear opacities. *B.* Selective right pulmonary angiogram demonstrates the aneurysm *(arrow)* of the right descending pulmonary artery.

sinuses and peripheral veins; it may be associated with Behçet disease. Larger aneurysms are usually seen secondary to atherosclerosis, thrombosis, or cystic medial necrosis.

Pulmonary aneurysms are often asymptomatic. They may present with signs and symptoms secondary to complications, such as rupture leading to hemoptysis or encroachment onto a bronchus.

On *chest radiograph*, a peripheral pulmonary artery aneurysm may present as a pulmonary nodule ranging in size from a few millimeters to a few centimeters. There may be surrounding hemorrhage noted as airspace disease. Hence, this could be easily overlooked. Centrally, it may appear as a large pulmonary artery (Fig. 21.32). *CT and MRI* both demonstrate central and peripheral pulmonary artery aneurysms and any internal thrombus well (Fig. 21.33). Calcification of the walls of the aneurysm may be seen (Fig. 21.34). The most valuable role of CT and MRI is to differentiate aneurysms from tumor. *Angiography* plays a dual role in both diagnosis (Fig. 21.32) and treatment of pulmonary aneurysms in the form of embolization with coils or balloons.

Pulmonary pseudoaneurysms are rare, the etiologies include trauma (Fig. 21.35), pneumonitis with consequent pulmonary vascular erosion (tuberculosis, mycotic) (Fig. 21.36), vasculitis such as Behçet syndrome, septic arterial seeding, and secondary to trauma. When an intensive care unit patient develops hemoptysis or a central enlarging mass with or without adjacent airspace disease on a chest radiograph, a Swan-Ganz catheter injury should be considered (56). The mass could represent a pulmonary artery pseudoaneurysm. When the pseudoaneurysm is peripheral, it can be treated with embolization, but when the pseudoaneurysm is central, surgical repair; allowing preservation of flow to the lung is preferred.

PULMONARY ARTERY APLASIA AND HYPOPLASIA

Pulmonary artery aplasia can be isolated or associated with hypogenetic lung or hypoplastic lung (Fig. 21.37). There are few if any clinical problems associated with isolated pul-

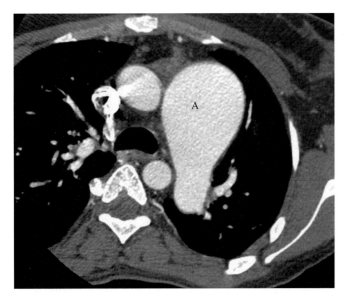

Figure 21.33 Pulmonary artery aneurysm. Computed tomography demonstrating pulmonary artery aneurysm (*arrow*) in a patient with congenital heart disease.

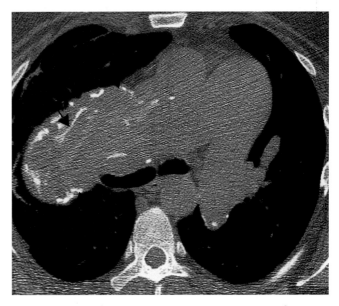

Figure 21.34 Pulmonary artery aneurysm. Computed tomography demonstrates peripherally calcified pulmonary artery aneurysm (*arrows*).

monary artery aplasia. The affected lung is normal in size or small, and there is marked decrease in pulmonary vasculature. The normal lung can demonstrate increased vasculature, as the cardiac output is diverted to that side. On chest radiograph, the affected lung is hyperlucent and may be small. Scintigraphy demonstrates normal ventilation but total absence of perfusion. CT and MRI may demonstrate absence of pulmonary artery and systemic to pulmonary collaterals (Fig. 21.37). Pulmonary artery hypoplasia can also occur secondary to radiation therapy (Fig. 21.38).

Swyer-James syndrome (Macleod syndrome) can mimic pulmonary artery hypoplasia or aplasia. It often occurs secondary to a viral infection in the immature developing lung that results in obliterative bronchiolitis. Pathologically, there may be the presence of bronchitis, bronchiolitis, constrictive obliterative bronchiolitis, and occasionally emphysema.

In pulmonary artery aplasia and hypoplasia, the pulmonary artery is absent or small and the lung small or normal in size but normally ventilated.

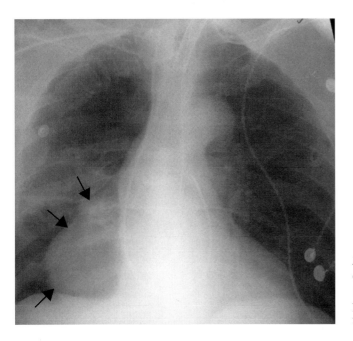

Figure 21.35 Pulmonary artery pseudoaneurysm. Chest radiograph demonstrates a right costophrenic angle smooth mass (*arrows*), secondary to Swan-Ganz catheter insertion, new from a prior normal chest radiograph and confirmed on computed tomography and angiography.

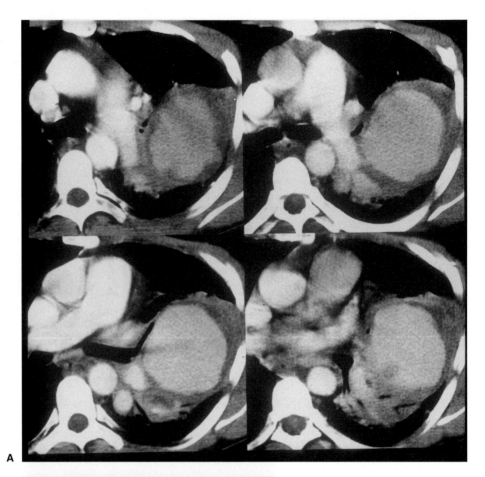

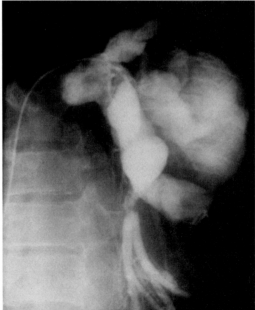

Figure 21.36 Mycotic pulmonary artery pseudoaneurysm. *A.* Computed tomography demonstrates an enhancing mass in the left mid-chest of almost equal attenuation to the pulmonary arteries, with surrounding low attenuation thrombus (*B*), confirmed on angiography.

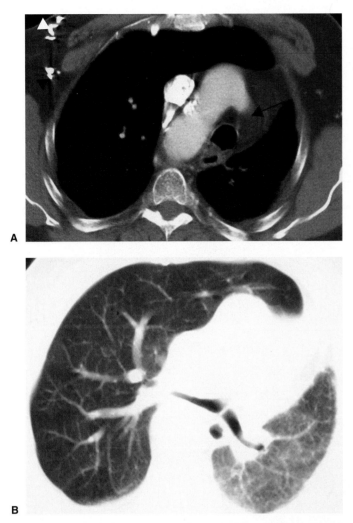

Figure 21.37 Pulmonary artery aplasia. *A.* Chest computed tomography demonstrates absent left pulmonary artery *(arrow)* and collateral chest wall vessels *(arrowheads). B.* Lung windows demonstrating hypoplastic left lung.

Patients are usually asymptomatic and detected incidentally. Less commonly, they present with recurrent respiratory infections and exertional dyspnea. On chest radiography, the abnormal lung is hyperlucent (Fig. 21.39), with diminished vasculature. Usually, an entire lung is affected, although there may be sparing of a segment or two or even patchy involvement of the opposite side. The pulmonary arteries are hypoplastic and reduced in number and caliber. The findings are well demonstrated on CT, which more commonly reveals the bilateral abnormalities. Air trapping is seen in the affected lung. Scintigraphy demonstrates decreased perfusion and abnormal ventilation. MRI demonstrates a small pulmonary artery on the affected side with decreased vasculature (Fig. 21.39).

In Swyer-James syndrome, the small pulmonary artery is associated with obliterative bronchiolitis and air trapping.

PULMONARY ARTERY TUMORS

Benign and malignant tumors of the pulmonary artery are rare and include leiomyosarcomas and fibrosarcomas. Benign tumors of the pulmonary artery are extremely rare. Almost all tumors arise centrally at the level of the pulmonary valve, pulmonary trunk, or right and left main pulmonary arteries. The artery may be completely occluded by tumor or by the tumor and adjacent thrombus, leading to distal atelectasis and infarction. Hematogenous spread with microscopic and macroscopic metastases is common. More commonly, a mediastinal or central bronchogenic tumor may invade the pulmonary artery.

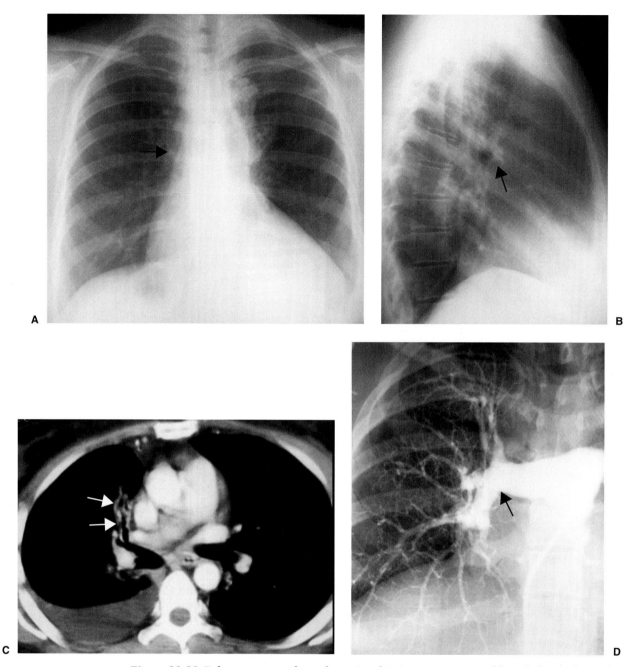

Figure 21.38 Pulmonary artery hypoplasia. *A and B.* Posteroanterior and lateral chest radiographs demonstrates diminutive right pulmonary artery *(arrows)*. *(C)* Computed tomography demonstrates right paramediastinal fibrotic changes secondary to radiation therapy *(arrows)*. *D.* Pulmonary angiogram demonstrates small right pulmonary artery *(arrow)* and small peripheral arteries.

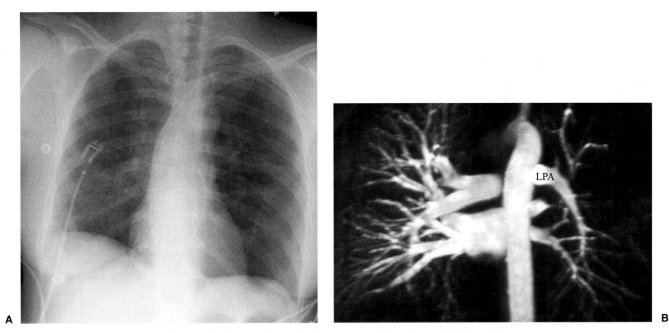

Figure 21.39 Swyer-James Syndrome. *A.* Chest radiograph demonstrates hypolucent left lung. *B.* Magnetic resonance angiography demonstrates small and decreased pulmonary vasculature on the left side. LPA, left pulmonary artery.

On *chest radiograph* there may be central pulmonary artery enlargement and multiple pulmonary nodules from hematogenous metastases. An intraluminal mass is seen on *CT or MRI*, sometimes associated with expansion of the pulmonary artery. Tumor may appear very similar to PE but may be differentiated by higher attenuation or finger-like projections or nodules invading adjacent vessel wall or extending into or outside the vessel wall (Fig. 21.40). In addition, tumor may enhance, whereas thrombus does not enhance (57). Angiography similarly demonstrates an intraluminal filling defect that can be indistinguishable from PE and may also demonstrate lobulation of the tumor or tumor blush and tumor vascularity.

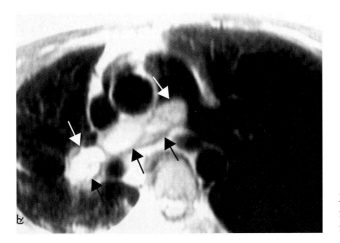

Figure 21.40 Pulmonary artery sarcoma. Gadolinium-enhanced magnetic resonance angiography demonstrates an enhancing tumor in the right pulmonary artery *(arrows)*.

REFERENCES

1. Dalen JE. When can treatment be withheld in patients with suspected pulmonary embolism? *Arch Intern Med* 1993;153:1415–1418.

2. Egermayer P, Town GI, Turner JG, et al. Usefulness of D-dimer, blood gas, and respiratory rate measurements for excluding pulmonary embolism. *Thorax* 1998;53:830–834.

3. Wells PS, Anderson DR, Rodger M, et al. Excluding pulmonary embolism at the bedside without diagnostic imaging: management of patients with suspected pulmonary embolism presenting to the emergency department by using a simple clinical model and d-dimer. *Ann Intern Med* 2001;135:98–107.

4. Schluger N, Henschke C, King T, et al. Diagnosis of pulmonary embolism at a large teaching hospital. *J Thorac Imaging* 1994;9:180–184.

5. Sostman HD, Gottschalk A. The stripe sign: a new sign for diagnosis of nonembolic defects on pulmonary perfusion scintigraphy. *Radiology* 1982;142:737–741.

6. Havig O. Deep vein thrombosis and pulmonary embolism. An autopsy study with multiple regression analysis of possible risk factors. *Acta Chir Scand* 1977;478[Suppl]:1–120.

7. Bell WR, Simon TL, DeMets DL. The clinical features of submassive and massive pulmonary emboli. *Am J Med* 1977;62:355–360.

8. Tourassi GD, Floyd CE, Coleman RE. Improved noninvasive diagnosis of acute pulmonary embolism with optimally selected clinical and chest radiographic findings. *Acad Radiol* 1996;3: 1012–1018.

9. The PIOPED Investigators. Value of the ventilation/perfusion scan in acute pulmonary embolism. Results of the prospective investigation of pulmonary embolism diagnosis (PIOPED) (see comments). *JAMA* 1990;263:2753–2759.

10. Anonymous. Value of the ventilation/perfusion scan in acute pulmonary embolism. Results of the prospective investigation of pulmonary embolism diagnosis (PIOPED). The PIOPED Investigators. *JAMA* 1990;263:2753.

11. Sostman HD, Coleman RE, DeLong DM, et al. Evaluation of revised criteria for ventilation-perfusion scintigraphy in patients with suspected pulmonary embolism (see comments). *Radiology* 1994;193:103–107.

12. Stein PD, Gottschalk A. Review of criteria appropriate for a very low probability of pulmonary embolism on ventilation-perfusion lung scans: a position paper. *Radiographics* 2000;20: 99–105.

13. Mills SR, Jackson DC, Older RA, et al. The incidence, etiologies, and avoidance of complications of pulmonary angiography in a large series. *Radiology* 1980;136:295–299.

14. Stein PD, Athanasoulis C, Alavi A, et al. Complications and validity of pulmonary angiography in acute pulmonary embolism. *Circulation* 1992;85:462–468.

15. Sostman HD, Ravin CE, Sullivan DC, et al. Use of pulmonary angiography for suspected pulmonary embolism: influence of scintigraphic diagnosis. *AJR Am J Roentgenol* 1982;139:673–677.

16. Stein PD, O'Connor JF, Dalen JE, et al. The angiographic diagnosis of acute pulmonary embolism: evaluation of criteria. *Am Heart J* 1967;73:730–741.

17. Newman GE. Pulmonary angiography in pulmonary embolic disease. *J Thorac Imaging* 1989;4: 28–39.

18. Remy-Jardin M, Remy J, Deschildre F, et al. Diagnosis of pulmonary embolism with spiral CT: comparison with pulmonary angiography and scintigraphy. *Radiology* 1996;200:699–706.

19. Remy-Jardin M, Baghaie F, Bonnel F, et al. Thoracic helical CT: influence of subsecond scan time and thin collimation on evaluation of peripheral pulmonary arteries. *Eur Radiol* 2000;10: 1297–1303.

20. Raptopoulos V, Boiselle PM. Multi-detector row spiral CT pulmonary angiography: comparison with single-detector row spiral CT. *Radiology* 2001;221:606–613.

21. Garg K, Welsh CH, Feyerabend AJ, et al. Pulmonary embolism: diagnosis with spiral CT and ventilation-perfusion scanning—correlation with pulmonary angiographic results or clinical outcome (see comments). *Radiology* 1998;208:201–208.

22. Remy-Jardin M, Remy J, Artaud D, et al. Peripheral pulmonary arteries: optimization of the spiral CT acquisition protocol (see comments). *Radiology* 1997;204:157–163.

23. Shah AA, Davis SD, Gamsu G, et al. Parenchymal and pleural findings in patients with and patients without acute pulmonary embolism detected at spiral CT. *Radiology* 1999;211:147–153.

24. Remy-Jardin M, Remy J, Artaud D, et al. Spiral CT of pulmonary embolism: technical considerations and interpretive pitfalls. *J Thorac Imaging* 1997;12:103–117.

25. Remy-Jardin M, Remy J, Artaud D, et al. Spiral CT of pulmonary embolism: diagnostic approach, interpretive pitfalls and current indications. *Eur Radiol* 1998;8:1376–1390.

26. Beigelman C, Chartrand-Lefebvre C, Howarth N, et al. Pitfalls in diagnosis of pulmonary embolism with helical CT angiography. *AJR Am J Roentgenol* 1998;171:579–585.

27. Teigen CL, Maus TP, Sheedy PF 2nd, et al. Pulmonary embolism: diagnosis with contrast-enhanced electron-beam CT and comparison with pulmonary angiography. *Radiology* 1995;194: 313–319.

28. Berry E, Kelly S, Hutton J, et al. A systematic literature review of spiral and electron beam computed tomography: with particular reference to clinical applications in hepatic lesions, pulmonary embolus and coronary artery disease. *Health Technol Assess* 1999;3:1–118.

29. Boonbaichaiyapruck S, Panpunnang S, Siripornpitak S, et al. Utilization of electron beam CT scan in diagnosis of pulmonary embolism. *J Med Assoc Thai* 1997;80:527–533.

30. Loud PA, Katz DS, Bruce DA, et al. Deep venous thrombosis with suspected pulmonary embolism: detection with combined CT venography and pulmonary angiography. *Radiology* 2001;219:498–502.

31. Loud PA, Katz DS, Klippenstein DL, et al. Combined CT venography and pulmonary angiography in suspected thromboembolic disease: diagnostic accuracy for deep venous evaluation. *AJR Am J Roentgenol* 2000;174:61–65.

32. Meaney JF, Weg JG, Chenevert TL, et al. Diagnosis of pulmonary embolism with magnetic resonance angiography. *N Engl J Med* 1997;336:1422–1427.

33. Gupta A, Frazer CK, Ferguson JM, et al. Acute pulmonary embolism: diagnosis with MR angiography. *Radiology* 1999;210:353–359.

34. Amundsen T, Kvaerness J, Jones RA, et al. Pulmonary embolism: detection with MR perfusion imaging of lung—a feasibility study. *Radiology* 1997;203:181–185.

35. Kauczor HU, Hofmann D, Kreitner KF, et al. Normal and abnormal pulmonary ventilation: visualization at hyperpolarized He-3 MR imaging. *Radiology* 1996;201:564–568.

36. Roberts HC, Kauczor HU, Schweden F, et al. Spiral CT of pulmonary hypertension and chronic thromboembolism. *J Thorac Imaging* 1997;12:118–127.

37. Schwickert HC, Schweden F, Schild HH, et al. Pulmonary arteries and lung parenchyma in chronic pulmonary embolism: preoperative and postoperative CT findings. *Radiology* 1994;191: 351–357.

38. King MA, Ysrael M, Bergin CJ. Chronic thromboembolic pulmonary hypertension: CT findings. *AJR Am J Roentgenol* 1998;170:955–960.

39. Bergin CJ, Sirlin CB, Hauschildt JP, et al. Chronic thromboembolism: diagnosis with helical CT and MR imaging with angiographic and surgical correlation (see comments). *Radiology* 1997; 204:695–702.

40. Sherrick AD, Swensen SJ, Hartman TE. Mosaic pattern of lung attenuation on CT scans: frequency among patients with pulmonary artery hypertension of different causes. *AJR Am J Roentgenol* 1997;169:79–82.

41. Remy-Jardin M, Remy J, Louvegny S, et al. Airway changes in chronic pulmonary embolism: CT findings in 33 patients. *Radiology* 1997;203:355–360.

42. Wolff K, Bergin CJ, King MA, et al. Accuracy of contrast-enhanced magnetic resonance angiography in chronic thromboembolic disease. *Acad Radiol* 1996;3:10–17.

43. Cervia JS, Caputo TA, Davis SD, et al. Septic pulmonary embolism complicating a central venous catheter (see comments). *Chest* 1990;98:1526.

44. Schraufnagel DE, Kay JM. Structural and physiologic changes in the lung vasculature in chronic liver disease. *Clin Chest Med* 1996;17:1–15

45. Woodruff WW 3rd, Hoeck BE, Chitwood WR Jr, et al. Radiographic findings in pulmonary hypertension from unresolved embolism. *AJR Am J Roentgenol* 1985;144:681–686.

46. Kanemoto N, Furuya H, Etoh T, et al. Chest roentgenograms in primary pulmonary hypertension. *Chest* 1979;76:45–49

47. McGoon MD. The assessment of pulmonary hypertension. *Clin Chest Med* 2001;22:493–508.

48. Powe JE, Palevsky HI, McCarthy KE, et al. Pulmonary arterial hypertension: value of perfusion scintigraphy. *Radiology* 1987;164:727–730.

49. Kuriyama K, Gamsu G, Stern RG, et al. CT-determined pulmonary artery diameters in predicting pulmonary hypertension. *Invest Radiol* 1984;19:16–22.

50. Resten A, Maitre S, Humbert M, et al. Pulmonary arterial hypertension: thin-section CT predictors of epoprostenol therapy failure. *Radiology* 2002;222:782–788.

51. Swensen SJ, Tashjian JH, Myers JL, et al. Pulmonary venoocclusive disease: CT findings in eight patients. *AJR Am J Roentgenol* 1996;167:937–940.

52. Chan CK, Hutcheon MA, Hyland RH, et al. Pulmonary tumor embolism: a critical review of clinical, imaging, and hemodynamic features. *J Thorac Imaging* 1987;2:4–14.

53. Shepard JA, Moore EH, Templeton PA, et al. Pulmonary intravascular tumor emboli: dilated and beaded peripheral pulmonary arteries at CT. *Radiology* 1993;187:797–801.

54. Rankin S, Faling LJ, Pugatch RD. CT diagnosis of pulmonary arteriovenous malformations. *J Comput Assist Tomogr* 1982;6:746–749.

55. Remy J, Remy-Jardin M, Wattinne L, et al. Pulmonary arteriovenous malformations: evaluation with CT of the chest before and after treatment. *Radiology* 1992;182:809–816.

56. Ferretti GR, Thony F, Link KM, et al. False aneurysm of the pulmonary artery induced by a Swan-Ganz catheter: clinical presentation and radiologic management. *AJR Am J Roentgenol* 1996;167:941–945.

57. Kauczor HU, Schwickert HC, Mayer E, et al. Pulmonary artery sarcoma mimicking chronic thromboembolic disease: computed tomography and magnetic resonance imaging findings. *Cardiovasc Intervent Radiol* 1994;17:185–189.

58. Gottschalk A, Stein PD, Henry JW, et al. Matched ventilation, perfusion and chest radiographic abnormalities in acute pulmonary embolism. *J Nuclear Med* 1996;37:1636–1638.

59. Stein PD, Relyea B, Gottschalk A. Evaluation of individual criteria for low probability interpretation of ventilation-perfusion lung scans. *J Nuclear Med* 1996;37:577–581.

60. Gottschalk A, Sostman HD, Coleman RE, et al. Ventilation-perfusion scintigraphy in the PIOPED study. Part II. Evaluation of the scintigraphic criteria and interpretations. *J Nuclear Med* 1993;34:1119–1126.

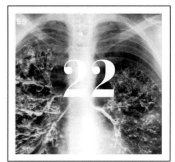

THORACIC INTERVENTIONAL TECHNIQUES

- Percutaneous Transthoracic Needle Biopsy
- Percutaneous Drainage Procedures
- Localization for Thoracoscopic Resection

PERCUTANEOUS TRANSTHORACIC NEEDLE BIOPSY

Image-guided percutaneous transthoracic needle biopsy (PTNB) of the lung is an important procedure in the diagnosis of thoracic and extrathoracic malignancies. It is also used, though less commonly, in the diagnosis of infectious and inflammatory disease. Suspected malignancies can be quickly and safely diagnosed, and sometimes staged, and appropriate therapies or surgical intervention can be planned. PTNB can also be used to evaluate potentially benign conditions. Although a benign entity such as hamartoma or infection is difficult to confirm, when it is obtained it may obviate the need for surgery. Fluoroscopically directed and ultrasound-directed procedures are fast and relatively inexpensive to perform and allow real-time imaging. Computed tomography (CT) and CT fluoroscopy have made it easier and more feasible to sample smaller and more awkwardly placed lesions with greater accuracy and efficiency.

METHODS

Performing needle biopsies with biplane fluoroscopic guidance can be faster and less expensive than performing the same procedure with CT guidance. When the lesion can be visualized in two planes, a fluoroscopic procedure may be preferred because the lung and lesion can be directly visualized in real-time (Fig. 22.1). Fluoroscopy, however, should not be used when the lesion cannot be reliably demonstrated on both the frontal and lateral chest radiographs or for lesions that are in difficult locations, such as adjacent to the hilum, mediastinum, or juxtavascular. For these lesions, CT is favored (Fig. 22.2). The main disadvantages of CT are its greater cost and longer procedure times. Detection of complications, such as pneumothorax, is frequently delayed because the patient is not imaged in real-time.

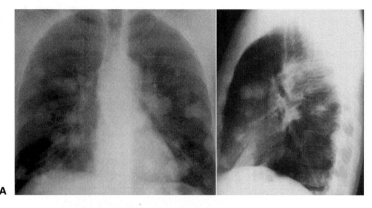

Figure 22.1 Multiple pulmonary nodules. Fine-needle aspiration and cytology confirmed metastatic melanoma. *A.* Posteroanterior and lateral chest x-ray shows numerous bilateral pulmonary nodules. *B.* Anteroposterior and *(C)* lateral fluoroscopic spot images confirm needle position in a right lower lobe nodule *(arrowheads)*.

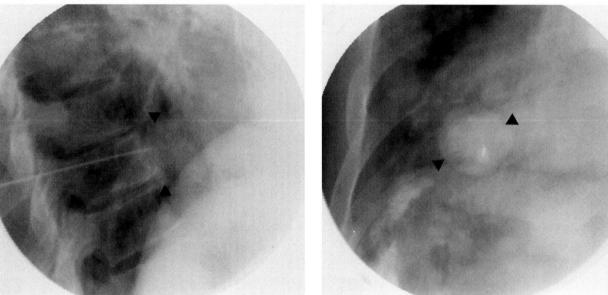

In recent years, CT fluoroscopy has become available. CT fluoroscopy provides a real-time cross-sectional image, updated about six times per second. X-ray tube cooling issues often limit the imaging time to 5 seconds per application, so it is most useful for brief looks rather than continuous real-time guidance.

Ultrasound is a very useful imaging modality for guiding interventional procedures. Several advantages include its real-time imaging, lack of ionizing radiation, low cost, and portability. For patients in the intensive care unit, intubated patients, or patients otherwise unable to be safely brought to the radiology department, ultrasound may be the only alternative. Ultrasound can be used to localize fluid collections for thoracentesis for guidance during drainage tube placement or for needle biopsies of lesions adjacent to the pleura or chest wall (1) (Fig. 22.3).

Methods for performing PTNB are use of a fine-caliber needle for aspiration sampling or use of a spring-loaded cutting needle to obtain larger and more intact core samples (Fig. 22.4). Fine-needle aspiration (FNA) is typically less traumatic on the surrounding tissue and has the benefit of allowing the cytopathologist to make a rapid diagnosis. It is best to have the cytopathologist present at the procedure to determine if the specimens are adequate for diagnosis rather than requiring a repeat biopsy. This is particularly helpful when the patient is in need of immediate treatment. Cutting needle systems are helpful when a larger amount of tissue is needed for histologic diagnosis or special staining. Core samples are also more accurate in the diagnosis of benign conditions and for certain

Aspirating needles obtain cells for cytology.

Core needles obtain tissue cores for histology.

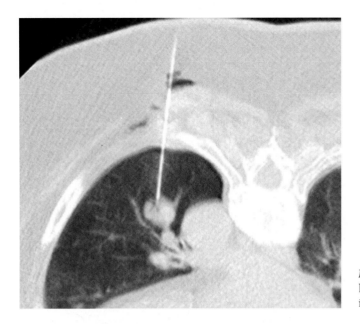

Figure 22. 2 Computed tomography-guided needle biopsy of a left lower lobe nodule. Note proximity of nodule to the descending thoracic aorta and left lower lobe pulmonary veins.

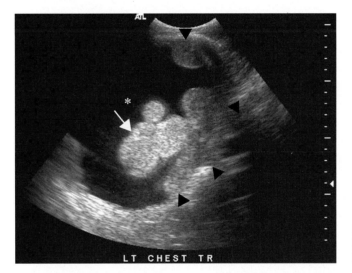

Figure 22.3 Prebiopsy ultrasound image demonstrating a lobulated pulmonary nodule (*arrow*), pleural thickening (*arrowheads*), and pleural effusion (*asterisk*).

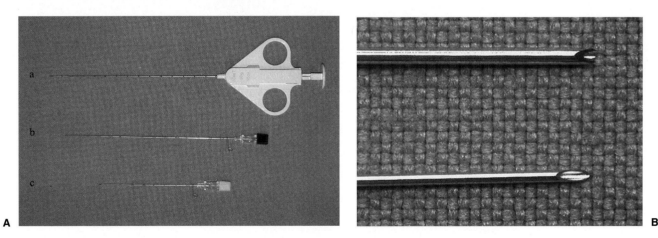

Figure 22.4 Examples of cutting and aspiration needles. *A. a.* Fifteen-centimeter 20-gauge cutting needle, *b.* 15 cm 22-gauge spinal needle, *c.* 9 cm 20-gauge coaxial introducing needle. *B.* Close-up view of a Franseen needle (*top*) and a spinal needle (*bottom*). Notice the toothed end of the Franseen needle, designed for macerating small bits of solid tissue to permit aspiration. The spinal needle has a smooth bevel for aspirations with less trauma to the tissue.

malignancies, such as lymphoma, where the relatively small amount of tissue obtained by FNA may be equivocal or nondiagnostic.

Either method can be performed via direct puncture or coaxial technique. In the latter, a larger caliber guiding needle, typically 19 gauge for lung and 17 gauge for chest wall, is first placed to the margin of the lesion and the biopsy device is passed through the center into the lesion. This allows multiple samples with only one pleural puncture; the risk of pneumothorax increases each time the pleural surface is transgressed. Coaxial systems are often advantageous when the need for multiple biopsy samples is anticipated or when the target lesion is small or difficult to reach.

Tissue sampling with FNA, regardless of the needle type used, can be performed in essentially the same way. By placing a syringe on the needle hub, gentile suction can be applied while agitating the needle tip within the lesion. It is best to release the suction as soon as there is a flash of blood at the needle hub to prevent obscuring cytopathologic visualization of abnormal cells with excessive blood. FNA and core needle systems should be positioned along the periphery of the lesion to reduce the amount of potentially necrotic tissue in the sample (Fig. 22.5). With either FNA or cutting needles, the patient should suspend respiration during the sampling process, particularly when the device is open to the atmosphere.

INDICATIONS

There are many indications for PTNB (Table 22.1), the most common of which is the presence of an indeterminate pulmonary nodule (2,3). Even in patients with a known history of extrathoracic malignancy, the presence of pulmonary metastasis can have significant impact on treatment. Presence of a new mediastinal or hilar mass are also valid indications for PTNB. PTNB can also be used for staging of known malignancies. It is also very useful in obtaining samples for culture and sensitivity testing in suspected infections, particularly in immunocompromised patients.

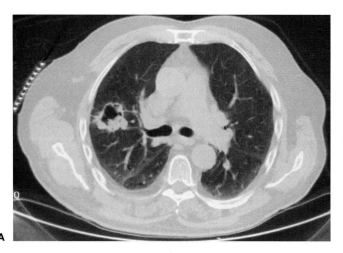 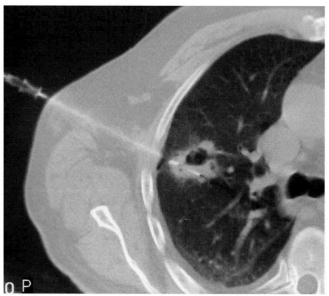

Figure 22.5 Right upper lobe cavitary mass. Fine-needle aspiration with cytology revealed squamous cell carcinoma. *A.* Localizing image from computed tomography-guided biopsy. *B.* Aspiration needle in place. Note the needle is positioned along the periphery of the lesion to reduce the chance of aspirating necrotic material.

Table 22.1: Indications for Percutaneous Transthoracic Needle Aspiration Biopsy

Indeterminate pulmonary nodule
Evaluation of suspected metastases
Mediastinal mass
Hilar mass
Staging of an extrathoracic neoplasm
Culture for infection

IMAGING AND SITE PREPARATION

Before performing any procedure, the patient's laboratory studies should be reviewed. Important tests include prothrombin time, partial thromboplastin time, and platelet count (4). When necessary, conscious sedation can be administered to the patient; however, it is important to keep any sedative light enough for the patient to follow commands appropriately, particularly breath-hold instructions. Patients with persistent coughing may have some temporary relief from a cough suppressant containing codeine, to help minimize motion while the needle is in place. Patients should be monitored with continuous pulse oxymetry and periodic blood pressure and heart rate measurements. Two liters of oxygen via nasal cannula is very helpful in making patients more comfortable and may be necessary for the patient with chronic obstructive pulmonary disease who has breathing difficulties while supine. Supplemental oxygen should be given to any patient receiving sedation.

The basic technique for either direct puncture or coaxial technique is similar. Based on scout imaging, the patient is placed on the CT table in an appropriate but secure position. The patient can be positioned in almost any orientation—supine, prone, lateral decubitus, or oblique. The two most important factors in choosing a position for the patient are (a) ease of lesion access across the shortest distance with avoidance of the fissures and (b) patient comfort, so they are more likely to remain motionless. For this reason, supine and prone positions are preferred. Easy needle trajectory is not helpful if the patient cannot maintain the position for the duration of the procedure. Once a position has been chosen, radiopaque markers are placed on the skin at the expected entry site and a scout image is obtained to select the level for needle placement. Small peripheral lesions can often present a problem due to their proximity to the ribs, which may prevent a direct trajectory. Angling the CT gantry a few degrees to be in-plane with the ribs is often helpful in displaying the intercostal spaces better and can help with biopsy planning. When imaging the lesion for biopsy planning, it is often helpful to have the patient breathe quietly instead of suspending respirations. This will give a good idea of how much the lesion can be expected to move during the procedure.

For procedures where the intercostal space must be traversed, the needle should be positioned so it remains as close to the superior surface of the adjacent rib as possible, because the neurovascular bundle runs directly below the inferior margin of each rib. Crossing the neurovascular bundle with a needle or catheter can result in significant pain and bleeding. The shortest path from skin to lesion should also be chosen. It is best to avoid crossing fissures, vessels, bronchi, and abnormal lung parenchyma, such as emphysema and bullae. Ideally, crossing as little aerated lung as possible is preferred (5) (Figs. 22.6 and 22.7).

After a proper entry site is selected, the site is cleaned and prepped with sterile technique, taking care to disinfect the entry site and surrounding region. A sterile operative field should be maintained at all times, and surgical-site drapes and covers should be used. Shaving any hair from the entry site is also recommended to maintain a clean skin surface. Local anesthesia can be achieved by using 1% to 2% lidocaine solution injected subcutaneously and then deeper into the soft tissues as needed.

Using periodic imaging either via axial CT images or real-time CT fluoroscopy, the biopsy device or introducing needle is carefully inserted through the chest wall to the margin of the target lesion. Ideally, the pleura should be crossed only once, because potential

Bleeding status should be evaluated before performing percutaneous lung biopsy.

Coaxial technique is preferred for lung biopsies, using one pleural puncture.

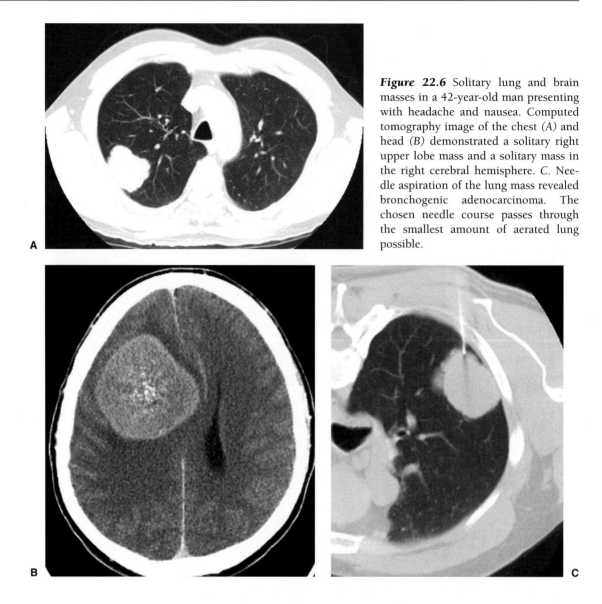

Figure 22.6 Solitary lung and brain masses in a 42-year-old man presenting with headache and nausea. Computed tomography image of the chest (*A*) and head (*B*) demonstrated a solitary right upper lobe mass and a solitary mass in the right cerebral hemisphere. *C.* Needle aspiration of the lung mass revealed bronchogenic adenocarcinoma. The chosen needle course passes through the smallest amount of aerated lung possible.

risk of pneumothorax increases with each pleura transgression. Ideally, the needle should be first positioned in the chest wall to establish the correct trajectory before any pleural punctures. When the chest wall is thin, the lidocaine needle can be used to assist with establishing the trajectory. The patient should be instructed to suspend respiration while crossing the pleura with the needle and to breathe quietly after the needle is across. This will help to prevent a large pleural puncture site and reduce the risk of pneumothorax. While the needle is within the lung or pleural space, the hub should remain closed to the atmosphere while the patient is breathing to limit the amount of air entering the thorax.

TECHNICAL FACTORS

Typically, three good core or FNA specimens are sufficient to make a diagnosis of malignancy, though more may be necessary if cultures or special pathologic stains are requested. In one study of 38 malignant lesions aspirated with a 25/22 gauge coaxial FNA system, 85% of the lesions were positive for malignancy with one, two, or three passes (6). Only 15% of lesions required up to six needle passes; 69% were positive with a single aspirate alone. When performing FNA, it is helpful to have cytopathology standing by to examine the specimens as they are obtained. This reduces the possibility of a nondiagnostic biopsy

In general, three tissue samples are sufficient for diagnosis.

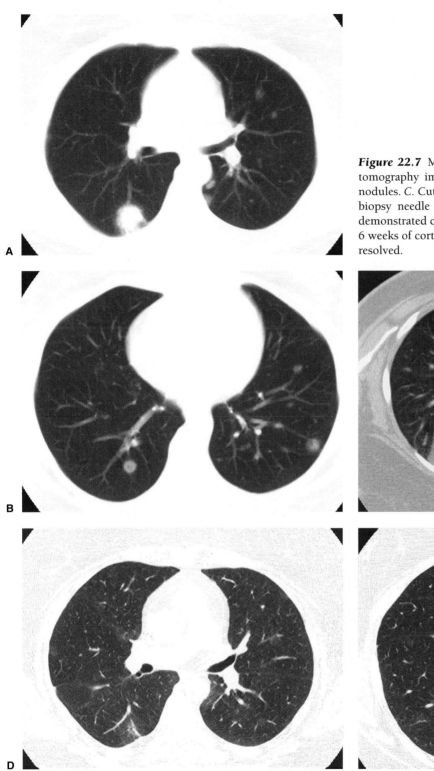

A

B

D

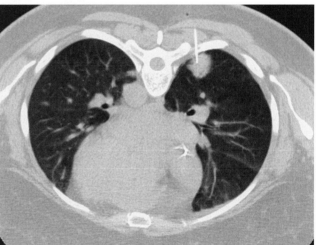

Figure 22.7 Multiple pulmonary nodules. *A and B.* Computed tomography images demonstrate multiple bilateral pulmonary nodules. *C.* Cutting needle biopsy of the largest nodule. Note the biopsy needle crosses through no aerated lung. Tissue cores demonstrated cryptogenic organizing pneumonia. *D and E.* After 6 weeks of corticosteroid therapy, the nodules nearly completely resolved.

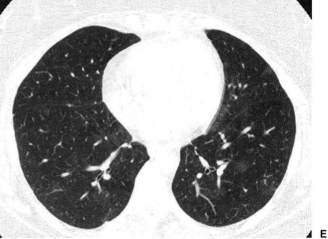

C

E

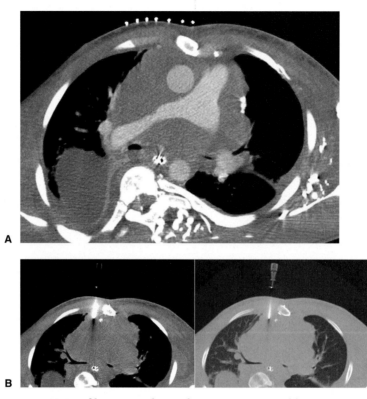

Figure 22.8 Infiltrating mediastinal mass in a 19 year-old man, 13 years after heart transplant. Histology revealed pericardial lymphoma. *A.* Localizing image through the main pulmonary artery from a contrast-enhanced computed tomography. *B.* Cutting needle biopsy of the mediastinal mass. Note the inability to visualize the aorta and pulmonary artery on the noncontrast images. The contrast-enhanced computed tomography was required to map the vital structures at the time of biopsy.

and gives an opportunity to obtain additional material if necessary. In a series of 896 malignant lesions, an 87% positive diagnostic rate after one procedure was shown, which rose to 96% after a second PTNB procedure in 75 patients (7). For patients in whom PTNB is indicated, particularly nonsurgical candidates, a second biopsy procedure should be considered if malignancy is suspected, rather than a more invasive open thoracotomy or thoracoscopic procedure.

PTNB of the chest wall, pleura, and mediastinum are performed in essentially the same manner as biopsies of the lung. Selecting a trajectory that avoids aerated lung reduces or eliminates the risk of pneumothorax (5). Percutaneous biopsy of pleural lesions has been shown to be quite effective (8), and in sampling a pleural lesion or a segment of pleural thickening, choosing a trajectory that passes tangentially to the pleura and lung is preferred. Additionally, careful contrast-enhanced CT may be necessary before the procedure to map locations of vital structures and vessels, which may not otherwise be adequately seen on noncontrast imaging (Fig. 22.8).

CONTRAINDICATIONS

Virtually all contraindications to PTNB are relative (Table 22.2). Coagulopathies should be corrected before the procedure. Aspirin, Coumadin, and other oral anticoagulant therapies should be discontinued for at least 5 days before the procedure. Heparin can be discontinued about 6 hours before the procedure. If necessary, platelet or fresh frozen plasma transfusions should be timed to be completed just before beginning the biopsy. For patients with severe emphysema, careful risk versus benefit discussions with both patient and consulting physician is suggested, because these patients can have significant respira-

Table 22.2: *Relative Contraindications to Percutaneous Transthoracic Needle Biopsy*

Coagulopathies
Emphysema
Contralateral pneumonectomy
Pulmonary hypertension
Intractable cough
Uncooperative patient

tory problems if they develop a pneumothorax and require a chest tube. Patients with contralateral pneumonectomy also face similar issues (Fig. 22.9). When a biopsy in a postpneumonectomy patient becomes necessary, it should only be attempted with appropriate medical personnel present in case it becomes necessary to emergently intubate the patient or place a large-caliber chest tube. In patients with pulmonary hypertension, deep lesions should be avoided due to risk of injury to the central pulmonary arteries and excessive bleeding. Biopsy of suspected malignant thymoma should be discussed with the thoracic surgeons before proceeding, because it is often desirable to have an intact capsule before surgery and prevent converting a noninvasive thymoma into an invasive one. Potential pulmonary arteriovenous malformations should not be biopsied, because it can lead to severe bleeding and potential air embolism.

A good contrast-enhanced CT and evaluation for feeding arteries or draining veins are important when planning a biopsy. Patients with intractable cough may make safe biopsy difficult due to repetitive motion with the needle in place. A patient who cannot maintain a stable position may be the only absolute contraindication.

A contrast-enhanced CT should be performed before biopsy of mediastinal masses to evaluate vascular anatomy.

For lung nodules, a contrast-enhanced CT should be taken to evaluate for possible arteriovenous malformation before biopsy.

POSTBIOPSY MANAGEMENT

Most postbiopsy pneumothoraces usually develop within the first hour after the procedure (9), therefore, imaging the patient with an upright chest radiograph is suggested at 1 and 3 hours after the procedure. Patients are monitored in a postprocedure recovery area for 4 hours after the procedure. Small pneumothoraces shown to be stable over several radiographs in asymptomatic patients usually resolve spontaneously, and outpatients may be discharged with detailed instructions about signs and symptoms of pneumothorax and

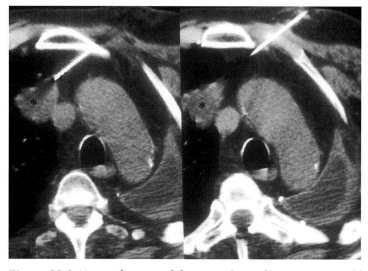

Figure 22.9 New right upper lobe mass *(asterisk)* in a 68-year-old man, status post–left pneumonectomy for lung carcinoma. The chosen trajectory passes obliquely through the mediastinum, into the lesion, without passing into any aerated right lung.

contact information in the event of symptoms, as well as activity instructions for the next few days. Positioning the patient with the biopsy site dependent and supplying nasal cannula oxygen can help speed resolution of a small pneumothorax. Development of a large or symptomatic pneumothorax may necessitate the placement of a chest tube or direct aspiration of air.

COMPLICATIONS AND TREATMENT

PTNB is a safe procedure, and most complications are minor and self-limited. There are, however, dangerous and potentially life-threatening complications that can arise (Table 22.3). Prompt identification and treatment can prevent significant morbidity and mortality.

Pneumothorax

Pneumothorax is the most common complication of lung biopsy, occurring in 10% to 60% of cases; it is more common with CT-guided procedures than fluoroscopy.

The risk of pneumothorax increases with each successive puncture of the pleura or a pleural fissure. A small asymptomatic pneumothorax often requires only observation, whereas large or symptomatic pneumothoraces may require evacuation. Several different treatment techniques are available, including needle aspiration, small caliber chest tube with a Heimlich valve (10), or the Tru-Close Thoracic Vent system (11) (Figs. 22.10 and 22.11) and larger surgical caliber chest tubes with continuous suction for a very large pneumothorax or a pneumothorax with a persistent air leak. A technique advocated by some to reduce the risk of pneumothorax during the procedure is to use about 10 mL of the patient's partially clotted blood to seal the needle tract. This "blood patch" technique has been shown by some to demonstrate no significant reduction in the pneumothorax rate (12,13), whereas other investigation of the blood patch technique in resected equine lungs suggested that the technique warrants further clinical evaluation (14). However, these results may not hold in living humans in which respiratory motion may be a confounding element.

Pneumothorax risk also increases with the severity of obstructive lung disease (Fig. 22.12), as demonstrated in several publications based on evaluation of chest radiographs both with and without spirometry (15–18). One study demonstrated a 52.5% pneumothorax rate for patients with severe obstructive disease as evidenced by spirometry, compared with 20.6% for patients with mild obstructive deficits (18). The chest tube rate was also higher, 22.5% in patients with severe obstructive disease and 2.9% in patients with mild disease. Arterial oxygenation also correlated with the incidence of pneumothorax. With arterial partial pressure of oxygen less than 50 mm Hg, the pneumothorax rate was 80%, as compared with a 0% rate with partial pressure of oxygen more than 80 mm Hg. Another study demonstrated a 46% pneumothorax rate when both chest radiograph and pulmonary function tests were consistent with emphysema (16). This study had a 19% chest tube rate. Compared with a 7% pneumothorax rate and 0% chest tube rate for patients with no chest radiograph or spirometric evidence of obstructive lung disease.

Once a pneumothorax develops, administering 2 to 3 L O_2 by nasal cannula will help speed resorption. In patients with severe emphysema, it may be better to perform a thoracoscopic resection or follow a lesion radiographically before attempting PTNB, because these patients can have significant morbidity and need for long-term drainage for persistent pneumothorax (19).

Table 22.3: Complications of Percutaneous Transthoracic Needle Biopsy

Pneumothorax
Bleeding
Air embolism
Infection or empyema
Bronchopleural fistula
Lung torsion
Pericardial tamponade
Death

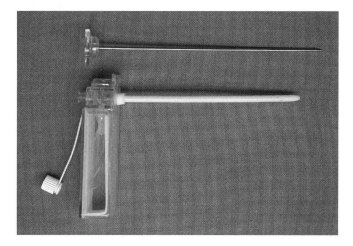

Figure 22.10 Tru-Close thoracic vent system and insertion trocar. The catheter is 14 French in diameter and has multiple side holes. A one-way Heimlich valve allows air to escape with the patient's respiratory motion, evacuating the pneumothorax. Adhesive wings holds the device onto the patient's chest.

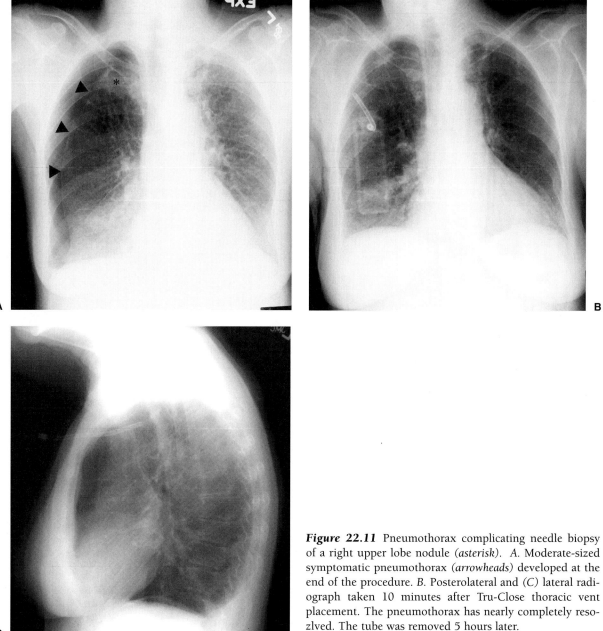

A

B

C

Figure 22.11 Pneumothorax complicating needle biopsy of a right upper lobe nodule (*asterisk*). *A.* Moderate-sized symptomatic pneumothorax (*arrowheads*) developed at the end of the procedure. *B.* Posterolateral and (*C*) lateral radiograph taken 10 minutes after Tru-Close thoracic vent placement. The pneumothorax has nearly completely resozlved. The tube was removed 5 hours later.

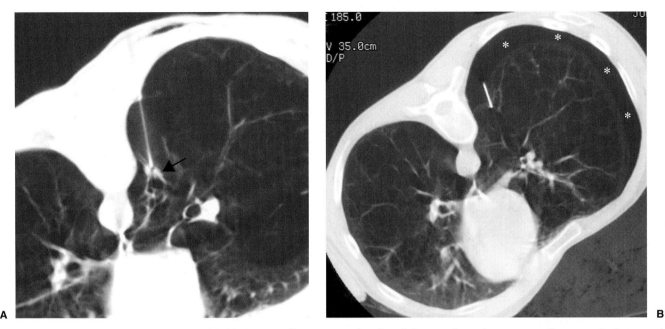

Figure 22.12 Seven-millimeter spiculated nodule in male with severe emphysema. *A.* Computed tomography-guided biopsy of RLL lobe lesion (*arrow*). *B.* Pneumothorax (*asterisks*) after the first aspiration.

Bleeding

Pulmonary parenchymal hemorrhage can occur at the biopsy site, particularly when the lesion is small or when multiple needle passes are necessary. Although a small amount of hemorrhage is usually asymptomatic for the patient, it can result in obscuration of the lesion, making additional samples difficult (Fig. 22.13). Some patients experience a small amount of self-limited hemoptysis. Patients should be coached before the procedure that this may happen to decrease anxiety if it occurs. Heavy hemoptysis during or after the biopsy, however, should be investigated, usually with CT angiography or catheter-directed angiography. Intercostal or internal mammary artery bleeding into pleural space (hemothorax) can be difficult to control percutaneously, can be life threatening, and requires surgical control (20). Massive life-threatening hemoptysis can occur with either bronchoarterial or bronchovenous fistula formation, especially when large-caliber or cutting needle devices are used, and may also require angiography. Excessive superficial bleeding can be treated with direct pressure but is uncommon during needle biopsy.

> Patients should be warned before lung biopsy that they may experience hemoptysis, because this can be a source of considerable patient anxiety if unexpected.

Air Embolism

Air embolism is a very rare complication that can occur when there is communication between a pulmonary vein and the atmosphere via the biopsy device or after formation of a bronchovenous fistula. Air embolism should be suspected if new neurologic symptoms or chest pain occur acutely during the procedure, which can lead to stroke, seizure, myocardial infarction, and death. To prevent further embolism, particularly to the central nervous system, the patient should be immediately placed in the left lateral decubitus position to prevent air from escaping the left atrium. Administering 100% O_2 by face mask may help speed resorption. Large emboli may require hyperbaric chamber treatment.

> Although air embolism is rare, it should be suspected if neurologic or cardiovascular symptoms develop during a lung biopsy.

> If air embolism is suspected, place the patient in the left lateral decubitus position and administer 100% oxygen by face mask.

Other Complications

Empyema is uncommon but may occur if infected material escapes into the pleural space. Rarer complications include tumor seeding along the needle tract (21), bronchopleural fistula formation, pericardial tamponade, lung torsion (22), and death. Of 28 cases of death

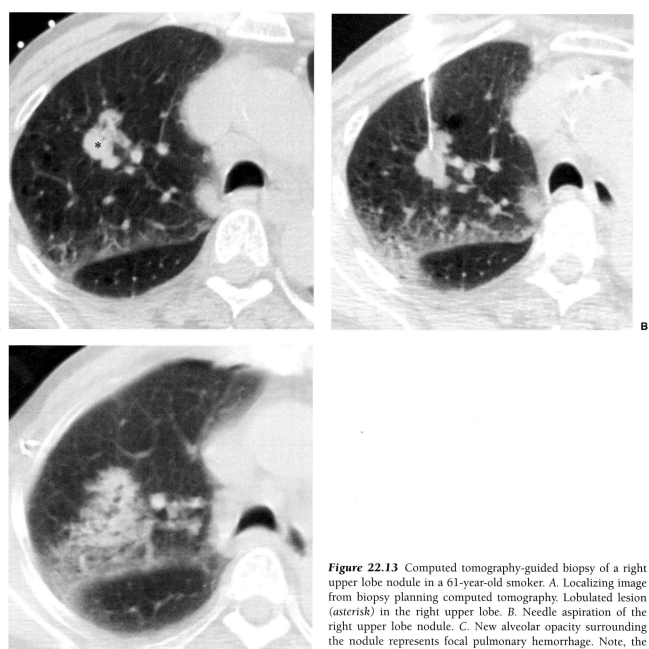

Figure 22.13 Computed tomography-guided biopsy of a right upper lobe nodule in a 61-year-old smoker. *A.* Localizing image from biopsy planning computed tomography. Lobulated lesion *(asterisk)* in the right upper lobe. *B.* Needle aspiration of the right upper lobe nodule. *C.* New alveolar opacity surrounding the nodule represents focal pulmonary hemorrhage. Note, the original lesion is significantly obscured.

related to PTNB in the literature, most were performed with large 16- to 18-gauge cutting needles. This includes 18 cases of pulmonary hemorrhage (1 severe pulmonary hypertension, 1 oversedated), 2 cases of tension pneumothorax, 5 cases of air embolism (3 proven; 1 performed with a 22-gauge needle on an intubated patient with acute respiratory distress syndrome), and 3 cases where deaths were temporally related to the procedure but without an identified reason (23,24).

PERCUTANEOUS DRAINAGE PROCEDURES

The radiologist is often called upon to help manage a large or loculated pleural effusion, empyema, or intrapulmonary abscess. Drainage procedures may be performed for either diagnostic or therapeutic purposes, and catheters can be placed to gravity drainage or continuous suction. Preintervention imaging is important to determine accessibility and to anticipate any potential complications. Essentially, any fluid collection in the chest wall, pleural space, lung, or mediastinum can be managed by a percutaneous image-guided drainage or aspiration as long as a safe and viable path to the fluid collection can be found (25).

METHODS

For CT-guided procedures, positioning the patient and prepping the entry site is typically done in the same manner as with needle biopsy. For diagnostic pleural fluid sampling, a long large-caliber angiocatheter may be all that is required. The angiocatheter can be placed into the fluid collection and the stylet removed. This will leave the softer and more flexible plastic sheath within the fluid. Tubing and a syringe are attached to the sheath, and fluid can be aspirated. Use of a soft sheath rather than leaving a sharp needle in place can reduce chances of further trauma to lung parenchyma or pleura should the fluid collection be drained completely.

When it is necessary to place a catheter for drainage, a multipurpose pigtail drainage catheter placed over a trocar is often the simplest device to insert (Fig. 22.14). These are usually available in sizes ranging from 8 to 16 French. It may be necessary to use serial dilatations over a short guidewire, however, when placing larger size drainage catheters, particularly in larger or muscular patients; the intercostal muscles can frequently impede direct placement of a larger size catheter. Once in place, the pigtail should be locked and the catheter affixed to the skin either with suture or an adhesive. Flushing the catheter with 5 to 10 mL of sterile heparinized saline two times daily can help reduce catheter clogging. Presence of pus or other infected material within a fluid collection may necessitate placement of a larger catheter for adequate drainage. This is often achievable by exchanging the catheter over a guidewire.

Superficial fluid collections may be amenable to ultrasound-guided procedures (26) (Fig. 22.15). The fluid collection can be marked and its depth determined. This can be done at a patient's bedside rather than transporting the patient to the radiology department. Ultrasound-guided procedures can be performed relatively quickly and often allow better characterization of fluid and potential septations than CT. However, conventional chest radiography is usually necessary because pneumothorax may be difficult to detect on ultrasound.

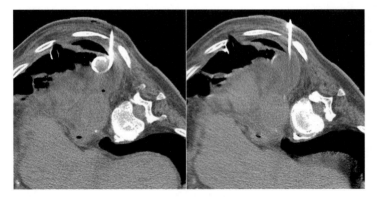

Figure 22.14 Pigtail catheter drainage of a mediastinal fluid collection. Drainage catheter placed with computed tomography guidance into infected fluid surrounding a descending aortic graft.

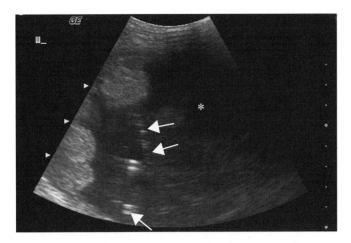

Figure 22.15 Ultrasound image demonstrating a pigtail catheter (*arrows*) within a pleural effusion (*asterisk*).

Loculated or fibrinous fluid collections are usually not amenable to a simple aspiration and drainage procedure. Often, they can be broken up by instilling 80,000 to 250,000 units of streptokinase (27–30) and leaving it in place for several hours before attempting drainage. The systemic effect of intracavitary thrombolytics is negligible (31). An alternate method is to use a C-shaped guidewire and torque it through the fluid collection for several minutes to break up any adhesions or thin septations before attempting further aspiration.

Complications of drainage procedures are similar to the risks of PTNB. Pneumothorax risk can be minimized by using stopcocks on tubing to keep the pleural space sealed from the atmosphere.

Consider streptokinase injection into loculated fluid collections to break down adhesions.

LOCALIZATION FOR THORACOSCOPIC RESECTION

There may be time where it is desirable to have a lesion completely excised without first obtaining histology. The use of video-assisted thoracoscopic surgery (VATS) has helped reduce the need for open thoracotomy in many cases (32). VATS allows visualization of nearly the entire hemithorax and the superficial surface of the lung (33,34). VATS is performed under general anesthesia, and the patient is intubated with a double-lumen endotracheal tube to allow ventilation of one lung and controlled deflation of the other. A fiberoptic video camera and other instrumentation are inserted via one or more intercostal spaces. Subpleural nodules are found at VATS when the lung is collapsed by physical deformation of the lung contour. Unfortunately, nodules deep to the pleural surface or very small nodules show no such contour deformities. In these cases, wire or dye localization can be performed before VATS to assist the surgeon in finding the lesion for resection (34). The radiologist can percutaneously anchor a wire in the lesion, place a small metallic coil at the lesion site (35), or stain the area of the lesion percutaneously with methylene blue dye (36). The blue stain or coil will be visible at the time of VATS and allows the surgeon to perform an appropriate wedge resection (Fig. 22.16). The main disadvantages of VATS are its need for general anesthesia and inability to be used in the presence of significant pleura adhesions. VATS also cannot be used in patients who will not tolerate single-lung ventilation (37).

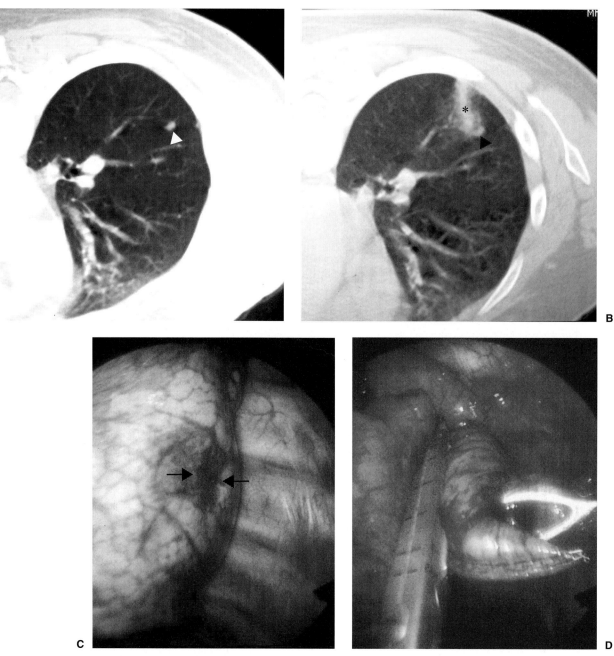

Figure 22.16 Methylene blue dye localization before video-assisted thoracoscopy. *A.* Localizing computed tomography image shows a 5 mm right lower lobe nodule *(arrowhead)*. *B.* After dye injection, the dye is seen as ground glass opacity *(asterisk)* adjacent to the nodule *(arrowhead)*. *C.* Image obtained during video-assisted thoracoscopic surgery. The blue stain *(arrows)* in the center of the image is the methylene blue dye used to mark the nodule. *D.* Wedge resection in progress. The blue dye and surrounding tissues are removed.

REFERENCES

1. Mathis G, Gehmacher O. Ultrasound-guided diagnostic and therapeutic interventions in peripheral pulmonary masses. *Wien Klin Wochenschr* 1999;111:230–235.
2. Polak J, Kubik A. Percutaneous thin needle biopsy of malignant and nonmalignant thoracic lesions. *Radiol Diagn* 1989;30:177–182.

3. Klein JS, Zarka MA. Transthoracic needle biopsy: an overview. *J Thorac Imaging* 1997;12: 232–249.
4. Klein JS, Zarka MA. Transthoracic needle biopsy. *Radiol Clin North Am* 2000;38:235–266, vii.
5. Haramati LB, Austin JH. Complications after CT-guided needle biopsy through aerated versus nonaerated lung. *Radiology* 1991;181:778.
6. Williams AJ, Santiago S, Lehrman S, et al. Transcutaneous needle aspiration of solitary pulmonary masses: how many passes? *Am Rev Respir Dis* 1987;136:452–454.
7. Sagel SS, Ferguson TB, Forrest JV, et al. Percutaneous transthoracic aspiration needle biopsy. *Ann Thorac Surg* 1978;26:399–405.
8. Scott EM, Marshall TJ, Flower CD, et al. Diffuse pleural thickening: percutaneous CT-guided cutting needle biopsy. *Radiology* 1995;194:867–870.
9. Perlmutt LM, Braun SD, Newman GE, et al. Timing of chest film follow-up after transthoracic needle aspiration. *AJR Am J Roentgenol* 1986;146:1049–1050.
10. Perlmutt LM, Braun SD, Newman GE, et al. Transthoracic needle aspiration: use of a small chest tube to treat pneumothorax. *AJR Am J Roentgenol* 1987;148:849–851.
11. Molina PL, Solomon SL, Glazer HS, et al. A one-piece unit for treatment of pneumothorax complicating needle biopsy: evaluation in 10 patients. *AJR Am J Roentgenol* 1990;155:31–33.
12. Bourgouin PM, Shepard JA, McLoud TC, et al. Transthoracic needle aspiration biopsy: evaluation of the blood patch technique. *Radiology* 1988;166:93–95.
13. Vine HS, Kasdon EJ, Simon M. Percutaneous lung biopsy using the Lee needle and a track-obliterating technique. *Radiology* 1982;144:921–922.
14. Moore EH, Shelton DK, Wisner ER, et al. Needle aspiration lung biopsy: reevaluation of the blood patch technique in an equine model. *Radiology* 1995;196:183–186.
15. Kazerooni EA, Lim FT, Mikhail A, et al. Risk of pneumothorax in CT-guided transthoracic needle aspiration biopsy of the lung. *Radiology* 1996;198:371–375.
16. Fish GD, Stanley JH, Miller KS, et al. Postbiopsy pneumothorax: estimating the risk by chest radiography and pulmonary function tests. *AJR Am J Roentgenol* 1988;150:71–74.
17. Miller KS, Fish GB, Stanley JH, et al. Prediction of pneumothorax rate in percutaneous needle aspiration of the lung. *Chest* 1988;93:742–745.
18. Quon D, Fong TC, Mellor J, et al. Pulmonary function testing in predicting complications from percutaneous lung biopsy. *Can Assoc Radiol J* 1988;39:267–269.
19. Kazerooni EA, Hartker FW 3rd, Whyte RI, et al. Transthoracic needle aspiration in patients with severe emphysema. A study of lung transplant candidates. *Chest* 1996;109:616–619.
20. Glassberg RM, Sussman SK. Life-threatening hemorrhage due to percutaneous transthoracic intervention: importance of the internal mammary artery. *AJR Am J Roentgenol* 1990;154:47–49.
21. Sinner WN, Zajicek J. Implantation metastasis after percutaneous transthoracic needle aspiration biopsy. *Acta Radiol Diagn (Stockh)* 1976;17:473–480.
22. Graham RJ, Heyd RL, Raval VA, et al. Lung torsion after percutaneous needle biopsy of lung. *AJR Am J Roentgenol* 1992;159:35–37.
23. Meyer JE, Ferrucci JT Jr, Janower ML. Fatal complications of percutaneous lung biopsy. Review of the literature and report of a case. *Radiology* 1970;96:47–48.
24. Pearce JG, Patt NL. Fatal pulmonary hemorrhage after percutaneous aspiration lung biopsy. *Am Rev Respir Dis* 1974;110:346–349.
25. Ghaye B, Dondelinger RF. Imaging guided thoracic interventions. *Eur Respir J* 2001;17:507–528.
26. Morrison MC, Mueller PR, Lee MJ, et al. Sclerotherapy of malignant pleural effusion through sonographically placed small-bore catheters. *AJR Am J Roentgenol* 1992;158:41–43.
27. Davies CW, Traill ZC, Gleeson FV, et al. Intrapleural streptokinase in the management of malignant multiloculated pleural effusions. *Chest* 1999;115:729–733.
28. Davies RJ, Traill ZC, Gleeson FV. Randomised controlled trial of intrapleural streptokinase in community acquired pleural infection. *Thorax* 1997;52:416–421.
29. Klein JS. Interventional techniques in the thorax. *Clin Chest Med* 1999;20:805–826, ix.
30. Lee KS, Im JG, Kim YH, et al. Treatment of thoracic multiloculated empyemas with intracavitary urokinase: a prospective study. *Radiology* 1991;179:771–775.
31. Davies CW, Lok S, Davies RJ. The systemic fibrinolytic activity of intrapleural streptokinase. *Am J Respir Crit Care Med* 1998;157:328–330.
32. Hazelrigg SR, Magee MJ, Cetindag IB. Video-assisted thoracic surgery for diagnosis of the solitary lung nodule. *Chest Surg Clin North Am* 1998;8:763–774, vii.
33. Lewis RJ, Caccavale RJ, Sisler GE. Imaged thoracoscopic lung biopsy. *Chest* 1992;102:60–62.
34. Bogot NR, Shaham D. Semi-invasive and invasive procedures for the diagnosis and staging of lung cancer. II. Bronchoscopic and surgical procedures. *Radiol Clin North Am* 2000;38:535–544.

35. Lizza N, Eucher P, Haxhe JP, et al. Thoracoscopic resection of pulmonary nodules after computed tomographic-guided coil labeling. *Ann Thorac Surg* 2001;71:986–988.

36. Lenglinger FX, Schwarz CD, Artmann W. Localization of pulmonary nodules before thoracoscopic surgery: value of percutaneous staining with methylene blue. *AJR Am J Roentgenol* 1994;163:297–300.

37. Thompson AB, Rennard SI. Diagnostic procedures not involving the pleura. In: Baum GL, Crapo JD, Celli BR, eds. *Textbook of pulmonary diseases*, 6th ed. Philadelphia: Lippincott-Raven, 1998: 239–253.

SUBJECT INDEX

Numbers followed by "f" indicate figures; those followed by "t" indicate tables.

A

Abdomen, chest radiography of, 51–53, 52f, 53f
Abdominal diseases, chest radiography of, 51–53, 52f, 53f
Abdominal injuries, upper, traumatic, 317–318, 318f
Abscess(es), lung, empyema vs., 462, 463f
Accessory paracardiac bronchus, 346f, 435
Achalasia, 201, 204t
　　NTMB in, 104
Acquired immunodeficiency syndrome (AIDS)
　　CD4 counts in, 117–118, 118t
　　pulmonary manifestations of, 117–125
　　　approach to, 117–118, 118t
　　　bacterial infections, 118–119, 119f
　　　fungal infections, 122, 122f
　　　lung cancer, 126–128, 127f
　　　lymphoma, 126, 126f, 127f, 128f
　　　mycobacterial infections, 119–121, 120f, 121f
　　　noninfectious, 125–128, 125f–128f
　　　Pneumocystis carinii pneumonia, 123–124, 123f, 124f
　　　tuberculosis, 119–120, 120f, 121f
　　　viral infections, 125
Actinomyces spp., aspiration pneumonia due to, 94–95, 94f
Acute interstitial pneumonitis, in critically ill patients, 225
Acute lymphocytic leukemia (ALL), invasive pulmonary aspergillosis in, 132f
Acute myelogenous leukemia (AML), invasive pulmonary aspergillosis in, 132f, 133f
Acute respiratory distress syndrome (ARDS)
　　in critically ill patients, 220–225
　　clinical presentation of, 221
　　CT of, 223–225, 224f
　　phases of, 221–223, 222f, 223t

radiography of, 221–223, 222f, 223t
risk factors for, 221, 221t
defined, 220–221, 221t
Acute traumatic aortic injury (ATAI), 295–299, 296f, 297t, 298f–300f
Adenocarcinoma
　　of lung, 148–149, 151f
　　as right upper lobe single pulmonary nodule, 152, 152f
Adenocarcinoma(s), esophageal, 190, 190f
Adenoid cystic carcinomas, of trachea, 450, 451f
Adenoma(s), parathyroid, 201, 204t
　　mediastinal, 212, 213f
Adenomatoid malformation, cystic, 175, 175f
Adult respiratory distress syndrome (ARDS), 244f
Age of onset
　　rheumatoid arthritis, 323
　　sarcoidosis, 350
　　scleroderma, 326
　　SLE, 325
AIDS. See Acquired immunodeficiency syndrome (AIDS)
Air bronchogram, 65, 65f
Air collections, thoracic, abnormal, in critically ill patients, 241–250, 241t, 242f–247f, 243t, 247t, 248t, 249f, 250f. See also Thoracic air collections, abnormal, in critically ill patients
Air embolism, PTNB and, treatment of, 628
Airspace disease
　　diffuse, in "butterfly" distribution, 358, 359f
　　in non-AIDS immunocompromised patients, 129–130
　　in pneumonia, 358, 358f
　　　in immunocompetent hosts, 82–83, 83f
Airway(s)
　　anatomy and physiology of, 2t, 10–12, 11f, 11t

central, 429–455. See also Central airways
devices used in, 256t, 279–284
　　endotracheal tube, 256t, 279–281, 279t, 280f, 281f
　　tracheostomy tube, 256t, 282–283, 282f, 282t
　　transtracheal oxygen catheter, 256t, 283–284, 283f
injuries to, chest radiograph findings of, 311t
metastases to, 188, 188f
Alveolar disease
　　chest radiography in, 358–362, 358f–362f, 358t, 360t, 362t
　　differential diagnosis of, 360t
　　mnemonic for, 360–362, 362t
Alveolar microlithiasis, 364f
Alveolar pulmonary edema, with bilateral alveolar opacity, 235f
American Joint Committee on Cancer, staging scheme for lung cancer, 160, 161t
American Journal of Roentgenology, 74
Amyloidosis, 442
　　classification of, 341–342, 341t
　　defined, 341
　　diffuse parenchymal disease in, 344f, 345
　　nodular parenchymal, 342, 343f
　　pulmonary manifestations of, 341–345, 341t, 342f–344f, 342t
　　thoracic manifestations of, 342, 342t
　　tracheobronchial, 342, 342f, 343f
Aneurysm(s)
　　aortic, 500–505. See also Aortic aneurysm
　　mycotic, aortic aneurysm due to, 502–503, 503f
　　posttraumatic, aortic aneurysm due to, 502
　　pulmonary artery, 606–608, 607t, 608f–610f
　　Rasmussen, 102
　　ruptured sinus of Valsalva, 522t, 525, 528, 528f, 529f

Angelchik reflux prosthesis, 288, 288f
Angiitis, necrotizing sarcoidal, pulmonary manifestations of, 331
Angiography
applications of, 44–45, 45f, 45t
of coarctation, 497
described, 44
indications for, 44–45, 45f, 45t
of pseudocoarctation, 499, 500
pulmonary, in pulmonary embolism, 586, 589, 589f
chronic, 597, 598f
Ankylosing spondylitis, pulmonary manifestations of, 328
Annuloaortic ectasia, aortic aneurysm due to, 501–502
Antiglomerular basement membrane disease, pulmonary manifestations of, 332, 333f
Antinuclear cytoplasmic antibody—associated vasculitides, manifestations of, 329–330, 330f, 331f
Antireflux devices, 256t, 288–289, 288f, 289f
Aorta, 482–512. *See also* Aortic dissection
anatomy and physiology of, 2t, 18–19, 18f, 19f
angiography of, indications for, 45t
anomalous coronary artery origins from, 514t, 520, 520f
ascending, normal synthetic interposition graft of, 507, 508f
coarctation of, 494–498. *See also* Coarctation
collapsed native, 507, 509f
devices used in, 256t, 267–269, 268f, 269f, 269t
MRI of, 39t, 485, 488f, 488t, 489f
repaired, 506–509, 506f–510f
thoracic
anomalies of, 514, 514t, 515f–519f, 517t
CT of, 35t
treatment of, surgical
CSGIT, 507, 507f
types of, 506f
Aortic aneurysm, 500–505
annuloaortic ectasia and, 501–502
atherosclerosis and, 501
causes of, 500t
chest radiography of, 504, 504f
classification of
cause-related, 501–503, 502f, 503f
integrity of aortic wall—related, 501
morphology-related, 500
site-related, 500
clinical manifestations of, 504
CT of, 504–505, 505f, 505t
cystic medial degeneration and, 501
defined, 500
Marfan syndrome and, 501, 502f
MRI of, 505
mycotic aneurysm and, 502–503, 503f
posttraumatic aneurysm and, 502

syphilis and, 502
Aortic arch
bovine, 8
cervical, 514, 519f
double, 514, 519f
mirror image right, 514
Aortic dissection, 483–490
aortography of, 489
chest radiography of, 62, 63f, 485, 485t, 486f
classification of, 484–485
clinical presentation of, 483–484
CT of, 485, 486t, 488t, 489f
follow-up care, 490
imaging of, 485, 486f–489f, 486t, 488t
management of, 490
pathogenesis of, 484
prevalence of, 483
risk factors for, 483, 484t
symptoms of, 483–484
transesophageal echocardiography of, 490
Aortic injuries, acute traumatic, 295–299, 296f, 297t, 298f–300f
Aortic stenosis, 552, 553f
Aortic valve, bicuspid, 513–514, 514t, 515f, 516f
prevalence of, 513–514, 514t, 515f, 516f
Aortic valve disease, 546t, 552–553, 553t, 554f
aortic stenosis, 552, 553f
aortic valve insufficiency, 552–553, 553t, 554f
Aortic valve insufficiency, 552–553, 553t, 554f
causes of, 553t
Aortography, of aortic dissection, 489
Aplasia, pulmonary artery, 608–609, 611f
Arteriovenous malformations (AVMs), pulmonary, 148, 150f, 605, 606f
Artery(ies), anatomy and physiology of, 2t, 18–19, 18f, 19f
Arthritis, rheumatoid. *See* Rheumatoid arthritis
Asbestosis, HRCT in, 384, 384t, 385f
Ascending aorta, normal synthetic interposition graft of, 507, 508f
Aspergilloma(s), 102, 102f, 110, 110f
Aspergillosis
allergic bronchopulmonary, 110–111, 111f
in immunocompetent hosts, 109–111, 110f, 111f
invasive, 110
tracheobronchial, in leukemia, 131, 134f
noninvasive, 110, 110f
pulmonary, invasive
in ALL, 132f
in AML, 132f, 133f
in multiple myeloma, 131, 131f
semiinvasive, 110
Aspergillus fumigatus, fungal infections due to, 109–111, 110f, 111f
Aspiration

categories of, 227, 227t
in critically ill patients, 226–228, 226t, 227f, 227t
foreign body, 447–448
Aspiration needles, types of, 618, 619f
Aspiration pneumonia
in critically ill patients, 226–228, 226t, 227f, 227t
in immunocompetent host, 94–103
Actinomyces and, 94–95, 94f
Chlamydia pneumoniae and, 95–96, 95f
described, 94, 94f
Mycobacterium tuberculosis and, 96–102, 97f–102f. *See also* Tuberculosis
Mycoplasma pneumoniae and, 96, 97f
Nocardia asteroides and, 95
Asthma, 404–407
chest radiography in, 405, 406f
clinical features of, 404–405
CT in, 405, 406f
defined, 404
pathophysiology of, 405
ATAI. *See* Acute traumatic aortic injury (ATAI)
Ataxia telangiectasia, pulmonary manifestations of, 346t, 348
Atelectasis
in critically ill patients, 228, 228f
in pneumonia in immunocompetent hosts, 83, 83f
Atherosclerosis, aortic aneurysm due to, 501
Atresia
bronchial, 434, 435f
pulmonary, 534t, 539, 540f
Atrial septal defect(s), 520, 521f, 522f, 522t
Atrial septal defect closure device, 256t, 278–279, 278f
Attenuation, lung parenchymal, HRCT in, 389–391, 390f, 390t, 391f, 391t
AVMs. *See* Arteriovenous malformations (AVMs)
Azygoesophageal recess, 7
Azygos fissure, 9
anatomy of, 479, 479f
Azygous continuation of inferior vena cava, 514t, 532, 533f

B
Bacillus anthracis, bacterial pneumonia due to, 91
Bacterial infections, AIDS-related, 118–119, 119f
Bacterial pneumonia
features of, 796
in immunocompetent hosts, 89–104, 91
Klebsiella and, 91–92
Legionella pneumophila and, 93, 93f
Pseudomonas aeruginosa and, 92–93, 92f

Staphylococcus aureus and, 89–91, 91f
Streptococcus pneumoniae and, 89, 90f
Barotrauma, radiologic manifestations of, 223, 223t
"Barrel-shaped" chest, 4
Basilar interstitial pneumonitis, scleroderma and, 326, 327f
Beam pitch, 32
Benign clear cell tumor, 176
Benign fibrous tumor of pleura, chest radiography of, 473–474, 473f–476f, 475b
Benign mesothelioma, chest radiography of, 473–474, 473f–476f, 475b
Bias
    lead time, defined, 148
    length time, defined, 148
    overdiagnosis, defined, 148
Bicuspid aortic valve, 513–514, 514t, 515f, 516f
    prevalence of, 513–514, 514t, 515f, 516f
"Big-rib" sign," 2, 3f
Blastoma(s), pulmonary, 179
Bleeding, PTNB and, treatment of, 628, 629f
Bone(s), chest radiography of, 53, 54f
Bourneville disease, pulmonary manifestations of, 346t, 348, 349f
Bovine aortic arch, 18
Bovine pericardial wrap, 507, 509f
Breast(s), symmetry of, chest radiography in, 50–51, 51f
Breast cancer, chest radiography of, 51
Bronchial atresia, 434, 435f
Bronchial gland carcinomas, 172
Bronchial gland tumors, 172
Bronchial segments, Jackson and Huber classification of, 434t
Bronchial stenosis, postoperative, 445, 445f
Bronchiectasis, 415–421
    causes of, 417–418, 417t
    chest radiography in, 419f, 4199–420
    clinical features of, 415–418, 417f–419f, 417t
    CT in, 102, 102f, 420–421, 420f, 421t
    cystic fibrosis and, 416–417, 417f
    defined, 416
    dyskinetic ciliary syndrome and, 418
    focal, 418, 419f
    HRCT in, 419
    imaging of, 419–420, 419f
    Kartagener syndrome and, 418
    Lady Windemere syndrome and, 418
    Mounier-Kuhn syndrome and, 418
    traction, 418
    tree-in-bud pattern of, 420, 420f, 421t
    tuberculosis and, 417
    Williams-Campbell syndrome and, 418, 418f
    Young syndrome and, 418
Bronchitis, chronic, diagnosis of, 407
Bronchoalveolar carcinoma

as airspace disease, 159, 159f
alveolar nodules caused by, 358, 359f
as large cavitary mass, 159, 159f
multiple, 158f, 159
Bronchoalveolar cell carcinoma, lymphangitis carcinomatosis from, 187, 187f
Bronchogenic cyst
    CT of, 205, 205f, 206f
    radiology of, 205, 206f
    with uniform high attenuation contents, 209, 212, 212f
Bronchogram(s), air, 65, 65f
Bronchography, applications of, 29, 29f
Broncholith(s), tuberculosis and, 102, 102f
Broncholithiasis, 108, 448
Bronchopneumonia, 84, 84f
Bronchoscopy, virtual, of central airways, 431–432, 431f
Bronchus(i)
    abnormalities of, chest radiography in, 368–369, 368f
    accessory paracardiac, 346f, 435
    diffuse enlargement of, 446–447, 447f
    intrapulmonary, anatomy and physiology of, 11–12, 11t
    main, anatomy and physiology of, 10–11, 11f
    rupture of, 445
Bulla(ae)
    defined, 414
    giant, diagnosis of, 414–415, 416f

C

Calcification(s)
    intracardiac, chest radiography of, 62, 62f
    in lung metastases, 185, 186f–187f
    metastatic pulmonary, pulmonary manifestations of, 340f, 341
    popcorn, hamartoma with, 148, 149f
Calcium, in mediastinal masses, CT in detection of, 209–212, 210t, 211f, 212f
Cancer
    breast, chest radiography of, 51
    colon, metastatic, calcification of, CT of, 372f
    esophageal, 189–193, 190f–193f, 190t. *See also* Esophageal cancer
    lung. *See* Lung cancer
    ovarian, pleural effusion and, 460, 460f
Caplan syndrome, 324–325
Carcinoid tumors, 169–171, 169t, 170f–172f
    atypical, 170f, 171
    histopathologic spectrum of, 169, 169t
    of trachea, 450–451, 452f
Carcinomatosis, lymphangitic, chest radiography in, 382–383, 382t, 383f
Carcinosarcoma, 179
Cardiac devices, 256t, 269–272, 270f–274f, 272t, 276f–278f

atrial septal defect closure device, 256t, 278–279, 278f
coronary artery bypass graft markers, 276–278, 277f
ICDs, 256t, 274–275, 274f
LVADs, 256t, 275, 276f
pacemakers, 256t, 269–271, 270f–274f, 272t
Cardiac disease
    acquired, 545–580. *See also specific disease, e.g.,* Aortic valve disease
    ischemic heart disease, 546t, 569–573, 569f–575f, 572t
    myocardial disease, 546t, 556–562
    neoplastic disease, 575, 575t, 576f–578f, 576t
    pericardial disease, 546t, 562–569
Cardiac echocardiography, 46f
Cardiac injuries, traumatic, 312–313, 312f
Cardiac mass, MRI of, 39t
Cardiac neoplasms, primary benign, 575t
Cardiac perfusion scan, applications of, 43, 44f
Cardiac tamponade, 313
Cardiac valve disease, 545–555. *See also specific disease, e.g.,* Mitral valve disease
    aortic valve disease, 546t, 552–553, 553t, 554f
    mitral valve disease, 545–552, 546f–552f, 546t
    myocarditis, 546t, 560, 561t, 562f
    pulmonic valve disease, 546t, 553–555, 554t, 555f, 556f
    tricuspid valve disease, 546t, 553–555, 554t, 555f, 556f
Cardiac viability, MRI of, 39t
Cardiogenic edema, *vs.* noncardiogenic edema, lung opacity in critically ill patients due to, 237–240, 237f, 238f, 239t, 240f, 241f
Cardiomegaly, chest radiography of, 60, 61f
Cardiomyopathy, 546t, 556–560, 556t, 557f–561f, 557t, 559t, 561t
    causes of, 556t
    dilated, 556–558, 557f–559f, 557t
    functional classifications of, 556t
    hypertrophic, 558, 559f
    prevalence of, 556
    restrictive, 558–560, 559t, 560f, 561f
Cardiopericardial silhouette, chest radiography of, 59–62, 59f–62f
Cardiovascular system, in critically ill patients, evaluation of, 229–236, 229t, 230f, 231t, 232t, 233f, 235f
Castleman disease, 182, 212, 213f
Catheter(s)
    central venous, 256t, 257–262, 258f–262f, 259t. *See also* Central venous catheter
    Hickman, 257
    percutaneous indwelling central, 255–257, 256f, 256t, 257f
    pulmonary artery, 256t, 263–264, 263f–266f, 265t

Catheter(s) (*contd*)
  malpositioned, traumatically
    inserted and, 319f
  transtracheal oxygen, 256t, 283–284,
    283f
  venous, 255–267, 256f–267f, 256t,
    259t, 265t
    central venous catheter, 256t,
      257–262, 258f–262f, 259t. *See*
      also Central venous catheter
    ECLS, 256t, 266–267, 267f
    PICC, 255–257, 256f, 256t, 257f
    pulmonary artery catheter, 256t,
      263–264, 263f–266f, 265t. *See*
      also Pulmonary artery catheter
Cavitary mass, upper lobe, right, 620,
  620f
Cavitary metastatic osteosarcoma, 370f
  pneumothorax due to, 468–469, 469f
Cavitary nocardiosis, in multiple
  myeloma, 135, 136f
Cavitary nodules, 369–371, 369f–372f,
  369t, 370b
  chest radiography in, 369–371
  differential diagnosis of, mnemonic
    for, 369t
Cavitation, in lung metastases, 185, 186f
CBV. *See* Circulating blood volume
  (CBV)
CD4 counts, in AIDS, 117–118, 118t
Central airways
  anatomy of, 433, 434t
  broncholithiasis of, 448
  congenital anomalies of, 434–435,
    435f, 436f
  CT of, 429–433, 430f–432f
  diffuse enlargement of, 446–447, 447f
  focal foreign bodies in, 447–448
  imaging of, 429–455
  infectious conditions of, 442–445
  inflammatory conditions of, 435–442
    amyloidosis, 442
    postintubation stenosis, 432f,
      435–436, 437f
    sarcoidosis, 441–442
    tracheobronchomalacia, 437–439,
      438f–439f
    tracheobronchopathia
      osteochondroplastica, 442
    ulcerative colitis, 442
    Wegener granulomatosis, 439–441,
      440f, 441f
  metastases of, 452–453, 452f
  postoperative stenosis and dehiscence
    of, 445, 445f
  saber sheath trachea of, 447
  stents in, 446, 446f
  tracheal diverticula of, 448
  tracheal masses, 448–452, 449f–452f
  tracheobronchomegaly of, 446–447,
    447f
  traumatic rupture of, 445
  ultrasonography of, 429
  virtual bronchoscopy of, 431–432,
    431f

Central venous catheter, 256t, 257–262,
    258f–262f, 259t
  arterial position of, 259, 261f
  complications associated with,
    258–262, 259t, 260f–262f
  malpositioned, 259, 260f
  positioning of, 257–258, 258f, 259f
  types of, 257, 258f
  uses of, 257
Central venous pressure (CVP)
  abnormal, causes of, 231–232, 231t
  in critically ill patients, evaluation of,
    229t, 231–232, 231t
Centrilobular emphysema, 407t, 408,
    408f, 408t, 409f
Cervical aortic arch, 514, 519f
Cervicothoracic sign, 66–67
Chemodectoma, of lung, 176–177
Chest
  "barrel-shaped," 4
  CT of, 35t
  flail, 300–301, 302f
  funnel, 4
Chest mass, MRI of, 39t
Chest radiography
  of abdomen, 51–53, 52f, 53f
  in abdominal diseases, 51–53, 52f, 53f
  in alveolar disease, 358–362,
    358f–362f, 358t, 360t, 362t
  aortic aneurysm and, 504, 504f
  of aortic dissection, 485, 485t, 486f
  applications of, 25–28, 26f–28f, 26t
  approach to, 49–67
    in PACS era, 67
  in asthma, 405, 406f
  of bones, 53, 54f
  in breast cancer, 51
  in bronchiectasis, 419f, 4199–420
  in cardiomegaly, 60, 61f
  of cardiopericardial silhouette, 59–62,
    59f–62f
  in chronic pulmonary embolism, 597,
    597f
  of coarctation, 496–497, 496f
  in critically ill patients, 219–220, 220t
  in diffuse lung disease, 357–371. *See*
    also Diffuse lung disease, chest
    radiography in
  in emphysema, 411–412, 411f, 411t
  empyema *vs.* lung consolidation on,
    217, 218f
  of extrathoracic soft tissues, 50–51,
    51f
  of great vessels, 62–63, 63f
  of honeycombing, 364–367, 365t,
    366f, 366t, 367f
  indications for, 26t
  of intracardiac calcifications, 62, 62f
  in lung cancer, 143–147, 144f–147f
  in lung cancer staging, 160
  of lungs, 64–67, 64f–67f. *See also*
    Lung(s), chest radiography of
  of mediastinal masses, 197–215. *See*
    also specific mass
  of mediastinum, 57–58, 57f–59f

of miliary nodules, 362–363,
    363f–365f, 363t, 365t
  in non-AIDS immunocompromised
    patients, 129–137, 130f–138f
  in PACS era, approach to, 67
  patient positioning for, 27–28, 27f,
    28f, 50
  of pleura, 54–57, 55f, 56f, 457–476.
    See also Pleura, abnormalities of
  of pleural effusion, 54, 55f, 56, 56f
  in pneumonia in immunocompetent
    hosts, 80–83, 81f–83f
  in pneumothorax, 54, 56f
  point sources in, 25, 27
  principles of, 25, 26f
  projection for, 50
  of pseudocoarctation, 498, 499f
  in pulmonary arterial hypertension,
    603, 603f
  in pulmonary embolism, 583–584,
    583t, 584f
  in sarcoidosis staging, 352t
  of small irregular opacities, 367, 367t,
    368f
  in splenomegaly, 52, 53f
  of tracheal deviation, 57–58, 59f
Chest tubes, 256t, 289–290, 289t, 290f,
    291f
Chest wall, 1–5, 2f–4f, 2t
  anatomy of, 2f–4f, 5
    ribs, 1–4, 3f
    sternum, 2f, 3f, 4–5, 4f
Chest wall chondrosarcoma, 476f
Chest wall invasion, in lung cancer,
    480
CHF. *See* Congestive heart failure (CHF)
Chickenpox pneumonia, in
    immunocompetent hosts, 112,
    112f
Chlamydia pneumoniae, aspiration
    pneumonia due to, 95–96, 95f
Chondroma(s), tracheal, 168, 449
Chondrosarcoma(s), 177, 178f
  chest wall, 476f
  tracheal, 450, 450f
Chronic bronchitis, diagnosis of, 407
Chronic obstructive pulmonary disease
    (COPD). *See also specific types,*
    e.g., Asthma
  asthma, 404–407
  bronchiectasis, 415–421
  chronic bronchitis, 407
  clinical history of, 402
  defined, 401
  emphysema, 407–413
  giant bulla, 414–415, 416f
  imaging of, impact of therapy on,
    421–422
  physical examination in, 402
  pulmonary function testing in,
    402–404, 403t
  radiologic studies in, 404
  spirometry in, 403
  symptoms of, 402
  types of, 401t

Chronic pulmonary embolism, 596–600, 597f–599f. *See also* Pulmonary embolism, chronic
Churg-Strauss syndrome, manifestations of, 330
Circulating blood volume (CBV)
  in critically ill patients, evaluation of, 229–230, 229t
  defined, 229
CMV. *See* Cytomegalovirus (CMV)
Coal worker's pneumoconiosis, HRCT in, 386–387, 387f
Coarctation, 494–498
  angiography of, 497
  appearance of, 495, 495f
  chest radiography of, 496–497, 496f
  clinical presentation of, 496
  CT of, 497
  defined, 494
  disorders associated with, 494, 495t
  MRI of, 497–498, 497f, 498f
  pathogenesis of, 495, 495f
Coccidioides immitis, fungal infections due to, 108–109, 109f
Colitis, ulcerative, 442
Collagen vascular diseases. *See also specific types*
  pulmonary manifestations of, 323–326
    rheumatoid arthritis, 323–325, 324f, 324t
    scleroderma, 326, 327f
    SLE, 325–326, 325t, 326f
Colon cancer, metastatic, calcification of, CT of, 372f
Comet-tail sign, 66, 67f
Communication, on radiographic report, 71–72
Complete transposition of great vessels, 537–538, 538f, 539f
Computed tomography (CT)
  aortic aneurysm and, 504–505, 505f, 505t
  of aortic dissection, 485, 486t, 488t, 489f
  applications of, 29–34, 30t, 31f–34f, 35t
  of ARDS, in critically ill patients, 223–225, 224f
  in asthma, 405, 406f
  in bronchiectasis, 420–421, 420f, 421t
  of bronchogenic cyst, 205, 205f, 206f
  of central airways, 429–433, 430f–432f
  in chronic pulmonary embolism, 597–600, 598f, 599f
  of coarctation, 497
  described, 31
  electron beam, in pulmonary embolism, 594
  in emphysema, 412–413, 412f, 413f
  in esophageal cancer, 191–193, 191f–193f
  helical, of central airways, 430–431, 431f, 433
  high-resolution
    in bronchiectasis, 419

  in interstitial lung diseases, 376–396
  indications for, 29, 30t
  of intramural hematoma, 491, 492f
  in lung cancer, 147–148, 148f–150f
  in lung cancer staging, 160, 162–164, 163f
  of mediastinal masses, 209–214, 210t, 211f–213f, 212t. *See also* Mediastinal masses, CT of
  of penetrating atherosclerotic ulcer, 493–494, 494f
  of pleura, 477–482
  in pneumonia in immunocompetent hosts, 80
  postprocessing steps, 32–34, 32f–34f
  principles of, 29, 31, 31f
  protocols for, 34, 35t
  of pseudocoarctation, 499, 499f
  in pulmonary arterial hypertension, 604
  in pulmonary embolism, 589
  in pulmonary thromboembolic disease, 581–582
  refinements in, 31–32
  thoracic, in critically ill patients, 217–219, 218f, 219f
  in Wegener's granulomatosis, 430f
Computed tomography angiography (CTA), 34
Computed tomography (CT)—guided needle biopsy, in lower lobe nodule, 617, 619f
Computed tomography (CT) pulmonary angiogram (CTPA), in pulmonary thromboembolic disease, 582
Computed tomography (CT) venography, in pulmonary embolism, 594, 595f
Congenital cystic adenomatoid malformation, 175, 175f
Congenital heart disease
  in adults, 513–543
  cyanotic, 533–541
    abnormal situs, 541, 541f, 541t
    complete transposition of great vessels, 537–538, 538f, 539f
    described, 533, 533t, 534t
    Ebstein anomaly, 534t, 536–537, 537f, 538f
    Eisenmenger physiology, 533t, 533–535, 534f, 535f
    pulmonary atresia, 534t, 539, 540f
    rare, 537–539, 538f–540f
    tetralogy of Fallot, 534t, 535–536, 535f, 536f
    truncus arteriosus, 533t, 538–539, 539f
  noncyanotic, 513–532. *See also specific disorder, e.g.,* Bicuspid aortic valve
    absent pulmonic valve, 514t, 528, 530f
    anomalous coronary artery origins, 514t, 520, 520f
    azygous continuation of inferior vena cava, 514t, 532, 533f

    bicuspid aortic valve, 513–514, 514t, 515f, 516f
    cor triatriatum, 514t, 528–529, 530f
    corrected transposition of great vessels, 514t, 529, 531, 531f
    left-to-right shunts, 514t, 520–528, 521f–529f, 522t
    persistent left superior vena cava, 514t, 532, 532f, 532t
    pulmonic valve stenosis, 514t, 528, 530f
    thoracic aorta anomalies, 514, 514t, 515f–519f, 517t
  types of, 514t
Congestive heart failure (CHF), pleural effusion and, 459
Constrictive pericarditis, 546t, 566–569, 566f–568f, 569t
Continuous suture graft inclusion technique (CSGIT), for aorta disorders, 507, 507f
Contusion(s)
  myocardial, 312
  pulmonary, 304–307, 304f–307f
    pneumothoraces with, 305f
    progression of, 305f
Conventional tomography, applications of, 29
COPD. *See* Chronic obstructive pulmonary disease (COPD)
Cor triatriatum, 514t, 528–529, 530f
Coronary artery(ies), imaging of, 569–571, 569f–571f
Coronary artery bypass graft markers, 276–278, 277f
Coronary artery disease, myocardial manifestations of, 546t, 571–573, 572f–575f, 572t
Corrected transposition of great vessels, 514t, 529, 531, 531f
Counting ribs, anatomy of, 480, 480f
Critically ill patients
  abnormal air collections in, 241–250, 241t, 242f–247f, 243t, 247t, 248t, 249f, 250f. *See also* Thoracic air collections, abnormal, in critically ill patients
  cardiovascular status evaluation in, 229–236, 229t, 230f, 231t, 232t, 233f, 235f
    central venous pressure, 229t, 231–232, 231t
    circulating blood volume, 229–230, 229t, 230f
    left ventricular function, 234–236, 235f
    pulmonary arterial pressure, 229t, 234
    pulmonary blood flow, 229t, 232–233, 232t, 233f
    pulmonary blood volume, 229t, 232–233, 232t, 233f
    systemic extravascular water, 236t
  lung opacity in, causes of, 237–240, 237f, 238f, 239t, 240f, 241f

Critically ill patients (*contd*)
pneumothorax in, 242–245,
242f–245f, 243t
thoracic imaging in, 217–254. *See also
specific modality and disorder*
acute interstitial pneumonitis, 225
ARDS, 220–225
aspiration, 226–228, 226t, 227f, 227t
aspiration pneumonia, 226–228,
226t, 227f, 227t
atelectasis, 228, 228f
in cardiovascular status evaluation,
229–236. *See also* Critically ill
patients, cardiovascular status
evaluation in
chest radiography, 219–220, 220t
clinical indications for, 217, 218f
CT, 217–219, 218f, 219f
infection, 225–226, 226t
nosocomial infections, 226, 226t
portable scanners in, 218–219
pulmonary parenchymal
opacification, 220–228, 221t, 222f,
223t, 224f, 226t, 227f, 227t, 228f
Cryptogenic organizing pneumonia,
HRCT in, 394–395, 394t, 395f
CSGIT. *See* Continuous suture graft
inclusion technique (CSGIT)
CT. *See* Computed tomography (CT)
CT of, 477–482
CTPA. *See* Computed tomography (CT)
pulmonary angiogram (CTPA)
Cutting instruments, types of, 618, 619f
CVP. *See* Central venous pressure (CVP)
Cyanosis
with shunt vascularity, 533t
without shunt vascularity, 534t
Cyclical hemothorax, 469, 469f
Cyst(s), bronchogenic
CT of, 205, 205f, 206f
radiology of, 205, 206f
with uniform high attenuation
contents, 209, 212, 212f
Cystic adenomatoid malformation, 175,
175f
Cystic fibrosis
bronchial pattern of, 368–369, 368f
bronchiectasis and, 416–417, 417f
Cystic medial degeneration, aortic
aneurysm due to, 501
Cytomegalovirus (CMV) pneumonia,
after renal transplant, 138f

D
Data pitch, 32
DeBakey classification, of aortic
dissection, 484–485
"Deep sulcus" sign, 308, 308f
Deep venous thrombosis (DVT)
causes of, 582–583, 582t
pathophysiology of, 582–583, 582t
in pulmonary thromboembolic disease,
582
Dermatomyositis, pulmonary
manifestations of, 327–328, 327f,
328f

Desquamative interstitial pneumonia
(DIP), HRCT in, 391–392, 392f,
392t
Diabetes mellitus, tracheobronchial
zygomycosis, 134, 135f
Diaphragm, anatomy and physiology of,
2t, 4f, 5–6
Diaphragm injuries, traumatic, 313–317,
313t, 314f–317f, 315t
Diaphragmatic inversion, 459
Dictation pointers, 70, 71, 72
Diffuse interstitial fibrosis, in rheumatoid
arthritis, 324
Diffuse lung disease, 357–399
chest radiography in, 357–371
alveolar disease, 358–362,
358f–362f, 358t, 360t, 362t
bronchial abnormality, 368–369,
368f
cavitary nodules, 369–371,
369f–372f, 369t, 370b
honeycombing, 364–367, 365t,
366f, 366t, 367f
miliary nodules, 362–363,
363f–365f, 363t, 365t
multiple nodules, 369–371,
369f–372f, 369t, 370b
nodular diseases, 385–389,
386f–388f, 386t, 389t
pulmonary edema, 381–382, 382t
small irregular opacities, 367, 367t,
368f
HRCT in
asbestosis, 384, 384t, 385f
characterized predominantly by
abnormally increased attenuation,
391–395, 392f, 392t–394t, 393f,
395f, 396f
characterized predominantly by
altered attenuation, 389–391,
390f, 390t, 391f, 391t
coal worker's pneumoconiosis,
386–387, 387f
cryptogenic organizing pneumonia,
394–395, 394t, 395f
desquamative interstitial
pneumonia, 391–392, 392f, 392t
hypersensitivity pneumonitis,
387–388, 388f
idiopathic pulmonary fibrosis,
383–384, 383t, 384f
lymphangitic carcinomatosis,
382–383, 382t, 383f
lymphoid interstitial pneumonia,
393–394, 394t
nonspecific interstitial pneumonia,
392–393, 393f, 393t
pulmonary alveolar proteinosis, 395,
396f
respiratory bronchiolitis—associated
interstitial lung disease, 389, 389t
reticular diseases, 381–384,
382t–384t, 383f–385f
sarcoidosis, 385–386, 386f, 386t,
387f
silicosis, 386–387, 387f

imaging of, goals of, 357
in non-AIDS immunocompromised
patients, 136–137, 138f
pattern recognition in, 357–371. *See
also* Pattern recognition, in
diffuse lung disease
Diffuse pulmonary hemorrhage
causes of, 332t
pulmonary manifestations of,
331–334, 332t, 333f
Diffusing capacity for carbon monoxide
(DL_{CO}), measurement of, in
COPD, 404
Dilated cardiomyopathy, 556–558,
557f–559f, 557t
Diverticulum(a), tracheal, 448
Double aortic arch, 514, 519f
"Double density" sign, in mitral valve
disease, 545, 546f
DVT. *See* Deep venous thrombosis (DVT)
Dyskinesia, primary ciliary,
bronchiectasis and, 418
Dyskinetic ciliary syndrome,
bronchiectasis and, 418
Dysplasia, MRI of, 39t

E
Ebstein anomaly, 534t, 536–537, 537f,
538f
Echinococcosis, 112–114, 113f
Echinococcus granulosis, parasitic
infections due to, in
immunocompetent hosts,
112–114, 113f
Echocardiography
cardiac, 46f
in pulmonary arterial hypertension,
603–604
transesophageal
of aortic dissection, 490
in pulmonary thromboembolic
disease, 582
transthoracic, in pulmonary
thromboembolic disease, 582
ECLS. *See* Extracorporeal life support
(ECLS)
Ectasia, annuloaortic, aortic aneurysm
due to, 501–502
Edema
cardiogenic, vs. noncardiogenic edema,
lung opacity in critically ill
patients due to, 237–240, 237f,
238f, 239t, 240f, 241f
interstitial, 235f
noncardiogenic, vs. cardiogenic, lung
opacity in critically ill patients
due to, 237–240, 237f, 238f, 239t,
240f, 241f
pulmonary. *See* Pulmonary edema
Effusion(s)
malignant, and mesothelioma, 481
pericardial, 59–60, 59f–61f, 563,
564f–566f, 564t
with classic "water bottle"
configuration, 59, 59f
pleural. *See* Pleural effusion

Eisenmenger physiology, 533t, 533–535, 534f, 535f
Electron beam CT, in pulmonary embolism, 594
Embolism
    air, PTNB and, treatment of, 628
    pulmonary, septic, 600–601, 600f
    pulmonary tumor, 604, 605f
Embolus(i), pulmonary, CT of, 35t
Emphysema, 407–413
    centrilobular, 407t, 408, 408f, 408t, 409f
    chest radiography of, 411–412, 411f, 411t
    CT in, 412–413, 412f, 413f
    defined, 407
    interstitial, in critically ill patients, 249–250, 250f
    panacinar, 407t, 408–409, 408t, 410f
    panlobular, 407t, 408–409, 408t, 410f
    paracicatricial, 407t, 409, 410f
    paraseptal, 407t, 408f, 409, 410f
    pathologic classification of, 407–408, 407t
    scintigraphy in, 413, 414f, 415f
    subcutaneous, 310f
    types of, 407–408, 407t, 408f
Empyema
    lung abscess *vs.*, 462, 463f
    lung consolidation *vs.*, on chest radiography, 217, 218f
    pleural effusion and, 461, 462f, 463f
    PTNB and, treatment of, 628
    tuberculous, 102f
Endobronchial benign granular cell tumor, 168, 168f
Endobronchial leiomyoma, 175–176, 176f
Endobronchial lesion, effects of, 144, 147f
Endobronchial metastasis, from teratocarcinoma, 188, 188f
Endobronchial squamous cell carcinoma, 153, 153f
Endometriosis, pulmonary, 177
Endoskeleton, thoracic, 2f
Endotracheal tube, malpositioned, 319f
Endotracheal tubes, 256t, 279–281, 279t, 280f, 281f
    complications associated with, 279t, 280–281, 281f
    positioning of, 279–280, 280f, 281f
Endovascular stent, percutaneous, 507, 510f
Eosinophilic granuloma, 366f
Eosinophilic pneumonia, 374f–375f
Epicardial coronary venous anatomy, 272f
Epithelial neoplasms, malignant, 169–172, 169t, 170f–172f
Epithelioid hemangioendothelioma, 177, 178f
Esophageal adenocarcinoma, 190, 190f
Esophageal cancer, 189–193, 190f–193f, 190t. *See also specific types*
    CT in, 191–193, 191f–193f

locally invasive, 191, 191f
    manifestations of, 190, 190f
    metastatic, 192f
    mortality associated with, 189–190
    MRI in, 193
    rare types of, 190t
    recurrent, 192f, 193f
    with tracheoesophageal fistula, 191f
Esophageal hiatus, 6
Esophageal injuries, traumatic, 311, 311t, 312f
Esophageal intubation, 318f–320f, 319
Esophageal tear, after trauma, 311, 311t, 312f
Esophageal varices, giant, 205, 205f
Esophagus
    anatomy and physiology of, 4f, 7, 7f, 7t
    devices used in, 256t, 284–289
        antireflux devices, 256t, 288–289, 288f, 289f
        feeding tubes, 256t, 284, 284f, 285f, 285t
        gastric banding, 256t, 289, 289f
        intraesophageal manometer, temperature probe, and pH probe, 256t, 286, 286f
        nasogastric tubes, 256t, 284, 284f, 285f, 285t
        orogastric tubes, 256t, 284, 284f, 285f, 285t
        pH probe, 256t, 286, 286f
        stents, 256t, 286–288, 287f
        temperature probe, 256t, 286, 286f
Ethnicity, as factor in SLE, 325
Eustachian valves, 14
Extracorporeal life support (ECLS), 256t, 266–267, 267f
    venoarterial, 267f
    venovenous, 267f
Extramedullary hematopoiesis, 206, 208f
    pulmonary manifestations of, 334, 335f
Extrapleural abnormalities, 475b
Extrapleural metastatic esophageal carcinoma, 476f
Extrapleural metastatic melanoma, 475f

F
"Fallen lung" sign, 310f, 311
Fat, in mediastinal masses, CT in detection of, 209–212, 210t, 211f, 212f
"Fat pad" sign, 563, 564f
Feeding tube, misplaced, 320f
Feeding tubes, 256t, 284, 284f, 285f, 285t
Felt enforcing ring, 507, 508f
Fibroma(s), tracheal, 168
Fibrosing mediastinitis, 108, 108f, 442–444, 443f
Fibrosis(es)
    cystic
        bronchial pattern of, 368–369, 368f
        bronchiectasis and, 416–417, 417f

idiopathic, pulmonary, HRCT in, 383–384, 383t, 384f
Fibrothorax, tuberculosis and, 471, 471f
Fissure(s)
    azygous, anatomy of, 479, 479f
    inferior accessory, 5, 9
        anatomy of, 478
    lung cancer crossing, 481, 481f
    pleural
        anatomy of, 8–9, 9f–10f, 477–479, 478f, 479f
        physiology of, 8–9, 9f–10f
    sagittal anterior minor, anatomy of, 479, 479f
    superior accessory, 9
        anatomy of, 477, 478f
Fistula(s), tracheoesophageal, esophageal cancer with, 191f
Flail chest, 300–301, 302f
Fluoroscopy, applications of, 29
Foramen for inferior vena cava, 6
Foreign body aspiration, 447–448
"Fourth mogul," 546–547, 547f
Fracture(s)
    rib, 300–302, 301f–303f, 303t
    spine, thoracic, 303, 303t, 304f
    sternal, 302–303
    vertebral, thoracic, 303, 303t, 304f
Free intraperitoneal gas, chest radiography of, 51–52, 52f
Friedlander pneumonia, 86, 86f
Fungal infections
    AIDS-related, 122, 122f
    in immunocompetent hosts, 105–111
        aspergillosis, 109–111, 110f, 111f
        Coccidioides immitis and, 108–109, 109f
        Histoplasma capsulatum and, 105–108, 105f–108f
        histoplasmosis, 105–108, 105f–108f. *See also* Histoplasmosis
Funnel chest, 4

G
Gallium (⁶⁷Ga) scan, applications of, 42
Gamuts in Radiology, 362
Gastric banding, 256t, 289, 289f
Gender
    as factor in rheumatoid arthritis, 323
    as factor in sarcoidosis, 350
    as factor in scleroderma, 326
    as factor in SLE, 325
Giant bulla, diagnosis of, 414–415, 416f
Golden S sign, 66, 67f
Goodpasture disease, pulmonary manifestations of, 332, 333f
Graft-*versus*-host disease
    acute, timing in, 338
    chronic, timing in, 338–339
Granular cell tumor, tracheal, 168, 168f
Granuloma(s)
    eosinophilic, 366f
    plasma cell, 182–183, 183f
Great vessels, chest radiography of, 62–63, 63f

H

Hamartoma(s), 148, 151f, 172–175, 173f–175f
  calcified, 173, 173f, 174f
  infantile, 175, 175f
  with popcorn calcification, 148, 149f
  tracheal, 449
Hamman-Rich syndrome, 225
Heart
  anatomy and physiology of, 2t, 14–17, 15f–17f
  angiography of, indications for, 45t
  CT of, 35t
    indications for, 30t
  devices used in, 256t, 269–279. *See also* Cardiac devices
  functioning of, imaging of, 43–44
  MRI of, indications for, 36t
  radionuclide imaging of, indications for, 41t
  ultrasound of, indications for, 47t
Heart disease, congenital, 513–543. *See also* Congenital heart disease
Heimlich Micro-Trach, 283
Helical CT pulmonary angiogram, in pulmonary embolism, 589–594, 590f–593f, 591t, 594t
Hemangioendothelioma, epithelioid, 177, 178f
Hemangioma(s), 175
  tracheal, 449
Hemangiopericytoma, 177
Hematologic disorders, pulmonary manifestations of, 334–339, 334t, 335f–340f
  extramedullary hematopoiesis, 334, 335f
  leukemias, 337–339, 338t, 339f, 339t
  lymphoproliferative of lung, 335–337, 336t, 337f, 338f
  multiple myeloma, 339, 340f
  sickle cell disease, 334–335, 334t, 335f
Hematoma(s), intramural, 490–493. *See also* Intramural hematoma
Hematopoiesis, extramedullary, 206, 208f
  pulmonary manifestations of, 334, 335f
Hemopericardium, 312f, 313
Hemorrhage, diffuse pulmonary
  causes of, 332t
  pulmonary manifestations of, 331–334, 332t, 333f
Hemosiderosis, idiopathic pulmonary, pulmonary manifestations of, 332–334, 333f
Hemothorax
  cyclical, 469, 469f
  rib fractures and, 300, 301f
Hereditary hemorrhagic telangiectasia, pulmonary manifestations of, 346t, 350, 351f
Hernia(s), diaphragmatic, 313, 313t, 314f–316f
Herniation, visceral, diaphragm rupture and, 313, 313t, 314f–316f
Hiatus, esophageal, 6

Hickman catheter, 257
High-riding scapula, 5
Hilum overlay sign, 64, 65f
Histiocytosis, Langerhans cell
  HRCT in, 389–391, 390t, 391f, 391t
  pulmonary manifestations of, 345, 345f, 346f
Histocytosis X, pulmonary manifestations of, 345, 345f, 346f
Histoplasma capsulatum, fungal infections due to, in immunocompetent hosts, 105–108, 105f–108f
Histoplasmoma(s), 107–108, 107f
Histoplasmosis
  acute, 105–106, 105f
  broncholithiasis in, 108
  chronic, 106–107, 107f
  delayed manifestations of, 107
  described, 105
  disseminated disease, 106, 106f
  fibrosing mediastinitis in, 108, 108f
  histoplasmomas in, 107–108, 107f
  in immunocompetent hosts, 105–108, 105f–108f
  miliary, 106, 106f
Hodgkin lymphoma, incidence of, 179
Honeycombing
  chest radiography in, 364–367, 365t, 366f, 366t, 367f
  differential diagnosis of, mnemonic for, 365t
  lower lobe, 366f
  upper lobe, 366f
HRCT. *See* Computed tomography (CT), high-resolution
Human immunodeficiency virus (HIV) infection, in immunocompromised hosts. *See also* Acquired immunodeficiency syndrome (AIDS), pulmonary manifestations of
Hydatid, parasitic infections due to, in immunocompetent hosts, 112–114, 113f
Hypersensitivity pneumonitis, HRCT in, 387–388, 388f
Hypertension
  pulmonary, 554, 555f, 556f
  pulmonary artery, 601–604. *See also* Pulmonary arterial hypertension (PAH)
Hypertrophic cardiomyopathy, 558, 559f
Hypoplasia, pulmonary artery, 609, 612f

I

IABP. *See* Intraaortic balloon pump (IABP)
Iatrogenic injuries, traumatic, 318f–320f, 319
ICDs. *See* Implantable cardiac defibrillators (ICDs)
Idiopathic interstitial pneumonias
  classification of, 378t
  definitions of, 378, 378t
  miliary metastases in
    in asbestosis, 384, 384t, 385f

characterized predominantly by abnormally increased attenuation, 391–395, 392f, 392t–394t, 393f, 395f, 396f
characterized predominantly by altered attenuation, 389–391, 390f, 390t, 391f, 391t
coal worker's pneumoconiosis, 386–387, 387f
in cryptogenic organizing pneumonia, 394–395, 394t, 395f
in desquamative interstitial pneumonia, 391–392, 392f, 392t
in hypersensitivity pneumonitis, 387–388, 388f
idiopathic pulmonary fibrosis, 383–384, 383t, 384f
in lymphangitic carcinomatosis, 382–383, 382t, 383f
in lymphoid interstitial pneumonia, 393–394, 394t
in nonspecific interstitial pneumonia, 392–393, 393f, 393t
patterns of abnormality with, 381, 381t
in predominantly nodular diseases, 385–389, 386f–388f, 386t, 389t
in predominantly reticular diseases, 381–384, 382t–384t, 383f–385f
in pulmonary alveolar proteinosis, 395, 396f
in pulmonary edema, 381–382, 382t
in respiratory bronchiolitis—associated interstitial lung disease, 389, 389t
in sarcoidosis, 385–386, 386f, 386t, 387f
in silicosis, 386–387, 387f
Idiopathic pulmonary fibrosis, HRCT in, 383–384, 383t, 384f
Idiopathic pulmonary hemosiderosis, pulmonary manifestations of, 332–334, 333f
Imaging modalities, 25–48. *See also specific type, e.g.,* Magnetic resonance imaging (MRI)
  applications of, 25–48
  effective radiation dose of, 30t
  spatial resolution of, 30t
Immune-complex vasculitis, manifestations of, 331–334, 332t, 333f
Immunocompetent hosts, pneumonia in, 79–115. *See also* Pneumonia(s), in immunocompetent hosts
Immunocompromised hosts
  infections in, 117–141. *See also specific infection and* Infection(s), in immunocompromised hosts
  non-AIDS, pulmonary manifestations of, 128–140
    airspace disease, 129–130
    approach to, 128–129
    chest radiography in, 129–137, 130f–138f
    diffuse lung disease, 136–137, 138f

nodules, 131–136, 131f–137f
noninfectious lung disease, 139–140, 139f
radiographic patterns of, 129
Implantable cardiac defibrillators (ICDs), 256t, 274–275, 274f
Infarct scan, applications of, 44
Infarction(s), myocardial, radiographic signs of, 546t, 572t
Infection(s). *See also specific infection*
of central airways, 442–445
in immunocompromised hosts, 117–141. *See also specific infection, e.g.,* Acquired immunodeficiency syndrome (AIDS)
AIDS, 117–128. *See also* Acquired immunodeficiency syndrome (AIDS)
bacterial infections, 118–119, 119f
fungal infections, 122, 122f
Kaposi sarcoma, 125–126, 125f
lung cancer and, 126–128, 127f
lymphoma, 126, 126f, 127f
mycobacterial infections, 119–121, 120f, 121f
non-AIDs patients, 128–140. *See also* Immunocompromised hosts, non-AIDS, pulmonary manifestations of
Pneumocystis carinii pneumonia, 123–124, 123f, 124f
viral infections, 125
pulmonary, in critically ill patients, 225–226, 226t
Inferior accessory fissure, 9
anatomy of, 478
Inferior pulmonary ligament, 8
Inferior triangle sign, 66
Inferior vena cava, azygous continuation of, 514t, 532, 533f
Inflammatory conditions
of central airways, 435–442. *See also specific disorder and* Central airways, inflammatory conditions of
pleural effusion and, 461–462, 462f, 463f
Inflammatory pseudotumor, thoracic, 182–183, 183f
Influenza, in immunocompetent hosts, 111, 112f
Intensive care unit (ICU)
lung parenchymal opacification in, 220, 220t
thoracic imaging of patients in, 217–254. *See also* Critically ill patients, thoracic imaging in
Interstitial edema, 235f
Interstitial emphysema, in critically ill patients, 249–250, 250f
Interstitial lung diseases
HRCT in, 376–396
anatomy on, 377, 377f
clinical indications for, 377–378, 378t

patterns of abnormality with, 381, 381t
pitfalls in, 378–379, 379f, 379t, 380f
technique of, 376–377
respiratory bronchiolitis—associated, HRCT in, 389, 389t
Interstitial pneumonia, 85, 85f
Interstitial pneumonitis, 366f
acute, in critically ill patients, 225
basilar, scleroderma and, 326, 327f
Interstitial pulmonary edema, chest radiography of, 62–63, 63f
Inter-sublobular septum, 8
Intraaortic balloon pump (IABP), 256t, 267–269, 268f, 269f, 269t
complications associated with, 268–269, 269t
described, 267
function of, 267
positioning of, 268, 268f, 269f
Intracardiac calcifications, chest radiography of, 62, 62f
Intraesophageal manometer, 256t, 286, 286f
Intramural hematoma, 490–493
clinical presentation of, 491
CT of, 491, 492f
historical background of, 490–491
imaging of, 491, 492f
management of, 491, 493
Intrapulmonary bronchi, anatomy and physiology of, 11–12, 11t
Intrathoracic devices, 255–293
Intrathoracic lines, 255–293
Intrathoracic splenosis, 317, 317f
Intrathoracic tubes, 255–293
Ischemic heart disease, 546t, 569–573, 569f–575f, 572t

J
Jackson and Huber classification of bronchial segments, 434t

K
Kaposi sarcoma, AIDS-related, 125–126, 125f
Kartagener syndrome, bronchiectasis and, 418
Kerley B lines, 381
Klebsiella spp., bacterial pneumonia due to, 91–92

L
Laceration(s), pulmonary, 307–309, 307f, 308f
Lady Windemere syndrome, bronchiectasis and, 417
Langerhans cell histiocytosis
HRCT in, 389–391, 390t, 391f, 391t
pulmonary manifestations of, 345, 345f, 346f
LAP-BAND adjustable gastric banding (LAGB) system, 289
Large cell carcinoma of lung, as large peripheral mass, 157, 157f
Larmor frequency, 36, 37, 38f

Larynx, sarcoidosis of, 352
Lead time bias, defined, 148
Left aortic arch with aberrant right subclavian artery, 514, 517f, 518f
Left atrial enlargement, signs of, 54t, 545
Left minor fissure, anatomy of, 478, 478f
Left ventricular assist devices (LVADs), 256t, 275, 276f
Left ventricular function, in critically ill patients, evaluation of, 234–236, 235f
Left-to-right shunts, 514t, 520–528, 521f–529f, 522t
atrial septal defects, 520, 521f, 522f, 522t
partial anomalous pulmonary venous return, 522t, 524, 526f, 527f
patent ductus arteriosus, 522t, 524, 524f, 525f
ventricular septal defects, 522, 522t, 523f
Legionella pneumophila, bacterial pneumonia due to, 93, 93f
Leiomyoma(s), 175–176, 176f
endobronchial, 175–176, 176f
tracheal, 449–450
Leiomyosarcoma(s), 176
duodenal, miliary metastases in, 363, 364f
Length time bias, defined, 148
Lesion(s), endobronchial, effects of, 144, 147f
Leukemia(s)
lymphocytic, acute, invasive pulmonary aspergillosis in, 132f
myelogenous, acute, invasive pulmonary aspergillosis in, 132f, 133f
myeloid, acute, 338, 339f
pulmonary manifestations of, 337–339, 338t, 339f, 339t
abnormal, 339t
T-cell, pulmonary manifestations of, 338
tracheobronchial invasive aspergillosis in, 131, 134f
types of, 338t
Ligament(s), inferior pulmonary, 8
Ligamentum arteriosum, 18
Lipoid pneumonia, 362f
Lipoma(s)
pleural, 473, 474f
tracheal, 167
Liver disease, pulmonary manifestations of, 341
Lobar pneumonia, 84f, 85, 85f
Louis-Bar syndrome, pulmonary manifestations of, 346t, 348
Luftsichel, 66, 66f
Lung(s)
abscess of, empyema *vs.*, 462, 463f
air bronchogram of, 65, 65f
anatomy and physiology of, 2t, 12
chemodectoma of, 176–177
chest radiography of, 64–67, 64f–67f
cervicothoracic sign in, 66–67

Lung(s), chest radiography of (*contd*)
    comet-tail sign in, 66, 67f
    golden S sign in, 66, 67f
    hilum overlay sign on, 64, 65f
    inferior triangle sign in, 66
    luftsichel in, 66, 66f
    silhouette sign on, 64, 64f
    superior triangle sign in, 66
    thoracoabdominal sign in, 66–67
    large cell carcinoma of, as large
        peripheral mass, 157, 157f
    left basilar cavity of, 154, 155f
    lymphoma of, with cavitary mass,
        153–154, 154f
    lymphoproliferative disorders of,
        manifestations of, 335–337, 336t,
        337f, 338f
    metastases to, 184–187, 184f–187f,
        184t
        calcification in, 185, 186f–187f
        cavitation in, 185, 186f
        hematogenous spread of, 184–185,
            184f, 185f
        lymphatic spread of, 187, 187f
        routes of metastatic dissemination,
            184t
        solitary nodule in, 186–187
    neurogenic tumors of, 176
    rheumatoid, 366f
    small cell carcinoma of. *See* Small cell
        carcinoma of lung
    squamous cell carcinoma of, 153, 154f
Lung cancer, 143–164. *See also specific*
        nodules and types of cancer, e.g.,
        Adenocarcinoma, of lung
    AIDS-related, 126–128, 127f
    chest radiography in, 143–147,
        144f–147f
    chest wall invasion in, 480
    crossing fissures, 481, 481f
    CT in, 35t, 147–148, 148f–150f, 160,
        162–164, 163t
    detection of, 143–148, 144f–147f
    diagnosis of, 148–152, 149f–151f
    large central mass in, 153–156,
        153f–157f
    large peripheral mass in, 157–158,
        157f
    morphology of, 160b
    multiple pulmonary nodules in, 159,
        159f, 160b
    non—small cell, calcified, 148, 149f
    peripheral infiltrate in, 158f, 159
    resectable, 162, 163f
    solitary pulmonary nodule in,
        152–153, 152f, 153b
    staging of, 160–163, 161t, 163f
        chest radiography in, 160
        CT in, 160, 162–164, 163t
    unresectable, 162, 163f
Lung consolidation, *vs.* empyema, on
        chest radiography, 217, 218f
Lung diseases
    cystic, abnormally reduced attenuation
        in, HRCT in, 389–391, 390f,
        390t, 391f, 391t

diffuse, 357–399. *See* Diffuse lung
        disease
    lower, 366t
    noninfectious, in non-AIDS
        immunocompromised patients,
        139–140, 139f
    obstructive, 401–428. *See also* Chronic
        obstructive pulmonary disease
        (COPD)
    in scleroderma, 367f
    upper, 365t
Lung injuries, traumatic, 304–309,
        304f–309f
Lung nodules. *See also* Pulmonary
        nodules
    calcified, 370f
    CT of, 35t
    missing, 143–144, 145f
Lung opacity, in critically ill patients,
        causes of, 237–240, 237f, 238f,
        239t, 240f, 241f
Lung parenchymal attenuation, altered,
        HRCT in, 389–391, 390f, 390t,
        391f, 391t
Lung perfusion scan, applications of,
        41–42
Lung transplantation, bilateral,
        pneumopericardium after,
        249–250, 250f
Lung ventilation scan, applications of,
        42
LVADs. *See* Left ventricular assist devices
        (LVADs)
Lymphangioleiomyomatosis (LAM),
        HRCT in, 390, 390f, 390t, 391t
Lymphangiomyomatosis, pulmonary
        manifestations of, 348, 349f,
        350f
Lymphangitic carcinomatosis
    bronchoalveolar cell carcinoma and,
        187, 187f
    HRCT in, 382–383, 382t, 383f
Lymphatic system, anatomy and
        physiology of, 2t, 21–22, 21f
Lymphoid interstitial pneumonia, HRCT
        in, 393–394, 394t
Lymphoid interstitial pneumonitis,
        pulmonary manifestations of,
        337, 337f, 338f
Lymphoma(s)
    AIDS-related, 126, 126f, 127f–128f
    with cavitary mass, of lung, 153–154,
        154f
    thoracic, 179–182, 179t, 180f–182f
        described, 179
        Hodgkin lymphoma, 179–180
        metastatic, 181f
        non-Hodgkin, 179–180, 180f
        prevalence of, 179
Lymphoproliferative diseases
    of lung, manifestations of, 335–337,
        336f, 337f, 338f
    thoracic, 179–183, 179t, 180f–183f
        Castleman disease, 182
        plasma cell granuloma, 182–183,
            183f

M
Macleod syndrome, 609, 611, 613f
Magnetic resonance angiography (MRA),
        40f
    in pulmonary thromboembolic disease,
        582
Magnetic resonance imaging (MRI)
    aortic aneurysm and, 505
    of aortic dissection, 485, 488f, 488t,
        489f
    applications of, 35–40, 36t, 35f–40f,
        39t
    in chronic pulmonary embolism, 600
    of coarctation, 497–498, 497f, 498f
    in esophageal cancer, 193
    examination time for, 39–40
    indications for, 35, 36t
    of mediastinal masses, 214
    of penetrating atherosclerotic ulcer,
        494
    precession in, 36, 37f
    principles of, 36, 36f
    protocols for, 39, 39t
    of pseudocoarctation, 499, 500
    in pulmonary arterial hypertension,
        604
    in pulmonary embolism, 594–596,
        596f
Malignant effusion, and mesothelioma,
        481
Malignant mesothelioma, pleural
        effusion and, 460–461, 461f, 462f
"M.A.L.P.", 11
MALToma, 182f
Manometer(s), intrasesophageal, 256t,
        286, 286f
Marfan syndrome, aortic aneurysm due
        to, 501, 502f
Mastectomy, prior right, chest
        radiography of, 51f
Measles, in immunocompetent hosts,
        111
Mediastinal contours, chest radiography
        of, 57, 58f
Mediastinal masses
    anterior, 200t
        disappearing, 201, 203f
        CT of, 209–214, 210t, 211f–213f, 212t
        in confirmation of location and
            extent, 209
        in detection of concurrent
            abnormalities, 214
        in enhancement of characteristics,
            212, 212t, 213f
        in identification of fat, water, and
            calcium, 209–212, 210t, 211f,
            212f
        specific diagnoses, 214
    differential diagnosis of, radiology of,
        199–206, 200f–208f, 200t, 204t,
        206t
    enhancing, 212, 212t, 213f
    localization of, radiology of, 197–198,
        198f, 199f
    middle, 204t
    MRI of, 214

radiology of, 197–215
Mediastinal parathyroid adenoma, 212, 213f
Mediastinitis, fibrosing, 108, 108f, 442–444, 443f
Mediastinum
  anatomy and physiology of, 2f, 2t, 6–8, 7f, 7t
    esophagus, 4f, 7, 7f, 7t
    thymus, 7f, 7t, 8
  chest radiography of, 57–58, 57f–59f
  compartments of, 199, 200f
Meig syndrome, 460, 460f
Melanoma, metastatic, extrapleural, 475f
Meningocele(s), bilateral lateral, 206, 207f
Mesothelioma(s)
  benign, chest radiography of, 473–474, 473f–476f, 475b
  malignant, pleural effusion and, 460–461, 461f, 462f
  malignant effusion and, 481
Metabolic diseases, pulmonary manifestations of, 341–345
  amyloidosis, 341–345, 341t, 342f–344f, 342t
  liver disease, 341
  metastatic pulmonary calcification, 340f, 341
  renal disease, 341
Metastatic pulmonary calcification, pulmonary manifestations of, 340f, 341
Microlithiasis, alveolar, 364f
Microscopic polyangiitis, manifestations of, 329
Miliary metastases, 363, 363f
Miliary nodules
  chest radiography in, 362–363, 363f–365f, 363t, 365t
  differential diagnosis of, mnemonic for, 363t
  metastatic, 363, 363f, 364f
Mirror image right aortic arch, 514
Mitral valve disease, 545–552, 546f–552f, 546t
  "double density" sign in, 545, 546f
  "fourth mogul" in, 546–547, 547f
  left atrial enlargement in, signs of, 54t, 545
  mitral valve insufficiency, 550–552, 551f, 552f
  mitral valve stenosis, 548–550, 548f–551f
  mortality associated with, 545
  prevalence of, 545
Mitral valve insufficiency, 550–552, 551f, 552f
Mitral valve stenosis, 548–550, 548f–551f
Moderator band, 15–16
Mounier-Kuhn syndrome, 446–447, 447f
  bronchiectasis and, 418
MRA. *See* Magnetic resonance angiography (MRA)

MRI. *See* Magnetic resonance imaging (MRI)
Mucoepidermoid tumors, 452
MUGA, 43
Multiple myeloma
  cavitary nocardiosis in, 135, 136f
  invasive pulmonary aspergillosis in, 131, 131f
  pulmonary manifestations of, 339, 340f
Mycobacteria
  atypical, AIDS-related, 121, 121f
  nontuberculous. *See* Nontuberculous mycobacteria (NTMB)
Mycobacterial infections, AIDS-related, 119–121, 120f, 121f
Mycobacterium tuberculosis, aspiration pneumonia due to, 96–102, 97f–102f. *See also* Tuberculosis
Mycoplasma spp.
  M. pneumoniae, aspiration pneumonia due to, 96, 97f
  pneumonia due to, 79
Mycotic aneurysm, aortic aneurysm due to, 502–503, 503f
Myeloma, multiple
  cavitary nocardiosis in, 135, 136f
  invasive pulmonary aspergillosis in, 131, 131f
  pulmonary manifestations of, 339, 340f
Myoblastoma, tracheal, 168, 168f
Myocardial contusion, 312
Myocardial disease, 546t, 556–562. *See also specific disease, e.g.,* Cardiomyopathy
Myocardial infarction, radiographic signs of, 546t, 572t
Myocarditis, 546t, 560, 561t, 562f
  infectious, 561t
  toxic, 561t

N

Nasogastric tubes, 256t, 284, 284f, 285f, 285t
Necrotizing sarcoidal angiitis, pulmonary manifestations of, 331
Needle(s), aspiration, types of, 618, 619f
Neoplasm(s). *See also* Tumor(s)
  pulmonary, benign, 166t
  tracheobronchial, 165–167, 166t, 167t. *See also* Tracheobronchial neoplasms
Neoplastic disease, 575, 575t, 576f–578f, 576t
Net magnetization vector, 37, 37f
Neurocutaneous disorders, 346–350, 346t, 347f, 349f–351f
Neurofibroma(s)
  apical, with neurofibromatosis, 206, 208f
  tracheal, 450
Neurofibromatosis
  neurofibroma in, apical, 206, 208f
  pulmonary manifestations of, 346–348, 346t, 347f

Neurogenic pulmonary edema, 360, 361f
Neurogenic tumors, of lung, 176
Nocardia asteroides, aspiration pneumonia due to, 95
Nocardiosis, cavitary, in multiple myeloma, 135, 136f
Nodular diseases, HRCT in, 385–389, 386f–388f, 386t, 389t
Nodule(s)
  cavitary, 369–371, 369f–372f, 369t, 370b
    chest radiography in, 369–371
    differential diagnosis of, mnemonic for, 369t
  miliary, 362–363, 363f–365f, 363t, 365t. *See also* Miliary nodules
  multiple, chest radiography in, 369–371, 369f–372f, 369t, 370b
  in non-AIDS immunocompromised patients, 131–136, 131f–137f
  pulmonary, 35t
    multiple, PTNB in, 617, 618f
Non—antinuclear cytoplasmic antibody—associated vasculitides, pulmonary manifestations of, 328–329
Noncardiogenic edema, *vs.* cardiogenic edema, lung opacity in critically ill patients due to, 237–240, 237f, 238f, 239t, 240f, 241f
Non-Hodgkin lymphoma, 179–180, 180f
Non—small cell lung cancer, calcified, 148, 149f
Nonspecific interstitial pneumonia (NSIP), HRCT in, 392–393, 393f, 393t
Nontuberculous mycobacteria (NTMB)
  in achalasia patients, 104
  in immunocompetent hosts, 103–104, 103f, 104f
  in immunocompromised patients, 104
Nosocomial infections, in ICU, 226, 226t
Nosocomial pneumonia, in ICU, risk factors for, 226, 226t
NTMB. *See* Nontuberculous mycobacteria (NTMB)
Nuclear medicine
  applications of, 40–44, 41t, 40f–44f
  described, 40
Nucleus(i), magnetic properties of, 36, 36f

O

Obstructive lung disease, 401–428. *See also* Chronic obstructive pulmonary disease (COPD)
  described, 401
Opacification, in pneumonia in immunocompetent hosts, 81, 81f
Opacity(s), small irregular, chest radiography in, 367, 367t, 368f
Orogastric tubes, 256t, 284, 284f, 285f, 285t
Osler-Weber-Rendu syndrome, pulmonary manifestations of, 346t, 350, 351f

Osseous injuries, traumatic, 300–303, 301f–304f, 303t
Osteosarcoma(s)
    cavitary metastatic, 370f
        pneumothorax due to, 468–469, 469f
    to lungs, metastatic, 186f
Ovarian cancer, pleural effusion and, 460, 460f
Overdiagnosis bias, defined, 148

P
"P" sign, 310f, 311
Pacemakers, 256t, 269–271, 270f–274f, 272t
    biventricular, 270, 271f
    complications associated with, 271, 272t, 273f, 274f
    described, 269
    dual-chamber, 270, 270f
    indications for, 270, 270f, 271f
    size of, 270, 270f
    temporary transvenous, 270, 270f
PAH. *See* Pulmonary arterial hypertension (PAH)
Panacinar emphysema, 407t, 408–409, 408t, 410f
Panlobular emphysema, 407t, 408–409, 408t, 410f
PAP. *See* Pulmonary arterial pressure (PAP)
Papilloma(s), squamous cell, of trachea, 448–449, 449f
Paracicatricial emphysema, 407t, 409, 410f
Paraseptal emphysema, 407t, 408f, 409, 410f
Parasitic infections, in immunocompetent hosts, 112–114, 113f
Parathyroid adenoma, 201, 204t
    mediastinal, 212, 213f
Partial anomalous pulmonary venous return, 522t, 524, 526f, 527f
Patent ductus arteriosus, 522t, 524, 524f, 525f
Pattern recognition, in diffuse lung disease, 357–371
    multiple patterns, 373f
    pointers in, 371–376
    two patterns in, 372b
PBV. *See* Pulmonary blood volume (PBV)
Pectus excavatum, 4
Penetrating atherosclerotic ulcer, 493–494, 494f
    CT of, 493–494, 494f
    imaging of, 493–494, 494f
    management of, 494
    MRI of, 494
    natural history of, 493
    pathophysiology of, 493
Percutaneous drainage procedures, 629–631, 630f, 631f
    methods of, 630–631, 630f, 631f
Percutaneous endovascular stent, 507, 510f

Percutaneous indwelling central catheter (PICC), 255–257, 256f, 256t, 257f
Percutaneous transthoracic needle biopsy (PTNB), 617–629
    air embolism due to, treatment of, 628
    bleeding due to, treatment of, 628, 629f
    complications of, 626–629, 626t, 627f–629f
    contraindications to, 624–625, 625f, 625t
    empyema due to, treatment of, 628
    imaging of, 621–622, 622f, 623f
    indications for, 617, 620, 621t
    methods of, 617–620, 618f–620f
    percutaneous drainage procedures, 629–631, 630f, 631f
    pneumothorax due to, treatment of, 626, 626t, 627f, 628f
    postbiopsy management, 625–626
    site preparation for, 621–622, 622f, 623f
    technical factors in, 622, 624, 624f
    thoracoscopic resection, localizations for, 631, 632f
Perfusion scintigraphy, in emphysema, 413, 414f, 415f
Peribronchial thickening, in pneumonia in immunocompetent hosts, 83
Pericardial disease, 546t, 562–569
    constrictive pericarditis, 546t, 566–569, 566f–568f, 569t
    pericardial effusion, 546t, 563, 5664f–566f
    types of, 563t
Pericardial effusion, 59–60, 59f–61f, 546t, 563, 564f–566f
    with classic "water bottle" configuration, 59, 59f
Pericardial neoplasms, primary benign, 575t
Pericardial wrap, bovine, 507, 509f
Pericarditis
    constrictive, 546t, 566–569, 566f–568f, 569t
    MRI of, 39t
Pericardium, anatomy and physiology of, 2t, 13, 13f
Persistent left superior vena cava, 514t, 532, 532f, 532t
PET. *See* Positron emission tomography (PET)
pH probe, 256t, 286
Phakomatosis(es), pulmonary manifestations of, 346–350
    ataxia telangiectasia, 346t, 348
    Bourneville disease, 346t, 348, 349f
    hereditary hemorrhagic telangiectasia, 346t, 350, 351f
    Louis-Bar syndrome, 346t, 348
    lymphangiomyomatosis, 348, 349f, 350
    neurofibromatosis, 346–348, 346t, 347f

Osler-Weber-Rendu syndrome, 346t, 350, 351f
    tuberous sclerosis, 346t, 348, 349f
PICC. *See* Percutaneous indwelling central catheter (PICC)
Pitch
    beam, 32
    data, 32
Planar radionuclide imaging, principles of, 40, 40f
Plasma cell granuloma, 182–183, 183f
Plasmacytoma(s), tracheal, 339, 340f
Pleura
    abnormalities of. *See also specific disorder, e.g.,* Pleural effusion
    chest radiography of, 457–476
        pleural effusion, 457–465, 458f–465f, 460b
        pleural implants, 470–472, 470f–472f
        pleural masses, 473–474, 473f–476f, 475b
        pleural plaques, 470–472, 470f–472f
        pneumothorax, 465–470, 466f–469f, 467b
    anatomic variants of, 477–480, 478f–480f
    anatomy of, 2t, 8–9, 477–480, 478f–480f
    benign fibrous tumors of, chest radiography of, 473–474, 473f–476f, 475b
    chest radiography of, 54–57, 55f, 56f
    CT of, 477–482
    fissures of, anatomy of, 477–479, 478f, 479f
    lipoma of, 473, 474f
    physiology of, 2t, 8–9
Pleural effusion, 47f
    causes of, 460b
        abdominal, 463–464, 464f
    chest radiography of, 54, 55f, 56, 56f, 457–465, 458f–465f, 460b
    CHF and, 459
    diagnosis of, 457–458
    empyema and, 461, 462f, 463f
    inflammatory disease and, 461–462, 462f, 463f
    inverting left hemidiaphragm, 459, 459f
    malignant mesothelioma and, 460–461, 461f, 462f
    ovarian carcinoma and, 460, 460f
    SLE and, 326, 326f, 463, 464f
    supine left, 458, 458f
    trauma and, 464–465, 465f
    unilateral left, 459–460, 460b
    vascular disease and, 464
Pleural fissures, 8–9, 9f–10f
Pleural implants, chest radiography of, 470–472, 470f–472f
Pleural injuries, traumatic, 304–309, 304f–309f
Pleural masses, chest radiography of, 473–474, 473f–476f, 475b

Pleural plaques, chest radiography of, 470–472, 470f–472f

Pneumatocele(s)
in critically ill patients, 249–250, 250f
pulmonary laceration/hematoma and contusion evolving into, 307f

Pneumococcal pneumonia, in immunocompetent hosts, 89, 90f

Pneumoconiosis, coal worker's, HRCT in, 386–387, 387f

Pneumocystis carinii pneumonia
AIDS-related, 123–124, 123f, 124f
with T-cell defect, 138f

Pneumomediastinum, 308, 308f
in critically ill patients, 245–248, 246f, 247f, 248t
causes of, 247t
defined, 245
subcutaneous emphysema and, 310f

Pneumonia(s)
airspace disease in, 358, 358f
aspiration
in critically ill patients, 226–228, 226t, 227f, 227t
in immunocompetent hosts, 94–103. *See also* Aspiration pneumonia, in immunocompetent hosts
atypical, in immunocompetent hosts, features of, 80b
bacterial
features of, 79b
in immunocompetent host, 89–104. *See also* Bacterial pneumonia, in immunocompetent host
chickenpox, in immunocompetent host, 112, 112f
CMV, after renal transplant, 138f
cryptogenic, organizing, HRCT in, 394–395, 394t, 395f
cryptogenic organizing, HRCT in, 394–395, 394t, 395f
desquamative interstitial, HRCT in, 391–392, 392f, 392t
diagnosis of, 79–80, 79b, 80b
eosinophilic, 374f–375f
Friedlander, 86, 86f
fungal, AIDS-related, 122, 122f
in immunocompetent host, 79–115.
See also specific types of pneumonia, e.g., Bacterial pneumonia
causes of, 79–80
clinical clues to, 80
radiologic clues to, 86–88, 87f, 88f
complications of, 88–89
differential diagnosis of, 86
fungal infections and, 105–111
imaging modalities in, 80
NTMB and, 103–104, 103f, 104f
parasitic infections and, 112–114, 113f
radiologic classification of, 84–85, 84f–86f
radiologic signs of, 81f–83f, 81–83

airspace disease, 82–83, 83f
atelectasis, 83, 83f
opacification, 81, 81f
peribronchial thickening, 83
silhouette sign, 82, 82f
viral infections and, 111–112, 112f
influenza, in immunocompetent hosts, 111, 112f
interstitial, 85, 85f
desquamative, HRCT in, 391–392, 392f, 392t
idiopathic. *See* Idiopathic interstitial pneumonias
lymphoid
HRCT in, 393–394, 394t
pulmonary manifestations of, 337, 337f, 338f
nonspecific, HRCT in, 392–393, 393f, 393t
lipoid, 362f
lobar, 84f, 85, 85f
lymphoid interstitial
HRCT in, 393–394, 394t
pulmonary manifestations of, 337, 337f, 338f
nonspecific interstitial, HRCT in, 392–393, 393f, 393t
nosocomial, in ICU, risk factors for, 226, 226t
pneumococcal, in immunocompetent hosts, 89, 90f
Pneumocystis carinii
AIDS-related, 123–124, 123f, 124f
with T-cell defects, 138f
round, 85, 86f
viral, in immunocompetent hosts, features of, 80b

Pneumonitis
hypersensitivity, HRCT in, 387–388, 388f
interstitial, 366f
acute, in critically ill patients, 225
basilar, scleroderma and, 326, 327f

Pneumopericardium, 312
after bilateral lung transplantation, 249–250, 250f
in critically ill patients, 248–249, 248t, 249f

Pneumoperitoneum, 318, 318f

Pneumothorax
bilateral balanced, 244, 244f
causes of, 467b
cavitary metastatic osteosarcoma and, 468–469, 469f
chest radiography of, 54, 56f, 465–470, 466f–469f, 467b
in critically ill patients, 242–245, 242f–245f, 243t
causes of, 242, 243t
defined, 242
diagnosis of, 465–468, 466f, 467b, 467f, 468f
ex vacuo, 245
large left, 307–308, 307f
left
moderate, 465–466, 466f

supine, 466, 466f
primary spontaneous, 243–244, 243f
PTNB and, treatment of, 626, 626t, 627f, 628f
pulmonary contusions and, 305f
rib fractures and, 300, 301f
right, 466, 467f
supine, 466, 467f
tension, 309, 309f

Polyangiitis, microscopic, manifestations of, 329

Polychondritis, relapsing, 438f

Polymyositis, pulmonary manifestations of, 327–328

Popcorn calcification, hamartoma with, 148, 149f

Port-A-Cath, 257, 258f

Positron emission tomography (PET)
applications of, 42–43, 43f
in lung cancer, 148–149, 151f
in lung cancer staging, 162
principles of, 41, 41f

Postintubation stenosis, tracheal, 431–433, 432f, 435–436, 437f

Postintubation tracheal stenosis, 432f, 435–436, 437f

Postoperative bronchial stenosis, 445, 445f

Posttransplant lymphoproliferative disorder, pulmonary manifestations of, 335

Posttraumatic aneurysms, aortic aneurysm due to, 502

Prebiopsy ultrasound image, 618, 619f

Precession, MRI, 36, 37f

Primary ciliary dyskinesia, bronchiectasis and, 418

Primary pulmonary sarcoma, 177, 178f

Progressive systemic sclerosis. *See* Scleroderma

Prosthesis(es), Angelchik reflux, 288, 288f

Proteinosis, pulmonary alveolar, HRCT in, 395, 396f

Pseudoaneurysm(s), 507, 508f
pulmonary, 608, 609t, 610t
pulmonary artery, 263–264, 266f

Pseudocoarctation, 498–500
angiography of, 499, 500
chest radiography of, 498, 499f
clinical features of, 498
CT of, 499, 499f
defined, 498
MRI of, 499, 500
pathogenesis of, 498

Pseudolymphoma(s), 181f, 337, 338f

Pseudomonas aeruginosa, bacterial pneumonia due to, 92–93, 92f

Pseudotumor(s)
of fluid in fissures, 457, 458f
inflammatory, thoracic, 182–183, 183f
tracheal, 183f

PTNB. *See* Percutaneous transthoracic needle biopsy (PTNB)

Pulmonary alveolar proteinosis, HRCT in, 395, 396f

Pulmonary angiography, in pulmonary embolism, 586, 589, 589f
  chronic, 597, 598f
Pulmonary arterial hypertension (PAH), 601–604
  chest radiography in, 603, 603f
  CT in, 604
  echocardiography in, 603–604
  MRI in, 604
  radiology in, 603–604, 603f
  V/Q scintigraphy in, 604
Pulmonary arterial pressure (PAP), in critically ill patients, evaluation of, 229t, 234
Pulmonary arteriovenous malformation, 148, 150f
Pulmonary artery(ies), angiography of, indications for, 45t
Pulmonary artery aneurysm, 606–608, 607t, 608f–610f
Pulmonary artery catheter, 256t, 263–264, 263f–266f, 265t
  complications associated with, 263–264, 265t, 266f
  design of, 263
  malpositioned, 263, 264f–265f
    traumatically inserted and, 319f
  positioning of, 263, 263f–265f
  uses of, 263
Pulmonary artery hypoplasia, 609, 612f
Pulmonary artery pseudoaneurysms, 263–264, 266f
Pulmonary artery sarcoma, 613, 613f
Pulmonary artery stenosis, 606, 606t, 607f
Pulmonary artery tumors, 611, 613, 613f
Pulmonary atresia, 534t, 539, 540f
Pulmonary blastoma, 179
Pulmonary blood flow, in critically ill patients, evaluation of, 229t, 232–233, 232t, 233f
Pulmonary blood volume (PBV)
  altered generalized, causes of, 232t
  in critically ill patients, evaluation of, 229t, 232–233, 232t, 233f
Pulmonary contusions, 304–307, 304f–307f
  pneumothoraces with, 305f
  progression of, 305f
Pulmonary edema
  alveolar, with bilateral alveolar opacity, 235f
  causes of, 239t
  distribution of, atypical, causes of, 239t
  HRCT in, 381–382, 382t
  interstitial, chest radiography of, 62–63, 63f
  negative-pressure, 218, 219f
  neurogenic, 360, 361f
  reexpansion, 241f
Pulmonary embolism, 581–601
  causes of, 582–583, 582t
  chest radiography in, 583–584, 583t, 584f
  chronic, 596–600, 597f–599f

chest radiography in, 597, 597f
  CT in, 597–600, 598f, 599f
  diagnosis of, radiology in, 597–600, 597f–599f
  MRI in, 600
  pulmonary angiography in, 597, 598f
  V/Q scintigraphy in, 597, 598f
  clinical presentation of, 583
  CT in, 589
  CT venography in, 594, 595f
  diagnosis of, 581–582
  electron beam CT in, 594
  helical CT pulmonary angiogram in, 589–594, 590f–593f, 591t, 594t
  incidence of, 581
  MRI in, 594–596, 596f
  pathophysiology of, 582–583, 582t
  pulmonary angiography in, 586, 589, 589f
  radiology in, 583–596, 583t
  radionuclide imaging in, 584, 585f, 586t, 587f, 588f
  septic, 600–601, 600f
Pulmonary embolus, CT of, 35t
Pulmonary endometriosis, 177
Pulmonary function tests, in COPD, 402–404, 403t
Pulmonary hypertension, 554, 555f, 556f
  causes of, 601–602, 601t
Pulmonary laceration, 307–309, 307f, 308f
Pulmonary lobule, line drawing of, 377f
Pulmonary neoplasms, 172–177, 173f–176f
  benign, 166t
    benign clear cell tumor, 176
    carcinosarcoma, 179
    chemodectomas, 176–177
    hamartomas, 172–175, 173f–175f
    hemangiomas, 175
    leiomyomas, 175–176, 176f
    neurogenic tumors, 176
    pulmonary endometriosis, 177
    teratomas, 176
  malignant, 167t, 177–179, 178f
    epithelioid hemangioendothelioma, 177, 178f
    hemangiopericytoma, 177
    primary pulmonary sarcoma, 177, 178f
    pulmonary blastoma, 179
Pulmonary nodules, 143–144, 144f–146f
  multiple, 159, 159f, 160b
    PTNB in, 617, 618f
  solitary, 152–153, 152f, 153b
Pulmonary parenchymal opacification, imaging of, 220–228, 221t, 222f, 223t, 224f, 226t, 227f, 227t, 228f. *See also specific disorders, e.g.,* Acute respiratory distress syndrome (ARDS)
Pulmonary pseudoaneurysms, 608, 609t, 610f
Pulmonary sarcomas, primary, 177, 178f
Pulmonary system, radionuclide imaging of, indications for, 41t

Pulmonary thromboembolic disease, 581–601. *See also specific disease, e.g.,* Pulmonary embolism
  causes of, 582–583, 582t
  chronic pulmonary embolism, 596–600, 597f–599f
  clinical presentation of, 583
  CT in, 581–582
  CTPA in, 582
  DVT in, 582
  MRA in, 582
  pathophysiology of, 582–583, 582t
  radiology in, 583t, 583–596
  risk factors for, 582, 582t
  transesophageal echocardiography in, 582
  V/Q scintigraphy in, 581–582
Pulmonary tumor embolism, 604, 605f
Pulmonary vascular disease, 581–616. *See also specific disease, e.g.,* Pulmonary thromboembolic disease
  pulmonary arterial stenosis, 606, 606t, 607f
  pulmonary artery aneurysm, 606–608, 607t, 608f–610f
  pulmonary artery aplasia, 608–609, 611f
  pulmonary artery tumors, 611, 613, 613f
  pulmonary AVMs, 605, 606f
  pulmonary tumor embolism, 604, 605f
Pulmonary vasculitides, manifestations of, 329t
  antinuclear cytoplasmic antibody—associated vasculitides, 329–330, 330f, 331f
  Churg-Strauss syndrome, 330
  immune-complex vasculitis, 331–334, 332t, 333f
  microscopic polyangiitis, 329
  non—antinuclear cytoplasmic antibody—associated vasculitides, 328–329
  Wegener granulomatosis, 329–330, 330f, 331f
Pulmonary veins, CT of, 35t
Pulmonary veno-occlusive disease, PAH due to, 602
Pulmonic valve, absent, 514t, 528, 530f
Pulmonic valve disease, 546t, 553–555, 554t, 555f, 556f
Pulmonic valve stenosis, 514t, 528, 530f
Pyrophosphate (99mTc-pyrophosphate), 44

R
Radiographic report, 69–77
  communication on, 71–72
  information on, 69–70
  pet peeves related to, 72–74, 76–77
  standards of practice for, 74–75
  style of, 70–71
Radiography, chest, applications of, 25–28, 26f–28f, 26t. *See also* Chest radiography

Radiologic studies, in COPD, 404
Radionuclide imaging
  indications for, 41t
  in pulmonary embolism, 584, 585f,
    586t, 587f, 588f
Radiopharmaceutical, components of, 40
Rasmussen aneurysms, 102
Red blood cell labeling (MUGA), 43
Renal cell carcinoma, miliary metastases
  in, 363, 363f
Renal disease, pulmonary manifestations
  of, 341
Renal transplantation, CMV pneumonia
  after, 138f
Respiratory bronchiolitis—associated
    interstitial lung disease, HRCT in,
    389, 389t
Restrictive cardiomyopathy, 558–560,
    559t, 560f, 561f
Reticular diseases, HRCT in, 381–384,
    382t–384t, 383f–385f
Rheumatoid arthritis
  age of onset of, 323
  bone abnormalities in, 325
  bronchial abnormalities in, 325
  described, 323
  diffuse interstitial fibrosis in, 324
  gender predilection for, 323
  miliary tuberculosis with, 138f
  necrobiotic nodules in, 324
  pleural abnormalities in, 323–324, 324f
  prevalence of, 323
  pulmonary manifestations of,
    323–325, 324f, 324t
  radiologic manifestations of, 324t
Rib(s)
  anatomy and physiology of, 1–4, 3f
  counting, 480, 480f
Rib fractures, 300–302, 301f–303f, 303t
  hemothorax with, 300, 301f
  pneumothorax with, 300, 301f
Right aortic arch with aberrant left
    subclavian artery, 514, 518f
Right middle lobe syndrome, 448
Round pneumonia, 85, 86f
Rubeola, in immunocompetent hosts,
    111
Ruptured sinus of Valsalva aneurysm,
    522t, 525, 528, 528f, 529f

S
Saber sheath trachea, 447
Sagittal anterior minor fissure, anatomy
    of, 479, 479f
Sarcoid, 366f
Sarcoidosis, 441–442
  age of onset of, 350
  described, 351
  gender predilection for, 350
  HRCT in, 385–386, 386f, 386t, 387f
  incidence of, 350
  of larynx, 352
  lymph node enlargement in, 352, 352f,
    353f
  pulmonary manifestations of,
    350–353, 352f, 352t, 353f

staging of, chest radiology in, 352t
Sarcoma(s)
  Kaposi, AIDS-related, 125–126, 125f
  pulmonary, primary, 177, 178f
  pulmonary artery, 613, 613f
Scapula, high-riding, 5
Schwannoma(s), 206, 207f
  of trachea, 450
Scimitar syndrome, 524
Scintigraphy
  in emphysema, 413, 414f, 415f
  perfusion, in emphysema, 413, 414f,
    415f
  ventilation/perfusion. *See*
    Ventilation/perfusion scintigraphy
Scleroderma
  age of onset of, 326
  basilar interstitial pneumonitis with,
    326, 327f
  clinical presentation of, 326
  gender as factor in, 326
  honeycombing in, 367f
  incidence of, 326
  pulmonary manifestations of, 326,
    327f
Sclerosis(es), tuberous, pulmonary
    manifestations of, 346t, 348, 349f
SCOOP model, 283, 283f
Septic pulmonary embolism, 600–601,
    600f
Shoulder girdle, anatomy and physiology
    of, 2f, 3f, 5
Shunt(s), left-to-right, 514t, 520–528,
    521f–529f, 522t. *See also* Left-to-
    right shunts
Sickle cell disease, pulmonary
    manifestations of, 334–335, 334t,
    335f
Sickle trait, 334
Silhouette sign, 64, 64f
  in pneumonia in immunocompetent
    hosts, 82, 82f
Silicosis, 374f
  HRCT in, 386–387, 387f
Sinus of Valsalva, ruptured aneurysm of,
    522t, 525, 528, 528f, 529f
Situs, abnormal, 541, 541f, 541t
SLE. *See* Systemic lupus erythematosus
    (SLE)
Small cell carcinoma of lung
  with rapid growth of lymph node
    metastases, 155, 156f
  with rapid response, 155, 156f–157f
  with SIADH, 154, 155f
Soft tissues, extrathoracic, chest
    radiography of, 50–51, 51f
Solitary pulmonary nodule (SPN),
    152–153, 152f, 153b
Spine, anatomy and physiology of, 2f–4f,
    5
Spine fractures, thoracic, 303, 303t, 304f
Spirometry, in COPD, 403
Splenomegaly, chest radiography of, 52,
    53f
Spondylitis, ankylosing, pulmonary
    manifestations of, 328

Sprengel's deformity, 5
Squamous cell carcinoma
  of lung, 153, 154f
  of trachea, 450, 451f
Squamous cell papilloma, of trachea,
    448, 449f
Stanford classification, of aortic
    dissection, 484
Staphylococcus aureus
  bacterial pneumonia due to, 89–91,
    91f
  pneumonia due to, 79
Stenosis(es)
  aortic, 552, 553f
  bronchial, postoperative, 445, 445f
  mitral valve, 548–550, 548f–551f
  postintubation, tracheal, 431–433,
    432f, 435–436, 437f
  pulmonary artery, 606, 606t, 607f
  pulmonic valve, 514t, 528, 530f
  tracheal, postintubation, 431–433,
    432f
Stent(s)
  in central airway disorders
    management, 446, 446f
  endovascular, percutaneous, 507, 510f
  esophageal, 256t, 286–288, 287f
  percutaneous endovascular, 507, 510f
Sternal fractures, 302–303
Sternum, anatomy and physiology of, 2f,
    3f, 4–5, 4f
Steroid(s), miliary tuberculosis in patient
    receiving, 138f
Streptococcus pneumoniae
  bacterial pneumonia due to, 89, 90f
  pneumonia due to, 79
Subcutaneous emphysema, 310f
Superior accessory fissure, 9
  anatomy of, 477, 478f
Superior triangle sign, 66
Superior vena cava, persistent left, 514t,
    532, 533f
Swyer-James syndrome, 609, 611, 613f
Syndrome of inappropriate antidiuretic
    hormone (SIADH), small cell
    carcinoma of lung in, 154, 155f
Syphilis, aortic aneurysm due to, 502
Systemic diseases, pulmonary
    manifestations of, 323–355. *See
    also Collagen vascular diseases;
    specific disease or type of disease,*
    e.g., Rheumatoid arthritis
  collagen vascular diseases, 323–326
  dermatomyositis, 327–328, 327f, 328f
  hematologic disorders, 334–339, 334t,
    335f–340f
  histiocytosis X, 345, 345f, 346f
  Langerhans cell histiocytosis, 345,
    345f, 346f
  metabolic diseases, 341–345
  phakomatoses, 346–350
  polymyositis, 327–328
  pulmonary vasculitides, 328–334, 329t
  sarcoidosis, 350–353, 352f, 352t, 353f
Systemic extravascular water, in critically
    ill patients, evaluation of, 236t

Systemic inflammatory response syndrome, 220–221, 221t
Systemic lupus erythematosus (SLE)
  age of onset of, 325
  ethnicity as factor in, 325
  gender as factor in, 325
  incidence of, 325
  pleural effusion and, 326, 326f, 463, 464f
  pulmonary manifestations of, 325–326, 325t, 326f
  radiologic manifestations of, 325, 325t
  zygomycosis in, 134, 134f

T
TBIs. *See* Tracheobronchial injuries (TBIs)
T-cell defect, *Pneumocystis carinii* pneumonia with, 138f
T-cell leukemias, pulmonary manifestations of, 338
Tear(s), esophageal, after trauma, 311, 311t, 312f
Telangiectasia
  ataxia, pulmonary manifestations of, 346t, 348
  hereditary hemorrhagic, pulmonary manifestations of, 346t, 350, 351f
Temperature probe, 256t, 286
Tension pneumothorax, 309, 309f
Teratocarcinoma, endobronchial metastasis from, 188, 188f
Teratoma(s), 176
  mediastinal, anterior, 209, 211f
Tetralogy of Fallot, 534t, 535–536, 535f, 536f
Thallium chloride (^{201}Tl), 43
Thebesian valves, 14
Thoracic air collections, abnormal, in critically ill patients, 241–250, 241t, 242f–247f, 243t, 247t, 248t, 249f, 250f
  interstitial emphysema, 249–250, 250f
  pneumatoceles, 249–250, 250f
  pneumomediastinum, 245–248, 246f, 247f, 248t
  pneumopericardium, 248–249, 248t, 249f
  pneumothorax, 242–245, 242f–245f, 243t
Thoracic aorta, 483–512. *See also* Aorta; Aortic dissection
  CT of, 35t
Thoracic endoskeleton, 2f
Thoracic imaging, in critically ill patients, 217–254. *See also* Critically ill patients, thoracic imaging in
Thoracic neoplasms, 165–195. *See also* specific type, e.g., Tracheobronchial neoplasms
  benign, 166t
  epithelial neoplasms, malignant, 169–172, 169t, 170f–172f

esophageal carcinoma, 189–193, 190f–193f, 190t
lymphoma, 179–182, 179t, 180f–182f. *See also* Lymphoma(s), thoracic
lymphoproliferative diseases, 179–183, 179t, 180f–183f
malignant, 166t
metastatic disease, 184–189, 184f–189f, 184t
  airway metastases, 188, 188f
  lung metastases, 184–187, 184f–187f, 184t
  pleural metastases, 189, 189f
  routes of, 184t
pulmonary neoplasms
  benign, 172–177, 173f–176f
  malignant, 177–179, 178f
tracheal neoplasms, benign, 167–168, 168f
tracheobronchial neoplasms, 165–167, 166t, 167t
Thoracic outlet, MRI of, 39t
Thoracic spine fractures, 303, 303t, 304f
Thoracic splenosis, 472, 472f
Thoracic trauma, 295–322
  aortic injuries, 295–299, 296f, 297t, 298f–300f
  biomechanics of, 295
  cardiac injuries, 312–313, 312f
  described, 295
  diaphragm injuries, 313–317, 313t, 314f–317f, 315t
  esophageal injuries, 311, 311t, 312f
  iatrogenic injuries, 318f–320f, 319
  lung injuries, 304–309, 304f–309f
  osseous injuries, 300–303, 301f–304f, 303t
  pleural injuries, 304–309, 304f–309f
  tracheobronchial injuries, 309–311, 310f, 311t
  types of, 320t
  upper abdominal injuries, 317–318, 318f
Thoracic vertebral fractures, 303, 303t, 304f
Thoracoabdominal sign, 66–67
Thoracoscopic resection, localizations for, 631, 632f
Thorax. *See also* Lung(s); specific components, e.g., Chest wall
  anatomy and physiology of, 1–23
  airways, 2t, 10–12, 11f, 11t
  aorta, 2t, 18–19, 18f, 19f
  arteries, 2t, 18–19, 18f, 19f
  chest wall, 1–5, 2f–4f, 2t
  diaphragm, 2t, 4f, 5–6
  heart, 2t, 14–17, 15f–17f
  lungs, 2t, 12
  lymphatic system, 2t, 21–22, 21f
  mediastinum, 2f, 2t, 6–8, 7f, 7t
  pericardium, 2t, 13, 13f
  pleura, 2t, 8–9
  pleural fissures, 8–9, 9f–10f
  veins, 19–20, 20f

CT of, indications for, 30t
interventional techniques of, 617–634. *See also specific modality, e.g.,* Percutaneous transthoracic needle biopsy (PTNB)
MRI of, indications for, 36t
ultrasound of, indications for, 47t
Thymolipoma, 197, 198f
Thymoma, 199, 201f, 209, 211f
Thymus, anatomy and physiology of, 7f, 7t, 8
Thyroid carcinoma, miliary metastases in, 363, 363f
Trachea
  anatomy of, 10–11, 11f, 433, 434t
  CT of, 35t
  deviation of, chest radiography of, 57–58, 59f
  diffuse enlargement of, 446–447, 447f
  diverticula of, 448
  physiology of, 10–11, 11f
  saber sheath, 447
  squamous cell carcinoma of, 450, 451f
  tuberculosis of, 444–445, 444f
Tracheal neoplasms, benign, 167–168, 168f
Tracheal plasmacytoma, 339, 340f
Tracheal pseudotumor, 183f
Tracheal stenosis, postintubation, 431–433, 432f
Tracheal web, 431f
Tracheobronchial amyloidosis, 342, 342f, 343f
Tracheobronchial injuries (TBIs), traumatic, 309–311, 310f, 311t
Tracheobronchial invasive aspergillosis, in leukemia, 131, 134f
Tracheobronchial neoplasms, 165–167, 166t, 167t, 448–452, 449f–452f
  adenoid cystic carcinomas, 450, 451f
  benign, 448–450, 449f
  carcinoid tumors, tracheal, 450–451, 452f
  chondromas, 449
  chondrosarcomas, 450, 450f
  hamartomas, 449
  hemangiomas, 449
  leiomyomas, 449–450
  malignant, 450–451, 450f–452f
  metastatic tumors, 452–453, 452f
  mucoepidermoid tumors, 452
  neurofibromas, 450
  schwannomas, 450
  squamous cell carcinoma, 450, 451f
  squamous cell papilloma, 448, 449f
  tracheobronchial papillomatosis, 448–449
Tracheobronchial papillomatosis, 448–449, 449f
Tracheobronchomalacia, 437–439, 438f–439f
Tracheobronchomegaly, 446–447, 447f
Tracheobronchopathia osteochondroplastica, 442

Tracheobronchopathia osteoplastica, 342, 343f
Tracheoesophageal fistula, esophageal cancer with, 191f
Tracheomalacia, 438f–439f
Tracheostomy tubes, 256t, 282–283, 282f, 282t
Transesophageal echocardiography
  of aortic dissection, 490
  in pulmonary thromboembolic disease, 582
Transplantation, renal, CMV pneumonia after, 138f
Transthoracic echocardiography, in pulmonary thromboembolic disease, 582
Transtracheal oxygen catheter, 256t, 283–284, 283f
Trauma
  pleural effusion and, 464–465, 465f
  thoracic, 295–322. *See also* Thoracic trauma
Tricuspid valve disease, 546t, 553–555, 554t, 555f, 556f
Truncus arteriosus, 533t, 538–539, 539t
Tube current, 27
Tube voltage (kVp), 27
Tuberculoma(s), 100, 100f
Tuberculosis
  AIDS-related, 119–120, 120f, 121f
  bronchiectasis due to, 417
  fibrothorax and, 471, 471f
  in immunocompetent host
    bronchogenic spread of, 101–102, 102f
    broncholiths in, 102, 102f
    complications of, 102, 102f
    incidence of, 96–97
    miliary, 97, 101f
    Mycobacterium tuberculosis and, 96–102, 97f–102f
    postprimary, 97, 99–101, 99f–101f
    primary, 97f, 97–99, 98f
    tuberculomas in, 100, 100f
  miliary
    in patient receiving steroids, 138f
    in rheumatoid arthritis patient receiving cytotoxic therapy, 138f
  tracheal, 444–445, 444f
    incidence of, 444
Tuberous sclerosis, pulmonary manifestations of, 346t, 348, 349f
Tumor(s). *See also specific types and* Neoplasm(s)

benign clear cell, 176
bronchial gland, 172
carcinoid. *See* Carcinoid tumors
endobronchial benign granula cell, 168, 168f
granular cell, tracheal, 168, 168f
mucoepidermoid, 452
neurogenic, of lung, 176
pulmonary artery, 611, 613, 613f
tracheobronchial, 448–452, 449f–452f
Twiddler syndrome, 271, 273f

U

Ulcer(s), penetrating atherosclerotic, 493–494, 494f. *See also* Penetrating atherosclerotic ulcer
Ulcerative colitis, 442
Ultrasonography
  applications of, 46, 46f, 47f, 47t
  of central airways, 429
  indications for, 46, 47t
  principles of, 46
Upper abdominal injuries, traumatic, 317–318, 318f
Upper lobe cavitary mass, right, 620, 620f

V

Varice(s), esophageal, giant, 205, 205f
Varicella-zoster, in immunocompetent hosts, 112, 112f
Vascular diseases
  pleural effusion and, 464
  pulmonary, 581–616. *See also* Pulmonary vascular disease
Vascular pedicle, measurement of, 229–230, 230f
Vascular system
  CT of, indications for, 30t
  MRI of, indications for, 36t
  ultrasound of, indications for, 47t
Vasculitis
  giant cell, manifestations of, 328
  immune-complex, manifestations of, 331–334, 332t, 333f
  medium-sized, manifestations of, 328–329
  pulmonary, manifestations of, 328–334. *See also* Pulmonary vasculitides, manifestations of
Vein(s), anatomy and physiology of, 19–20, 20f
Vena cava

inferior, azygous continuation of, 514t, 532, 533f
superior, persistent left, 514t, 532, 532f, 532t
Venography, CT, in pulmonary embolism, 594, 595f
Venous catheters, 255–267, 256f–267f, 256t, 259t, 265t. *See also* Catheter(s), venous
Ventilation/perfusion scintigraphy
  in chronic pulmonary embolism, 597, 598f
  in pulmonary arterial hypertension, 604
  in pulmonary thromboembolic disease, 581–582
Ventricular septal defects, 522, 522t, 523f
Viral infections
  AIDS-related, 125
  in immunocompetent host, 111–112, 112f
    influenza, 111, 112f
    rubeola, 111
    varicella-zoster, 112, 112f
Virtual bronchoscopy, of central airways, 431–432, 431f
Visceral herniation, diaphragm rupture and, 313, 313t, 314f–316f
von Recklinghausen disease, pulmonary manifestations of, 346–348, 346t, 347f

W

Water
  in mediastinal masses, CT in detection of, 209–212, 210t, 211f, 212f
  systemic extravascular, in critically ill patients, evaluation of, 236t
Wegener granulomatosis, 439–441, 440f, 441f
  CT of, 430f
  manifestations of, 329–330, 330f, 331f
  organs involved in, 439
Williams-Beuren syndrome, 606
Williams-Campbell syndrome, bronchiectasis and, 418, 418f

Y

Young syndrome, bronchiectasis and, 418

Z

Zygomycosis, in SLE, 134, 134f